Dermatological Signs of Internal Disease

4th Edition

Jeffrey P. Callen MD

Professor of Medicine (Dermatology)
Chief, Division of Dermatology
University of Louisville School of Medicine
Louisville KY
USA

Joseph L. Jorizzo MD

Professor and Former (Founding) Chair
Department of Dermatology
Wake Forest University School of Medicine
Medical Center Boulevard
Winston-Salem NC
USA

Jean L. Bolognia MD

Professor of Dermatology
Department of Dermatology
Yale University
New Haven CT
USA

John J. Zone MD

Professor and Chair
Department of Dermatology
University of Utah
Salt Lake City UT
USA

Warren W. Piette MD

Professor and Chairman
Department of Dermatology
John H. Stroger Hospital of Cook County
and Professor of Dermatology
Rush University Medical Center
Chicago IL
USA

SAUNDERS

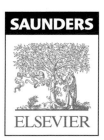

ELSEVIER

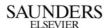

SAUNDERS
ELSEVIER

an imprint of Elsevier Inc.

© 2009, Elsevier Inc. All rights reserved.

© Harcourt Brace Jovanovich 1988
© Harcourt Brace & Company 1995
© 2003, Elsevier Science Limited. All rights reserved

First edition 1988
Second edition 1995
Third edition 2003

ISBN 978-1-4160-6111-3

British Library Cataloguing in Publication Data

A catalogue record for this book is available from the British Library

Library of Congress Cataloging in Publication Data

A catalog record for this book is available from the Library of Congress

Notice
Medical knowledge is constantly changing. Standard safety precautions must be followed, but as new research and clinical experience broaden our knowledge, changes in treatment and drug therapy may become necessary or appropriate. Readers are advised to check the most current product information provided by the manufacturer of each drug to be administered to verify the recommended dose, the method and duration of administration, and contraindications. It is the responsibility of the practitioner, relying on experience and knowledge of the patient, to determine dosages and the best treatment for each individual patient. Neither the Publisher nor the author assume any liability for any injury and/or damage to persons or property arising from this publication.

The Publisher

ELSEVIER your source for books,
journals and multimedia
in the health sciences

www.elsevierhealth.com

Working together to grow
libraries in developing countries

www.elsevier.com | www.bookaid.org | www.sabre.org

ELSEVIER   BOOK AID International   Sabre Foundation

The
publisher's
policy is to use
**paper manufactured
from sustainable forests**

Printed in China
Last digit is the print number: 9 8 7 6 5 4 3 2 1

Commissioning Editor: *Claire Bonnett*
Development Editor: *Nani Clansey*
Editorial Assistant: *Rachael Harrison*
Project Manager: *Alan Nicholson*
Design: *Charles Gray*
Illustration Manager: *Gillian Richards*
Marketing Manager(s) (UK/USA): *Clara Toombs/Courtney Ingram*

Contents

Preface

In this fourth revision of our book we selected co-authors to completely revise many of the chapters. We rearranged, shortened, or expanded other chapters to enhance our goal of providing the practicing physician, academic physician, or resident with a teaching text that explores the relationship of the skin to internal diseases or conditions. Although colleagues aided us in this revision, we continued to serve as contributing editors to ensure that the spirit of the book continues, and that important entities are covered and that duplication is avoided. As in the first three editions, we chose to provide suggested readings rather than an extensive reference list. These suggested readings have been updated so that the interested reader may delve into the most current literature. We have continued the use of color photographs throughout this edition, and in many cases have found new photographs for inclusion.

Acknowledgments

Dr Callen thanks Ms Sandra Lingle, who typed many drafts for previous editions and assisted with the many administrative complexities involved in the production of this text. He thanks the following physicians: L.G. Owen, MD; M.W. McCall, MD; Carol L. Kulp-Shorten, MD; Jyoti B. Burruss, MD; Kristin O. Donovan, MD; Shannon M. McAllister, MD; Alfred L. Knable, MD; Timothy S. Brown, MD; David Daniels, MD; Janine Malone, MD; Anna Hayden, MD; and Soon Bahrami, MD, for allowing him the time to write by providing care for his patients in his absence. Dr Callen dedicates this book to his wife Susan, his children and grandchildren Amy, Dan, Liam and Aviva, and David, Laura, Judah and Noa.

Dr Jorizzo thanks his faculty, residents, and staff for their ongoing support. Dr Jorizzo dedicates this book to Irene Carros, to John, Michael and Melina, to Margaret and the late Joseph, and to Johanna and Paul.

List of Contributors

Jean L. Bolognia MD
Professor of Dermatology
Department of Dermatology
Yale University
New Haven CT
USA

Anneli R. Bowen MD
Assistant Professor of Dermatology
Department of Dermatology
University of Utah
Salt Lake City UT
USA

Susan Burgin MD
Assistant Professor of Dermatology
Harvard Medical School, Boston
and Attending Dermatologist
Beth Israel Deaconess Medical
Center, Boston
BIDMC Dept of Dermatology
Boston MA
USA

Jeffrey P. Callen MD
Professor of Medicine
(Dermatology)
Chief, Division of Dermatology
University of Louisville School of
Medicine
Louisville KY
USA

Charles Camisa MD
Chief
Division of Dermatology
Medical Surgical Specialists
Naples FL
USA

Lisa M. Cohen MD
Clinical Assistant Professor
Tufts University School of
Medicine, Boston
and Co-Director, Caris Cohen DX
Newton MA
USA

Dennis L. Cooper MD
Professor of Internal Medicine
(Oncology)
Department of Internal Medicine
Yale University
New Haven CT
USA

Edward W. Cowen MD,
MHSc
Staff Clinician
Dermatology Branch, CCR
National Cancer Institute
National Institutes of Health
Bethesda MD
USA

Thomas G. Cropley MD,
FAAD
Professor and Chairman
Department of Dermatology
University of Virginia Health
System
Charlottesville VA
USA

Mark D.P. Davis MD
Professor of Dermatology
Mayo Clinic
Rochester MN
USA

Boni E. Elewski MD
Professor of Dermatology
Department of Dermatology
University of Alabama at
Birmingham
The Eye Foundation
Birmingham AL
USA

Joseph C. English III MD
Associate Professor of
Dermatology
Clinical Vice Chairman for Quality
and Innovation
Department of Dermatology
University of Pittsburgh
Pittsburgh PA
USA

Vincent Falanga MD, FACP
Professor and Chairman
Department of Dermatology and
Skin Surgery
Roger Williams Medical Center
Boston University
Boston MA
USA

Steven R. Feldman MD, PhD
Professor of Dermatology and
Pathology
Wake Forest University
School of Medicine
Winston-Salem NC
USA

David Fiorentino MD, PhD
Professor of Dermatology
Associate Professor of Medicine
(Rheumatology)
Department of Dermatology
Stanford University School of
Medicine
Stanford CA
USA

Raechele Cochran Gathers
MD, FAAD
Senior Staff Physician
Henry Ford Health System
Department of Dermatology
Detroit MI
USA

Gary Goldenberg MD
Assistant Professor of Dermatology
Director, Dermatopathology
Laboratory
University of Maryland School of
Medicine
Baltimore MD
USA

Kenneth E. Greer MD
Professor of Dermatology
Department of Dermatology
University of Virginia Medical
Center
Charlottesville VA
USA

Marc E. Grossman MD, FACP
Professor of Clinical Dermatology
Columbia University
College of Physicians and
Surgeons
White Plains NY
USA

Christopher B. Hansen MD
Assistant Professor of Dermatology
Department of Dermatology
University of Utah
Salt Lake City UT
USA

Christina L. Haverstock MD
Resident Physician
Department of Dermatology
Wake Forest University
Baptist Medical Center
Winston-Salem NC
USA

Mark D. Herron MD
Private Practice
Montgomery AL
USA

Warren R. Heymann MD
Clinical Professor of Medicine and
Pediatrics
Head, Division of Dermatology
University of Medicine and
Dentistry
Robert Wood Johnson Medical
School at Camden
Clinical Associate Professor of
Dermatology
University of Pennsylvania School
of Medicine
Philadelphia PA
USA

J. Mark Jackson MD
Associate Clinical Professor
Medicine/Dermatology
University of Louisville
Division of Dermatology
Dermatology Specialists PSC
Louisville KY
USA

Joseph L. Jorizzo MD
Professor and Former (Founding)
Chair
Department of Dermatology
Wake Forest University School of
Medicine
Winston-Salem NC
USA

George Kroumpouzos MD, PhD
Clinical Assistant Professor of Dermatology
Brown Medical School
Boston MA
USA

Andrew D. Lee MD
Chief Resident
Department of Dermatology
Wake Forest University
School of Medicine
Winston-Salem NC
USA

Clive M. Liu MD
Board Certified Dermatologist
Dermatology Associates of Seattle
Seattle WA
USA

Cheryl L. Lonergan MD
Dermatopathology Fellow
University of Virginia Health System
Department of Pathology
Charlottesville VA
USA

B. Asher Louden MD
Private Practice Dermatologist
Mountain State Dermatology
Vienna WV
USA

Aaron M. Loyd MD
Resident Physician
Department of Dermatology
Wake Forest University
Baptist Medical Center
Winston-Salem NC
USA

Susannah E. McClain MD
Dermatology Resident
Department of Dermatology
University of Maryland School of Medicine
Baltimore MD
USA

Amy J. McMichael MD
Associate Professor of Dermatology
Department of Dermatology
Wake Forest University School of Medicine
Winston-Salem NC
USA

Mary Gail Mercurio MD
Assistant Professor of Dermatology
University of Rochester Medical Center
Department of Dermatology
Rochester NY
USA

Drew W. Miller MD
Resident in Dermatology
Department of Dermatology
Wake Forest University School of Medicine
Winston-Salem NC
USA

Mohammad Reza Namazi MD
Assistant Professor of Dermatology
Department of Dermatology
Shiraz University of Medical Sciences
Faghihi Hospital
Shiraz
Iran

Julia R. Nunley MD
Professor
Department of Dermatology
Virginia Commonwealth University
Richmond VA
USA

Manisha J. Patel MD
Assistant Professor
Department of Dermatology
Johns Hopkins School of Medicine
Baltimore MD
USA

Daniel J. Pearce MD
Chief Resident
Department of Dermatology
Wake Forest University School of Medicine
Winston-Salem NC
USA

Warren W. Piette MD
Professor and Chairman
Department of Dermatology
John H. Stroger Hospital of Cook County
Chicago IL
USA

Ted Rosen MD
Professor of Dermatology
Department of Dermatology
Baylor University Medical School
Houston TX
USA

Julie V. Schaffer MD
Assistant Professor of Dermatology and Pediatrics
Department of Dermatology
New York University
New York NY
USA

Kathryn Schwarzenberger MD
Associate Professor of Medicine and Director, Dermatology Residency Program
Division of Dermatology
Fletcher Allen Health Care
University of Vermont College of Medicine
Burlington VT
USA

Sarah L. Taylor MD, MPH, DABFM
Fellow
Department of Dermatology
Wake Forest University
School of Medicine
Winston-Salem NC
USA

Michael D. Tharp MD
The Clark W. Finnerdi Professor and Chair
Department of Dermatology
Rush University Medical Center
Chicago IL
USA

Ruth Ann Vleugels MD
Harvard Medical School
Department of Dermatology
Boston MA
USA

Stephen E. Wolverton MD
Professor of Clinical Dermatology
Vice Chair of Clinical Affairs
Department of Dermatology
Indiana University School of Medicine
Indianapolis IN
USA

Gary S. Wood MD
Johnson Professor and Chairman
Department of Dermatology
University of Wisconsin
Madison WI
USA

Christopher B. Yelverton MD, MBA
Resident
Department of Dermatology
Wake Forest University School of Medicine
Winston-Salem NC
USA

Brad Alan Yentzer MD
Senior Clinical Research Fellow
Department of Dermatology
Wake Forest University School of Medicine
Winston-Salem NC
USA

Gil Yosipovitch MD
Professor
Department of Dermatology, Neurobiology and Anatomy, and Regenerative Medicine
Wake Forest University School of Medicine
Winston-Salem NC
USA

John J. Zone MD
Professor and Chair
Department of Dermatology
University of Utah
Salt Lake City UT
USA

Jeffrey Paul Zwerner MD, PhD
Clinical Instructor in Dermatology
Department of Dermatology
Stanford University Medical Center
Stanford CA
USA

Christopher B. Hansen
and Jeffrey P. Callen

Chapter | 1 |

Lupus Erythematosus

Lupus erythematosus (LE) is a multisystem disorder whose spectrum runs from a relatively benign, self-limited cutaneous eruption to a severe, often fatal, systemic disease. Prior to Hargraves' recognition of the LE cell, lupus erythematosus was diagnosed by a constellation of clinical findings. Ultimately, the American College of Rheumatology (ACR) developed a set of criteria that could be used for the classification of systemic lupus erythematosus (SLE). The criteria were revised in 1982 (Table 1–1). When a patient fulfills four or more of the ACR criteria, either concurrently or serially, during any period of observation, that patient can be classified as having SLE.

In the 1940s and 1950s, dermatologists first recognized that most of their patients with chronic, scarring discoid lupus erythematosus (DLE) lesions had few, if any, systemic findings, whereas those with photosensitivity and/or malar erythema frequently had systemic disease. They also recognized a middle group in whom the cutaneous lesions were more transient than in patients with systemic disease, but for whom the prognosis was not as poor as that for patients with SLE. These patients were later categorized as having subacute cutaneous LE. The classification of cutaneous subsets was stressed by Gilliam and his coworkers. Gilliam proposed that cutaneous manifestations characterized by an interface dermatitis (histopathologically specific LE) be classified into one of three groups based on clinical features. An individual LE patient can present with more than one subtype of disease. He also recognized that LE patients can have skin disease that is not histopathologically specific (Table 1–2). Although each subset listed in Table 1–2 is generally predictive of outcome, it must be remembered that the full spectrum of LE-associated organ dysfunction is possible in any individual patient.

The prevalence of SLE is reported to be 17–48/100 000 people. The prevalence of cutaneous LE is not well established, but it may be two to three times more common than systemic LE. SLE has a strong female preponderance, with a 12:1 female-to-male ratio in the childbearing years. In patients with cutaneous LE this ratio appears to decrease to 3.6:1.

CHRONIC CUTANEOUS LUPUS ERYTHEMATOSUS

Chronic cutaneous LE can have several clinical manifestations. The most common subset is patients with discoid lupus erythematosus (DLE) lesions. These patients may be classified as having localized DLE, when the lesions are only on the head and neck, or widespread DLE, when the lesions are on other body surfaces as well as the head and neck. DLE can also occur as one manifestation of SLE in approximately 20% of patients. Other, less common forms of chronic cutaneous LE include hypertrophic or verrucous (wart-like) lesions, lesions on the palms and/or soles, oral DLE, lupus tumidus, and lupus erythematosus panniculitis (LEP, or lupus profundus).

Discoid Lupus Erythematosus

The DLE lesion is characterized by erythema; telangiectasia; adherent scale, which varies from fine to thick; follicular plugging; dyspigmentation; and atrophy and scarring (Fig. 1–1). The lesions are usually sharply demarcated and can be round, thereby giving rise to the term discoid (or disc like). The presence of scarring and/or atrophy is the characteristic that separates these lesions from those of subacute cutaneous LE (SCLE). The differential diagnosis most often includes papulosquamous diseases such as psoriasis, lichen planus, secondary syphilis, superficial fungal infection, polymorphous light eruption, and sarcoidosis. A histopathologic examination is usually helpful in confirming the diagnosis, and only rarely is immunofluorescence microscopy necessary.

Patients with localized discoid lesions of LE have lesions located solely on the head, neck, or both. These appear to represent the majority of cases of discoid lesions of LE. These patients differ from those with widespread discoid lesions of LE in a number of ways. They have fewer manifestations that suggest systemic disease, and they less frequently demonstrate a positive antinuclear antibody (ANA) titer or leukopenia. It

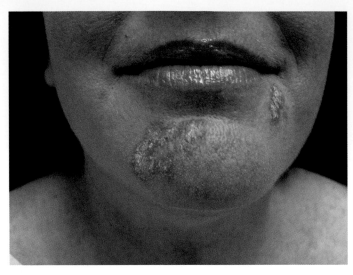

Figure 1–1 Discoid lesion of lupus erythematosus. Erythematous to violaceous lesion with adherent scale, slight atrophy, and early scar formation.

Table 1–1 Revised ACR criteria for the diagnosis of systemic lupus erythematosus

If four or more of the following criteria are present serially or simultaneously during any observation, the patient is said to have systemic lupus erythematosus:

1. Malar rash
2. Discoid lupus erythematosus lesions
3. Photosensitivity, by history or by observation
4. Oral ulcers, usually painless, observed by the physician
5. Arthritis, nonerosive, involving two or more joints
6. Serositis, pleuritis or pericarditis
7. Renal disorder with proteinuria (>500 mg/day) or cellular casts
8. Central nervous system disorder with seizures or psychosis (absence of known cause)
9. Hematologic disorder, such as hemolytic anemia, leukopenia ($<4000/mm^3$) or thrombocytopenia ($<100\,000/mm^3$)
10. Immunologic disorder, detected by positive lupus erythematosus preparation, abnormal titers of anti-native DNA and anti-Sm, and false-positive VDRL or RPR results
11. Positive antinuclear antibody titers

From Tan EM, Cohen AS, Fries JF, et al. The 1982 revised criteria for the classification of systemic lupus erythematosus. Arthritis Rheum 1982; 25: 1271–1277, with permission.

Table 1–2 A classification of mucocutaneous lesions in lupus erythematosus

I.   LE-specific histopathologic findings
    A.   Chronic cutaneous LE
        1.   DLE (widespread versus localized)
        2.   Hypertrophic/verrucous LE
        3.   Palmar/plantar LE
        4.   Oral DLE
        5.   LE panniculitis
    B.   SCLE
        1.   Polymorphous light eruption-type lesions
        2.   Annular lesions (often found in Asian patients with SCLE [annular erythema of primary Sjögren's syndrome])
        3.   Papulosquamous lesions (? photosensitive psoriasis)
        4.   Neonatal LE
        5.   C2-deficient LE-like syndrome
        6.   Drug-induced SCLE
    C.   ACLE
        1.   Malar erythema
        2.   Photosensitivity dermatitis
        3.   Generalized erythema
II.   LE-nonspecific histopathologic findings
    A.   Vasculopathy
        1.   Urticaria
        2.   Vasculitis
        3.   Livedo reticularis/leg ulcerations
    B.   Mucosal lesions
    C.   Nonscarring alopecia
    D.   Bullous LE or epidermolysis bullosa acquisita
    E.   Associated mucocutaneous problems
        1.   Mucinous infiltrations
        2.   Porphyrias
        3.   Lichen planus
        4.   Psoriasis
        5.   Sjögren's syndrome
        6.   Squamous cell carcinomas

LE = lupus erythematosus, DLE = discoid LE, SCLE = subacute cutaneous LE, ACLE = acute cutaneous LE.

appears that the rare patient with discoid lesions of LE who progresses to develop more of the criteria for SLE is generally not in the subset with localized discoid lesions of LE. Those patients with disease localized to the head and neck will frequently (roughly 50%) have a remission, whereas in those with widespread involvement the disease rarely becomes clinically inactive (less than 10%). Lastly, it also appears that those with widespread disease respond less well to antimalarial treatment. Thus, it seems that it is prognostically worthwhile to separate the patients with localized discoid lesions of LE and those with widespread discoid lesions of LE into different subsets.

Hypertrophic Lupus Erythematosus

Hypertrophic or verrucous DLE (HLE) is a unique subset in which an unusual lesion occurs. The thick, adherent scale is replaced by massive hyperkeratosis, and the lesions look like warts or squamous cell carcinomas (Fig. 1–2). These lesions usually occur in the setting of other, more typical DLE lesions. These patients tend to have chronic disease, to have little in the way of systemic symptoms or abnormal laboratory findings, and to be extremely difficult to treat with conventional therapy. They may respond to oral retinoids.

Palmar/Plantar Discoid Lupus Erythematosus

The lesions of DLE can occur on the palms and/or soles (Fig. 1–3). The frequency of this subset is low, and there is no specific clinical or serologic correlation. These patients can have chronic cutaneous disease, or the lesions can be present in

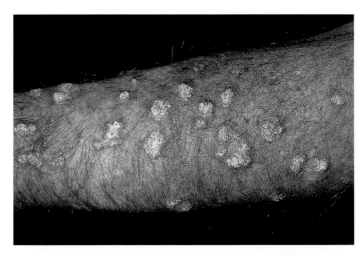

Figure 1–2 Hypertrophic (verrucous) lupus erythematosus. These wart-like lesions were present in a patient with typical discoid lupus erythematosus elsewhere. They simulate warts, keratoacanthoma, or squamous cell carcinoma.

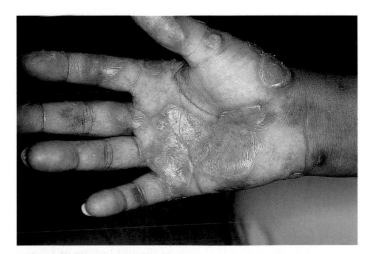

Figure 1–3 Erosive lesions of discoid lupus erythematosus involving the palms. Typical lesions of discoid lupus erythematosus are present elsewhere.

patients with SLE. Palmar and/or plantar lesions are often difficult to treat.

Oral Discoid Lupus Erythematosus

Oral discoid lesions of LE are histopathologically and clinically similar to cutaneous discoid lesions of LE. These lesions are different from the oral and nasal ulcerations that occur in SLE. Those occurring in the patient with SLE are associated with active systemic disease and are histopathologically nonspecific. Lesions that look like those of discoid lesions of LE in the oral mucosa have associations similar to those seen with localized or widespread discoid lesions of LE.

Lupus Tumidus

Lupus tumidus is characterized by erythematous to violaceous plaques or nodules, usually on sun-exposed surfaces. The lesions typically have no epidermal changes, and when they heal they leave little if any residual scarring or atrophy. Patients with lupus tumidus are photosensitive. Serologic abnormalities are distinctly uncommon in these patients. The pathology of tumid LE reveals an increase in mucin and a periappendigeal and perivascular dermal infiltrate composed of lymphocytes, but there is little if any change at the dermal–epidermal interface. It is possible that both clinically and histologically there is overlap with reticulated erythematous mucinosis and tumid LE. There are several controversies regarding this entity: (1) some authorities believe that this is not a variant of lupus erythematosus; and (2) as there is no residual scarring or atrophy it could be argued that it is better classified as a variant of subacute cutaneous lupus erythematosus. Patients with tumid LE are usually responsive to antimalarials.

Lupus Panniculitis

LEP is a lobular panniculitis that occurs rarely in patients with DLE or with SLE (Fig. 1–4). Whether LEP is histopathologically distinct is controversial; thus, in the authors' opinion the patient should have documented SLE or DLE to be classified as having LEP. LEP is often chronic, and it can lead to cutaneous and subcutaneous atrophy and occasional ulceration. Twice as many patients with LEP do not have systemic disease as have systemic disease. It has been postulated that renal disease in the patient with LEP is rarely present, and when present, it is among the more benign forms.

Chilblains Lupus

Chilblains lupus is a rare manifestation of LE that typically develops as red or dusky plaques in acral locations (Fig. 1–5) that are exacerbated by cold and may improve – but do not always resolve – in warmer weather. This entity can be difficult to distinguish from 'common' pernio in the absence of other features of LE, but lesions should have histological changes of LE, such as vacuolated interface changes. These lesions are often recalcitrant to typical treatments of cutaneous LE, such as antimalarials. Over time, lesions may take an appearance of more typical DLE. In half of patients, chilblains may be the

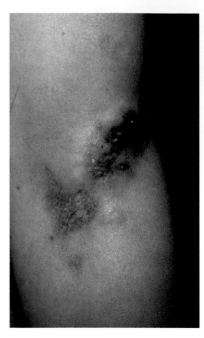

Figure 1–4 Lupus profundus (panniculitis). This woman has inflammatory, subcutaneous nodular lesions that have resulted in subcutaneous atrophy with calcification on the lateral aspect of the arm. Typical lesions of discoid lupus erythematosus were present on other body sites.

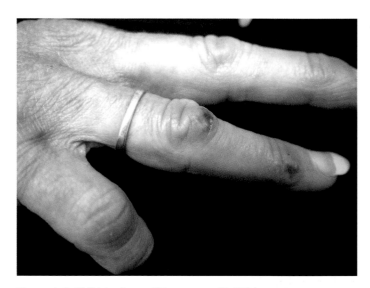

Figure 1–5 Chilblains lupus. This woman with SLE has cutaneous nodules that develop on her hands.

only presenting manifestation of LE. Long-term follow-up of these patients for signs of systemic disease is warranted.

DLE–SLE Subset

The DLE–SLE subset defines a small group of patients (about 5–10%) who, by the nature of their selection, have systemic disease in association with scarring cutaneous disease. Patients whose disease progresses from being purely cutaneous into this group are characterized by widespread DLE, the presence of clinically appreciable periungual telangiectasias, persistent

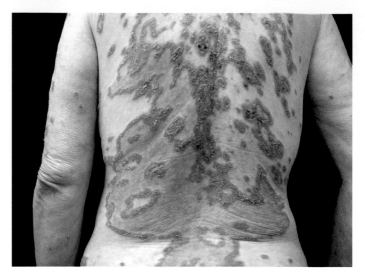

Figure 1–6 Widespread annular scaly lesions of subacute cutaneous lupus erythematosus.

elevated erythrocyte sedimentation rates, leukopenia, and positive ANA titers. Patients in this group may have DLE alone at the onset, DLE with other symptoms or signs, or systemic disease without cutaneous lesions. The time frame is variable, but most patients in this group develop the criteria for SLE within 1.3 years of diagnosis. These patients rarely have renal disease, and even when they do it is most often transient and mild. DLE–SLE is a distinct LE subset because of its relatively benign, albeit chronic, course.

SUBACUTE CUTANEOUS LUPUS ERYTHEMATOSUS

The predominant skin lesion in some patients with subacute LE has all the features of the DLE lesion but without the scarring or atrophy. Follicular plugging is rarely observed in the subacute cutaneous lesion. Patients with such lesions as their major cutaneous manifestation have been classified as having a subset of LE called subacute cutaneous LE (SCLE). It is important to understand, however, that the patient in the SCLE subset can also have the scarring lesions of DLE or the lesions generally associated with SLE, such as a malar rash or vasculitic lesions. Many of the patients with SCLE fulfill four or more of the ACR criteria for SLE; thus, some authorities have not recognized these patients as forming a distinct subset. However, these patients do differ from patients with DLE and are still on the benign end of the LE spectrum. Therefore, we feel that SCLE should be considered a distinct LE subset.

SCLE skin lesions are of at least two types: annular and papulosquamous. Annular SCLE (SCLE-A) lesions are characterized by erythematous rings with central clearing (Fig. 1–6). Often there is a slight scale. The lesions of SCLE-A must be differentiated from other figurate erythemas, such as erythema annulare centrifugum or erythema multiforme. Papulosquamous SCLE (SCLE-P) lesions are characterized by plaques and papules with scale (Figs 1–7 and 1–8). The differential diagnosis of SCLE-P lesions includes psoriasis and lichen planus.

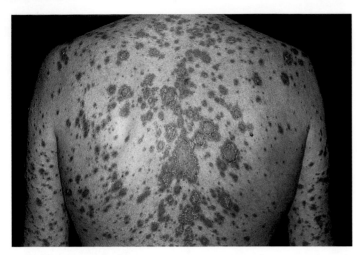

Figure 1–7 Subacute cutaneous lupus erythematosus, papulosquamous variant. This patient developed an exquisitely photosensitive eruption after minimal sun exposure.

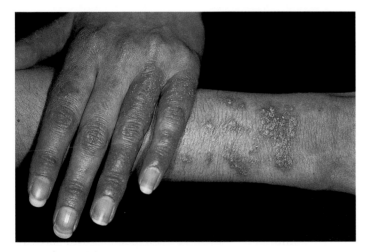

Figure 1–8 Lichen planus-like lesions of subacute cutaneous lupus erythematosus.

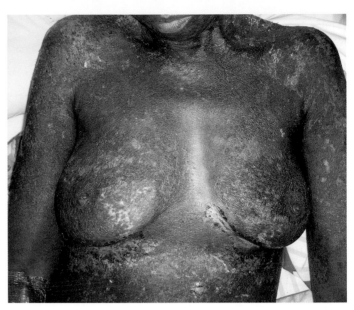

Figure 1–9 Toxic epidermal necrolysis-like lesions in a patient with SLE.

Several patients with presumed psoriasis who have shown flaring with ultraviolet light therapy have in fact had SCLE. In both SCLE-A and SCLE-P the lesions often begin as erythematous papules or plaques in a photosensitive distribution. At the early stage the process may be difficult to distinguish clinically from polymorphous light eruption, and this characteristic histopathologic finding may not be observed. The usual patient has only one type of SCLE lesion, but in about 10% both annular and papulosquamous lesions can be present. DLE skin lesions, generally limited in number, can occur in up to 35% of patients in the SCLE subset. Rare cutaneous patterns include an erythroderma, a pityriasis rubra pilaris-like disease, a disease mimicking toxic epidermal necrolysis (Fig. 1–9) and an erythema gyratum repens-like disease.

About 50% of patients with SCLE have four or more of the ACR criteria for SLE. This takes into account the skin lesions as one criterion and photosensitivity as a second (more than 90% of patients with SCLE have these two criteria). Those with SCLE also frequently have serologic abnormalities, in particu-

lar the presence of anti-Ro (SS-A) antibody. Approximately 40–50% have arthralgias or a nondeforming arthritis. Serositis, central nervous system disease, and renal disease are possible, but are uncommon in SCLE. The type of clinical skin lesion (annular versus papulosquamous) has not been related to specific organ system involvement.

Patients with SCLE have been described in association with other conditions. They may have Sjögren's syndrome, idiopathic thrombocytopenic purpura, urticarial vasculitis, other cutaneous vasculitic syndromes, and/or deficiency of the second component of complement (C2d). Recently, an annular erythema has been described in Asian or Polynesian patients with Sjögren's syndrome. In the authors' opinion this is a clinical variant of SCLE. Anti-Ro (SS-A)-positive SCLE has been induced by hydrochlorothiazide, calcium channel blockers, terbinafine, angiotensin-converting enzyme (ACE) inhibitors, and a growing list of other drugs (Table 1–3). Drug-induced disease may account for as many as one-fifth of patients with new-onset SCLE. Drug-induced SCLE may be reversible upon cessation of the triggering/exacerbating agent; however, some patients' lesions persist after withdrawal of the offending drug.

Laboratory studies in patients with SCLE have focused on the finding of anti-Ro (SS-A) and anti-La (SS-B) antibodies. These antibody systems are poorly represented in rodent tissue substrates, and thus many of these patients were believed previously to have 'ANA-negative LE.' However, with the widespread use of HEp-2 (human epithelium) as a substrate, it has become apparent that many anti-Ro-positive patients are not ANA negative. On a single determination in patients with SCLE, anti-Ro (SS-A) is present in 35–60% of cases. There is some controversy regarding the special relationship of anti-Ro (SS-A) with SCLE-A, several studies suggesting a stronger relationship than with SCLE-P. Repeated testing will demonstrate a positive anti-Ro (SS-A) test result in 60–95% of patients with SCLE. Despite this high percentage, we must keep in mind that

Table 1–3 Drugs reported to cause or exacerbate subacute cutaneous lupus erythematosus

Thiazides – chlorothiazide, hydrochlorothiazide and triamterene*
Terbinafine*
Biologic therapy – etanercept, infliximab

Antihypertensive therapies
    Calcium channel-blocking agents – diltiazem,nifedipine,
        nitrendipine
    Verapamil

ACE inhibitors – captopril, cilazapril, enalapril, lisinopril
Griseofulvin
PUVA therapy
Cinnarizine
Interferon-β
Statins – pravastatin, simvastatin
Leflunomide
Docetaxel
Phenytoin
COL-3
Gold
Naproxen
Aldactone
Fertilizer and pesticide containing hay
Ranitidine
Bupropion
Doxorubicin
Efalizumab
Ticlodipine

*Hydrochlorothiazide is the most frequently associated agent; however, in the literature there are more reports associating terbinafine with drug-induced SCLE.

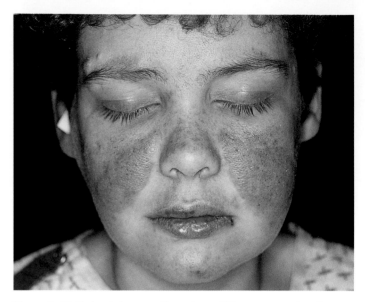

Figure 1–10 Systemic lupus erythematosus. This young man has the typical butterfly eruption of systemic lupus erythematosus.

(often SCLE-A), which begins shortly after birth and spontaneously resolves over a period of 4–6 months. In addition, neonates may have cytopenia, hepatitis and neurologic disease as manifestations of NLE. Data from a registry of NLE have demonstrated that the cutaneous eruption may be delayed in its onset and may not resolve for up to a year. The heart block is usually permanent and can result in fatal outcomes. NLE has been linked to the presence of anti-Ro (SS-A) or, on rare occasions, anti-U_1RNP in the mother and infant. However, some babies with anti-Ro (SS-A) can be normal; thus, the presence of this antibody is not the only determining factor. The mother of a baby with NLE may be asymptomatic, may have photosensitivity, or may have a connective tissue disease (e.g., LE, rheumatoid arthritis, or Sjögren's syndrome). In one study, at the time of follow-up half of those mothers who had initially been asymptomatic developed a connective tissue disease (usually SCLE or SLE). Women with anti-Ro(SS-A) antibodies who have not had a neonate with one of the manifestations of LE have roughly a 1% risk of having a baby with one or more manifestations of NLE; however, once a mother has one child with NLE, the risk for a subsequent pregnancy is 25% and it is not predictable what the manifestation(s) of the NLE will be, therefore patients should be followed by a high-risk obstetrician. There is some risk of the affected neonate developing a collagen vascular disease later in life.

the marker of the disease is not this serologic result but rather the clinical skin lesion. Also, anti-Ro (SS-A) is found in many non-SCLE situations; thus, it is neither a sensitive nor a specific marker of SCLE.

NEONATAL LUPUS ERYTHEMATOSUS

Neonatal LE (NLE) is a syndrome in which cutaneous disease is frequently present. NLE can also manifest as congenital heart block. In addition, transient hemolytic anemia, thrombocytopenia, leukopenia, and hepatitis may be observed in NLE. For unknown reasons, patients with NLE uncommonly have both cutaneous disease and heart block. However, families in which one baby has had heart block can subsequently have normal infants, infants with heart block, or infants with cutaneous disease. These neonates have photosensitive cutaneous disease

ACUTE CUTANEOUS LUPUS ERYTHEMATOSUS

Acute cutaneous lupus erythematosus (ACLE) produces malar erythema, the classic 'butterfly' rash from which the term LE (wolf-like redness) was coined (Fig. 1–10). The rash is induced by sun exposure, or by exposure to other sources of ultraviolet light. Patients with a butterfly rash usually have active systemic disease, but there is no specific correlation between the rash and the organ system involved.

Several cutaneous abnormalities had been part of the ACR criteria but have been found to be less specific than photosensitivity. Diffuse hair loss (alopecia) was one of the original criteria. Patients with SLE can develop a diffuse hair thinning, but this is most likely related to the presence of a severe episode of systemic illness. This type of hair loss is seen after major surgery, or can follow systemic infections or pregnancy. It is known as telogen effluvium because the trauma of the associated disease forces most hairs to cycle into the same phase, and they then all go through the telogen (resting) phase 3–6 months later, at which time the hair loss occurs. This hair loss is different from the alopecic lesion of DLE.

Photosensitivity is a major factor in all types of cutaneous LE. It is one of the 11 ACR criteria for the classification of SLE. Photosensitivity implies that there is an abnormal reaction to sunlight. An abnormal reaction to sunlight occurs in all patients with LE; however, in general, most of those with DLE are not considered to have 'true' photosensitivity, despite a worsening of their clinical disease in the spring and summer. Almost all patients with SCLE are photosensitive, and about 60–75% of those with SLE demonstrate photosensitivity. Studies have demonstrated that either UVB, UVA, or both may exacerbate cutaneous disease in the lupus patient. In addition, polymorphous light eruption may be more common in LE patients, and appears to be more common in their family members.

OTHER CUTANEOUS CHANGES ASSOCIATED WITH LUPUS ERYTHEMATOSUS

Any mucosal surface (oral, nasal, or vaginal) may be affected in LE. Occasionally the lesions may be histologically specific, but nonspecific erosions or ulcerations are seen in roughly 5–10% of patients with SLE. The presence of oral ulcers may correlate with active systemic disease.

Raynaud's phenomenon was one of the original 14 criteria for SLE. It occurs in otherwise healthy patients and in those with scleroderma, cold-associated disorders, or other collagen–vascular diseases. There has been some suggestion that the presence of Raynaud's phenomenon is associated with a more benign SLE course, but this is controversial.

Palmar erythema and periungual telangiectasias occur as nonspecific signs of SLE. Periungual telangiectasias are an important finding in DLE because they occur only in patients who are likely to have or to develop SLE. Nailfold capillaroscopy has also demonstrated abnormalities, but the use of this procedure to differentiate LE from other collagen–vascular diseases is controversial.

Secondary Sjögren's syndrome occurs in LE, and its incidence varies from 5% in chronic cutaneous LE to 10–30% in SCLE and SLE. The presence of Sjögren's syndrome has been linked to cutaneous vasculitis and central nervous system disease in patients with LE. Furthermore, a recent link of primary Sjögren's syndrome with an annular erythema probably represents a variant of SCLE.

Cutaneous vasculitis can complicate LE. It can be manifested as urticaria-like lesions, nailfold infarcts, or palpable purpura. The presence of vasculitis in the patient with SCLE has been correlated with a positive anti-Ro (SS-A) titer, but not with active systemic disease. However, the presence of vasculitis in patients with SLE correlates with active disease and a poor prognosis. In particular, active renal disease or central nervous system disease has been reported in patients with vasculitis.

Livedo reticularis and/or pyoderma gangrenosum-like leg ulcerations may occur in patients with antiphospholipid antibodies (anticardiolipin and lupus anticoagulant). Many of these patients have LE, but some have a primary antiphospholipid antibody syndrome (Fig. 1–11). These patients are characterized by arterial occlusions that can result in transient ischemic attacks, cerebrovascular accidents, and recurrent fetal loss; by venous occlusion that can result in thrombophlebitis, renal or hepatic vein occlusion, and/or pulmonary embolism; by thrombocytopenia; and by cardiac valvular vegetations and dysfunction.

Bullous (or vesicular) lesions can complicate LE. Often, these lesions are present in the patient with active systemic disease. The lesions are often grouped (Fig. 1–12) and do not occur in a photodistribution. Bullous LE can simulate dermatitis herpetiformis or epidermolysis bullosa acquisita, both clinically and histopathologically. Furthermore, some patients with epidermolysis bullosa acquisita either have or develop SLE. Both patients with epidermolysis bullosa acquisita and those with bullous LE have antibodies directed against type VII collagen, thereby leading to the speculation that these disorders are closely related, if not identical. Patients with bullous LE are usually exquisitely responsive to therapy with dapsone.

Various other cutaneous changes or diseases occur more commonly in patients with LE. Squamous cell carcinoma can complicate the longstanding lesions of DLE. Cutaneous mucin deposition occurs in LE, but in some patients' nodules, mucinous plaques or reticular erythematous mucinosis may occur. Various porphyrias can occur in those with LE. Lichen planus, psoriasis, and autoimmune bullous disorders may occur with an increased frequency.

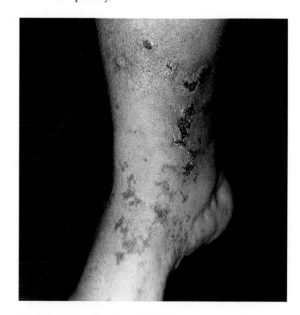

Figure 1–11 Necrosing livedo reticularis in a patient with antiphospholipid antibody syndrome.

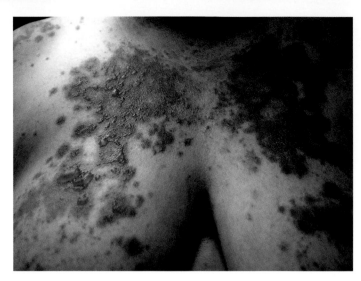

Figure 1–12 Grouped vesicular lesions on an erythematous base on photoexposed and photoprotected skin of a patient with active systemic lupus erythematosus.

LABORATORY PHENOMENA IN PATIENTS WITH CUTANEOUS LUPUS ERYTHEMATOSUS

The full gamut of systemic disease manifestations of SLE can occur in patients with cutaneous disease, and thus these individuals can have any or all of the laboratory associations of the disorder. Serologic abnormalities are common in LE. They are rarer in patients with 'pure' cutaneous disease, such as DLE or HLE. The presence of abnormalities in these patients correlates with progressive disease or with the criteria for SLE.

ANA is a system that represents many antibodies to multiple substrates. The frequency of a positive ANA titer correlates with the substrate used. The reported pattern of the ANA titer may also correlate with specific antibodies; however, except when interpreted by experts, the ANA pattern is not specific. Table 1–4 lists the antibody subsets and their clinical correlates. Table 1–5 presents the frequency of these antibodies in the subsets discussed. Anti-native DNA (double-stranded) correlates with active SLE and, in particular, active renal disease. However, we must be certain that the testing method used does not detect anti-single-stranded DNA, which is not SLE-specific. Anti-Ro (SS-A) was initially described in ANA-negative LE and Sjögren's syndrome. However, it is also present in NLE, vasculitis, SCLE, and C2-deficient LE syndromes. Thus, it is not specific for any one subset. Antibody testing must be carefully correlated with other laboratory findings and with clinical abnormalities. Neither diagnosis nor therapy should be based solely on these laboratory abnormalities.

Circulating immune complexes can be found often in patients with SLE and SCLE, but rarely are they detected in patients with pure cutaneous disease. Circulating immune complexes tend to correlate with vasculitis, active renal disease, arthritis, or serositis. They may be pathogenetically important in vasculitis and renal involvement, but are probably not involved in the pathogenesis of the nonvasculitic cutaneous lesion. Complement activation is also a feature of SLE, and hypocomplementemia correlates with active systemic disease.

Table 1–4 Antibody subsets in lupus erythematosus

Positive titer/finding	Clinical disorder
Antinuclear antibody	Wide array of collagen–vascular diseases and some normal patients
HEp-2 (substrate)	Less specific
Mouse liver (substrate)	More specific
Anti-single-stranded DNA	Nonspecific presence in patients with cutaneous LE suggests systemic disease
Anti-double-stranded DNA (anti-native DNA)	SLE, active nephritis
Antihistone antibody	Drug-induced SLE
Anti-U$_1$RNP	Mixed connective tissue disease
Anti-Sm	SLE
Anti-Ro (SS-A)	SCLE, neonatal LE, Sjögren's syndrome, vasculitis, C2 deficiency-associated LE, drug-induced SCLE
Anti-La (SS-B)	Sjögren's syndrome
Antiphospholipid antibody–anticardiolipin antibody, and/or lupus anticoagulant	Thromboses (venous or arterial), cerebrovascular accidents, transient ischemic attacks, recurrent fetal loss, livedo reticularis, pyoderma gangrenosum-like leg ulcers, cutaneous necrosis, cardiac valvular vegetations, thrombocytopenia

LE = lupus erythematosus, SLE = systemic LE, SCLE = subacute cutaneous LE.

Table 1–5 Frequency of antinuclear antibody and other antibodies in various clinical subsets of lupus erythematosus (%)

Test	DLE	HLE	DLE/SLE	SCLE	NLE	ACLE
ANA	5–10	5	75	50–75	60–90	95+
Anti-ssDNA	35	25	75	20–50	?	90
Anti-nDNA	5	5	10	10	10–50	70
Anti-U$_1$RNP	<5	<5	?	10	?	40
Anti-Sm	<5	<5	25	10	?	25
Anti-Ro (SS-A)	5	5–10	5	40–95	90	30
Anti-La (SS-B)	<5	<5	5	15	15–20	10

ANA = antinuclear antibody, ss = single stranded, n = native, RNP = ribonucleoprotein, DLE = discoid LE, HLE = hypertrophic LE, SLE = systemic LE, SCLE = subacute cutaneous LE, NLE = neonatal LE, ACLE = acute cutaneous LE.

Patients with persistent hypocomplementemia should be evaluated for complement component deficiencies, of which C2 deficiency is the most common.

Cutaneous immunofluorescence applied as a diagnostic and prognostic tool has led to a better understanding of LE.

Lesional immunofluorescence may be helpful when the clinical and histopathologic diagnosis is in question. However, we must realize that normal facial skin can demonstrate false-positive reactions in 10–20% of cases. The use of noninvolved, 'nonexposed' skin in the lupus band test is believed to correlate with active renal disease. Refined antibody testing has reduced the need for immunofluorescence testing.

TREATMENT OF CUTANEOUS LUPUS ERYTHEMATOSUS

Before therapy is begun, it is necessary to evaluate the patient thoroughly to note the extent of disease and to be able to reassure them about the benign nature of the process. Table 1–6 lists the testing that should be ordered. This testing is costly, but if all results are negative the value of the assurance that can be given is inestimable.

The goals of management of cutaneous LE are to suppress disease activity, improve the patient's appearance, and prevent the development of deforming scars, atrophy or dyspigmentation. Few randomized clinical trials have been performed, and hence the response to all therapies has largely been determined only by a global assessment by the treating physician. Recently, an outcomes measure specific to cutaneous lupus has been developed by Werth and colleagues, named the Cutaneous Lupus Erythematosus Disease Area and Severity Index (CLASI). This tool can be used to quantify disease activity and damage over time, and is a step towards more evidence-based treatment.

The most important therapeutic manipulation (Table 1–7) is the use of sunscreens and sun avoidance. This is a basic aspect of therapy that is frequently overlooked. Sunscreens with a sun protective factor of at least 15 are to be used every day. Some patients also react to ultraviolet A light and require a broader-spectrum sunscreen. The patient should be encouraged to apply the sunscreen each morning, and then again prior to sun exposure. Sunbathing, whether active or passive, is strongly discouraged. The use of sunbeds in tanning parlors should also be strongly discouraged. Artificial tanning from chemicals that do not involve UV activation is safe. Protective clothing and intelligent planning (e.g., early morning or late afternoon) with regard to sun exposure are encouraged. In addition, there are several companies that make clothing which has been demonstrated to have photoprotective properties.

Although topical corticosteroids have been shown to be effective under experimental conditions, when prescribed in the clinic or office they may not be highly effective. Probably because of their expense, messiness, and the time involved in their application, they are not always used as directed. Despite these failures, topical corticosteroids should be prescribed in conjunction with other agents. The choice of a specific agent is based on the clinical lesion and the area of the body that is affected. The prescribing physician must bear in mind that these agents can produce atrophy, which is also a sign of the disease. Other topical immunomodulators, such as tacrolimus ointment and pimecrolimus cream, have also been used with some success, particularly in ACLE, but additional studies are warranted. These agents may prove to be a reasonable choice for longer-term treatment of lesions on the face in particular, to avoid atrophy, telangiectasias and steroid-induced acne.

Lesions that do not respond to topical agents can be injected with a corticosteroid, such as triamcinolone acetonide (3–

Table 1–6 Evaluation of the patient with cutaneous lupus erythematosus

I.	History
II.	Physical examination
III.	Standard tests
	A. Skin biopsy for routine processing
	B. Complete blood count with differential
	C. Tests of renal function
	D. Urinalysis
	E. Serologic tests – ANA, anti-nDNA, anti-Sm, anti-Ro (SS-A)
	F. Total hemolytic complement (if abnormal C2, C3, C4 levels)
	G. Serum protein electrophoresis
IV.	Optional tests
	A. Immunofluorescence microscopy
	B. Antiphospholipid antibodies

Table 1–7 Agents used to treat cutaneous lupus erythematosus

Standard therapy
Sunscreens
Smoking cessation
Topical corticosteroids
Intralesional corticosteroids
Antimalarials
Hydroxychloroquine
Chloroquine
Quinacrine
Alternative therapy
Topical agents – tretinoin, tazarotene, tacrolimus, pimecrolimus
Dapsone
Auranofin
Cytotoxic/immunosuppressive agents – azathioprine, methotrexate, mycophenolate mofetil
Thalidomide
Efalizumab
Systemic corticosteroids

4 mg/mL). Hypertrophic lesions, scalp lesions, palmar lesions, and recalcitrant DLE lesions are well suited to therapy with intralesional corticosteroids. Again, it is important to recognize that atrophy is dose related, and that there is a fine line between effectiveness and this complication. Secondary infection can occur at the injection site.

Antimalarials form a mainstay of systemic therapy of cutaneous LE. The mechanism of action of these agents is unknown, but may relate to photoprotection and/or to immunomodulation. The agents available include hydroxychloroquine sulfate, chloroquine phosphate, and quinacrine HCl (quinacrine is available, but only from a compounding pharmacy.) Antimalarial agents have been shown to be less effective in patients who smoke. Smoking cessation has resulted in improved efficacy in individual patients. It is not known whether smoking is associated with a worsening of the LE, or whether it inactivates or blocks the action of the antimalarial. Chloroquine and hydroxychloroquine may be associated with retinopathy, whereas the major side effect of quinacrine is bone marrow suppression, and an orange-yellow discoloration of the skin. The authors' first choice is hydroxychloroquine because, despite possibly being less efficacious, it has less ocular toxicity than chloroquine. Hydroxychloroquine is given by mouth in a dose of 200–400 mg/day. Regular ophthalmologic examinations are scheduled. When this regimen is less effective than desired, either quinacrine 100 mg once or twice daily can be added, or the patient can be switched to chloroquine (250–500 mg/day). Antimalarials are effective for DLE, SCLE, LEP, and the arthritis, malaise and aches associated with LE, but are less effective for patients with hypertrophic, palmar, or vasculitic lesions. Patients with the DLE–SLE subset respond more poorly to antimalarials than do those without systemic manifestations.

The number of patients with cutaneous LE who respond well to antimalarials has not been systematically studied but has been estimated at 75–90%. However, there is clearly a subset of patients who remain recalcitrant to the above-mentioned therapies. Many other systemic agents have been used for recalcitrant cutaneous LE syndromes. Systemic corticosteroids are less effective for the cutaneous disease, despite their dramatic effect on systemic symptoms and signs. Immunosuppressants such as azathioprine, mycophenolate mofetil, and methotrexate have been reported to be effective in recalcitrant cases. Perhaps the most dramatic clinical response to treatment comes from thalidomide at doses of 50–150 mg/day. Thalidomide prescribing is associated with a program to prevent pregnancy (STEPS program), and the physician and pharmacy must be registered with the company. In addition, there is real concern about the possibility of thalidomide-induced peripheral neuropathy that may not be reversible upon cessation of the drug. Additionally, several other cytotoxic/immunosuppressive agents have been used in individual patients with some success. Dapsone 100–200 mg/day has been reported to be effective. It may be helpful in the rare patient with SCLE, those with LE and cutaneous vasculitis syndromes, and individuals with bullous LE. High-dose intravenous immunoglobulin has provided good but short-lived results in some patients. Lastly, there are newer biologic agents that have been used off label for recalcitrant cutaneous LE. Efalizumab 1 mg/kg/week has been reported to be effective in a case series, and a randomized trial may be forthcoming. Lastly, the use of biological TNF-α inhibitors has been more controversial, and they are currently not widely recommended owing to reports of induction of antinuclear antibodies and lupus-like syndromes in some patients with rheumatoid arthritis and psoriasis using these medications.

SUGGESTED READINGS

Albrecht J, Berlin JA, Braverman IM, et al. Dermatology position paper on the revision of the 1982 ACR criteria for systemic lupus erythematosus. Lupus 2004; 13: 839–849.

Callen JP. Management of 'refractory' skin disease in patients with lupus erythematosus. Best Pract Res Clin Rheumatol 2005; 19: 767–784.

Callen JP. Cutaneous lupus erythematosus: a personal approach to management. Australas J Dermatol 2006; 47: 13–27.

Krathen MS, Dunham J, Gaines E, et al. The cutaneous lupus erythematosus disease activity and severity index: Expansion for rheumatology and dermatology. Arthritis Rheum 2008; 59: 338–344.

Kuhn A, Sticherling M, Bonsmann G. Clinical manifestations of cutaneous lupus erythematosus. J Dtsch Dermatol Ges 2007; 5: 1124–1137.

Lee HJ, Sinha AA. Cutaneous lupus erythematosus: understanding of clinical features, genetic basis, and pathophysiology of disease guides therapeutic strategies. Autoimmunity 2006; 39: 433–444.

Lin JH, Dutz JP, Sontheimer RD, Werth VP. Pathophysiology of cutaneous lupus erythematosus. Clin Rev Allergy Immunol 2007; 33: 85–106.

Rothfield N, Sontheimer RD, Bernstein M. Lupus erythematosus: systemic and cutaneous manifestations. Clin Dermatol 2006; 24: 348–362.

Sticherling M, Bonsmann G, Kuhn A. Diagnostic approach and treatment of cutaneous lupus erythematosus. J Dtsch Dermatol Ges 2008; 6: 48–59.

Tebbe B. Clinical course and prognosis of cutaneous lupus erythematosus. Clin Dermatol 2004; 22: 121–124.

Usmani N, Goodfield M. Efalizumab in the treatment of discoid lupus erythematosus. Arch Dermatol 2007; 143: 873–877.

Ruth Ann Vleugels
and Jeffrey P. Callen

Chapter | **2** |

Dermatomyositis

DEFINITION AND CLASSIFICATION

Dermatomyositis is a condition that combines an inflammatory myopathy with a characteristic cutaneous disease. A closely related disease, polymyositis, has all the clinical features of the muscular disease of dermatomyositis but lacks the characteristic cutaneous findings. A third idiopathic inflammatory myopathy, inclusion body myositis, also lacks cutaneous disease, but has a unique pattern of weakness with prominent involvement of the wrist and finger flexors and quadriceps. The pathogenesis of these disorders is only partially understood, but immune-mediated muscle damage is believed to be important as a pathogenetic mechanism. Both polymyositis and dermatomyositis may occur in the presence of other collagen–vascular diseases, such as lupus erythematosus, scleroderma, Sjögren's syndrome, and various vasculitides. Dermatomyositis appears to be characterized by an increased frequency of internal malignancy, whereas the association of polymyositis with malignancy is less well resolved. There is a female to male preponderance of approximately 2 : 1, with a peak incidence in the fifth and sixth decades, and it appears that the incidence of both myopathies is increasing. Both dermatomyositis and polymyositis may also occur in children. Because both disorders are associated with morbidity and occasional deaths, a prompt and aggressive approach to therapy is indicated.

Bohan and Peter first suggested the use of five criteria to define polymyositis and dermatomyositis. These include (1) proximal symmetric muscle weakness that progresses over a period of weeks to months; (2) elevated serum levels of muscle-derived enzymes; (3) an abnormal electromyogram; (4) an abnormal muscle biopsy; and (5) the presence of cutaneous disease compatible with dermatomyositis. These criteria are useful for patient evaluation, but it is not necessary to perform all the muscle testing in patients with characteristic skin disease, particularly those who have proximal muscle weakness and elevated muscle-derived enzymes.

The inflammatory myopathies may be subclassified into eight groups. The following system of classification has been useful in differentiating groups of patients with regard to their prognosis, potential for an associated process, and potential to respond to various therapies: (1) dermatomyositis; (2) polymyositis; (3) myositis in association with malignant disease; (4) juvenile myositis (most often diagnosed before age 16); (5) myositis in association with another collagen–vascular disease; (6) inclusion body myositis; (7) dermatomyositis sine myositis (amyopathic dermatomyositis); and (8) drug-induced disease (either a myopathy or drug-induced cutaneous lesions).

Given that the incidence and prevalence of amyopathic dermatomyositis appear to be increasing, Sontheimer has proposed a revised classification system that recognizes the cutaneous manifestations of the inflammatory myopathies (Table 2–1).

PATHOGENESIS

The pathogenesis of the idiopathic inflammatory myopathies is not well understood. The pathogenetic mechanisms involved in the muscular disease are better understood than are those involved in the induction of cutaneous disease. Many agents and events have been associated with the appearance of dermatomyositis and/or polymyositis, including various infections (particularly viral or parasitic infections), vaccination, neoplasms, drug-induced disease, various types of stress, and trauma. In addition, dermatomyositis and polymyositis have been linked with various diseases associated with immunologic phenomena. The demonstration of the Jo-1 antibody in patients with myositis further supports a viral etiology because the antigen for the Jo-1 antibody has characteristics similar to those of viral and muscle proteins. On numerous occasions dermatomyositis has been linked to penicillamine therapy for other conditions. Patients with active dermatomyositis or polymyositis have been demonstrated to have upregulation of type I interferon-α/β-inducible genes in blood samples, and the level of type I interferons has been shown to be correlated with disease activity. Despite having this upregulation of type I interferons in common, it is thought that the immunopathogenesis of dermatomyositis and polymyositis is different. In polymyositis, clonally expanded autoreactive CD8-positive T cells invade myocytes expressing major histocompatibility complex (MHC) class I antigens and cause necrosis via the

Table 2–1 The idiopathic inflammatory myopathies
Dermatomyositis (DM)
Adult-onset DM
Classic DM
DM with malignancy
DM in a patient with another connective tissue disease
Clinically amyopathic DM (also known as DM sine myositis)
Juvenile-onset DM (JDMS)
Clinically amyopathic JDMS
Classic JDMS
Polymyositis
Inclusion body myositis
Adapted from Sontheimer RD, Cutaneous features of classical dermatomyositis and amyopathic dermatomyositis. Curr Opin Rheumatol 1999; 11: 475–482.

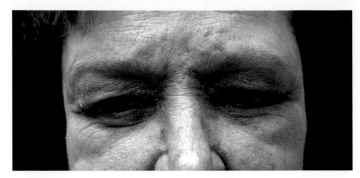

Figure 2–1 Heliotrope eruption with mild edema and violaceous, scaly patches.

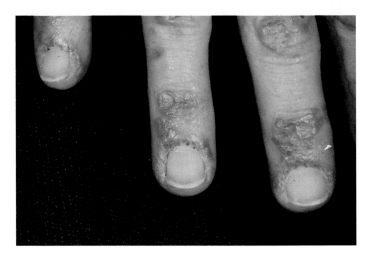

Figure 2–2 Gottron's papules. This shows typical erythematous to violaceous papules and plaques over the bony prominences on the extensor surfaces of the hands.

perforin pathway. In dermatomyositis, autoantigens activate a humoral immune process in which complement is deposited in capillaries, causing capillary necrosis and ischemia. For both diseases, a genetic predisposition has also been suggested. Thus, under appropriate circumstances in a possibly immuno-genetically predisposed individual, an infection, drug, trauma, or neoplasm may be able to initiate an inflammatory reaction in the muscle and skin. Through a complex set of reactions involving immunologic phenomena, muscle damage and cutaneous disease may occur.

MANIFESTATIONS

Cutaneous Manifestations

The characteristic and possibly pathognomonic cutaneous features of dermatomyositis are the heliotrope cutaneous eruption and Gottron's papules. Several other cutaneous features that occur in patients who have dermatomyositis are characteristic of the disease but are not pathognomonic. These include malar erythema, poikiloderma in a photosensitive distribution, a violaceous erythema on the extensor surfaces, alopecia with or without scaly poikilodermatous changes, and periungual and cuticular changes. These signs may occur in other collagen–vascular diseases, in particular lupus erythematosus, and they are also used to differentiate dermatomyositis from polymyositis. The cutaneous disease in dermatomyositis is photodistributed and often photoaggravated. In addition, pruritus may be a prominent feature in dermatomyositis, and may be helpful in clinically distinguishing this entity from lupus erythematosus. Quality-of-life impairment in dermatomyositis is greater than in other skin diseases, including both psoriasis and atopic dermatitis, based on its cutaneous manifestations alone.

The heliotrope cutaneous eruption consists of a dark lilac discoloration or a violaceous to dusky erythematous cutaneous eruption with or without edema in a symmetric distribution involving the periorbital skin (Fig. 2–1). Often only the upper lid is involved. Sometimes this sign is subtle and may involve only a mild discoloration along the eyelid margin. The heliotrope cutaneous eruption can follow the course of the myositis, or it can wax and wane in discordance with disease activity, i.e., the rash may or may not follow the course of the disease. Reactivation of the heliotrope eruption or of any other cutaneous manifestation of dermatomyositis in a patient otherwise considered to be in remission may signify a relapse of the myositis. Most often, however, the activity of the muscle disease in not reflected by that of the cutaneous disease.

Gottron's papules are found over bony prominences, particularly the metacarpophalangeal joints, the proximal interphalangeal joints, and/or the distal interphalangeal joints. They may also be found over bony prominences such as the elbows, knees, and feet. The lesions consist of slightly elevated violaceous papules and plaques (Figs 2–2 and 2–3); they often contain telangiectasias, and there may be hyper- and/or hypopigmentation. These lesions can be clinically confused with those of lupus erythematosus or, at times, with those of papulosquamous disorders such as psoriasis or lichen planus. In instances in which differentiation is difficult, a biopsy for routine histologic examination and immunofluorescence microscopy may be helpful.

Nailfold changes consist of periungual telangiectasias, a characteristic cuticular change with hypertrophy of the cuticle, and small hemorrhagic infarcts within this hypertrophic area

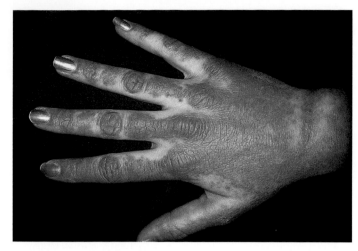

Figure 2–3 Photosensitivity dermatitis found in dermatomyositis. Note the sparing of the interdigital webs and the prominence of the lesions occurring over the joints.

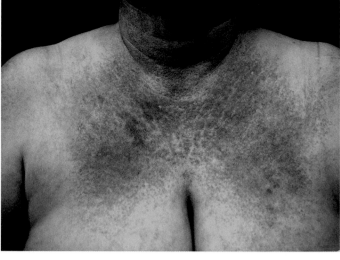

Figure 2–5 Poikilodermatous eruption in the photosensitive distribution in a woman with malignancy and dermatomyositis.

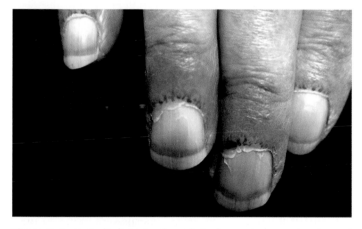

Figure 2–4 Cuticular hypertrophy, splinter hemorrhages, and periungual telangiectases in a patient with dermatomyositis.

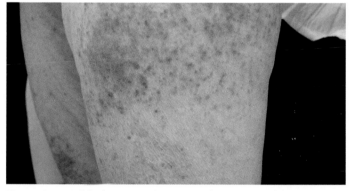

Figure 2–6 Poikilodermatous changes on the lateral thighs, known as the 'holster sign'.

(Fig. 2–4). The periungual telangiectases may be clinically apparent or may be appreciated only by capillary microscopy. Clinically, they are indistinguishable from those seen in other connective tissue diseases. The cuticular overgrowth may be similar to that seen in scleroderma.

Poikiloderma can occur within Gottron's papules or in a photodistribution including the extensor surfaces of the arms or the upper back and the 'V' of the neck (aka the Shawl sign) (Fig. 2–5). These changes are seen in about one-third to half of patients with dermatomyositis. This photosensitive poikilodermatous eruption must be differentiated from lupus erythematosus and from other diseases that cause poikilodermatous skin changes. In addition, poikilodermatous changes may also occur on the lateral thighs, known as the 'holster sign' (Fig. 2–6).

Scalp involvement in dermatomyositis is relatively common. Mild to moderate nonscarring alopecia (Fig. 2–7) can occur in some patients and often follows a flare of the systemic disease. The scalp is usually diffusely affected by a psoriasis-like process with poikilodermatous features. Clinical distinction from seborrheic dermatitis or psoriasis is difficult at times, but histopathologic evaluation is helpful.

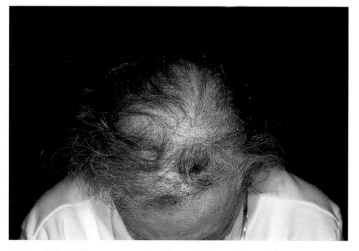

Figure 2–7 Diffuse nonscarring alopecia in a patient with dermatomyositis.

Less common cutaneous findings include an exfoliative erythroderma as well as vesiculobullous, erosive, and ulcerative lesions. Patients with myositis can also develop the lesions of other collagen–vascular diseases. The presence of these types of lesions allow physicians to classify the patients into an overlap category. In general, sclerodermatous skin changes have been the most frequently seen in patients with overlap syndrome. However, cutaneous vasculitis, discoid lupus erythematosus, and rheumatoid nodules have also been known to occur in patients with dermatomyositis.

Skin biopsy may aid in differentiating dermatomyositis from other papulosquamous or eczematous diseases, but cannot be used to reliably distinguish dermatomyositis from lupus erythematosus. In addition, direct immunofluorescence microscopy is usually not helpful in differentiating LE and DM. Classically, skin biopsy in dermatomyositis demonstrates a vacuolar interface dermatitis with mucin deposition in the dermis. Cutaneous lesions of dermatomyositis that do not demonstrate the interface change classically observed with the pathognomonic and characteristic skin lesions include mechanic's hands (hyperkeratosis of the lateral fingers and palms), panniculitis, cutaneous vasculitis, urticaria, a flagellate erythema, and follicular hyperkeratosis.

Although cutaneous lesions precede muscle disease in 30–56% of patients with classic dermatomyositis, myositis follows within 3–6 months in most cases. In a significant portion of these patients the myositis resolves with therapy, and the cutaneous disease becomes the most important feature. Amyopathic dermatomyositis is diagnosed when typical cutaneous disease is present for at least 6 months without clinical weakness, with repeatedly normal serum muscle enzyme levels, and in patients who have not been treated with systemic corticosteroids or immunomodulatory agents. Predictive factors for progression to classic dermatomyositis with muscle involvement have not yet been identified in this subset of patients.

Muscle Disease

Clinical and laboratory abnormalities that suggest muscle disease are characteristic features of polymyositis and dermatomyositis. Even in patients who have only cutaneous disease at presentation, myositis often follows at some point. Myositis precedes the cutaneous findings in less than 10% of patients. The myositis occurring in dermatomyositis is indistinguishable from that occurring in polymyositis as assessed by clinical, histopathologic, and laboratory features. Also, when considered alone, the individual features of myositis are not diagnostic of dermatomyositis or polymyositis; rather, the diagnosis is one of exclusion.

Clinically, the myopathy affects mainly the proximal muscle groups of the shoulder and pelvic girdle. In severe progressive disease all muscles may become involved. The disease is usually symmetric. The initial complaints include weakness, fatigue, an inability to climb stairs, an inability to raise the arms for actions such as hair grooming or shaving, an inability to rise from a squatting or sitting position, or a combination of these features. The progression of disease is variable, but usually occurs over a period of weeks to months. Muscle aching is a common subjective complaint, but frank tenderness on palpation is variable. An inability to swallow and symptoms of aspiration may reflect the involvement of striated muscle of the pharynx or upper esophagus. Dysphagia often signifies a rapidly progressive course and may be associated with a poor prognosis.

The associated laboratory abnormalities include enzyme level elevations, disturbances of electrical action, histopathologic changes and/or abnormalities on magnetic resonance imaging (MRI) or spectroscopy. Muscle enzyme levels are frequently elevated in patients with inflammatory myopathy. The enzymes that are commonly elevated are creatine kinase, aldolase, lactic dehydrogenase, and/or serum transaminases. A creatine kinase determination seems to be the most practical test available for measuring the activity of the muscle disease.

Electromyography (EMG) characteristically shows sharp or positive waves, insertional irritability and fibrillation, and short polyphasic motor units. Innervation remains intact; thus there is a lack of neuropathic changes. The muscle biopsy shows typical features, including type II fiber atrophy, necrosis, regeneration, a centralization of the nuclei, and a lymphocytic infiltrate in a perifascicular and/or perivascular region. Other tests that may be used are various imaging techniques, in particular MRI, which may improve yield and demonstrate clinically inapparent inflammation. In children, levels of Factor VIII-related antigen or neopterin may predict a more severe dermatomyositis variant with vasculopathy.

Systemic Features

Dermatomyositis and polymyositis are multisystem disorders. This is reflected by the high frequency of other clinical features in patients with these diseases.

Arthralgias and/or arthritis may be present in up to one-quarter of patients with inflammatory myopathy. This percentage rises in patients with overlap syndromes. The usual picture is one of generalized arthralgias accompanied by morning stiffness. The small joints of the hands, wrists, and ankles may be involved with symmetric nondeforming arthritis. Patients with arthritis may have a lower frequency of malignancy than do those who do not have arthritis.

Esophageal disease as manifested by dysphagia is estimated to be present in 15–50% of patients with inflammatory myopathy. The dysphagia can be of two types: proximal or distal. Proximal dysphagia is caused by the involvement of striated muscle in the pharynx or proximal esophagus. This involvement correlates well with the severity of the muscle disease and is corticosteroid responsive. Distal dysphagia is related to the involvement of nonstriated muscle and appears to be more frequent in patients who have overlap syndromes. Distal dysphagia may also be accompanied by symptoms of reflux esophagitis. In general, dysphagia portends a poor prognosis and is often associated with pulmonary involvement.

Pulmonary disease occurs in approximately 15–30% of patients with dermatomyositis and polymyositis. It can be characterized by a primary diffuse interstitial fibrosis that may be manifested radiologically, or by abnormalities seen on pulmonary function testing. Pulmonary disease may also occur as a direct complication of the muscular disease, such as hypoventilation or aspiration in patients with dysphagia, or it may be a result of treatment, such as with opportunistic infections or drug-induced hypersensitivity pneumonitis. It is important to note that patients with amyopathic dermatomyositis may have aggressive lung disease even in the absence of myositis. Overall, pulmonary complications have been associated with a poor prognosis. Data have suggested that patients with myositis who have Jo-1 antibodies are at a greater risk for pulmonary involvement. In fact, 70% of patients with Jo-1 antibodies have interstitial lung disease. The antisynthetase syndrome is the constellation of interstitial lung disease, myositis, polyarthritis, Raynaud's phenomenon, fever, and mechanic's hands in a patient with anti-transfer RNA autoantibodies.

Cardiac disease may also occur in patients with inflammatory myopathy, as manifested by myocarditis or pericarditis. Pericarditis appears to be more common in patients with overlapping features of other connective tissue diseases. Myocarditis can result in conduction defects, arrhythmias, or, when severe, congestive heart failure.

Calcinosis of the skin or muscle is unusual in adults but may occur in up to 40% of children with dermatomyositis. Calcinosis cutis is manifested by firm, yellow-white, or skin-colored nodules, often over bony prominences. Occasionally, these nodules can extrude through the surface of the skin, in which case secondary infections may occur. Calcification of the muscles is often asymptomatic and may be seen only on radiologic examination. In severe forms the calcinosis can cause loss of function, and rarely, bone formation is possible.

Pregnancy has been shown to have an effect on the inflammatory myopathy. In addition, the inflammatory myopathy may produce profound effects on the neonate and/or the mother. Studies suggest that dermatomyositis and/or polymyositis may be activated during pregnancy, or that the initial manifestations may be appreciated during pregnancy. In addition, in a large group of women with multiple pregnancies, premature delivery, spontaneous abortions, perinatal deaths, and fetal loss were more common in patients with active myositis.

AMYOPATHIC DERMATOMYOSITIS

An evolving topic in the realm of dermatomyositis is how to classify and refer to patients with only or predominantly cutaneous disease. It is becoming more widely accepted that a subset of patients will have skin-limited disease, similar to patients with lupus limited to the skin rather than with systemic involvement. This is a change from the previous notion that all patients with dermatomyositis would by definition have some degree of muscle involvement if physicians simply investigated sufficiently to find it. In the current nomenclature, clinically amyopathic dermatomyositis includes patients with both amyopathic and hypomyopathic dermatomyositis, subgroups which are estimated to comprise 10–20% of the total population of dermatomyositis patients seen by academic dermatology departments.

Amyopathic dermatomyositis has been recognized to include a unique subset of patients with typical cutaneous biopsy-proven disease for at least 6 months without weakness or abnormal muscle enzymes. By definition, these patients must not have received 2 consecutive months or more of systemic immunosuppressive therapy in the first 6 months after skin disease onset, and must not have received medications known to cause dermatomyositis-like skin changes, including hydroxyurea and statins. These patients can be referred to as having provisional amyopathic dermatomyositis until 2 years after diagnosis, at which point their disease can be called confirmed amyopathic dermatomyositis. Although it presents with cutaneous disease indistinguishable from that of classic dermatomyositis, amyopathic dermatomyositis is a distinct entity rather than a group of patients in whom muscle abnormalities are not yet detectable. In the largest systematic review of adult-onset clinically amyopathic dermatomyositis, most patients had a normal EMG, muscle biopsy, and/or muscle MRI when performed.

Hypomyopathic dermatomyositis includes cutaneous findings and subclinical myositis evident on laboratory tests, EMG, biopsy, and/or MRI, but no clinical weakness or muscle tenderness. Importantly, these findings do not reliably predict the onset of clinically significant muscle disease at a later time, and should therefore not necessarily warrant more aggressive therapeutic intervention. Sontheimer reported that no patients with hypomyopathic dermatomyositis had developed clinically significant muscle weakness at the time of follow-up, despite an average duration of skin disease of 5.4 years.

Cutaneous lesions and histopathology are indistinguishable from those of classic dermatomyositis. Similar to classic dermatomyositis, there is a female preponderance, a peak onset in the fifth and sixth decades, and a pediatric population affected by amyopathic dermatomyositis. Laboratory results in amyopathic dermatomyositis are similar to those in classic dermatomyositis except for a relative lack of anti-Jo-1 antibodies, including in patients with pulmonary disease. Finally, similar to classic dermatomyositis, amyopathic dermatomyositis has associations with both pulmonary disease and cancer, mandating that these patients be followed for manifestations of both interstitial lung disease and malignancy.

MYOSITIS AND MALIGNANCY

The issue of the relationship between dermatomyositis–polymyositis and malignancy has been clarified. The frequency of malignancy in dermatomyositis has varied from 6% to 60% in various studies. This variation is probably related to differing methods, and the best data suggest that 18–32% of patients with dermatomyositis have or will develop a malignancy. In 1992, Swedish investigators first documented the increased frequency of malignancy in patients with dermatomyositis over that in the general population. Although patients with polymyositis had a slight increase in cancer frequency, it was not highly significant and could be explained by a more aggressive cancer search creating a diagnostic suspicion bias. Subsequent studies from other Scandinavian countries have demonstrated similar findings. A more recent Australian study demonstrated a relative risk of malignancy three to six times that of the general population in patients with dermatomyositis. This study also found an increased risk of malignancy with polymyositis, but less so than with dermatomyositis, again possibly pointing to diagnostic suspicion bias. Although this risk declines over time, it is highest in the first 3 years after diagnosis, and remains elevated for at least 5 years. Heightened surveillance for malignancy must therefore continue for at least 3 years from the onset of the disease.

Malignancies may occur prior to, concurrently with, or after the onset of dermatomyositis. In addition, the myositis may follow the course of the malignancy (a paraneoplastic course) or follow its own course, independent of treatment of the malignancy. Studies demonstrating the benefits of cancer surgery on the myositis and studies showing no relationship of cancer surgery to the myositis have been reported. Relapse of myositis may indicate cancer recurrence and warrants careful investigation. A wide variety of malignancies have been reported in patients with dermatomyositis and polymyositis. Gynecologic malignancy, in particular ovarian carcinoma, is overrepresented in published reports. Lung, pancreatic, colon, non-Hodgkin's lymphoma, and breast cancer are also over-represented. Furthermore, in a Southeast Asian population it seems that carcinoma of the nasopharynx is overrepresented.

Another issue is whether age is a factor in the frequency of malignancy in patients with myositis. Reports of young adults and children have suggested that age alone is not a factor in the presence of an underlying malignancy. Malignancy in younger age groups occurs in tissues that are more commonly affected by malignancy in the absence of myopathy (e.g., a 30-year-old man would be more likely to harbor a testicular tumor, whereas a 70-year-old man would be more likely to have colon cancer). Overall, young age should not dissuade a clinician from completing a careful malignancy work-up.

Finally, the issue of whether the use of immunosuppressive medications is associated with an increased risk of subsequent malignancy in patients with myositis remains controversial. In several studies there has been no demonstrated increased risk of malignancy associated with the immunosuppressive therapy commonly given to control the inflammatory myopathy in dermatomyositis and polymyositis. On the other hand, there are several reports of Epstein–Barr virus-associated lymphomas arising in patients with systemic rheumatic diseases, including dermatomyositis, on immunosuppressive medications such as methotrexate. In some of these cases the lymphoma resolved after discontinuation of immunosuppressive therapy without requiring the initiation of radiation therapy or chemotherapy.

EVALUATION OF THE PATIENT WITH MYOSITIS

The diagnosis of myositis is one of exclusion (Table 2–2). A complete history should be conducted, with particular attention to drugs or toxins that may be involved. It should include a history of previous malignancies, previous travel, changes in the diet, and any symptoms of associated phenomena, such as dysphagia, dyspnea, or arthritis. A thorough review of systems is necessary to aid in the evaluation of patients with dermatomyositis for malignancies.

Table 2–2 Evaluation of the patient with myositis

I. History
A. Previous malignancy
B. Associated symptoms
C. History of toxins, infections, travel, vaccinations, or drug intake
II. Physical examination
A. Dermatologic evaluation
B. Women: pelvic and breast examination
C. Men: rectal and prostate examination
III. Evaluation of muscle disease
A. Creatine kinase, aldolase, and urinary creatine
B. Electromyography (if A is normal)
C. Muscle biopsy (if A and B are normal)
D. MRI (particularly if A is normal and B and C are declined)
IV. Skin disease evaluation
A. Lesional biopsy for routine histopathologic evaluation
B. Immunofluorescence in selected patients
V. Routine studies
A. Complete blood count, comprehensive metabolic panel, and urinalysis
B. Thyroid function
C. Stool occult blood testing
D. Electrocardiogram
E. Women: Papanicolaou smear, CA-125
F. Gastrointestinal endoscopy (age-appropriate)
G. Fasting glucose and lipids (in children)
VI. Radiographic examination
A. Chest X-ray, consider high-resolution chest CT
B. CT scan chest/abdomen
C. Women: pelvic ultrasound, pelvic CT scan, mammography
VII. Pulmonary function tests (with diffusion studies)
VIII. Esophageal studies, e.g., barium swallow, manometry, or cineradiography
IX. Optional
A. Holter monitor
B. Echocardiogram
C. Autoantibody studies; e.g., Jo-1, Mi-2, PM, SRP, etc.
D. Viral serologic testing
X. Further testing is based on abnormalities discovered in steps I–V. Malignancy screening should be performed at the time of diagnosis and annually for at least 3 years

A complete history and physical examination should be conducted, even if the examining physician is a specialist. In women a careful breast and pelvic examination should be included. These examinations should not be deferred. If the examiner does not feel confident in these areas, it is necessary to obtain a gynecologic consultation. Similarly, in men, examination of the rectum and prostate is necessary.

The routine evaluation includes a complete blood count and comprehensive metabolic panel, urinalysis, stool occult blood testing, tests for thyroid function, an electrocardiogram, chest X-ray, age-appropriate gastrointestinal endoscopic studies, chest and abdominal computed tomography (CT) scans, and in women, mammography, pelvic ultrasound, pelvic CT scan, CA-125, and a Papanicolaou smear. Children should have a fasting glucose and lipid screening because of an increased risk of insulin resistance and lipoatrophy. Pulmonary function tests, including diffusion studies, should be performed regardless of whether there are symptoms or abnormalities on the chest X-ray. Given that chest X-rays have a false-negative rate of up to 10% in diagnosing pulmonary disease in dermatomyositis, high-resolution chest CT scans are occasionally warranted. An esophageal study is necessary to evaluate the possibility of dysmotility. Optional studies include a Holter monitor, echocardiography, and serologic tests. Malignancy screening should take place annually for 3 years, in addition to careful investigation of any new signs or symptoms. In addition to the tests above, screening should include age-, race-, and ethnicity-related testing. For example, Asian patients residing in Southeast Asia should have a careful ear, nose, and throat examination to evaluate for nasopharyngeal cancer.

Although they may be positive in pure cases of dermatomyositis–polymyositis, tests of antinuclear antibody have not traditionally been shown to influence the prediction of the course of the disease or its therapy. Antinuclear antibody is positive in approximately two-thirds of cases. Newer serologic studies, including myositis-specific autoantibodies (MSAs), have become available. A variety of such tests has been found and includes Jo-1, Mi-2, PL-7, PL-12, EJ, OJ, KS, Zo, YRS, and SRP. Three others, U_1RNP, Ku, and PM-Scl, have been found in myositis-overlap syndromes. Anti-MJ and -PMS1 have been found to correlate to cases of juvenile dermatomyositis. Although these tests correlate with subsets of patients, the correlations are imperfect. For example, anti-Jo-1 antibodies are linked to pulmonary disease and the antisynthetase syndrome, yet are not uniformly present in these circumstances. Most recently, novel autoantibodies have been identified in clinically amyopathic dermatomyositis, anti-CADM-140, and in malignancy-associated myositis, anti-p155 and anti-p155/p140, which may allow a redefined classification of idiopathic inflammatory myopathies. Widespread use of autoantibody testing is currently discouraged because it neither confirms nor excludes the diagnosis, is an imperfect predictor of the prognosis, and is not helpful in monitoring therapy. The novel autoantibodies in malignancy-associated myositis may, however, help identify patients requiring more aggressive malignancy work-up and surveillance in the future.

A subsequent evaluation is necessary following the initiation of therapy. Repeat testing of each abnormality is advised.

Follow-up of the myositis generally includes a combination of the clinical examination with muscle enzyme determinations. Repeat muscle biopsy or electromyography is reserved for unusual circumstances. The use of biomechanical assessment to quantify muscle strength may be of benefit in following a patient's course. Careful questioning with regard to new symptoms should occur at each follow-up visit, and if a symptom develops, careful evaluation is necessary. On at least a yearly basis, a repeat chest X-ray, urinalysis, complete blood count, comprehensive metabolic panel, stool guaiac, rectal, pelvic, and breast examinations, mammography, and a Papanicolaou smear should be conducted. It is important to note that the current recommendations for malignancy screening are an evolving concept.

COURSE AND TREATMENT

Several general measures are helpful in treating patients with dermatomyositis and polymyositis. Bed rest is often valuable in those with progressive weakness; however, this must be combined with an aggressive but passive range-of-motion exercise program to prevent contractures. Any patient with muscle disease should have an appropriate physical therapy regimen. Nutrition is important because of the negative nitrogen balance that exists in inflammatory myopathy. This is particularly important in children. Patients who have evidence of dysphagia should have the head of the bed elevated and should avoid eating meals before retiring. Pruritus can interfere with sleep patterns and overall quality of life, and should therefore be treated accordingly.

The overall therapeutic plan is determined primarily by the presence or absence of myositis or other internal organ involvement. The mainstay of therapy for myositis is the use of systemic corticosteroids. There has been debate over low-dose versus high-dose therapy and alternate-day therapy. Traditionally, prednisone is given in a dose of 1–2 mg/kg/day as the initial therapy. This treatment should continue for at least 1 month and until after the myositis has become clinically and enzymatically inactive. At this point, the dose is slowly tapered, generally over a period 1.5–2 times as long as the period of active treatment. Approximately 25–30% of patients with dermatomyositis and/or polymyositis will not respond to systemic corticosteroids or will develop significant steroid-related side effects. In these patients, immunosuppressive agents (methotrexate, azathioprine, cyclophosphamide, chlorambucil, mycophenolate mofetil, intravenous immunoglobulin, or cyclosporine) may be an effective means of inducing or maintaining remission. Roughly half to three-quarters of patients treated with an immunosuppressive agent respond, as evidenced by an increase in strength, a reduction in enzyme levels, or a reduction in steroid dosage.

Methotrexate can be used on a weekly basis, given either orally or intravenously. It is administered in an empiric dose of 25–50 mg/week. The drug usually becomes effective in 4–8 weeks and is therefore not recommended for rapid control of a fulminant disease process.

Azathioprine has been used in a double-blind controlled trial with prednisone versus a group with prednisone and placebo. In a short-term analysis of 3 months, there were no differences between these two groups. However, in the open follow-up study 3 years later, a significantly lower steroid dosage was needed and significantly greater muscle strength was found in the patients who had been treated with azathioprine. Azathioprine is administered orally in a dosage of 1–2 mg/kg/day, depending on the results of thiopurine methyl transferase (TPMT) testing in order to achieve efficacy yet avoid bone marrow suppression.

The use of immunosuppressive agents is to be undertaken with caution. A complete evaluation prior to prescribing immunosuppressive therapy is necessary, as are the usual measures for follow-up of these patients. The need for liver biopsy in patients taking methotrexate is controversial, but if chronic therapy is planned, liver biopsy should accompany this therapy.

Some patients fail to respond to these agents, and in these individuals various other measures have been suggested. Single-case or open-trial reports support the benefits of pulse methylprednisolone therapy, combination immunosuppressive therapy, chlorambucil, cyclosporine, rituximab, and total body irradiation. High-dose intravenous immunoglobulin (IVIg) is the only therapy that has been tested in a randomized, placebo-controlled clinical trial. It is given at a dose of 1 g/kg on 2 consecutive days monthly for 6 months. This therapy has been beneficial for both the myositis as well as the cutaneous disease. A placebo-controlled study showed no benefit from plasmapheresis. Despite case reports demonstrating benefits from anti-tumor necrosis factor-α (anti-TNF-α) medications, a pilot study of infliximab for patients with refractory inflammatory myopathies demonstrated radiological and clinical worsening of muscle disease and activation of the type I interferon system in several cases. A series of patients treated with etanercept all had exacerbation of muscle disease.

Therapy for cutaneous disease in patients with dermatomyositis is often difficult because, even though the myositis may respond to treatment with corticosteroids and/or immunosuppressants, the cutaneous lesions often persist. In one study, 50% of patients who received immunosuppressive therapy for muscle involvement showed no improvement in cutaneous manifestations. Although cutaneous disease may be of minor importance in patients with serious fulminant myositis, in many patients the cutaneous disease becomes the most important aspect of the disorder. Most patients with cutaneous lesions are photosensitive; thus, as in patients with lupus erythematosus, the daily use of a broad-spectrum sunscreen with a sun protective factor of at least 30 is recommended. Topical modalities include corticosteroids, tacrolimus, or pimecrolimus. Hydroxychloroquine in doses of 200–400 mg/day is effective in approximately 80% of patients, partially controlling the cutaneous disease and allowing a reduction in corticosteroid dosage. Patients who do not respond well or fully to hydroxychloroquine can be switched to chloroquine 250–500 mg/day, or they can receive quinacrine 100 mg twice daily in addition. (Quinacrine may not be available in all locations.) The usual precautions regarding antimalarial therapy should be taken, including a careful ophthalmologic examination and follow-up. It appears that patients with dermatomyositis have a greater potential to develop morbilliform drug reactions with hydroxychloroquine, and a pre-treatment warning is helpful. Open-label studies support the usefulness of methotrexate in doses between 10 and 40 mg/week and of mycophenolate mofetil for the skin disease. Observations regarding retinoids, dapsone, thalidomide, adjuvant leflunomide, antiestrogens, sirolimus, total body irradiation, infliximab, etanercept, and efalizumab are anecdotal, but intravenous immunoglobulin appears to be effective and safe, albeit expensive. Patients with amyopathic dermatomyositis may respond to one-tenth the usual dose of IVIg. Although case reports and one small trial have shown improvement in skin manifestations of dermatomyositis with rituximab, the largest open trial to date demonstrated modest improvement of muscle disease but limited effects on cutaneous disease. Finally, studies have suggested that aggressive corticosteroid therapy is not warranted in patients without clinical evidence of myositis. Therefore, treatment for amyopathic dermatomyositis can differ significantly from that of classic dermatomyositis.

Patients with established calcinosis may require more than supportive therapy. Occasionally the calcinosis will regress without therapy. However, various therapies have been tried, including low-dose warfarin, colchicine, diltiazem, and probenecid. Aggressive corticosteroid therapy does seem to reduce the risk of development of calcinosis in children.

Given the frequently refractory nature of skin disease in dermatomyositis compared to muscle disease, it is necessary to develop methods to assess the severity of cutaneous disease accurately in order to design clinical trials that can reliably evaluate the efficacy of therapeutic interventions. A Dermatomyositis Skin Severity Index (DSSI) has been developed as a modified version of the Psoriasis Area and Severity Index (PASI) and validated as a severity measure in cutaneous disease. It incorporates the average redness, induration, and scaliness of the cutaneous lesions of dermatomyositis on the head, trunk, and upper and lower extremities. A study found that the DSSI correlated well with the physician's global assessment, poikiloderma score, and pruritus, and supported its use as both a valid and a reliable measure of severity of skin disease in dermatomyositis. An additional index, the Cutaneous Dermatomyositis Area and Severity Index (CDASI), has also been designed and involves the assessment of erythema, scale, excoriation, ulceration, poikiloderma, and calcinosis at 18 anatomical locations. The CDASI may be more sensitive than the DSSI to changes in disease severity over time, but this has yet to be fully elucidated. The Cutaneous Assessment Tool (CAT) measures skin involvement in cases of juvenile dermatomyositis with activity and damage scores that have been shown to have moderate to good reliability. Validated outcome measures will have a significant role in future clinical trials for cutaneous disease associated with dermatomyositis.

The prognosis of dermatomyositis and polymyositis varies greatly depending on the series of patients studied. Factors that affect the prognosis include the patient's age, the type and severity of the myositis, the presence of dysphagia, the presence of an associated malignancy, the presence of lung disease or clinically apparent cardiac disease, and the response to corticosteroid therapy. The concept that therapy alters the prognosis seems to be well established by retrospective reports on the benefits of corticosteroids and immunosuppressants.

SUGGESTED READINGS

Bohan A, Peter JB, Bowman RL, Pearson CM. A computer-assisted analysis of 153 patients with polymyositis and dermatomyositis. Medicine 1977; 56: 255.

Buchbinder R, Forbes A, Hall S, et al. Incidence of malignant disease in biopsy-proven inflammatory myopathy. Ann Intern Med 2001; 134: 1087–1095.

Callen JP, Wortmann RL. Dermatomyositis. Clin Dermatol 2006; 24: 363–373.

Carroll CL, Lang W, Snively B, et al. Development and validation of the Dermatomyositis Skin Severity Index. Br J Dermatol 2008; 158: 345–350.

Dalakas M, Hohlfeld R. Polymyositis and dermatomyositis. Lancet 2003; 362: 971–982.

Edge JC, Outland JD, Dempsey J, Callen JP. Mycophenolate mofetil as an effective corticosteroid-sparing therapy for recalcitrant dermatomyositis. Arch Dermatol 2006; 142: 65–69.

Gerami P, Schope J, McDonald L, et al. A systematic review of adult-onset clinically amyopathic dermatomyositis (dermatomyositis sine myositis): a missing link within the spectrum of the idiopathic inflammatory myopathies. J Am Acad Dermatol 2006; 54: 597–613.

Iorizzo LJ 3rd, Jorizzo JL. The treatment and prognosis of dermatomyositis: an updated review. J Am Acad Dermatol 2008; 59: 99–112.

Hill CL, Zhang Y, Sigurgeirsson B, et al. Frequency of specific cancer types in dermatomyositis and polymyositis: a population-based study. Lancet 2001; 357: 96–100.

Huber AM, Dugan EM, Lachenbruch PA, et al. The Cutaneous Assessment Tool: development and reliability in juvenile idiopathic inflammatory myopathy. Rheumatology 2007; 46: 1606–1611.

Mimori T, Imura Y, Nakashima R, Yoshifugi H. Autoantibodies in idiopathic inflammatory myopathy: an update on clinical and pathophysiological significance. Curr Opin Rheumatol 2007; 19: 523–529.

Peloro TM, Miller OF 3rd, Hahn TF, Newman ED. Juvenile dermatomyositis: a retrospective review of a 30-year experience. J Am Acad Dermatol 2001; 45: 28–34.

Rider LG, Miller FW. Idiopathic inflammatory muscle disease: clinical aspects. Baillières Best Pract Res Clin Rheumatol 2000; 14: 37–54.

Sontheimer RD. Cutaneous features of classic dermatomyositis and amyopathic dermatomyositis. Curr Opin Rheumatol 1999; 11: 475–482.

Sontheimer RD. Would a new name hasten the acceptance of amyopathic dermatomyositis (dermatomyositis sine myositis) as a distinctive subset within the idiopathic inflammatory dermatomyopathies spectrum of clinical illness? J Am Acad Dermatol 2002; 46: 626–636.

Walsh R, Kong S, Yao Y, et al. Type I interferon-inducible gene expression in blood is present and reflects disease activity in dermatomyositis and polymyositis. Arthritis Rheum 2007; 56: 3784–3792.

Susannah E. McClain,
Gary Goldenberg,
Vincent Falanga,
and Joseph L. Jorizzo

Chapter | **3** |

Scleroderma, Raynaud's Phenomenon, and Related Conditions

SCLERODERMA

Cutaneous fibrosis may result from many different conditions. A partial list includes porphyria cutanea tarda, chronic graft-versus-host disease, Werner's syndrome, carcinoid syndrome, phenylketonuria, scleroderma, exposure to chemical and environmental agents (e.g., vinyl chloride, bleomycin, silica), and gadolinium exposure (i.e., nephrogenic systemic fibrosis). However, the term scleroderma is generally reserved for a more specific clinical spectrum, and it represents a group of disorders manifested by cutaneous and multisystem disease of unknown cause. Scleroderma is classified into two major categories: localized scleroderma and systemic sclerosis (Table 3–1).

Localized Scleroderma

Clinical Manifestations

There are three main morphologic subvariants of localized scleroderma: plaque morphea, generalized morphea, and linear scleroderma. However, further clinical subdivisions are possible.

Morphea

Morphea can appear as an indurated plaque, as guttate (droplike) lesions, and as subcutaneous varieties. Plaque-like morphea is by far the most common form of localized scleroderma. It occurs more commonly in females than in males, and primarily in young adults. The lesions of plaque morphea, which are usually single or few in number, begin as flesh-colored to erythematous plaques, which may be slightly edematous. In time, the plaque expands and its center may become white to yellow and is often sclerotic. During the active phase, plaques of morphea often have a violaceous border ('lilac ring') (Fig. 3–1). Plaques on the trunk – the preferred site – are frequently oval and vary from a few to many centimeters in diameter. Hyperpigmentation and gradual softening may develop over a period of years. Guttate morphea is a less common subvariant characterized by multiple, 2–5-mm indurated lesions.

Morphea is often confused clinically with lichen sclerosus et atrophicus (LS&A). Lesions of LS&A are not nearly as sclerotic as morphea plaques, but they may coexist with morphea (Fig. 3–2). Generalized morphea cannot be precisely defined except that, by contrast with plaque morphea, its lesions are larger, more numerous, and rapidly progressive, often coalescing to involve extensive portions of the body (Fig. 3–3). This diffuse cutaneous involvement can result in muscular constriction and immobility, leading to severe dyspnea. It is often refractory to aggressive treatment.

Linear scleroderma

Linear scleroderma is most common in young girls. It can occur as a single lesion, usually on an extremity, can be widespread (Fig. 3–4), or can be limited to the forehead or scalp, where is it known as en coup de sabre (Fig. 3–5). There is controversy about whether en coup de sabre is truly a variant of linear scleroderma. Patients may display facial hemiatrophy (Parry–Romberg syndrome).

The hallmark of linear scleroderma is a band-like area of sclerosis that, when crossing joint lines, can limit the motion of the underlying joint. Moreover, linear scleroderma and its en coup de sabre subvariant are often associated with atrophy either of the affected area or of the underlying tissues. In its most severe form in children, linear scleroderma can cause partial or complete growth arrest of the affected extremity, disabling contractures, and disfigurement. On occasion, amputation has been necessary.

All three main morphologic variants of localized scleroderma exhibit an added level of severity when the involvement extends to the underlying tissues. Thus, fasciitis and muscle and bone involvement can be part of the clinical picture. In general, fasciitis is more common in linear scleroderma and generalized morphea. A clinical picture of unilateral fasciitis, with minimal if any overlying skin involvement, can occur in patients with a history of morphea at other skin sites. Subgroups of patients with thoracic paraspinal morphea and

Table 3–1 Classification of scleroderma

Localized scleroderma
Morphea (plaque, guttate, or subcutaneous)
Generalized morphea
Linear scleroderma
Systemic sclerosis
Limited (no truncal involvement)*
Diffuse (widespread skin involvement)*

*Both limited and diffuse disease can exhibit CREST features. (CREST = calcinosis, Raynaud's phenomenon, esophageal dysmotility, sclerodactyly, and telangiectasia)

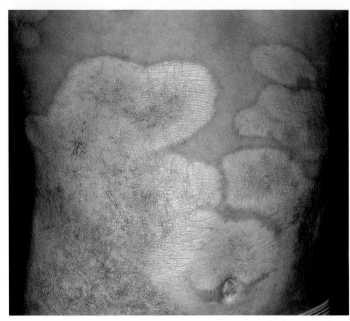

Figure 3–2 Lichen sclerosus et atrophicus/morphea overlap. This child has widespread disease, and after several years he developed pulmonary fibrosis.

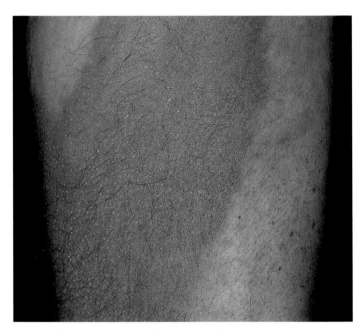

Figure 3–1 Sclerotic plaque of morphea with hyperemic border.

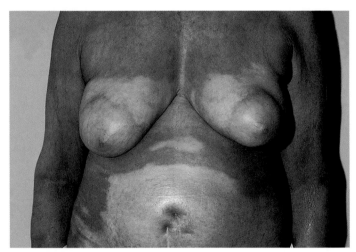

Figure 3–3 Generalized morphea. The lesions are widespread and coalescent.

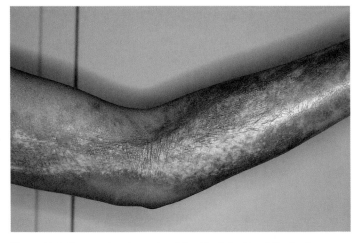

Figure 3–4 Linear scleroderma involving the left side of the body.

pansclerotic morphea involving the head have also been reported. Morphea lesions exhibit a characteristic tumor-like exuberant appearance with profound extension to the underlying tissue. Blisters and bullae occasionally arise within lesions of localized scleroderma.

Diagnosis and Differential Diagnosis

The diagnosis of morphea and other variants of localized scleroderma is based on the clinical appearance of the lesion. Histologic studies are useful in excluding other pathologic processes and in confirming the presence of fibrosis. It should be noted that the term fibrosis refers to an excessive accumulation of collagen in addition to an increased number of fibroblasts. Conversely, sclerosis is defined as excessive collagen accumulation with either a normal or a diminished number of fibroblasts. In general, however, fibrosis is often used as a general term to describe the basic pathologic process of increased collagen deposition. Biopsy specimens from

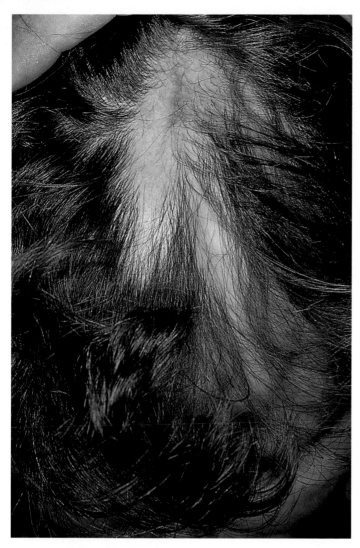

Figure 3–5 En coup de sabre involvement of the face, forehead, and scalp. Atrophy of the skin and subcutaneous structures is the key feature of this condition.

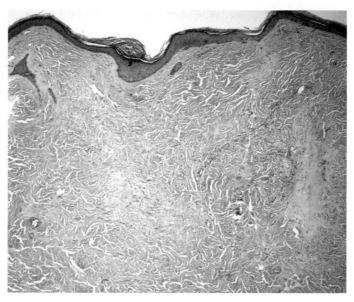

Figure 3–6 Histologic examination of morphea, ×10. Thickened and densely packed collagen bundles in the dermis, with atrophy or absence of the skin appendages.

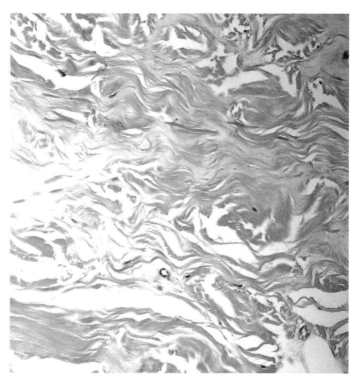

Figure 3–7 Histologic examination of morphea, ×40. Thickened and densely packed collagen bundles in the dermis.

well-developed lesions should include underlying subcutaneous tissue and histologically are square in appearance (the so-called 'square biopsy'). The epidermis may be normal or atrophic, with thickened and densely packed collagen bundles in the dermis, atrophy or absence of the skin appendages, adnexal trapping, and – not infrequently – replacement of the fat cells in the subcutaneous tissue by pale-staining hyalinized collagen bundles. This histologic picture is often identical to the change seen in the skin in systemic sclerosis. In the early inflammatory stages of morphea, a predominantly lymphocytic infiltrate, with or without plasma cells, is seen in the dermis and superficial subcutaneous fat (Figs 3–6 and 3–7).

The differential diagnosis of localized scleroderma is relatively straightforward, and it is not difficult to separate it from systemic sclerosis or eosinophilic fasciitis. The major disorder considered in the differential diagnosis of the plaque lesions of morphea is atrophoderma of Pasini and Pierini. This condition may be an incomplete clinical expression of morphea, and it is characterized by hyperpigmented, depressed, nonin-durated lesions, most commonly on the posterior trunk. Lichen sclerosus et atrophicus is another entity commonly confused with morphea. Indeed, morphea and lichen sclerosus et atrophicus can coexist in the same patient and even in the same biopsy specimen. The atrophic stage of linear scleroderma resembles acrodermatitis atrophicans clinically. Acrodermatitis atrophicans may result from infection with *Borrelia* organisms, which have also been implicated – albeit not convincingly – in the pathogenesis of localized scleroderma. Other entities to include in the differential diagnosis are toxic oil syndrome, drug reaction (especially bleomycin), silicosis, chemical exposure (vinyl chloride, organic solvents, pesticides, epoxy resin), graft-versus-host disease, and nephrogenic systemic psoriasis.

There is no recognized internal organ involvement in localized scleroderma, despite the common occurrence of serum autoantibodies (occasionally a positive ANA). In rare instances a clinical association has been reported between localized scleroderma and lupus erythematosus, dermatomyositis, and other systemic autoimmune disorders.

Treatment

Treatment of localized scleroderma is currently unsatisfactory. Many different medications have been used, including aminobenzoate potassium (Potaba), phenytoin, penicillamine, vitamin E, oral colchicine, topical calcipotriene under occlusion, psoralens and ultraviolet A light (PUVA), and UVA-1 light (available primarily in Europe). A recent case series reported on the efficacy of combined calcipotriol–betamethasone dipropionate ointment. Antimalarials have been effective in some patients. Treatment with low-dose weekly methotrexate may arrest the progression of the disease and leads to eventual softening of the skin over a period of months. Several recent reports suggested that weekly methotrexate combined with monthly pulses of intravenous methylprednisolone or low-dose, rapidly tapering prednisone results in control of disease in children with en coup de sabre and even Parry–Romberg syndrome. So far no controlled therapeutic trials have been possible with localized scleroderma.

Systemic Sclerosis

Clinical Manifestations

Systemic sclerosis is characterized by cutaneous and internal organ fibrosis. Almost all patients have Raynaud's phenomenon, which generally precedes the other clinical manifestations. The cause of systemic sclerosis is unknown, but important steps in its pathogenesis include excessive synthesis of collagen and other matrix macromolecules, endothelial cell injury, and dysregulation of the immune system. Additionally, increased levels of vascular endothelial growth factors have been identified, contributing to vascular malformations and the vasculopathies inherent to this disease. Systemic sclerosis affects women up to 15 times more commonly than it does men, with onset between ages 30 and 50. Family members are more commonly affected than the general population, pointing to a genetic component.

Depending on the extent of the cutaneous involvement, patients with systemic sclerosis are classified as having either limited or diffuse disease. By contrast with the diffuse disease, which is characterized by extensive proximal and truncal skin involvement, limited systemic sclerosis includes clinical induration confined to the hands, forearms, face, and legs. There is general agreement that diffuse disease portends a worse progression in terms of cutaneous and systemic complications. However, it should be recognized that no simple rules exist

and that patients with limited disease can also develop systemic life-threatening complications. The morbidity and mortality from systemic sclerosis are related primarily to pulmonary, renal, cardiac, and gastrointestinal involvement. With the use of potent antihypertensive drugs, particularly angiotensin-converting enzyme (ACE) inhibitors, renal failure is less common now than it was a decade ago. Increasing evidence points to pulmonary fibrosis as a more common cause of death.

The skin may be edematous and slightly erythematous at the onset, but pale, waxy, taut skin eventually ensues (Fig. 3–8). A disturbance of the normal pigmentation of the skin is often remarkable in patients with systemic sclerosis (Fig. 3–9). Patients may develop widespread hyperpigmentation that simulates Addison's disease, but more commonly there is a patchy and often follicular hypo- or hyperpigmentation. Particularly during the late stages of the disease, hypertrichosis may develop in the most affected areas of the forearms and hands. Telangiectatic mats (Fig. 3–10) on the lips and palms especially, and capillary nailfold abnormalities with areas of

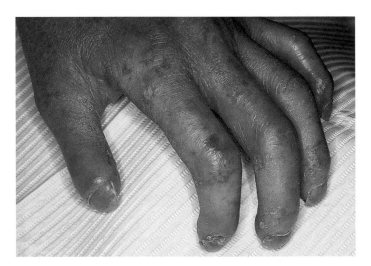

Figure 3–8 Taut, bound-down skin on the digits and hands in systemic sclerosis. This symmetrical involvement of the digits is a clinical feature that helps distinguish systemic sclerosis from eosinophilic fasciitis.

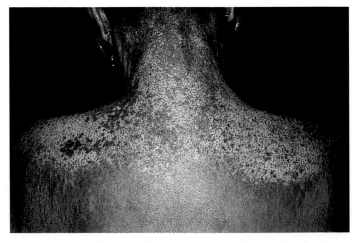

Figure 3–9 Patchy hypo- and hyperpigmentation in systemic sclerosis.

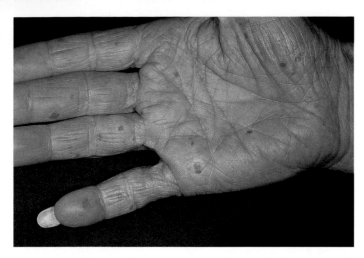

Figure 3–10 Telangiectatic mat in systemic sclerosis. The designation of CREST syndrome (i.e. calcinosis, Raynaud's phenomenon, esophageal dysmotility, sclerodactyly, and telangiectasia) is appropriate for the form of scleroderma in this patient.

vascular atrophy or enlarged and tortuous capillaries, are common.

There has been some confusion concerning the term CREST syndrome, which is apparently classified by some authors as an entity separate from systemic sclerosis. The acronym CREST refers to calcinosis, Raynaud's phenomenon, esophageal dysmotility, sclerodactyly, and multiple telangiectasias. Most of these features are hallmarks of systemic sclerosis. Patients with CREST have systemic sclerosis. Thus, patients with either limited or diffuse disease may exhibit all the features of CREST. There are patients with exaggerated CREST features that are quantitatively different from features observed in other patients with systemic sclerosis; it is not clear how best to define these patients. Patients with exaggerated CREST features have an increased occurrence of pulmonary hypertension and gastrointestinal complications and a high frequency of anticentromere antibodies.

Cutaneous sclerosis in patients with systemic sclerosis is typically most severe on the fingers, producing hyperpigmented, bound-down skin (see Fig. 3–8). Ultimately, contractures and tapering of the distal portions of the fingers occur. The vascular lesions, known as telangiectatic mats, occur on the hands (both dorsal and palmar aspects), central face, and oral mucous membrane.

Systemic Involvement

A substantial proportion of patients with systemic sclerosis have abnormal pulmonary function tests, which may include reduced vital capacity, impaired carbon monoxide diffusion, and pulmonary hypertension. The pulmonary dysfunction is generally the result of interstitial lung disease and pulmonary arterial hypertension, and not of restricted movement of the chest wall by the cutaneous sclerosis, as had originally been hypothesized. Radiographs of the chest often show abnormalities with advanced disease, and may show features of fibrosis, cyst formation, and pulmonary calcification.

Renal failure was a leading cause of death in patients with systemic sclerosis until the availability of hemodialysis and ACE inhibitors. A hypertensive crisis may develop suddenly in patients with systemic sclerosis, and may quickly precipitate renal failure. Pericarditis is a potentially devastating complication in systemic sclerosis. Myocardial fibrosis and asymptomatic myocardial infarction due to obliterative vascular changes may occur.

Esophageal disease occurs in the majority of patients with systemic sclerosis, leading to dysphagia, reflux esophagitis, and ultimately, strictures and obstructions. Severe esophageal disease may lead to weight loss and aspiration pneumonia. The loss of normal peristaltic function in the distal portion of the esophagus and the replacement of the smooth muscle by collagen produce the esophageal disease. Dysfunction of the stomach, small bowel, colon, and rectum is a late but disabling complication.

Primary muscle, joint, and nervous system diseases occur in systemic sclerosis, but are relatively uncommon and may be seen more frequently in patients with overlap syndromes, such as mixed connective tissue disease.

Diagnosis, Course, Prognosis, and Treatment

The diagnosis of systemic sclerosis is primarily clinical. The criteria established by the American College of Rheumatology (formerly called the American Rheumatic Association) are primarily for clinical trial purposes, but may be helpful in establishing a diagnosis. Diagnostic criteria include one major or two minor criteria. The single major criterion is bilateral sclerosis proximal to the metacarpophalangeal or metatarsophalangeal joints. Sclerodactyly, digital pitting scars, and bibasilar pulmonary fibrosis are the three minor criteria.

Characteristically, patients have a symmetrical induration of the fingers and hands with variable symmetrical extension to proximal areas. The early edematous phase of systemic sclerosis is followed by cutaneous fibrosis over several weeks or months. Partial resolution for variable periods is not uncommon. The transition from the edematous to the fibrotic phase, a time when the cutaneous involvement and stiffness may seem improved, should not mislead the clinician. The absence of sclerodactyly in the presence of cutaneous fibrosis elsewhere virtually excludes the diagnosis of systemic sclerosis and should lead to a consideration of localized scleroderma, scleredema, eosinophilic fasciitis, or other sclerotic conditions.

Laboratory studies are helpful both diagnostically and prognostically. They include baseline and follow-up tests for pulmonary, renal, cardiac, and muscular disease. Serum autoantibody testing is an important part of the evaluation. Anticentromere antibodies are generally more frequent in limited disease, whereas anti-topoisomerase I (formerly Scl 70) antibodies are more common in diffuse disease and generally portend a poor prognosis. X-ray studies of the hands to show calcifications or of the teeth to show widening of the periodontal spaces have been used on rare occasions to confirm the diagnosis. The barium swallow, although not as sensitive or precise a test, is more readily available than are motility studies for the evaluation of esophageal disease.

The course of systemic sclerosis is largely unpredictable, but patients with diffuse disease and anti-topoisomerase I antibodies generally fare worse, developing systemic complications sooner than do patients with limited disease. Esophageal involvement can lead to strictures and the need for frequent dilatations. Esophageal reflux and aspiration probably aggravate the pulmonary involvement and represent one more reason for controlling gastric acidity. Severe sclerodactyly limits hand function, and disabling contractures lead to progressive loss of independence.

There is no cure for systemic sclerosis, and the treatment is directed primarily towards complications. Pharmacologic agents that are used for systemic sclerosis can be grouped into various categories (Table 3–2). Some of the drugs listed, such as nifedipine and captopril, help prevent complications. No medication has been shown to consistently improve the cutaneous sclerosis and internal organ involvement. D-Penicillamine has been reported to improve the cutaneous involvement in retrospective studies. Aggressive therapy with daily oral cyclophosphamide is gaining favor to treat patients with severe disease, particularly when there is pulmonary involvement. Autologous bone marrow transplantation following high-dose chemotherapy is being tested, and beneficial results have been observed. Newer research targeting endothelin receptors is also promising.

Digital ulcers are a major cause of disability and morbidity in patients with systemic sclerosis. Ulcers on the distal portion of the digits are generally the result of poor blood supply; vasodilators should be tried in such cases. Additional therapeutic agents worth trying are pentoxifylline and stanozolol, but their effectiveness is unclear. Recent trials have observed the efficacy of bosentan in preventing new digital ulcerations. Ulcers over bony prominences, such as the interphalangeal joints (Fig. 3–11), are mainly caused by trauma and can be improved by local care and protective dressings and devices. Occlusive dressings can stimulate the formation of granulation tissue, but care must be taken that they do not macerate or injure the extremely fragile wound edges. Occlusive dressing use can be limited to the initial phase of digital ulcer treatment to stimulate painless debridement and granulation tissue. Thereafter, the wound can be kept moist with topical antibiotics. Recently, it was found that chemical debriding agents are helpful and are used with success throughout the treatment of digital ulcers. Sympathetic blocks are generally used when all else fails, but are inconsistently helpful. Endothelial cell injury and intimal proliferation lead to a fixed defect in the vasculature that is generally not amenable to vasodilatation.

Table 3–2 Some pharmacologic agents that may be useful in systemic sclerosis
Immunosuppressive drugs
Azathioprine
Cyclophosphamide
Cyclosporine
Tacrolimus
Mycophenolate mofetil
Anti-inflammatory agents
Methotrexate
Nonsteroidal anti-inflammatory drugs
Collagen modulators
D-Penicillamine
Interferons
Colchicine
Vasoactive agents
Captopril
Nifedipine
Pentoxifylline
Others
Endothelin-1 antagonist
Photopheresis
Aminobenzoate potassium
Autologous bone marrow transplantation following high-dose ablative chemotherapy

EOSINOPHILIC FASCIITIS

Eosinophilic fasciitis was first described in 1974. Classically, patients develop symmetrical lower or upper extremity edema after strenuous exertion. This is followed by hyperpigmentation and progressive induration in the edematous areas, giving rise to the development of disabling contractures. A 'groove sign' may be present, referring to linear indurated depressions in which veins may appear sunken. Monoclonal gammopathy and multiple myeloma have been associated with eosinophilic fasciitis, causing some experts to advocate bone marrow biopsies in patients with coexistent eosinophilic fasciitis and hematologic abnormalities. Several features distinguish eosinophilic fasciitis from both localized scleroderma and systemic sclerosis (Table 3–3). The absence of Raynaud's phenomenon, sclerodactyly, and autoantibodies (at least initially) sets this entity apart from systemic sclerosis. The symmetrical nature of the eosinophilic fasciitis, its primary fascial involvement, and the

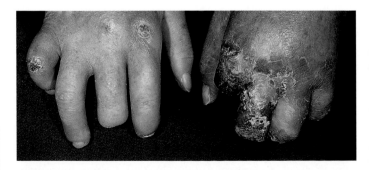

Figure 3–11 Multiple ulcers on interphalangeal and metacarpophalangeal joints as well as autoamputation in a patient with systemic sclerosis.

Table 3–3 Distinguishing features of several disorders manifested by cutaneous fibrosis

Features	LS	SSc	EF	Sd	Sm	NSF
Primarily children	++	−	−	+	−	−
Primarily women	++	++	+	−	−	−
Rapid onset	−	−	++	+	−	+
Symmetrical	−	++	++	+	+	+
Extremities	+	+	++	−	−	++
Face	+	+	++	−	−	−
Trunk	+	+	−	++	+	−
Raynaud's phenomenon	−	++	−	−	−	−
Sclerodactyly	−	++	−	−	−	−
Pigment changes	++	+	−	−	−	+
Telangiectasia	−	+	−	−	−	−
Calcinosis	+	+	−	−	−	−
Systemic disease	−	++	+	+	+	+
Blood eosinophilia	+	−	++	−	−	−
Fascial involvement	+	+	++	−	−	−
Autoantibodies	+	++	−	−	−	−
Monoclonal spike	−	−	−	+	++	−
Steroid responsiveness	+	−	++	−	−	−
Resolution in time	++	−	++	++	−	+/−

LS = localized scleroderma; SSc = systemic sclerosis; EF = eosinophilic fasciitis; Sd = scleredema; Sm = scleromyxedema; NSF = nephrogenic systemic fibrosis; − = rare; + = common; ++ = very common.

infrequent pigmentary changes help separate it from localized scleroderma. However, patients with otherwise classic eosinophilic fasciitis may subsequently develop patches of morphea. The reverse does not seem to be true, although it is certainly possible for an extensive lesion of localized scleroderma to extend down to the fascia and result in histologic fasciitis.

A syndrome characterized by peripheral blood eosinophilia, myalgia, neuropathy, cutaneous sclerosis, and systemic involvement was reported in 1989 in patients taking a contaminated preparation of L-tryptophan. This clinical entity, occasionally fatal and often causing substantial morbidity, was labeled eosinophilia myalgia syndrome (EMS). Its clinical features resembled those described in the Spanish toxic oil syndrome, an epidemic resulting from the ingestion of adulterated cooking oil. The nature of the exact contaminant responsible for EMS is still a source of dispute, and multiple contaminants may have played a role. It is of interest that some patients with EMS have a clinical presentation indistinguishable from that of eosinophilic fasciitis, and that some patients with eosinophilic fasciitis described before the EMS epidemic were taking L-tryptophan, presumably before the alleged contamination of this amino acid preparation. In addition to the possible role of a contaminant, abnormalities in the metabolism of L-tryptophan have been implicated in some patients with EMS and other fibrotic disorders. Other possible triggers include trauma, arthropod bites, and borreliosis.

RAYNAUD'S PHENOMENON AND DISEASE

Raynaud's phenomenon (uncommon, associated with other diseases) and disease (a common, isolated, idiopathic finding) are generally the result of paroxysmal vasospasm. The conditions are seen mainly in women and primarily involve the digits, occurring after abrupt exposure to cooler temperatures or as a result of emotional stress. In many cases, the typical changes of Raynaud's phenomenon or disease are manifest because of vasospasm in an already compromised vasculature. This occurs with systemic sclerosis, atherosclerosis, thromboangiitis obliterans, neurovascular compression syndromes, use of vasoconstricting drugs (e.g., methylsergide or ergot preparations), or occupational exposures (e.g., jackhammer operation or vinyl chloride). The presence of a fixed vascular obstruction is particularly evident in systemic sclerosis, in which intimal proliferation is present early in the clinical course.

The classic Raynaud's phenomenon is the triphasic cutaneous color reaction of pallor, followed by cyanosis, and then reactive hyperemia. The majority of patients, however, experience only one or two phases of the reaction, and the episodes usually occur over a period of a few minutes, at least initially. In some patients, the only clue to the underlying vascular spasm is numbness in one or more digits. Raynaud's phenomenon initially appears on the digits of one or both hands, but may eventually involve the feet, nose, and tongue. Involvement of the digits is often splotchy or segmental. As the disorder progresses, vascular insufficiency frequently produces cutaneous ulcers, scars, and gangrenous lesions of the digits. In such cases a repairable vascular defect proximally should be sought, and referral to a vascular surgeon is indicated. Angiodynography, thermography, and angiography may be necessary for further evaluation of the patient.

Management of Raynaud's phenomenon is directed at symptomatic relief. Avoidance of trigger factors is of paramount importance. Cessation of smoking should be strongly advised, and patients should avoid cold environments or situations, vasoconstricting drugs, and trauma as much as possible. Topical vasodilators (such as nitroglycerin) may only shift the blood supply to more vascularized areas. Vasodilating medications, such as nifedipine, nicardipine, prazosin, or reserpine, may be helpful, the dosage generally being dictated by the patient's therapeutic response and the medication's effect on systemic arterial pressure. Additionally, patients receiving the phosphodiesterase inhibitor sildenafil and the angiotensin receptor blocker losartan showed significant improvement from baseline in the frequency and severity of their attacks of Raynaud's phenomenon, as well as in their capillary flow velocity. Reports have also surfaced of successful treatment of Raynaud's phenomenon with the longer-acting tadalafil. However, the ACE inhibitor captopril has not been shown to be of significant benefit. There is evidence that digital perfusion may actually worsen when the blood pressure is substantially reduced. Biofeedback and relaxation techniques are worth trying in some cases. Pentoxifylline and stanozolol have also been used with variable success. A very promising therapeutic approach for patients with severe Raynaud's phenomenon is botulinum toxin A, as a recent case series illuminated its ability to dramatically improve pain and promote healing of digital ulcerations, thereby preventing the need for surgical sympathectomy. Every attempt should be made to find a treatable cause for Raynaud's phenomenon.

MIXED CONNECTIVE TISSUE DISEASE (MCTD)

MCTD is classified as one of the overlap syndromes because it has features of several connective tissue disorders, especially lupus erythematosus and systemic sclerosis. MCTD is believed by most to be a distinct overlap syndrome that is defined by the presence of unusually high titers of a circulating antibody with specificity for a nuclear ribonucleoprotein antigen (U_1RNP), which is known as extractable nuclear antigen. Anti-DNA antibodies are present in only a minority of patients, and the positive antinuclear antibody titer in their sera produces a speckled immunofluorescence pattern. Overlapping features of two or three connective tissue disorders is not rare. The most frequent overlap syndromes include systemic sclerosis and dermatomyositis (rarely, with lupus erythematosus and dermatomyositis). Patients with such overlap syndromes do not have elevated titers of extractable nuclear antigen and are not labeled as having MCTD. MCTD is much more common in women than in men, and has a mean age of onset of 37 years.

The clinical features of MCTD include Raynaud's phenomenon, swelling or puffiness of the fingers and hands, sclerodactyly, arthralgia and arthritis, abnormal esophageal motility, and polymyositis. Lupus erythematosus-like cutaneous eruptions, capillary dilatation of periungual vessels, Gottron's papules, and heliotrope discoloration of the eyelids are not uncommon cutaneous changes in MCTD, but widespread scleroderma and ulceration of the fingertips are rare.

The significance of separating MCTD from lupus erythematosus, systemic sclerosis, and dermatomyositis is based on studies of early series of patients suggesting that individuals with MCTD have a more benign course and a better response to prednisone than do patients with those other connective tissue diseases. Those with MCTD have a low incidence of renal and central nervous system disease, but not all patients have a benign course, especially those with an early age of onset. Mild disease may be controlled with nonsteroidal anti-inflammatory drugs or low doses of systemic corticosteroids, but larger doses of prednisone, such as 1 mg/kg/day, are necessary in patients with more serious involvement of internal organs. The changes least likely to respond to therapy appear to be the scleroderma-like features, especially pulmonary fibrosis. The ultimate prognosis in this clinical entity is not known, and large series of patients followed for extensive periods are needed.

NEPHROGENIC SYSTEMIC FIBROSIS (NSF)
(see also Chapter 32)

First identified in 1997 as 'nephrogenic fibrosing dermopathy', this relatively recently described entity must be considered in the differential diagnosis of scleroderma-like disorders. It is seen most commonly in patients with renal insufficiency (the majority of whom are on hemodialysis), occurring equally in both sexes and all races. Cutaneous findings include a relatively acute onset of symmetric indurated plaques with a peau d'orange or papulonodular appearance. The extremities are most commonly affected, with rare truncal involvement and no facial involvement. Bullous lesions have also been described. Thickened skin may involve joints, leading to debilitating contractures over a short period (days to weeks). Associated diseases include hypercoagulability, cardiomyopathy, liver dysfunction, idiopathic pulmonary fibrosis, systemic lupus erythematosus, and brain tumors. Although the majority of patients with NSF do have renal disease, there does *not* appear to be a relationship between the etiology or severity of renal dysfunction and the severity of NSF. The etiology of NSF has yet to be defined, despite consistent associations between NSF and exposure to gadolinium-based contrast media. Diagnosis is based on clinical and histopathologic findings, with a history of renal disease aiding the diagnosis. Unfortunately, no one specific therapy has proved effective in the treatment of NSF. Case reports have been published which point to the efficacy of extracorporeal photophoresis, plasmapheresis, UV phototherapy, and IVIg, but no controlled trials exist to date.

SUGGESTED READINGS

Bischoff L, Derk CT. Eosinophilic fasciitis: demographics, disease pattern and response to treatment: report of 12 cases and review of the literature. Int Soc Dermatol 2008; 47: 29–35.

Blauvelt A, Falanga V. Idiopathic and L-tryptophan-associated eosinophilic fasciitis before and after L-tryptophan contamination. Arch Dermatol 1991; 127: 1159–1166.

Clements PJ. Systemic sclerosis (scleroderma) and related disorders: clinical aspects. Best Pract Res Clin Rheumatol 2000; 14: 1–16.

Denton CP, Black CM. Scleroderma and related disorders: therapeutic aspects. Best Pract Res Clin Rheumatol 2000; 14: 17–35.

Dytoc MT, Kossintseva I, Ting PT. First case series on the use of calcipotriol-betamethasone dipropionate for morphoea. Br J Dermatol 2007; 157: 615–617.

Fleming JN, Nash RA, McLeod DO, et al. Capillary regeneration in scleroderma: stem cell therapy reverses phenotype? PLoS ONE 2008; Jan 16; 3(1): e1452.

Galan A, Cowper S, Bucala R. Nephrogenic systemic fibrosis (nephrogenic fibrosing dermopathy). Curr Opin Rheumatol 2006; 18: 614–617.

Henness S, Wigley F. Current drug therapy for scleroderma and secondary Raynaud's phenomenon: evidence-based review. Curr Opin Rheumatol 2007; 19: 611–618.

Kreuter A, Gambilcher T, Breukmann F, et al. Pulsed high-dose corticosteroids combined with low-dose methotrexate in severe localized scleroderma. Arch Dermatol 2005; 141: 847–852.

Sfikakis PP, Papamichael C, Stamatelopoulos KS, et al. Improvement of vascular endothelial function using the oral endothelin receptor antagonist bosentan in patients with systemic sclerosis. Arthritis Rheum 2007; 56: 1985–1993.

Tuffanelli DL. Localized scleroderma. Semin Cutan Med Surg 1998; 17: 27–33.

White B, Moore WC, Wigley FM, et al. Cyclophosphamide is associated with pulmonary function and survival benefit in patients with scleroderma and alveolitis. Ann Intern Med 2000; 132: 947–954.

Zandman-Goddard G, Tweezer-Zaks N, Shoenfeld Y. New therapeutic strategies for systemic sclerosis – a critical analysis of the literature. Clin Dev Immunol 2005; 12: 165–173.

Chapter | 4 |

*Jeffrey P. Zwerner,
Jeffrey P. Callen,
and David F. Fiorentino*

Vasculitis

Vasculitis is a multisystem disorder with frequent involvement of the skin. The organs with the richest vascular supply are those most commonly affected by the disease process. Severity can range from self-resolving, skin-limited disease to progressive multiorgan failure and death.

Understanding of the vasculitides has been difficult owing to the considerable overlap in the clinical and histologic features of the various causes of vessel inflammation. In addition, there is a general lack of 'pathognomonic' signs, symptoms, or laboratory values of the individual vasculitic disorders. It is imperative, however, for the practicing dermatologist to have a working knowledge of the vasculitides in order to correctly assess patients for possible underlying diseases, to correctly evaluate for end-organ damage, and to determine the most appropriate treatment plan.

CLASSIFICATION

In 1952, Zeek offered a classification of vasculitis based primarily on variations in the size of involved blood vessels and end-organ involvement that still serves as a framework today. Since that time multiple classification systems have been proposed, most notably by the American College of Rheumatology (ACR) and the Chapel Hill Consensus Conference (CHCC).

We prefer to subclassify these disorders based solely on vessel size (Table 4–1). Small vessels, the arterioles and post-capillary venules that reside in the papillary and mid dermis, are involved in Henoch–Schönlein purpura, urticarial vasculitis, and the disease variably known as 'hypersensitivity vasculitis'/cutaneous leukocytoclastic angiitis. The latter is sometimes inaccurately referred to as leukocytoclastic vasculitis (LCV); leukocytoclastic vasculitis is simply the histopathologic description of neutrophilic vasculitis, and is found in all clinical forms of vasculitis. Medium vessels, the medium-sized arteries and veins located in the deep dermis and subcutis, are involved in the antineutrophil cytoplasmic antibody (ANCA)-associated vasculitides and polyarteritis nodosa (PAN). The diseases in the latter category are typically associated with a mix of small-vessel and medium-vessel involvement, with the possible exception of PAN (which, by some definitions, is strictly limited to medium-sized vessels). Large vessels, the aorta and large arteries and veins, are involved in giant cell arteritis and its variants; however, this group of diseases does not have cutaneous manifestations secondary to the vasculitis. The clinician can determine the size of vessel involved based on the type of cutaneous lesion seen: purpura (palpable or not), urticaria, and vesicles characterize small-vessel vasculitis, whereas nodules, ulcers, necrosis, and livedo reticularis are found in medium-sized vessel disease.

It is necessary to perform a thorough evaluation in patients with cutaneous disease as a manifestation of vasculitis in order to offer reliable prognostic advice. Systemic involvement associated with small-vessel vasculitis is distinct from that of medium-vessel disease: glomerulonephritis and pulmonary hemorrhage characterize the former, whereas arterial aneurysms, hypertension, mononeuritis multiplex, and bowel ischemia are more typically seen in the latter.

PATHOGENESIS

There is strong experimental and clinical evidence suggesting that most cutaneous vasculitides, especially those affecting the small vessels, are associated with circulating immune complexes (CIC). This is supported by the high frequency of in situ antibody deposition detected by direct immunofluorescence of organ biopsies in these patients. Although the initiating trigger for these CICs may vary from one disease to the next, the deposition of the CICs in the vessel wall, and the subsequent inflammatory cascade that is triggered, is similar for all members of this group of diseases.

Figure 4–1 is a schematic representation of the pathogenesis of leukocytoclastic vasculitis first proposed by Sams et al. in 1976. This schema remains relevant today. After antigenic exposure, soluble antigen–antibody complexes (CIC) are formed which can lodge in the vessel wall. This leads to activation of the complement cascade, resulting in the release of vasoactive proteins (i.e., histamine), recruitment of inflammatory cells, and cytokine release, with the end result of vessel wall damage, leakage of fluid (urticarial lesions), leakage of erythrocytes (purpura), and ischemia (necrosis or ulceration).

31

Table 4–1 Proposed classification of cutaneous vasculitis

Vessel caliber	Classification	Subclassification
Small	Henoch–Schönlein purpura Acute hemorrhagic edema of infancy Erythema elevatum diutinum Urticarial vasculitis	
Small and medium	Cryoglobulinemic	
	ANCA	Wegener's granulomatosis Granulomatous vasculitis of Churg–Strauss Microscopic polyangiitis
	Secondary	Infection Neoplasm Inflammatory disorder Drug exposure
Medium	PAN Cutaneous PAN	

Adapted from Chung L, Kea B, Fiorentino DF. Cutaneous vasculitis. In: Bolognia JL, Jorizzo JL, Rapini RP, et al., eds. Dermatology, 2nd edn. London: Mosby, 2008; 347–367.

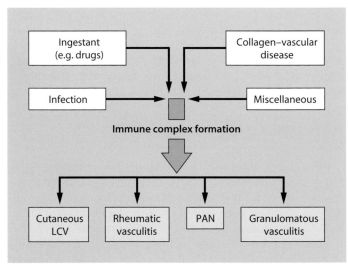

Figure 4–1 Schematic representation of multiple antigenic exposures leading, through the mechanisms of immune complex formation and deposition, to the varying manifestations of vasculitis. LCV = leukocytoclastic vasculitis; PAN = polyarteritis nodosa.

A different pathogenic mechanism appears to play a role in the ANCA-associated vasculitides. ANCA are autoantibodies that are directed against neutrophil-derived products, and include the cytoplasmic (cANCA) antibody, which is directed against proteinase 3 (PR3), and perinuclear (pANCA) antibody, which is directed primarily against myeloperoxidase (MPO). Proinflammatory molecules such as TNF-α and IL-1, released in response to local or systemic infection, induce PR3 and MPO translocation to the neutrophil cell surface. This may then allow these antigens to bind ANCA, which activates neutrophils and increases their adherence to endothelial cells – the end result is vessel damage.

ETIOLOGIC ASSOCIATIONS

Many etiologic agents have been implicated in the various vasculitic syndromes. In general, the lists of etiologic factors or associated conditions are similar for all the syndromes and involve infections, drugs, protein (i.e., complement) abnormalities, and inflammatory disease. Genetic predisposition may also play a role in selected vasculitides – these include complement deficiencies as well as polymorphisms in various cytokines, such as IL-8 and IL-1. Medications are implicated in roughly 20% of vasculitis cases. The resulting vasculitis can affect vessels of various sizes and so the resulting clinical picture can be quite variable, although small-vessel disease is by far the most common. Certain medications, most notably propylthiouracil, hydralazine, allopurinol, and minocycline, may induce an ANCA-associated vasculitis, typically with high-titer ANCA. Recent reports have also observed that drug-induced vasculitis affecting small vessels is commonly associated with dermal eosinophila.

The incidence of systemic or cutaneous vasculitis in adults with malignancy is estimated to be 2.5–5%. Paraneoplastic vasculitis is more commonly associated with hematologic rather than solid tumors, the exception being Henoch–Schönlein purpura (HSP), where multiple reports have suggested that the converse is true. Vasculitis has been reported to occur prior to the discovery of the neoplasm, concurrently with it, or after it has been recognized. In addition, the development of vasculitis has been associated with the recurrence of malignancy.

Overall, in only roughly half of cutaneous vasculitis cases can a known underlying etiology be determined (Table 4–2).

Rheumatic disease can be associated with small or medium-sized vasculitis, accounting for around 12% of cutaneous vasculitis cases. Cutaneous vasculitis is most commonly linked to systemic lupus erythematosus (SLE), rheumatoid arthritis (RA) and Sjögren's syndrome (SS). In RA, vasculitis typically occurs in patients with end-stage disease and is associated with high titers of rheumatoid factor. Vasculitis in SLE patients generally reflects a systemic flare in their underlying rheumatic disease.

CLINICAL MANIFESTATIONS

Small-Vessel Vasculitis

Small-vessel vasculitis involves predominantly the postcapillary venule, so the lesions represented are most often urticaria-like or palpable purpura (Fig. 4–2). Vesiculobullous lesions, pustules, cutaneous necrosis, and/or ulceration (Fig. 4–3) can occur, but are much less common – ulceration or necrosis may often be due to concurrent medium-sized vessel involvement. The purpuric lesions occur most frequently on the legs or over dependent areas, whereas the urticaria-like lesions often are generalized. It is written that the urticarial lesions are different from typical urticaria in that they tend to resolve over a prolonged period, may leave a bruised appearance, and are often described as burning instead of pruritic. These findings are not always reliable, and any patient with unexplained fixed or unusual urticarial lesions deserves a skin biopsy to evaluate for possible vasculitis.

About 40–50% of patients with cutaneous small-vessel vasculitis do not have clinically evident systemic manifestations. In patients with Henoch–Schönlein purpura (HSP), symptoms of abdominal pain, arthritis, and signs of renal involvement are frequent. HSP is more common in children, but can also occur in adults. Urticarial vasculitis is another predominantly small-vessel vasculitis that may be associated with significant systemic features. Patients with urticarial vasculitides, especially those with low complement levels, may exhibit low-grade fever, angioedema, joint complaints, abdominal pain, and/or obstructive lung disease.

Almost any organ system can be involved in patients with small-vessel vasculitis. Gastrointestinal symptoms include colicky pain, hemorrhage, ulceration, and perforation. Pulmonary involvement includes pleuritis, effusions (particularly in patients with lupus erythematosus), nodules, infiltrates, or cavitations. Nervous system involvement can be manifested by neuropathy, cephalalgia, or intracranial hemorrhage. Rare patients can have pancreatitis or myocarditis.

The prognosis of cutaneous vasculitis is directly dependent on the presence or absence of major organ involvement. In patients with HSP, renal disease occurs in 50–80% of adults and less often in children. End-stage renal disease occurs in 10–20% of adult HSP patients. Adverse renal outcome is associated with spread of purpura above the waist, elevated erythrocyte sedimentation rate, fever, and adult onset. Long-term follow-up studies of patients with HSP suggest that hypertension and proteinuria often complicate future pregnancies. In most patients in whom drugs or infections have caused the vasculitis, the disease is self-limited. There appears to be a higher incidence of associated rheumatic diseases and abnormal circulating proteins (e.g., cryoglobulins or hyperglobulinemia) in those patients with chronic disease. Additionally, the risk of visceral disease and recurrence appears to correlate with disease severity during the initial episode.

Medium-Sized Vessel Vasculitis

Medium-sized vessel vasculitis involves arterioles and arteries. Patients with medium-sized vessel disease can also have cutaneous small-vessel vasculitis (Fig. 4–4), which complicates the

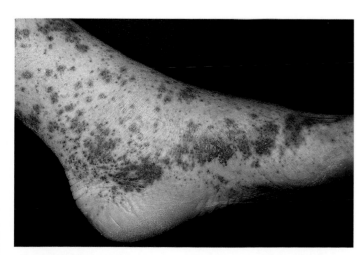

Figure 4–2 Typical palpable purpuric lesions seen in a patient with hypersensitivity vasculitis/small-vessel vasculitis.

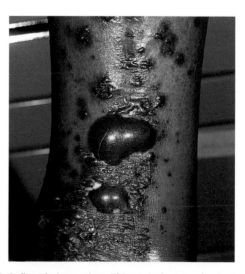

Figure 4–3 Bullous lesions exist within typical areas of palpable purpura in this patient with cutaneous small-vessel vasculitis.

Table 4–2 Secondary vasculitis

Association	Incidence	Agent/disease
Infection	15–20%	Bacterial
		Group A β-hemolytic *Streptococcus*
		Staphylococcus aureus
		Mycobacterium leprae
		*Mycobacterium tuberculosis**
		*Neisseria menigococcus**
		Rickettsiae*
		Spirochetal (e.g., syphilis)*
		Viral
		Hepatitis A, B, and C
		Herpes simplex virus*
		Varicella zoster*
		Influenza virus
		HIV/AIDS
		Fungal
		Candida albicans
		Mucormycosis*
		Protozoan
		Plasmodium malariae
		Helminthic
		Schistosoma haematobium
		Schistosoma mansoni
		Onchoncerca volvulus
Neoplasms	2–5%	Paraproteinemia
		Lymphoproliferative disorders
Inflammatory disorders	15–20%	Sarcoidosis
		Inflammatory bowel disease
		Connective tissue disease
Drug exposure	10–15%	Medications
		Aspirin Oral contraceptives
		Insulin Phenothiazines
		Penicillins Phenylbutazone
		Sulfonamides Allopurinol
		Quinolones Thiazides
		Streptomycin Retinoids
		Streptokinase Anti-influenza vaccines
		Hydantoins Leukotriene inhibitors
		Tamoxifen Interferons
		Quinine Nutritional supplements
		Serum Vitamins
		Foods
		Milk Gluten
		Proteins

Modified from Lotti T, Ghersetich I, Comacchi C, Jorizzo JL. Cutaneous small-vessel vasculitis. J Am Acad Dermatol 1998; 39: 667–687; quiz 688–690.
*Can be due to direct infection of vessels.

classification. Cutaneous manifestations of medium-vessel disease include livedo reticularis, purpura, necrosis, ulceration of the skin, and nodules. The types of medium-sized vessel vasculitis include PAN, ANCA-associated vasculitides, cryoglobulinemic vasculitis, and vasculitis associated with rheumatic syndromes.

In general, PAN is a systemic vasculitis that, technically speaking, involves solely the medium-sized vessels. However, it is our experience that patients can present with lesions typical of PAN but also have evidence of small-vessel disease, at least in the skin. Classic PAN is associated with multisystem involvement, and those who have it have significant morbidity

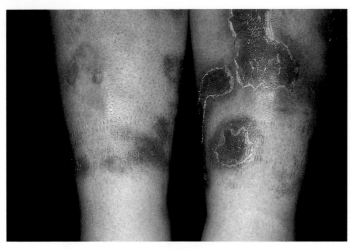

Figure 4–4 Cutaneous small-vessel vasculitis was the first evidence of recurrence in this patient with Wegener's granulomatosis.

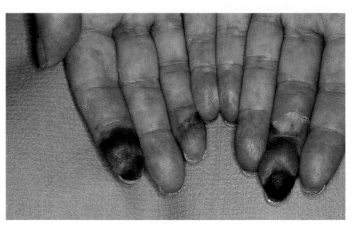

Figure 4–6 Ischemic necrosis of the fingertips in a patient with polyarteritis nodosa secondary to hepatitis B antigenemia. (Courtesy of Dr Neil A. Fenske, Tampa, FL.)

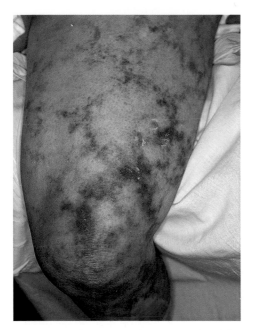

Figure 4–5 Cutaneous polyarteritis nodosa as manifested by a livedo pattern with purpuric and necrotic lesions.

and potentially fatal outcomes. The skin is involved in 40–50% of patients with classic PAN. This involvement may be palpable purpura, livedo reticularis (Fig. 4–5), nodules, necrosis, ulcerations (Fig. 4–6), or atrophie blanche. Systemic disease frequently involves the kidneys and may result in renal failure and/or hypertension. Peripheral neuropathy, arthritis, and muscle weakness are also common. Of note, neither glomerulonephritis nor pulmonary involvement is associated with PAN and, if present, should raise the possibility of ANCA-associated vasculitis.

Patients can also have disease limited to the skin (cutaneous PAN), although this 'cutaneous' form is often associated with fever and neurologic involvement (especially mononeuritis multiplex) of the involved extremities. Cutaneous PAN is classically manifest by localized necrosing livedo reticularis with or without nodules. Associated diseases can be present, namely arthritis and/or inflammatory bowel disease.

ANCA-associated vasculitides have predominantly small-vessel and medium-vessel involvement and often similar cutaneous manifestations. Conditions include Wegener's granulomatosis, microscopic polyangiitis, and Churg–Strauss syndrome. All of the diseases have frequent cutaneous and systemic involvement, and all are associated with ANCA in the majority of cases. PR3 antibodies are present in Wegener's granulomatosis (75–80%), whereas MPO antibodies are present in Churg–Strauss syndrome (55–60%) and microscopic polyangiitis (50–60%). Caution must be exercised in placing too much diagnostic importance on ANCA, as for each disease patients can produce ANCA with either specificity or none at all. In addition, ANCA is not specific for the ANCA-associated vasculitides, as they can be seen in response to medications, inflammatory bowel disease, chronic active hepatitis, and rheumatic disorders such as RA and SLE.

Cryoglobulinemic vasculitis is associated with circulating, cold-precipitable antibodies, termed 'mixed' cryoglobulins. Mixed cryoglobulins consist of monoclonal IgM (type II) or polyclonal IgM (type III) directed against IgG. Clinical manifestations include palpable purpura, arthralgias, and weakness. Peripheral neuropathy and renal involvement may also be present. The vast majority of cryoglobulinemic vasculitis is associated with hepatitis C virus (HCV). Because cryoglobulin production is related to chronic B-cell lymphocyte stimulation by HCV, the incidence of non-Hodgkin's lymphoma in these patients is estimated to be 35 times greater than that of the general population. Other causes of cryoglobulinemic vasculitis include other infections (HIV, hepatitis B), connective tissue diseases (Sjögren's syndrome, SLE, systemic sclerosis), and lymphoproliferative disorders (B-cell non-Hodgkin's lymphoma, CLL, primary and secondary macroglobulinemia). Rheumatoid factor (RF) is found in 70% of patients, and the presence of hypocomplementemia correlates with systemic involvement.

Rheumatic Vasculitis

Rheumatic vasculitis refers to any of the vasculitides in a patient with one of the collagen–vascular diseases, such as rheumatoid arthritis, lupus erythematosus, Sjögren's syndrome, scleroderma (progressive systemic sclerosis), or dermatomyositis–polymyositis.

Patients with lupus erythematosus can have various presentations of vasculitis. Small-vessel vasculitis limited to the skin is the most common presentation and typically manifests as purpuric lesions on the legs, or, less commonly, small, tender purpuric macules or depressed punctate scars over the palmar surfaces of the hands and fingertips. It appears that the majority of hand/finger lesions in SLE patients are actually discoid lupus erythematosus or pernio, and not a vasculitis.

Rheumatoid arthritis may be complicated by vasculitis Rheumatoid vasculitis is also characterized by palpable purpura, digital infarcts, nodules, ulcerations, or necrosis. It has been correlated with high titers of rheumatoid factor and with the presence of rheumatoid nodules. In a large study, Scott and colleagues reported that cutaneous lesions complicated rheumatoid vasculitis in 88% of the 50 patients. It is frequently a systemic vasculitis with an associated mortality rate of 30–40%. The prognosis appears to be worse in rheumatoid vasculitis when neuropathy is present, or when the vasculitis is an early manifestation of systemic disease.

Inflammatory vascular disease (vasculitis) has been recognized as a complication of Sjögren's syndrome. In general, SS patients with vasculitis are more likely to have an extraglandular disease such as arthritis, peripheral neuropathy, CNS vasculitis, Raynaud's phenomenon, or renal disease.

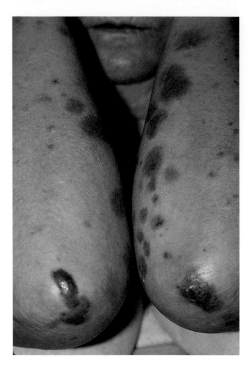

Figure 4–7 Erythema elevatum diutinum. These violaceous nodular lesions on the extensor surfaces and over bony prominences represent a localized leukocytoclastic vasculitis. (Courtesy of Dr Neil A. Fenske, Tampa, Florida.)

VASCULITIS VARIANTS

An unusual cutaneous vasculitic syndrome, known as erythema elevatum diutinum (EED), is worthy of special mention. It is rare, but its major manifestation is cutaneous disease. The lesions begin as red-purple papules that coalesce to form red-yellow plaques (Fig. 4–7). The lesions are most prominent over points of trauma, such as the elbows, knees, dorsum of the hands, and buttocks. Systemic disease is rare. EED is said to be responsive to the antileprosy agent dapsone, whereas most cases of the other cutaneous vasculitides may be less responsive to this drug.

DIFFERENTIAL DIAGNOSIS AND EVALUATION

Purpura (whether palpable or not) is the most common finding in cutaneous small-vessel vasculitis, and the differential diagnosis of purpura is discussed in Chapter 11. Macular purpura may also be representative of thrombocytopenia, disseminated intravascular coagulation, Rocky Mountain spotted fever, or hemorrhagic disorders (see Chapter 11). In addition, if pustules are present, the differential diagnosis must be expanded to include infections such as disseminated gonor-

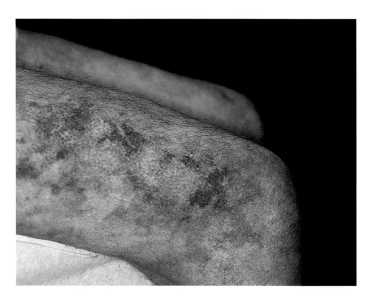

Figure 4–8 Livedo reticularis with cutaneous necrosis in a patient with atheromatous emboli.

rhea and bacterial or fungal endocarditis. Palpable purpura can also occur in embolic disorders, such as endocarditis, artheromatous emboli (Fig. 4–8), or left atrial myxoma, as well as in LCV. Lichenoid eruptions as can occur with lupus erythematosus, dermatomyositis, and lichen planus, or drug reactions can also closely resemble the lesions of cutaneous vasculitis and require biopsy for differentiation.

Biopsy plays a critical role in the diagnosis of cutaneous vasculitis. In the majority of patients who present with palpable purpura limited to the lower extremities and lack of visceral involvement, biopsy can be deferred. In these cases, we see our patients again in 2–3 weeks to reassess the course of the disease. Skin biopsy is indicated in patients with diffuse, severe (ulcerative, nodules), persistent disease or in the presence of systemic involvement. The timing of the biopsy is critical, as lesions more than 24–48 hours old will often demonstrate nonspecific histologic changes. When evaluating lesions of small-vessel disease, a punch biopsy will suffice. Incisional biopsies are often required, especially when attempting to diagnose medium-sized vessel disease. In ulcerative lesions, a recent study suggests that the yield of detecting the affected vessel may be increased by including the center of the ulcer in the biopsy specimen. When biopsing livedo reticularis, the white center of the circular livedo segment should be the focus, as the erythema is due to venous congestion caused by the involved artery. Although not always indicated, direct immunofluorescence (DIF) should be performed whenever one is considering a diagnosis of HSP.

After the diagnosis has been confirmed, the clinician must consider the extent of systemic involvement and potentially associated conditions. The basic evaluation should be thorough and comprehensive (Table 4–3).

TREATMENT

The treatment of vasculitis is based on the organs involved and on the severity of disease. All agents used in treating vasculitides have anti-inflammatory effects as part of their mode of action. Treatment of cutaneous vasculitis is empiric, as large, well-controlled studies are lacking.

Any factor causing or exacerbating vasculitis should be treated or removed. This may occur in the vasculitis that complicates drug therapy, treatable infections, drug abuse, or tumors. Often, the patient has recognized certain drugs as a cause and has stopped using them. Patients should also be informed that tight-fitting clothing, cold exposure, and extended periods of standing can all exacerbate the disease.

In limited cutaneous disease little therapy may be required. Both colchicine and/or dapsone, used either individually or in combination, can be very effective in controlling many cases of chronic cutaneous vasculitis. Colchicine may also improve the joint symptoms associated with small-vessel disease. Antihistamines may be helpful, especially in urticarial vasculitis. In nonresponsive cases low doses of systemic corticosteroids can be used, although the use of immunosuppressive agents to treat chronic disease is preferred over chronic use of corticosteroids.

Systemic disease is treated with a variety of anti-inflammatory agents. Corticosteroid therapy is the first line of treatment for many patients, especially with severe or life-threatening disease, but long-term use is associated with multiple side effects.

Thus, many immunosuppressive and cytotoxic agents have been used in the treatment of vasculitis. The agents used most frequently are the alkylating agents, such as cyclophosphamide or chlorambucil; the antimetabolites azathioprine or mycophenolate mofetil; and the folic acid antagonist methotrexate. Cyclophosphamide use is complicated by predictable bone

marrow suppression as well as the risk of hemorrhagic cystitis, bladder cancer, and azoospermia. In light of these serious potential toxic effects, cyclophosphamide is only rarely used for primarily cutaneous vasculitis. In systemic vasculitides, cyclophosphamide is generally used with high-dose glucocorticosteroids to induce remission, and then an agent with a more favorable side-effect profile is used as maintenance therapy. Chlorambucil is similar to cyclophosphamide and has been used in severe disease. The use of chlorambucil is hampered by its bone marrow suppression, which is not as predictable as that induced by cyclophosphamide.

Azathioprine, mycophenolate mofetil, and low-dose methotrexate (5–20 mg/week) have been shown to have some success in the treatment of both cutaneous and systemic vasculitis. Although we have had different patients respond to each of the agents, we have had the most success with azathioprine and it is generally our first-line immunomodulator for patients with persistent cutaneous vasculitis unresponsive to dapsone and colchicine. In terms of dosing, we advocate

Table 4–3 Evaluation of patients with vasculitis

I. History
  A. Infections
  B. Drugs, other ingestants or exposures
  C. Other symptoms: Raynaud's phenomenon, musculoskeletal, neurologic, cardiorespiratory, etc.
  D. Previous history of associated disorders
II. Physical examination
  A. General appearance
  B. Type of cutaneous lesion
III. Skin biopsy
IV. Laboratory studies
  A. Necessary
    1. Complete blood count
    2. Erythroctye sedimentation rate
    3. Urinalysis
    4. Cryoglobulin, serum/urine protein and immunofixation electrophoresis
    5. Hepatitis C antibody, possibly B surface antigen, HIV antibody
    6. ANCA
    7. Serum multiphasic analysis, which includes tests of renal and hepatic function
  B. Optional
    1. C3,C4,total hemolytic complement
    2. Antinuclear antibody, anti-Ro (SS-A)
    3. Skin biopsy for direct immunofluorescence
V. Radiographic examination
  A. Chest X-ray

dosing azathioprine based on the patient's thiopurine 5-methyltransferase (TPMT) activity level along with their weight. Plasmapheresis and intravenous immunoglobulin (IVIg) have a role in the treatment of severe, typically systemic, vasculitis. Plasmapheresis removes circulating agents, such as CIC or antigens. IVIg is thought to work by increasing the catabolism of immunoglobulins and leads to a dramatic decrease in the titer of pathologic antibodies. Compared to the other agents discussed in this chapter, plasmapheresis and IVIg have a much more rapid onset of action. With both agents, however, the improvement is short term, and these agents are best used as temporizing measures.

Various targeted agents have begun to be used to treat vasculitis. The anti-tumor necrosis factor-α (TNF-α) agents were the first to be tested, mostly in ANCA-associated vasculitides. Etanercept does not appear to be effective for Wegener's granulomatosis, although infliximab appears to be more promising for various forms of vasculitis, including the ANCA-associated vasculitides, cryoglobulinemic vasculitis, cutaneous PAN, and vasculitis associated with RA. In the trial of etanercept and Wegener's granulomatosis, not only was there a lack of effect, but the investigators observed an increased number of solid malignancies. Rituximab, a monoclonal anti-CD20 antibody that depletes mature B lymphocytes, has also demonstrated significant efficacy in various vasculitides, most notably ANCA-associated vasculitis and cryoglobulinemic vasculitis. In HCV-related cryoglobulinemic vasculitis, rituximab is added to antiviral agents and has the added benefit of treating the underlying B-cell lymphoproliferative disorder seen in these patients. We have had positive experience with rituximab in treating several patients with cutaneous vasculitis. One note of caution: both the anti-TNF-α agents and (less often) rituximab have also been shown to induce vasculitis, and caution should therefore be exercised.

SUGGESTED READINGS

Bahrami S, Malone JC, Webb KG, Callen JP. Tissue eosinophilia as an indicator of drug-induced cutaneous small-vessel vasculitis. Arch Dermatol 2006; 142: 155–161.

Blanco R, Martinez-Taboada VM, Rodriguez-Valverde V, Garcia-Fuentes M. Cutaneous vasculitis in children and adults. Associated diseases and etiologic factors in 303 patients. Medicine (Baltimore) 1998; 77: 403–418.

Bloch DA, Michel BA, Hunder GG, et al. The American College of Rheumatology 1990 criteria for the classification of vasculitis. Patients and methods. Arthritis Rheum 1990; 33: 1068–1073.

Callen JP. Colchicine is effective in controlling chronic cutaneous leukocytoclastic vasculitis. J Am Acad Dermatol 1985; 13: 193–200.

Callen JP. Cutaneous vasculitis: what have we learned in the past 20 years? Arch Dermatol 1998; 134: 355–357.

Diaz-Perez JL, De Lagrán ZM, Díaz-Ramón JL, Winkelmann RK. Cutaneous polyarteritis nodosa. Semin Cutan Med Surg 2007; 26: 77–86.

Fiorentino DF. Cutaneous vasculitis. J Am Acad Dermatol 2003; 48: 311–340.

Jennette JC, Falk RJ, Andrassy K, et al. Nomenclature of systemic vasculitides. Proposal of an international consensus conference. Arthritis Rheum 1994; 37: 187–192.

Lotti T, Ghersetich I, Comacchi C, Jorizzo JL. Cutaneous small-vessel vasculitis. J Am Acad Dermatol 1998; 39: 667–687; quiz 688–690.

Prins C, Gelfand EW, French LE. Intravenous immunoglobulin: properties, mode of action and practical use in dermatology. Acta Dermatol Venereol 2007; 87: 206–218.

Sams WM Jr, Thorne EG, Small P, et al. Leukocytoclastic vasculitis. Arch Dermatol 1976; 112: 219–226.

Saulsbury FT. Henoch–Schönlein purpura in children. Report of 100 patients and review of the literature. Medicine (Baltimore) 1999; 78: 395–409.

Solans-Laque R, Bosch-Gil JA, Pérez-Bocanegra C, et al. Paraneoplastic vasculitis in patients with solid tumors: report of 15 cases. J Rheumatol 2008; 35: 294–304.

Stone JH, Nousari HC. 'Essential' cutaneous vasculitis: what every rheumatologist should know about vasculitis of the skin. Curr Opin Rheumatol 2001; 13: 23–34.

Zeek PM. Periarteritis nodosa: a critical review. Am J Clin Pathol 1952; 22: 777–790.

Brad A. Yentzer,
Joseph L. Jorizzo,
Kenneth E. Greer,
and Jeffrey P. Callen

Chapter | 5 |

Miscellaneous Disorders With Prominent Features Involving the Skin and the Joints

RHEUMATOID ARTHRITIS

Definition, Diagnosis, and Epidemiologic Data

Rheumatoid arthritis (RA) is a multisystemic disease of unknown cause characterized primarily by synovitis, which in many cases produces typical erosive joint deformity. There is a remarkable heterogeneity from patient to patient with respect to the clinical manifestations and course of RA. Extra-articular manifestations commonly involve the skin and/or the lungs, but may also involve the hematologic, cardiovascular, and neurologic systems. Occasionally the extra-articular manifestations dominate the clinical picture, but most often RA is a disease of the joints. It is found worldwide, and affects females two to three times more often than males. Although it occurs in all ages, it is most prominent between the fourth and sixth decades of life.

The diagnosis is relatively easy to make in the advanced stages but is challenging early in the course of the disease. Criteria have been developed by the American College of Rheumatology for the diagnosis of classic, definite, probable, and possible RA, primarily to standardize patients for the purposes of clinical research. Criteria also are available for clinical remission, disease progression, and the functional capacity of patients with the disease. Information regarding these criteria is available from the Arthritis Foundation or the American College of Rheumatology (Atlanta, Georgia). The diagnosis of RA is based on a combination of clinical, radiographic, and laboratory findings, including the serum rheumatoid factor titer. A newer test for anti-cyclic citrullinated peptide (CCP) antibodies is more specific for RA than rheumatoid factor, but less sensitive. Histologic changes in the synovium and the presence of skin nodules are additional criteria. The rheumatoid factor, measured primarily as IgM with specificity against altered IgG, is positive in approximately 75% of patients with RA and in 1–5% of normal subjects. High titers of rheumatoid factor are generally associated with more severe, erosive forms of the disease, with rheumatoid nodules and with a higher incidence of systemic complications.

Cutaneous Manifestations

A number of cutaneous findings are reported in patients with RA, but there are no pathognomonic manifestations (Table 5–1). Few of these conditions are characteristic for RA, with the notable exception of the rheumatoid nodule. Pyoderma gangrenosum and a wide spectrum of vasculitic lesions are not uncommon in patients with RA, but they occur more commonly in association with other disorders. The cutaneous eruption of juvenile idiopathic arthritis (JIA), formerly known as juvenile rheumatoid arthritis (JRA), is helpful in establishing the diagnosis of the disease, but is not specific. A large group of miscellaneous dermatoses have been described in patients with RA. Finally, there are a wide variety of cutaneous changes associated with various therapeutic agents used to treat the disease.

Rheumatoid Nodules

Rheumatoid nodules are firm, nontender, freely movable subcutaneous masses that occur in approximately 20–25% of adult patients with RA. They are the most characteristic extra-articular manifestations of the disease and are more common in patients with severe arthritis, high-titer rheumatoid factor, and/or rheumatoid vasculitis. The dome-shaped flesh-colored nodules usually vary from 0.5 cm to several centimeters in diameter. They tend to occur near the elbows and in areas subject to trauma, particularly over bony prominences (Fig. 5–1). Any subcutaneous site can be affected, however, and histologically identical lesions have been found in the sclerae, larynx, heart, lungs, and abdominal wall. The lesions develop insidiously and are usually persistent, but may regress spontaneously. The clinical differential diagnosis of rheumatoid nodules includes gouty tophi, xanthomas, deep or nodular granuloma annulare, and ganglion and epidermal inclusion cysts.

Histologically, three distinct zones are observed in well-developed rheumatoid nodules: (1) a central zone of fibrinoid

Table 5–1 Cutaneous findings in rheumatoid arthritis

Common skin lesions
   Rheumatoid nodules
   Superficial ulcerating rheumatoid necrobiosis
   Rheumatoid papules
   Palmar erythema
   Nail ridging
   Onycholysis
   Dilated nailfold capillaries
   Atrophic or transparent skin over bony prominences

Vasculitic lesions
   Capillaritis
   Livedo reticularis
   Petechiae
   Purpura
   Gangrenous/ulcerating plaques

Leg ulcers
   Felty's syndrome
   Pyoderma gangrenosum
   Vasculitis

Miscellaneous associations
   Urticaria-like lesions of Still's disease
   Amyloidosis
   Bullous diseases

Skin changes secondary to medications
   Corticosteroids
     Cushingoid facies
     Tinea pedis
     Bruising or striae
   TNF-α blockers
     Leukocytoclastic vasculitis
     Psoriasiform exanthem
     Palmoplantar pustulosis
     Injection site reaction
   Leflunomide
     Focal epidermal necrolysis

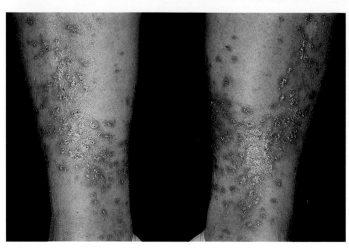

Figure 5–2 Multiple papules in a patient with rheumatoid arthritis, the so-called rheumatoid papule.

necrosis; (2) a middle zone of palisading histiocytes; and (3) a peripheral zone of highly vascularized granulation tissue with a chronic, mononuclear inflammatory cell infiltrate. Early lesions are composed primarily of the granulation tissue but have focal areas of leukocytoclastic vasculitis that are believed to be relevant in the pathogenesis of the nodules. Histologically the differential diagnosis includes the transient nodules seen in acute rheumatic fever, deep granuloma annulare, and necrobiosis lipoidica diabeticorum.

Rheumatoid nodules occur in disorders other than RA, including systemic lupus erythematosus and scleroderma. They may also occur independently of other diseases and in a disorder reported as benign rheumatoid nodulosis. The nodules in the latter disorder are now believed to be the subcutaneous or nodular lesions of granuloma annulare and not those of RA. Granulomas also occur in RA in a condition called palisaded neutrophilic granulomatous dermatitis (PNGD), formerly known as rheumatoid papules or superficial ulcerating rheumatoid necrobiosis (Fig. 5–2).

Rheumatoid Vasculitis

The spectrum of clinical lesions reported to be rheumatoid vasculitis is wide and varies with the size and location of the vessels involved and with the extent of the disease. Leukocytoclastic change can occur most commonly in the small arterioles and venules of the skin, but this same necrotizing process may occur in larger vessels of the mesentery, heart, and central nervous system. Cutaneous lesions include petechiae, palpable purpura, gangrenous plaques, digital infarcts, and large ischemic ulcerations of the lower extremities, especially over the malleoli. Vasculitis usually occurs in patients with severe forms of RA and has been classified as mild, moderate, or severe. The cutaneous lesions of mild rheumatoid vasculitis include small digital infarcts, especially of the nailfolds and digital pulp (often called Bywater's lesions), and petechiae and livedo reticularis. Palpable purpura of the lower extremities and buttocks is typical in moderate disease (Fig. 5–3). This syndrome is clinicopathologically indistinguishable from cutaneous small-vessel vasculitis from other causes. Severe disease

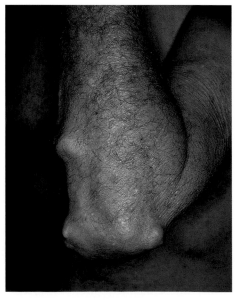

Figure 5–1 Rheumatoid nodules on the elbow.

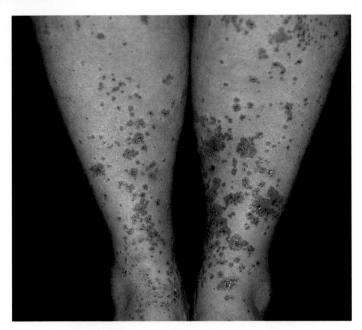

Figure 5–3 Multiple palpable purpuric lesions typical of cutaneous small-vessel vasculitis in a patient with circulating immune complexes and high-titer rheumatoid factor.

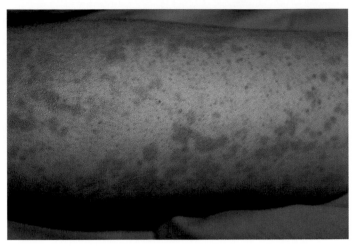

Figure 5–5 Transient faint erythema of juvenile idiopathic arthritis. (Courtesy of Kenneth E. Greer, MD, Charlottesville, VA.)

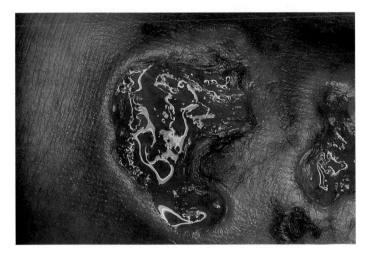

Figure 5–4 Rheumatoid vasculitis manifest as large ulcers on the dorsal foot.

can occur in an explosive fashion, involving cutaneous and systemic organs and having a mortality rate approaching 30%. Larger vessels, including muscular arteries, are affected. The cutaneous lesions may include the changes seen in mild or moderate rheumatoid vasculitis, in addition to large ulcers from necrosing livedo reticularis (retiform purpura) and digital gangrene (Fig. 5–4). Most evidence suggests that the vasculitic lesions are related to circulating immune complexes.

Miscellaneous Dermatologic Conditions Associated with RA

Several nonspecific cutaneous lesions have been reported in patients with RA, including such changes as palmar erythema,

focal or generalized hyperpigmentation, thinning of the skin (especially over the joints), Raynaud's phenomenon, yellow skin and the yellow nail syndrome, and nails with dusky red lunulae. There are numerous reports linking RA to pyoderma gangrenosum, as well as blistering diseases, particularly epidermolysis bullosa acquisita.

Both children with JIA and patients with adult-onset Still's disease often have a characteristic pink to salmon-colored urticarial or measles-like eruption associated with a high, spiking fever. The cutaneous eruption and fever peak in the late afternoon. The eruption is minimally pruritic to asymptomatic and is most obvious on the chest, abdomen, and extensor surfaces of the arm (Fig. 5–5). It is usually transitory, but may persist for several days. It is helpful diagnostically when evaluating a patient with arthralgias, fever, and negative laboratory parameters, including rheumatoid factor.

Treatment

The mainstay of RA therapy is the early institution of disease-modifying antirheumatic drugs (DMARDs) (Table 5–2). Methotrexate is often still a first choice for moderate to severe disease. Corticosteroids are often given in short bursts for flare control, but are sometimes used chronically in low doses. Biological therapies include those that block tumor necrosis factor (TNF)-α (etanercept, adalimumab, and infliximab), those that modulate T-cell activation (abatacept), those that inhibit type I receptors of interleukin (IL)-1 (anakinra), and agents that affect B-cell activation (rituximab). The TNF antagonists have been demonstrated to prevent progression of erosive disease and may prevent deformities associated with RA. It is not clear whether any of the agents are effective in the treatment of the skin manifestations of RA, and some patients have been reported in whom vasculitis or accelerated nodulosis has been associated with the use of methotrexate or TNF therapies. Rheumatoid vasculitis should be viewed as an extra-articular manifestation of RA that dictates more stable control of the underlying disease.

Table 5–2 A pharmacologic approach to RA (adapted from the ACR guidelines)

First choice
  NSAIDs
  DMARD(s) – methotrexate
  Local corticosteroid injections
  Low-dose systemic corticosteroid

Second-line
  Other DMARD(s)
    Hydroxychloroquine
    Sulfasalazine
    Leflunomide
    Azathioprine
  Biologics (+/– methotrexate)
    Etanercept
    Infliximab
    Adalimumab
    Anakinra
    Abatacept
    Rituximab
  Systemic corticosteroids
  Combination therapy

Adjuncts
  Fish oil
  Bisphosphonates
  Calcium + vitamin D

Table 5–3 Classification of psoriatic arthritis

Types	Incidence	Major characteristics
Asymmetrical oligoarthritis	70	Usually one or a few small joints of the hands and feet
Symmetrical polyarthritis	15	Clinically indistinguishable from rheumatoid arthritis, yet more benign
Primarily distal interphalangeal joints	5	So-called classic pattern; marked nail involvement and 'sausage digits'
Arthritis mutilans	5	Severe, rapid development that is destructive, telescoping
Psoriatic spondylitis	5	Not an uncommon accompaniment of other forms (uncommon alone)

PSORIATIC ARTHRITIS

General and Epidemiologic Aspects

Psoriatic arthritis is an erosive inflammatory joint disease with widely variable clinical manifestations that occurs in approximately 6–10% of patients with arthritis, 20–35% of patients with psoriasis, and 0.02–0.1% of the general population. Epidemiologic, genetic, clinical, serologic, and radiologic data have established that psoriatic arthritis is a distinctive group of diseases. The overall sex ratio is equal. The male preponderance reported in some studies is probably based on series dealing with specific clinical subtypes, such as distal joint psoriatic arthritis, which appears to be more common in men. Psoriatic arthritis is typically an adult-onset disease with a peak age of onset between 35 and 45 years. It may occur in childhood, however, and may be difficult to distinguish from JIA. The pathogenesis is unknown, but genetic factors are important. The genetic marker HLA-B27 has a high incidence in patients with psoriatic spondylitis, but not in individuals with the other subtypes of psoriatic arthritis.

Classification and Clinical Manifestations

Several classification systems have been proposed, including that listed in Table 5–3. All five types of arthritis in this classification can occur independent of psoriasis. At least 70% of patients with psoriatic arthritis are classified as having the asymmetric oligoarticular pattern, in which the arthritis is restricted to one or a few small joints of the hands and feet

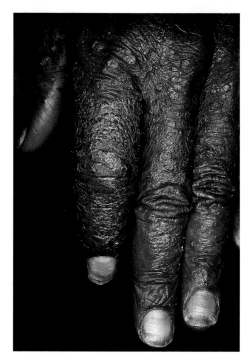

Figure 5–6 Deforming asymmetrical oligoarticular arthritis of the hands in a patient with plaque psoriasis.

(Fig. 5–6). The metatarsophalangeal and interphalangeal joints are most frequently affected, and the disease develops acutely in 50% of these cases. Fifteen percent of patients with psoriatic arthritis develop a pattern of disease that is clinically indistinguishable from RA – the so-called symmetric polyarthritis. The distal interphalangeal joints may be involved along with the proximal interphalangeal joints, but the rheumatoid factor titer is negative. Patients with psoriasis who have arthritis, rheumatoid nodules, and positive tests for rheumatoid factors are said to have RA and coincidental psoriasis, and are not classified as having psoriatic arthritis. Rheumatoid nodules are never considered to be part of the clinical spectrum of psoriatic arthritis.

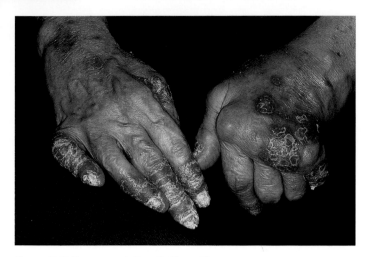

Figure 5–7 Severe psoriatic arthritis mutilans.

Each of the three remaining types – arthritis mutilans, psoriatic spondylitis, and classic distal interphalangeal arthritis – accounts for approximately 5% of cases. Arthritis mutilans is the most destructive and disabling type of psoriatic arthritis (Fig. 5–7).

At least 75% of patients with psoriatic arthritis will have cutaneous psoriasis before the onset of the arthritis. Dystrophic nails eventually develop in at least 85% of cases, a higher frequency than in psoriasis without arthritis. The nail dystrophy appears to be especially common in patients with distal joint disease.

Diagnosis and Differential Diagnosis

The diagnosis of psoriatic arthritis is based on clinical, laboratory, and X-ray findings. The major laboratory finding is the negative test for rheumatoid factor in a psoriatic patient with arthritis whose disease fits the clinical definition of psoriatic arthritis. Many of the X-ray changes occur in both RA and psoriatic arthritis. Several radiological features, however, appear to be more characteristic of, but not specific for, psoriatic arthritis: (1) destructive changes of isolated small joints, especially the interphalangeal joints of the fingers and toes, with erosion and expansion of the base of the terminal phalanx; (2) arthritis mutilans, producing the so-called pencil-in-cup changes; (3) terminal phalangeal osteolysis, predominantly of the hallus; (4) periostosis and ankylosis of the small bones of the hands and feet; and (5) atypical spondylitis or sacroiliitis. In addition, a resorptive osteolysis with soft-tissue atrophy of the digits has been seen in association with acral pustular psoriasis, and is to be distinguished from psoriatic arthritis mutilans.

Early in the course of psoriatic arthritis the radiographic appearance is usually normal or shows nonspecific changes such as soft-tissue swelling. The destructive changes, which result from more severe joint inflammation, appear with time. The differential diagnosis includes Reiter's syndrome (which shares many features with psoriatic spondylitis and other HLA-B27 spectrum diseases), RA, acute arthritis, and osteoarthritis.

Treatment and Prognosis

The majority of patients with psoriatic arthritis have mild disease characterized by periods of remission and exacerbation, and a more benign course than that seen in patients with RA. Aspirin and other nonsteroidal anti-inflammatory drugs are often sufficient to control the disease. Systemic corticosteroids are relatively contraindicated, owing to their adverse effects, which in some patients include a marked 'rebound' exacerbation of their cutaneous disease. Improvement of the skin lesions, especially with nonsystemic forms of therapy, is not generally associated with improvement in the joint disease. The oral retinoid acitretin has been used successfully to control cutaneous disease and occasionally improves the arthritis. The adverse effects from the long-term administration of retinoids, especially the production of bone hyperostoses, limit the usefulness of these drugs for chronic diseases, including psoriatic arthritis. In severe or progressive forms of the disease, oral methotrexate or cyclosporine may be beneficial for both skin and joint disease in carefully selected patients. Three TNF-α blockers are now FDA approved for the treatment of psoriatic arthritis, including etanercept, infliximab, and adalimumab. All of the TNF-α agents are approved for use in conjunction with methotrexate and low doses of prednisone, and their effects are longer lasting when administered in combination with methotrexate. Other biologic agents that are currently approved for the treatment of psoriasis vulgaris (efalizumab and alefacept) and those with approval pending (anti-IL-12/23 agents) either have little effect on psoriatic arthritis or have been associated with flares of joint disease. Antimalarials, commonly used in the treatment of RA, are not generally used in patients with psoriasis, but in some patients the arthritis responds well to these agents. Physical or occupational therapy, including rest, splinting, range-of-motion exercises, and adaptive devices, is an essential aspect of patient care. In patients with severe disease that produces functional limitation, reconstructive surgery, similar to that used in RA, can be remarkably effective.

The long-term prognosis of psoriatic arthritis is unpredictable, and there may be periods of acute inflammation followed by months or years of disease inactivity. A recurrence of joint disease occurs spontaneously and without any known provoking stimulus. Fortunately, only a small percentage of patients with psoriatic arthritis develop severe crippling disease.

BEHÇET'S DISEASE

Clinical Manifestations

Behçet's disease is a complex multisystem disorder described by the Turkish dermatologist Hulusi Behç in the late 1930s. Although relatively common in the Middle East and Asia, it is uncommon in northern Europe, Great Britain, and the United States. Behçet's occurs in both sexes and is primarily a disease of young adults.

Because there is no pathognomonic laboratory test, the diagnosis is based on clinical criteria (Table 5–4). The oral aphthae experienced by these patients are like those seen in patients with simple aphthosis (i.e., canker sores). They are

Table 5–4 Clinical criteria for Behçet's disease

Recurrent oral aphthosis
AND
At least two of the following:
  Recurrent genital aphthosis
  Uveitis
  Synovitis
  Cutaneous pustular vasculitis
  Meningoencephalitis

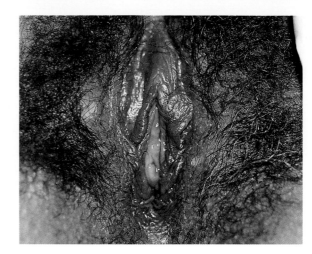

Figure 5–10 Vulvar aphthae in Behçet's disease.

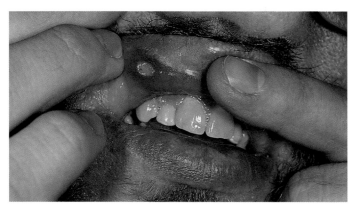

Figure 5–8 Oral aphthous lesions in a patient with Behçet's disease.

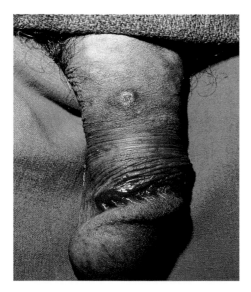

Figure 5–9 Aphthae on the penis in a patient with Behçet's disease.

usually multiple and occur in crops (Fig. 5–8). The genital aphthae are similar, except that they occur less frequently (Figs 5–9 and 5–10). Pathergy – the development of cutaneous papulopustular lesions 24 hours after cutaneous trauma (e.g., by needle prick or intradermal injection) – is a characteristic feature seen in many patients with Behçet's disease. The term pustular vasculitis excludes the often-confused acneiform or follicle-based lesions from diagnostic considerations. Deeper

lesions, occurring in subcutaneous fat, may mimic those of erythema nodosum or superficial migratory thrombophlebitis. Skin lesions that mimic the neutrophilic dermatoses, including Sweet's syndrome and pyoderma gangrenosum, may also occur in Behçet's disease.

Behçet's disease is a multisystem disorder. Posterior uveitis (i.e., retinal vasculitis) is the most classic ocular lesion seen in Behçet's disease. The arthritis seen in patients with Behçet's disease is nonerosive and inflammatory, and affects both large and small joints. Patients with HLA-B27-positive sacroiliitis should be considered as part of the Reiter's/HLA-B27 spectrum of disease and not as having Behçet's disease. Meningoencephalitis may be more common in patients with Behçet's disease than was previously appreciated. Neurologic manifestations have a late onset in patients with Behçet's disease and are remarkably variable in their presentation. A vasculitis of the vasovasorum, with a propensity to affect large arteries and veins, can be a cause of death in patients with Behçet's disease. The kidney may be relatively spared in these patients. Inflammatory bowel disease and other autoimmune disorders that can be associated with recurrent oral aphthosis and synovitis must be excluded.

Pathogenesis

Behçet's is considered an autoinflammatory disorder, often causing an immune-mediated occlusive vasculitis. Cellular immunity has been evaluated extensively in patients with Behçet's disease. The earliest mucocutaneous lesions in Behçet's disease represent a neutrophilic vascular reaction or fully developed leukocytoclastic vasculitis, and there is some support for a role for immune complex-mediated vessel damage in the pathogenesis of lesions. Studies of neutrophil function show that a heat-stable serum factor (present in the serum of patients with Behçet's disease) dramatically enhances the migration of patient and control neutrophils. The characteristic pustular vasculitic lesions, the aphthae, and possibly the systemic lesions in this disease may well result from an enhanced accumulation of neutrophils in sites of immune complex-mediated vessel damage. The histologic appearance of late-established lesions is dominated by a lymphocytic infiltrate in various tissues.

A role for cytokines and adhesion molecules also seems certain. The role of IL-8 in particular appears to play an important role in the pathogenesis of lesions, as well as functioning as a marker for disease activity. A role for heat shock protein, TNF-α, and other cytokines has also been suggested.

The etiology of Behçet's disease remains unknown, but various studies have implicated genetic factors, environmental pollution, viral and bacterial agents, and immunologic factors. The genes indicating disease susceptibility are HLA-B51 and HLA-DRW52, and have been associated with more severe disease. A genetic predisposition that triggers immunologic disease in response to viral or other infection is one theory of disease pathogenesis. Evidence supports *Streptococcus sanguinis*, *Mycoplasma fermentans*, herpes simplex (HSV-1), and bowel flora antigens as possible triggers.

Histology

Most studies of lesions of internal organs in Behçet's disease are of autopsy material. It is not surprising that the major finding reported is a lymphocytic 'perivasculitis.' This same histologic pattern is seen in late mucocutaneous lesions. Earlier lesions (more accessible to study in the skin) show leukocytoclastic vasculitis or a milder, neutrophilic vascular reaction.

Course and Treatment

The clinical course of Behçet's disease is extremely variable. Many patients suffer frequent, painful bouts of oral and genital aphthae and arthritis for years. The progression of posterior uveitis to ultimate blindness is the major cause of morbidity. Death in Behçet's disease is usually the result of central nervous system involvement, bowel perforation, or large arterial or venous occlusion.

Therapy for mucosal lesions may be supportive, with topical viscous lidocaine, potent topical corticosteroids, or intralesional corticosteroid injections. Oral colchicine therapy may be associated with a reduced severity and frequency of aphthae. Oral thalidomide therapy is extremely effective for mucocutaneous involvement, but use of this drug requires care regarding prevention of pregnancy and for the possible development of a sensory neuropathy. Adherence to a safety program designed by the manufacturer of the drug and monitored by Boston University is imperative. Low-dose weekly methotrexate therapy may be beneficial in selected patients. Oral dapsone may be substituted or added. Systemic corticosteroid therapy, alone or with azathioprine, is a mainstay of treatment for more severe ocular and systemic disease. Oral chlorambucil therapy and cyclosporine are more toxic therapies for patients with resistant ocular or neurologic disease. There are case reports of successful treatment of uveitis associated with Behçet's disease using biologic agents such as infliximab, etanercept, adalimumab, and rituximab. In most case reports where biologics were initiated, the extraocular manifestations also improved, but tended to recur when the drug was withdrawn.

SWEET'S SYNDROME (ACUTE FEBRILE NEUTROPHILIC DERMATOSIS)

Clinical Manifestations

Sweet described a group of patients with one or more attacks of painful, erythematous plaques accompanied by fever, arthralgias, and leukocytosis. This syndrome is more frequent in women (female:male 4:1) between the ages of 30 and 60 years. The cutaneous lesions are regarded as distinctive, but may simulate several other processes. The characteristic lesion is a well-defined erythematous plaque with a mamillated surface, which may give the clinical impression of microvesiculation (Fig. 5–11). There is rarely any accompanying epidermal change or ulceration, and the lesions heal without scar formation. Pustules may stud the surface or may be initiated by a variety of traumatic injuries (pathergy), such as a needlestick, wound debridement, or burn. The lesions are accompanied by fever and malaise in most patients, and by myalgias and/or arthralgias in about half. Untreated lesions resolve over 6–8 weeks; however, many patients continue to produce lesions either chronically or recurrently. There have been several reports of neutrophilic infiltration of organs other than the skin. Most frequently reported is pulmonary involvement, followed by bone infiltrates (multifocal sterile osteomyelitis), eye disease (peripheral ulcerative keratitis), and infiltration of the heart, muscles, nervous system, and gastrointestinal system.

Histology and Laboratory Findings

Histopathologically there is a dense dermal infiltrate composed of mature polymorphonuclear leukocytes. The infiltrate may be more pronounced in perivascular areas, and leukocytosis is frequent, but, classically, the vessel walls are spared. Minor vascular inflammation has been shown in several reports, and so a careful clinical correlation is often needed. In patients with an associated leukemia the infiltrate may

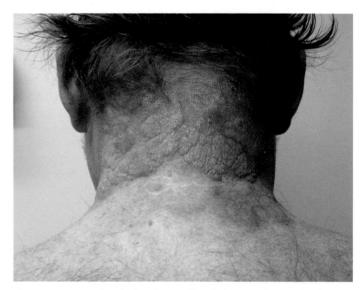

Figure 5–11 Pseudovesiculated, mamillated plaques of acute febrile neutrophilic dermatosis.

consist entirely of mature neutrophils or may include leukemic cells. The laboratory findings include a leukocytosis composed of mature neutrophils. White blood cell counts generally range from 10 000 to 20 000 cells/mm³. A careful examination of the peripheral smear is warranted in any patient with leukocytosis, anemia, or thrombocytopenia.

Associated Conditions

Sweet's syndrome has been described with a variety of diseases, but the most frequent association is with myelogenous leukemia or pre-leukemia. Sweet's syndrome is not clinically or histopathologically different in the presence of leukemia, but the patients more frequently tend to be anemic or thrombocytopenic. This syndrome has also been reported in conjunction with lupus erythematosus, RA, Sjögren's syndrome, Behçet's disease, inflammatory bowel disease, pregnancy, benign monoclonal gammopathy, lymphoma, myelodysplastic disorders, and several solid tumors, as well as after infection with streptococcus.

Treatment

Sweet's syndrome is usually an acute, steroid-responsive, self-limiting disease. In general, a 2–3-week tapering course of oral prednisone (40–60 mg/day) is effective. One or more exacerbations, requiring a brief reinstitution of corticosteroids, are common. In individual reports, dapsone, potassium iodide, indometacin, clofazimine, colchicine, thalidomide, isotretinoin, methotrexate, chlorambucil, and pulse dosing of methylprednisolone have been used successfully. There are new case reports of successful treatment of Sweet's with biologic agents, including TNF-α antagonists.

PYODERMA GANGRENOSUM

Clinical Manifestations

Pyoderma gangrenosum is an uncommon, ulcerative, cutaneous condition with distinctive clinical characteristics. In roughly 50% of patients with pyoderma gangrenosum there is an associated systemic disease. The diagnosis is made by the exclusion of other processes that may cause cutaneous ulcers. The diagnostic evaluation of the patient presumed to have pyoderma gangrenosum has two objectives: (1) to exclude other causes of cutaneous ulceration, as this is a diagnosis of exclusion; and (2) to determine whether there is an associated treatable systemic disorder. In patients with other underlying disease, such as inflammatory bowel disease, RA, or myelodysplastic disorders, treatment of the pyoderma gangrenosum is directed to treatment of these underlying conditions.

The ulceration(s) of classic pyoderma gangrenosum are often clinically characteristic. The border is well defined with a deep erythematous to violaceous color (Fig. 5–12). The lesion extends peripherally, and often the border overhangs the ulceration (undermined) as the inflammatory process spreads within the dermis, only secondarily causing necrosis of the epidermis. Pain is a prominent feature and is sometimes severe. As the lesion heals, scar formation occurs, and the

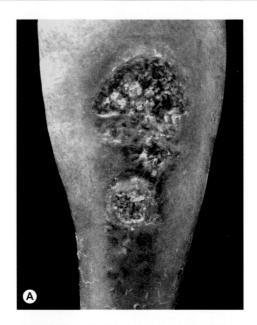

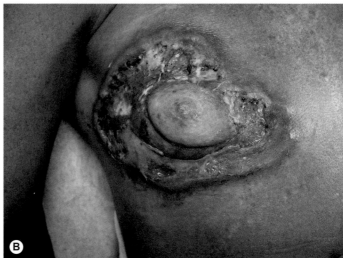

Figure 5–12 (A) Classic pyoderma gangrenosum in a patient with partially controlled Crohn's disease. (B) Pyoderma gangrenosum developed following a breast biopsy performed at the same time as abdominal surgery in this patient with Crohn's disease.

resulting scar is often described as cribriform. As described with Sweet's syndrome, patients with pyoderma gangrenosum may also have neutrophilic infiltration of internal organs, including the lung, liver, heart, and bone. Several variants of pyoderma gangrenosum have been described.

Pustular Eruption of Ulcerative Colitis

In this process, the patient is acutely ill with fever and develops multiple sterile pustules. These lesions often resemble the pustular vasculitis seen in patients with Behçet's disease.

Pyostomatitis Vegetans

This process is one in which chronic, pustular, and eventually vegetative erosions develop on the mucous membranes, most notably in the mouth.

Atypical or Bullous Pyoderma Gangrenosum

In this variant, the ulcerations are more superficial than in classic pyoderma gangrenosum. There is often a bullous, blue-gray margin, and the upper extremities and face are the most commonly affected sites (Fig. 5–13). This variant has been reported in patients with hematologic disease, specifically, pre-leukemia, myeloid metaplasia, or acute myelogenous leukemia.

Peristomal Pyoderma Gangrenosum

These patients often have a stoma created after surgery for inflammatory bowel disease or for cancer (Fig. 5–14). Some patients have no evidence of active bowel disease, whereas in others careful study reveals active disease, in particular Crohn's disease. These patients are often thought to have an infection, and surgeons will often debride the ulcer or relocate the stoma – approaches that often result in a recurrence of the disease. Treatment of the underlying process is often helpful, otherwise the treatments listed below are used.

Histopathology

The histopathologic features of pyoderma gangrenosum are not specific, but they are useful in ruling out other causes of cutaneous ulceration. There is controversy over what is the initial histopathologic change, with most classifying the process as a neutrophilic dermatosis and others believing that the initial changes involve lymphocytic infiltration.

Associated Conditions

Although associated conditions are common (Table 5–5), perhaps approximately half of the patients have 'idiopathic' disease. The most common associated conditions are inflammatory bowel disease, arthritis, paraproteinemia, and hematologic malignancy.

Arthritis is a frequent finding in patients with pyoderma gangrenosum. In general, the arthritis associated with pyoderma gangrenosum is a symmetrical polyarthritis, which may be seronegative or seropositive. As with Sweet's syndrome, patients with pyoderma gangrenosum may also have neutrophilic infiltrates in other organs.

Treatment

In mild cases, local measures such as dressings, rest, topical agents, or intralesional injections may be sufficient to control the disease process. In patients with severe disease or those who do not respond to local therapies, systemic agents such as sulfonamides, sulfones, thalidomide, or corticosteroids have been the most commonly used. Systemic corticosteroids have been used extensively in patients with pyoderma gangrenosum and its variants, and are generally believed to be effective.

Immunosuppressive agents have been suggested for use in patients who fail to respond to other therapies, particularly systemic corticosteroids, or who develop steroid-related side effects. Individual reports of the use of azathioprine, mycophenolate mofetil, cyclophosphamide, chlorambucil, or cyclosporine have suggested that these agents may be beneficial, at least in some patients. Infliximab and adalimumab have both been shown to be effective in patients with pyoderma gangrenosum, the former in a randomized placebo-controlled trial. Both agents appear to be effective regardless of the presence or absence of inflammatory bowel disease. Intravenous immunoglobulin has also been reported to be effective.

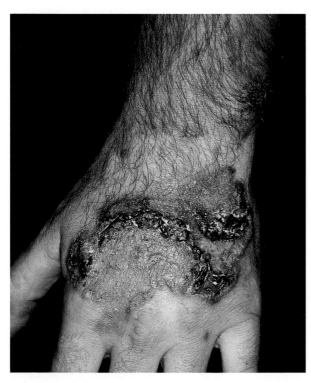

Figure 5–13 Atypical pyoderma gangrenosum.

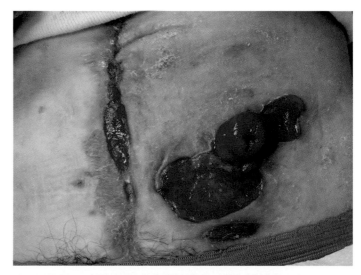

Figure 5–14 Several peristomal ulcerations developed following colectomy in this young woman with Crohn's disease. Also of note is the ulceration in the midline incision created during surgery.

Table 5–5 Diseases associated with pyoderma gangrenosum

Common associations

Inflammatory bowel disease
　Chronic ulcerative colitis
　Regional enteritis, granulomatous colitis (Crohn's disease)

Arthritis
　Seronegative with inflammatory bowel disease
　Seronegative without inflammatory bowel disease
　Rheumatoid arthritis
　Spondylitis
　Osteoarthritis

Hematologic diseases
　Myelocytic leukemias
　Hairy cell leukemia
　Myelofibrosis, agnogenic myeloid metaplasia
　Monoclonal gammopathy (IgA)

Rarely reported associations

Chronic active hepatitis
Myeloma
Polycythemia rubra vera
Paroxysmal nocturnal hemoglobinuria
Takayasu's arteritis
Primary biliary cirrhosis
Systemic lupus erythematosus
Wegener's granulomatosis
Hidradenitis suppurativa
Acne conglobata
Malignancy
Thyroid disease
Pulmonary disease
Sarcoidosis
Diabetes mellitus
Other pustular dermatoses

BOWEL BYPASS–BOWEL-ASSOCIATED DERMATOSIS–ARTHRITIS SYNDROME

Clinical Manifestations

Approximately 20% of patients who underwent jejunoileal bypass surgery for morbid obesity developed a serum sickness-like illness characterized by cutaneous pustular vasculitis, synovitis, fever, and flu-like symptoms. An identical syndrome has been reported in patients who have not had bypass surgery but who have had Billroth II surgery for peptic ulcer disease, or who have had inflammatory bowel disease. The concept of pustular vasculitis has been proposed to link the similar clinicopathologic features with the proposed immunopathogenetic features seen in patients with Behçet's disease, bowel bypass–bowel-associated dermatosis–arthritis syndrome, and an idiopathic cutaneous pustular vasculitis.

The pathomechanism of lesions in patients with bowel bypass syndrome may have involved circulating immune complexes that contain bacterial peptidoglycans of presumed bowel origin as the circulating antigens. Bacterial overgrowth in the blind loop of the bowel could result in the formation of immune complexes that enter the circulation and deposit

in target tissues, such as the skin and synovium, producing the clinical features of this syndrome.

Patients experience the onset of the serum sickness-like illness 2–3 months or more after bypass surgery or Billroth II surgery, or at some point in the course of their inflammatory bowel disease. An increased frequency of diarrhea and gastrointestinal disturbance accompanies the systemic disease. Polyarticular arthralgias, myalgias, and a nonerosive arthritis that affects peripheral joints are frequent findings. Cutaneous pustular vasculitis occurs in a truncal distribution. Erythema nodosum-like lesions may also occur. Bouts may occur every 4–6 weeks.

Histopathology

Early reports of the histopathologic findings of cutaneous lesions in bowel bypass syndrome described leukocytoclastic vasculitis. Subsequent reports have corrected this to a neutrophilic vascular reaction indistinguishable from the vessel changes seen in the cutaneous lesions of Behçet's disease.

Treatment

Systemic corticosteroid therapy controlled the signs and symptoms of bowel-associated dermatosis–arthritis syndrome. The bowel bypass patients were cured by restoration of normal bowel anatomy. Systemic antibiotics (e.g., tetracycline, metronidazole, and erythromycin) are efficacious, perhaps owing to their effect on the reduction of bowel bacterial overgrowth. Thalidomide, colchicines, and dapsone have been successfully used in individual patients. Patients with inflammatory bowel disease need better control of their underlying disease.

REACTIVE ARTHRITIS (REITER'S SYNDROME)

Clinical Manifestations

The term reactive arthritis (ReA) has replaced Reiter's syndrome to encompass a broader group of patients, in whom inflammatory arthritis develops after an infection. The genitourinary (GU) or gastrointestinal (GI) tracts are common sources of infection associated with ReA. Reiter's syndrome is a multisystem disease of uncertain pathogenesis that is clinically characterized by the triad of nongonococcal urethritis, arthritis, and conjunctivitis (Table 5–6). The psoriasis-like skin lesions are called keratoderma blennorrhagicum (palms, soles) and circinate balanitis (penis) (Figs 5–15 and 5–16). The oral lesions are pustular and psoriasis-like, not aphthae, as in Behçet's disease. The association of ankylosing spondylitis with the histocompatibility antigen HLA-B27 has expanded the concept of HLA-B27-associated spondyloarthropathy to a spectrum of diseases that includes Reiter's syndrome, ankylosing spondylitis, enteropathic arthritis, and psoriasis with spondyloarthritis.

The evidence for a genetic predisposition to reactive arthritis and the HLA-B27 spectrum of diseases is strong, with a convincing HLA association. Reactive arthritis has been well known to develop following nongonococcal urethritis (the venereal form, caused by *Chlamydia* or *Ureaplasma urealyticum*) or dysentery (the dysenteric form, after shigellosis or infection with other

Table 5–6 Description and treatment of Reiter's syndrome

Signs and symptoms	Treatments
Mucocutaneous	Skin lesions
	Topical corticosteroids
Circinate balanitis	Tar
Keratoderma blennorrhagicum	UV light
Pustular oral lesions	
General	Mild disease
	NSAIDs
Hallmarks	Antibiotics
Nongonococcal urethritis	Moderate/severe disease
Arthritis	Methotrexate
Conjunctivitis	Sulfasalazine
Other	Systemic
Fever	corticosteroids
Malaise	(rebound risk)
Weight loss	TNF-α inhibitors
Gastrointestinal distress	Other biologics
Seronegative, erosive, axial arthropathy	
Achilles tendonitis	
Plantar fasciitis	
Iritis and/or keratitis	
Meningoencephalitis, psychotic episodes, seizures, or cranial or peripheral neuropathies	
Cardiac conduction abnormalities	

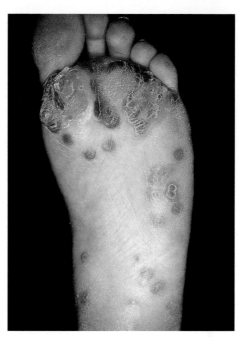

Figure 5–16 Keratoderma blennorrhagicum seen in a patient with Reiter's syndrome.

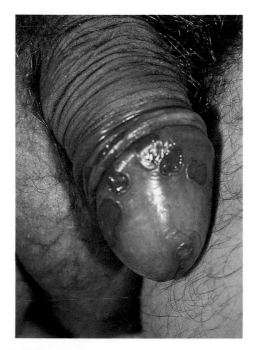

Figure 5–15 Circinate balanitis present in a patient with Reiter's syndrome.

enteric pathogens). It has been proposed that the complex multisystem immunologic response to the infections mentioned occurs in genetically predisposed individuals. The disease has also been well described in patients with human immunodeficiency virus (HIV) infection.

The post-venereal form of reactive arthritis is a disease primarily of young men. The disease process usually occurs in bouts that often last from 1 to 12 months, and which recur in

about half of patients. Fever, malaise, weight loss, and gastrointestinal distress are almost always accompanied by seronegative, erosive axial arthropathy. Achilles tendonitis and plantar fasciitis are prototypic manifestations that occur in about one-fifth of patients. The urethritis is nonspecific and is a feature of the post-venereal form. The ocular findings include conjunctivitis, iritis, and keratitis. The neurologic manifestations are varied and include meningoencephalitis, psychotic episodes, seizures, or cranial or peripheral neuropathies. Cardiac conduction abnormalities may occur.

The mucocutaneous manifestations of Reiter's syndrome and the HLA-B27 spectrum of reactive arthritis are clinicopathologically similar to those of psoriasis. Characteristic patterns of cutaneous disease exist in patients with Reiter's syndrome. Circinate balanitis is a psoriasis-like dermatitis of the head of the penis (see Fig. 5–15). Keratoderma blennorrhagicum is the name given to the psoriasis-like lesions that may be particularly thick (i.e., oyster shell-like) on the soles (see Fig. 5–16). The oral lesions resemble the pustular, geographic tongue-like lesions of acute pustular psoriasis. Patients with HLA-B27-positive enteropathic arthritis also may have aphthae, creating confusion with Behçet's disease. These patients are best considered with the HLA-B27 spectrum of disease.

More than 50% of patients with reactive arthritis may experience a relapsing course of the disease. Death occurs in less than 1% of patients; a significant percentage (about one-third) acquire some disability.

Histopathology

The histopathologic findings of cutaneous lesions from patients with Reiter's syndrome are indistinguishable from those of the lesions of psoriasis. The hallmark is the intraepidermal spongiform pustule. Neutrophils migrate into the epidermis to form these pustules. The epidermis is thickened (acanthosis), and nuclei are retained in the stratum corneum (i.e., parakeratosis).

Treatment

Although not curable, the disease is treatable. Nonsteroidal anti-inflammatory agents and topical regimens (corticosteroids, tar derivative, and ultraviolet light, as for psoriasis) are the mainstays of treatment for the mild musculoskeletal and cutaneous manifestations of Reiter's syndrome. Systemic methotrexate given in low weekly doses is an important therapeutic option for severe disease. Systemic corticosteroids are beneficial, but as in psoriasis, they may produce severe pustular flares of the cutaneous disease when tapered. Biologic agents, especially TNF-α antagonists, are used in Reiter's disease. Patients with HIV disease receiving antiretroviral therapy have a better prognosis than untreated HIV patients.

KAWASAKI'S DISEASE (MUCOCUTANEOUS LYMPH-NODE SYNDROME)

Clinical Manifestations

Kawasaki, a Japanese pediatrician, first described an acute febrile mucocutaneous syndrome with striking lymphadenopathy occurring in Japanese children in the late 1960s. This syndrome has now been reported worldwide. Diagnostic criteria have been described (Table 5–7), five or six of which must be present for the diagnosis to be made.

The cause of Kawasaki's disease remains unknown. Epidemiologic factors suggest an infectious cause, but no rickettsial, viral, or toxic agent has been identified. Kawasaki's disease is most common in children between 6 months and 4 years of age. Asian ancestry is a high-risk factor, although the syndrome occurs in all races. There is no clear HLA association.

High fevers (up to 40.5°C) are described as being 'hectic,' and may last up to 3 weeks. Within the first week of fever, edema and erythema develop on the hands and feet, a macular erythematous eruption begins, and oral erythema and conjunctival congestion occur (Fig. 5–17). A strawberry tongue may develop. During the resolution stage, brawny change and desquamation occur acrally (post-erythemal desquamation) (Fig. 5–18). The cervical lymphadenopathy may be dramatic.

The most important clinical complication is the development of coronary aneurysms, which may result from coronary artery vasculitis, and can produce death from myocardial infarction. Recently, adult coronary artery disease has been recognized as a complication of Kawasaki's disease. Cardiac changes are indistinguishable from the changes seen in juvenile polyarteritis nodosa.

The cutaneous lesions represent a scarletiform erythema and may show simple vasodilation and a perivascular lymphocytic reaction. They may occasionally resemble lesions of erythema multiforme. A number of other acute syndromes may mimic some features of Kawasaki's disease. The differential diagnosis includes Stevens–Johnson syndrome, toxic shock syndrome, scarlet fever, infantile polyarteritis nodosa, Rocky Mountain spotted fever, leptospirosis, mononucleosis, viral exanthems, the phenytoin syndrome, and collagen–vascular diseases.

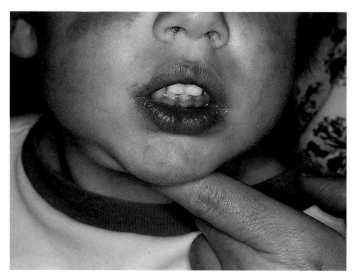

Figure 5–17 Kawasaki's syndrome.

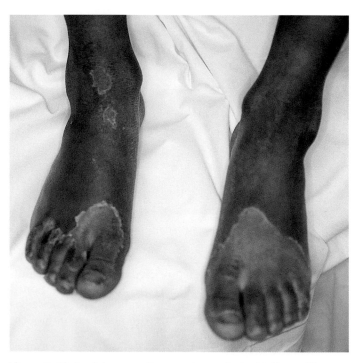

Figure 5–18 Acral desquamation seen in a patient with Kawasaki's syndrome.

Table 5–7 Description and treatment of Kawasaki's disease

Signs and symptoms	Treatments
Must have at least 5: High fever (unresponsive to antibiotics) Strawberry tongue Edematous hands and feet Exanthem Cervical lymphadenopathy	Mild disease High-dose salicylate Moderate/severe disease Intravenous immunoglobulin *Avoid corticosteroids

Treatment

Patients usually recover spontaneously in 1–3 weeks. Up to one-third may have coronary artery involvement. The mortality rate in Kawasaki's syndrome may be as high as 1–2%. Studies suggest that high-dose salicylate treatment (80–180 mg/kg/day) may be efficacious in reducing the coronary involvement in this syndrome. Intravenous immunoglobulin therapy has become the treatment of choice. The data suggest that systemic corticosteroid therapy should be avoided.

GOUT

A detailed discussion of gout, which is a systemic disorder characterized by recurrent arthritis and hyperuricemia with urate deposition in synovial and nonarticular tissues, is beyond the scope of this chapter. The cutaneous manifestations of gout are intradermal or subcutaneous nodules called tophi. They occur in avascular tissue over the ears, olecranon, and prepatellar bursae, or in acral sites, often associated with tendons (Fig. 5–19). They may discharge a chalky material. Microscopic

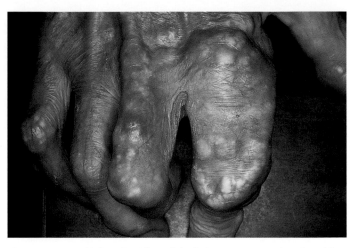

Figure 5–19 Multiple yellowish nodular lesions representative of tophi.

examination of this material reveals the typical crystals, which also can be seen in biopsy specimens fixed in alcohol, but not in formaldehyde. Therapy includes oral colchicine and/or allopurinol as a prophylactic measure, and indometacin for acute attacks.

SUGGESTED READINGS

Bennett ML, Jackson JM, Jorizzo JL, et al. Pyoderma gangrenosum. A comparison of typical and atypical forms with an emphasis on time to remission. Case review of 86 patients from 2 institutions. Medicine (Baltimore) 2000; 79: 37–46.

Brooklyn TN, Dunnill MG, Shetty A, et al. Infliximab for the treatment of pyoderma gangrenosum: a randomised, double blind, placebo controlled trial. Gut 2006; 55: 505–509.

Burns JC. Kawasaki disease. Adv Pediatr 2001; 48: 157–177.

Douglas KM, Ladoyanni E, Treharne GJ, et al. Cutaneous abnormalities in rheumatoid arthritis compared with non-inflammatory rheumatic conditions. Ann Rheum Dis 2006; 65: 1341–1345.

Gelfand JM, Gladman DD, Mease PJ, et al. Epidemiology of psoriatic arthritis in the population of the United States. J Am Acad Dermatol 2005; 53: 573.

Gladman DD, Antoni C, Mease P, et al. Psoriatic arthritis: epidemiology, clinical features, course, and outcome. Ann Rheum Dis 2005; 64: ii14–17.

Kalayciyan A, Zouboulis C. An update on Behçet's disease. J Eur Acad Dermatol Venereol 2007; 21: 1–10.

Kavanaugh A, Ritchlin C, Boehncke WH. Quality indicators in psoriatic arthritis. Clin Exp Rheumatol 2007; 25: 98–101.

Majithia V, Geraci SA. Rheumatoid arthritis: diagnosis and management. Am J Med 2007; 120: 936–939.

Savage C, St Clair EW. New therapeutics in rheumatoid arthritis. Rheum Dis Clin North Am 2006; 32: 57–74, viii.

Taylor W, Gladman D, Helliwell P, et al., and the CASPAR Study Group. Classification criteria for psoriatic arthritis: development of new criteria from a large international study. Arthritis Rheum 2006; 54: 2665–2673.

Tognon S, Graziani G, Marcolongo R. Anti-TNF-alpha therapy in seven patients with Behçet's uveitis: advantages and controversial aspects. Ann N Y Acad Sci 2007; 1110: 474–484.

Weenig RH, Davis MD, Dahl PR, Su WP. Skin ulcers misdiagnosed as pyoderma gangrenosum. N Engl J Med 2002; 347: 1412–1418.

Wollina U, Hansel G, Koch A, et al. Tumor necrosis factor-alpha inhibitor-induced psoriasis or psoriasiform exanthemata: first 120 cases from the literature including a series of six new patients. Am J Clin Dermatol 2008; 9: 1–14.

Yazici H, Ben-Chetrit E, Bang D, et al., eds. Behçet's disease and other autoinflammatory conditions. Clin Exp Rheumatol 2007; 25: S1–S119.

Yeung RS. Pathogenesis and treatment of Kawasaki's disease. Curr Opin Rheumatol 2005; 17: 617–623.

Chapter 6

Andrew D. Lee
and Joseph L. Jorizzo

Urticaria

Urticaria is a cutaneous vascular reaction pattern characterized by well-circumscribed areas of dermal edema and erythema, commonly associated with pruritus (Fig. 6–1). The lesions resolve within 24 hours. Lesions that simulate urticaria and can be proved to last for more than 24 hours (e.g., by drawing circles around individual lesions and observing their duration) are properly termed urticarial lesions. Angioedema is the name given to the clinicopathologic process that is identical to urticaria, except that the subcutaneous tissue rather than the dermis is affected, it may be associated with pain rather than pruritus, and it may take longer to resolve. As many as one in five people is affected by urticaria and/or angioedema at some point. Acute urticaria, which is urticaria that has resolved spontaneously in less than 1 month, affects primarily young adults. Chronic urticaria – the occurrence of urticaria for more than 6 consecutive weeks – is most common in middle-aged women.

PATHOGENESIS

Urticaria and urticarial lesions may be a final common pathway for a number of immunologic or nonimmunologic reactions that lead to cutaneous vasodilatation with extravasation of edema fluid in response to perivascular inflammation. Although the mechanisms involved in the various types of urticaria are not completely understood, it is believed that the vascular reaction in most patients with urticaria results from the release of mediators from cells such as mast cells and basophilic leukocytes. These mediators affect vascular permeability and result in extravasation of plasma into the dermis or subcutaneous tissue, with resultant urticaria or angioedema, respectively.

One classic mechanism of mast cell activation with resultant mediator release that is involved in some cases of urticaria is IgE-mediated (i.e., immediate hypersensitivity reaction) mast cell degranulation. IgE antibody is produced by B cells and plasma cells in response to an array of antigens. IgE then binds to mast cells or basophils through Fc receptors on those cells. Exposure to antigen results in antigen bridging of two IgE molecules. A calcium-requiring process that ultimately leads to histamine release follows. Immunologically mediated urticaria may also occur via C3a- or C5a-mediated mast cell degranulation. This is most probably the mechanism involved in the mast cell effects from circulating immune complexes (i.e., serum sickness-like reaction) that activate complement after their deposition in cutaneous blood vessels.

Evidence suggests that many patients with chronic idiopathic urticaria may have histamine-releasing autoantibodies. In many patients chronic idiopathic urticaria may therefore be an autoimmune disease.

Direct or indirect pharmacologic mechanisms (i.e., nonimmunologic) may also lead to mast cell degranulation. Medications, such as the opiate derivatives, have a direct effect on mast cells. Nonsteroidal anti-inflammatory agents (NSAIDs) have indirect effects on blood vessels, possibly by inducing the lipoxygenase pathway of arachidonic acid metabolism.

Other inflammatory mediators in addition to histamine are probably involved in urticaria. These include eosinophil chemotactic factor of anaphylaxis, neutrophil chemotactic factor, serotonin, slow-reacting substances of anaphylaxis, prostaglandins, proteases, and thromboxanes. The immediate sequelae include smooth muscle effects, vascular leakage, and pruritus. The delayed consequences of mast cell degranulation include infiltration with eosinophils, neutrophils, and mononuclear cells.

CLASSIFICATION

One method for the classification of urticarial reactions is presented in Table 6–1. The classification of urticarial lesions within one of these categories requires a combination of information obtained from the patient's history, physical examination, laboratory assessment, and occasionally histopathologic findings.

IgE-dependent urticaria and angioedema may occur in a number of different settings. Unfortunately, a provable association between urticaria and a specific antigen can be established in only a minority of patients with chronic urticaria (probably <5%).

Patients with an atopic diathesis (a personal or family history of asthma, hay fever, allergic rhinitis, and/or atopic dermatitis) have an increased prevalence of urticaria. Although scratch test evaluation and radioallergosorbent test results to specific

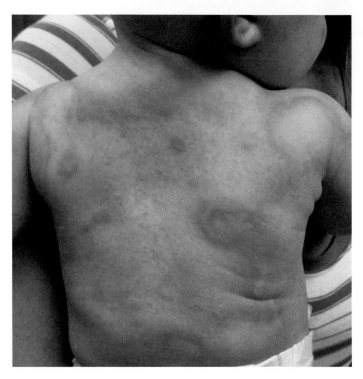

Figure 6–1 Acute urticaria.

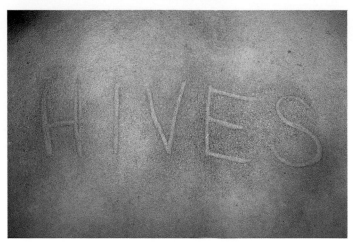

Figure 6–2 Dermatographism. Stroking of the skin leads to the urticarial reaction.

Table 6–1 Classification of urticarial reactions

I. IgE-dependent urticaria and angioedema
   A. Specific antigen sensitivities
   B. Some physical urticarias in which an IgE-mediated pathogenesis is suspected
      1. Symptomatic dermatographism
      2. Cholinergic urticaria
      3. Solar urticaria
      4. Essential acquired cold urticaria

II. Non-IgE-dependent urticaria and angioedema
   A. Direct mast cell effects
   B. Effects by the alteration of arachidonic acid pathways

III. Angioedema related to complement
   A. Hereditary angioedema
   B. Acquired angioedema

IV. Urticarial reactions probably related to circulating immune complexes
   A. Serum sickness–like reactions
   B. Urticarial vasculitis

V. Contact urticaria
VI. Idiopathic urticaria

antigens may correlate with asthma, hay fever, and allergic rhinitis, they seldom correlate with the cause of urticaria. Urticaria seldom accompanies an exacerbation of the other atopic conditions, such as asthma. Categories of antigen that may produce urticaria by a presumed IgE-dependent mechanism include foods (especially those that contain salicylate, tartrazine, or azo dyes; nuts; seafood; and fruits), infections (e.g., bacterial, fungal, and viral), infestations (e.g., scabies and intestinal parasites), drugs and chemicals (e.g., penicillin and sulfa drugs), inhalants, physical stimuli, and systemic disease.

The physical urticarias are an important subgroup of the chronic urticarias and may account for as many as 10% of all cases. The lesions of physical urticaria are induced by various physical stimuli. In several of these physical urticarias, an IgE-mediated pathogenesis has been strongly supported by clinical laboratory passive transfer experiments. The mechanisms involved in the other types of physical urticaria remain speculative. Symptomatic dermatographism (Fig. 6–2), cholinergic urticaria, solar urticaria, and essential acquired cold urticaria are four well-studied physical urticarias that may involve IgE-mediated immunologic reactions. The physical stimulus (e.g., stroking the skin, general increase in body temperature, sun exposure, and cold contact, respectively) may produce antigens that react with IgE and lead to the release of mast cell-derived mediators, with the subsequent production of urticarial lesions.

The lesions of urticaria or angioedema that are otherwise indistinguishable from those produced by an IgE-mediated mechanism may be produced by nonimmunologic mechanisms. Examples include urticaria from radiocontrast media, opiates, and tubocurarine, all of which have direct effects on mast cells. Also, the NSAIDs, including aspirin, may exacerbate urticaria, possibly by increased generation of arachidonic acid metabolites such as leukotrienes (some of which were formerly called slow-reacting substances of anaphylaxis).

Hereditary angioedema occurs as an autosomal dominant genodermatosis. Urticaria and angioedema may be associated with systemic histaminic effects, such as wheezing, diarrhea, and laryngeal edema that may even result in asphyxiation. The lesions result from a qualitative or quantitative C1 esterase inhibitor deficiency. Complement cascade activation results in mast cell degranulation by C3a, C4a, and C5a; however, the episodic nature of the attacks remains unexplained.

A deficiency of C1 esterase inhibitor may also occur as an acquired defect in association with lymphomas, monoclonal gammopathies, or systemic lupus erythematosus. Family members are not affected in this acquired form.

Schnitzler syndrome is a rare variant of chronic urticaria manifested by nonpruritic wheals, recurrent fevers, bone and joint pain, and a monoclonal IgM gammopathy. Histologically, superficial edema with a neutrophil-predominant infiltrate is seen. This urticarial eruption is generally resistant to treatment, including systemic corticosteroids and antihistamines. Thalidomide and anakinra, an IL-1 receptor antagonist, have both been reported as effective treatments for refractory disease. NSAIDs are helpful for fevers, and bone and joint pain.

In contrast to typical urticaria (in which individual lesions last for less than 24 hours), urticarial lesions lasting for more than 24 hours may occur in a serum sickness-like reaction (Fig. 6–3). These reactions are most probably circulating immune complex-mediated reactions that occur 1–2 weeks after exposure to antigens, such as heterologous serum (classic reaction) or certain infectious agents or drugs. The systemic signs and symptoms may include fever, arthralgias, arthritis, myalgias, lymphadenopathy, elevated liver function tests, and possibly proteinuria.

Urticarial vasculitis is another type of urticarial lesion associated with serum sickness-like signs and symptoms, lasts for 24–72 hours, and often resolves with residual purpura. Histologic evaluation reveals leukocytoclastic vasculitis, which is considered to be a marker for circulating immune complex-mediated vessel damage. Urticarial vasculitis was originally reported as a lupus erythematosus-like syndrome and as hypocomplementemic vasculitis. The normocomplementemic end of the urticarial vasculitis spectrum may be associated with less systemic disease. The severe end of the spectrum may feature patients with fully developed systemic lupus erythematosus. In addition to persistent urticarial wheals, patients may present with transient arthralgias, gastrointestinal symptoms, renal disease, and obstructive pulmonary disease, especially in smokers. It is important to distinguish urticarial vasculitis from usual urticaria because of these systemic implications, and because therapy for urticarial vasculitis may involve oral dapsone, colchicine, thalidomide, or systemic corticosteroids and/or immunosuppressive agents rather than antihistamines.

In general, urticaria should be viewed as a cutaneous reaction to substances that are distributed systemically, often after oral intake or inhalation. Contact urticaria is the term applied to urticarial lesions occurring on the skin or mucous membranes after simple contact with eliciting substances. The reaction occurs within 30–60 minutes and resolves within 24 hours. This reaction may occur by immunologic or nonimmunologic mechanisms, depending on the offending agent.

Unfortunately, in up to 25% of patients with acute urticaria and in up to 90–97% of patients with chronic urticaria the cause may never be found. These patients with idiopathic urticaria appear well despite their cutaneous malady. Of patients with chronic urticaria that lasts for 6 months, about 50% will have active disease 10 years later, exemplifying the chronic frustration that some of these patients experience.

DIFFERENTIAL DIAGNOSIS

The diagnosis of a cutaneous eruption as urticaria is not usually difficult, owing to the characteristic appearance and short duration of the lesions. Other dermatologic diseases may have diagnostic lesions that occur in association with or are superimposed on urticarial eruptions (i.e., urticarial lesions that last more than 24 hours), such as bullous pemphigoid with tense blisters and an urticarial eruption, and erythema multiforme with target lesions and urticarial lesions. Insect bites often appear urticarial but last for several days, and close examination usually discloses a central punctum. The lesions of mast cell disease, such as urticaria pigmentosa lesions, are persistent dermal mast cell infiltrates that urticate when firmly stroked.

The cutaneous lesions in urticaria result from infiltration of the dermis with fluid, giving the tissue an orange-peel appearance like that produced by intradermal injection (e.g., intradermal skin tests). Unless the history suggests that the lesions have lasted for longer than the 24 hours allowed by the definition of urticaria, other dermal infiltrates can be confused with urticaria on cursory cutaneous examination. These longstanding infiltrative conditions include granulomatous infiltrates (e.g., sarcoidosis, leprosy, and cutaneous tuberculosis), malignant infiltrates (e.g., cutaneous T-cell lymphoma, and metastatic disease), fibrous processes (e.g., morphea), metabolic deposits (e.g., amyloidosis and mucinosis), and nonurticarial inflammatory infiltrates (e.g., tumid lesions of lupus erythematosus, and lymphocytoma cutis).

PATIENT EVALUATION

After a diagnosis of urticaria has been made, further evaluation of the patient begins with a thorough history, including details

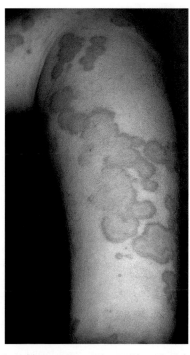

Figure 6–3 Urticarial lesions in a patient with urticarial vasculitis. These lesions may take several days to resolve.

of the present illness; a medical history, including medications and social and family history; and a review of systems. The patient must understand that urticaria may result from a newly developed allergy to a medication or other substance to which they have been exposed for years. With this in mind, the patient should relate possibly relevant exposures for the 12–24 hours prior to each outbreak of urticaria. Are clues provided by the time of onset, or association with work, meals, medications, or environmental exposures? The clinician should inquire specifically about certain exposures typically associated with urticaria (Table 6–2).

In addition to questions directed at possibly related exposures, the clinician must also ask questions aimed at distinguishing urticaria from urticarial lesions resulting from circulating immune complex-mediated vessel damage (i.e., urticarial vasculitis, and the urticarial lesions of serum sickness-like reactions). To this end, the clinician should inquire about the duration of individual lesions (i.e., less than or more than 24 hours), and about the presence of serum sickness-like signs and symptoms. These signs, symptoms, and findings may include fever, arthralgias, arthritis, myalgias, lymphadenopathy, proteinuria, and elevated liver function test results.

The patient may be encouraged to keep a personal diary. If the patient records possibly relevant exposures occurring during the 12–24 hours prior to the onset of each outbreak of lesions, a pattern may emerge to provide clues as to the cause of the urticaria.

A comprehensive physical examination is important for all patients with chronic urticaria. This can be conducted by the patient's primary care physician. Not only might systemic signs associated with the urticaria be revealed, but also clues as to etiologic systemic disease might be unveiled. During the cutaneous examination, the clinician might draw a circle with a pen around a new lesion and ask the patient to report later on the duration of that individual lesion. As mentioned, a lesion that lasts for more than 24 hours is urticarial, not urticaria. Also on cutaneous examination the clinician can assess for dermatographism by firmly stroking the skin on the patient's back. Although this test is positive in 5% of normal individuals, it is useful in patients with urticaria to assess patient compliance with antihistamine therapy and the adequacy of that therapy. If the dermatographic response is not blocked, the antihistamine dose must be increased if the urticaria itself is to be controlled. Urticarial lesions should also be examined for purpura. If purpura is present on the lower legs, it may be of no significance. If it is present on nonexcoriated truncal lesions, it may be a sign of urticarial vasculitis.

Histopathologic examination of lesional skin is not required in the patient with routine urticaria. If an examination is performed, a dermal mixed cellular, perivascular infiltrate is usually observed. An identical reaction occurring in the deep dermis and subcutaneous tissue is a sign of angioedema. When urticarial vasculitis is suspected, biopsy of a lesion is indicated. The characteristic histologic finding is leukocytoclastic vasculitis with the following features: fibrinoid necrosis of blood vessel walls, infiltration of vessel walls with neutrophils showing karyorrhexis (breaking up of nuclei), extravasation of erythrocytes, and endothelial swelling.

Although the clinical laboratory can be an invaluable adjunct to the evaluation of the patient with acute urticaria, a cost-effective approach is mandatory. Because the list of associations of urticaria is vast, the 'shotgun' approach to laboratory evaluation would not be complete, even after many thousands of dollars' worth of tests had been ordered. In general, tests should be ordered when suggested by the history and physical examination. A complete blood count with differential, Westergren sedimentation rate, urinalysis, and chemistry profile might be a screening approach for the patient with urticaria of unknown cause that lasts for more than 1–2 weeks. These tests might provide leads for obtaining supplemental information from the history and physical examination, and suggest additional evaluation. For example, a patient with urticaria who has intermittent diarrhea and peripheral blood eosinophilia should undergo multiple stool evaluations for ova and parasites. Table 6–3 suggests additional laboratory tests.

A detailed summary of the special evaluations required in the patient with suspected physical urticaria is beyond the scope of this chapter. However, Table 6–4 provides an overview of the physical urticarias.

TREATMENT

The treatment of acute or chronic urticaria consists of two aspects: removal of the cause, and treatment of the signs and symptoms. Acute urticaria is, by definition, self-limiting. An evaluation aimed at uncovering the cause of acute urticaria is warranted to permit avoidance of the offending precipitant to prevent future attacks. Therapy of urticaria is aimed at controlling signs and symptoms (Fig. 6–4).

Removal of the Cause

In many patients identification of the causative factors in chronic urticaria is frustrating, and a reversible factor may be isolated in as few as 2–10% of patients. Most studies suggest a poor correlation between positive scratch test results and the antigens responsible for urticaria. As part of the treatment approach, many clinicians advocate empiric trials with elimination diets, even if a careful history excludes the common precipitants listed in Table 6–2. The chemicals contained in many foods that produce urticaria relatively commonly are azo dyes, tartrazine, and salicylates. Diets that exclude these substances are well known to nutritional consultants and have been widely published. Diets excluding yeasts also have been well described. Another approach is to use a very restrictive diet, such as rice and water, for 3–4 days. If the patient has urticaria while eating only rice and water, the urticaria is almost certainly not food related. However, if the urticaria resolves on this diet, foods can be reintroduced gradually until the urticaria recurs. In this way, the offending substance may be identified. Other general points of therapy include the avoidance of dairy products in penicillin-sensitive individuals (dairy products from penicillin-treated cattle may contain traces of penicillin) and the avoidance of nonsteroidal anti-inflammatory agents (NSAIDs), opiate derivatives, or

Table 6–2 Some causes of urticaria*

Infections	Contactants

Bacterial infections
    Dental abscess
    Sinusitis
    Otitis
    Cholecystitis
    Pneumonitis
    Cystitis
    Hepatitis
    Vaginitis
	Wool

	Silk
	Occupational exposure
	Potatoes
	Antibiotics

Fungal infections
    Tinea
    Candida
	Cosmetics
	    Dyes
	    Hairspray
	    Nail polish
	    Mouthwash
	    Toothpaste
	    Perfumes
	    Hand cream
	    Soap

Other infections/infestations
    Scabies
    Helminth
    Protozoa
    Trichomonas	

	Insect repellent
Drugs and chemicals	**Endocrinopathies**
Salicylates	Thyroid disease
Indometacin and other, newer nonsteroidal anti-inflammatory agents	Diabetes mellitus
Opiates	Pregnancy
Radiocontrast material	Menstruation
Penicillin (medication, milk, blue cheese)	Menopause
Sulfonamides	**Physical stimuli**
Sodium benzoate	Dermatographism
Douches	Light
Ear drops or eyedrops	Pressure
Insulin	Heat
Menthol (cigarettes, toothpaste, iced tea, hand cream, lozenges, candy)	Cold
Tartrazine (vitamins, birth control pills, antibiotics, FDC yellow #5)	Water
Foods	Vibration
Nuts	**Systemic disease**
Berries	Rheumatic fever
Fish	Juvenile rheumatoid arthritis
Seafood	Leukemia
Bananas	Lymphoma
Grapes	Connective tissue disease (lupus erythematosus, rheumatoid arthritis, Sjögren's syndrome, other)
Tomatoes	
Eggs	Acquired immunodeficiency disease
Cheese	**Familial disorders**
Inhalants	Hereditary angioedema
Animal danders	Muckle–Wells syndrome
Pollen	
*Partial list of most frequently described causes in each category.	

Table 6–3 Laboratory tests that may be helpful in the evaluation of urticaria

Complete blood count
Erythrocyte sedimentation rate
Syphilis serology
Renal function tests
Liver function tests
Hepatitis B and C serology
Mononucleosis serology
Thyroid function tests (thyroid-stimulating hormone and thyroid)
Antinuclear antibody test
C3 and C4 tests
Anti-DNase B or the streptococcal serology
Urinalysis
Vaginal smear
Stool specimen examination for ova and parasites
Pulmonary function tests
Sinus radiographs
Dental radiographs
Chest radiograph
Skin biopsy
Other specific tests as directed by history and physical examination

angiotensin-converting enzyme (ACE) inhibitors that may exacerbate urticaria of any cause by nonimmunologic mechanisms.

Treatment of Signs and Symptoms

The patient with acute urticaria and/or angioedema may present to the primary care physician or to the emergency department in acute distress, with wheezing, anaphylactoid signs and symptoms, or laryngeal edema with airway obstruction. Emergency measures include the administration of epinephrine (adrenaline) (1 : 1000, 0.3–0.5 mL subcutaneously), which reduces the release of histamine from mast cells by increasing cyclic adenosine monophosphate levels within the cells, and which also directly affect smooth muscle. Tracheostomy may rarely be required. Patients prone to develop laryngeal edema, such as those with hereditary angioedema, should be given commercially available kits containing preloaded epinephrine (adrenaline) syringes with instructions for intramuscular injection.

Antihistamines with a specificity for H_1 receptors are the treatment of choice for almost all types of urticaria. These agents competitively inhibit histamine at the H_1 receptor of blood vessels. Antihistamines do not prevent the release of histamine from mast cells; therefore, they must be given to the patient around the clock. Simply taking the antihistamine 'when I get hives' is practically useless because the histamine will have already bound to H_1 receptors and have induced its pathologic effects. In most studies, hydroxyzine (Atarax), a piperazine-class antihistamine, is the most effective traditional antihistamine. The dosage can be low initially (10 mg orally every 6 hours, with 20–30 mg at bedtime), with a relatively prompt increase to the maximal dosage to control lesions (50–100 mg four times daily). The major side effects are sedation and anticholinergic effects, such as dry mouth, tachycardia, double vision, urinary retention, and constipation. If hydroxyzine is ineffective, an H_1 antihistamine from another class may be added (Table 6–5).

Controlling signs and symptoms of chronic urticaria can be much more challenging. First-line therapy includes the second-generation H_1 antihistamines such as loratadine, cetirizine, and fexofenadine. These antihistamines are safe, effective, and associated with less sedation than the classic antihistamines. Newer nonsedating antihistamines, such as desloratadine and levocetirizine, may offer greater clinical improvement. If symptomatic improvement is not fully achieved with initial licensed doses, additional benefit may be obtained from increasing to 2–3 times the daily dose. However, caution is advised with high doses of fexofenadine, as it is an active metabolite of terfenadine, an antihistamine associated with arrhythmias and no longer available. Finally, adding a sedating H_1 antihistamine to the regimen at bedtime can also be helpful, especially if symptoms interfere with sleep.

Doxepin is a particularly potent agent with H_1 and H_2 antihistaminic effects that is commonly used to treat urticaria. The side effects from doxepin are not insignificant (e.g., agranulocytosis, hallucinations, ataxia, cardiac effects, and photosensitization), but are generally controllable with lower dosing. Reports of synergistic therapeutic benefits from combining H_1 antihistamines and H_2 antagonists, such as cimetidine or ranitidine, have been balanced by reports showing no added benefit.

Patients with hereditary angioedema may have a dramatic reduction in the frequency and severity of attacks and may benefit during acute attacks from systemic treatment with attenuated androgens, such as danazol or stanozolol. These agents stimulate the synthesis of the deficient C1 esterase inhibitor.

Systemic corticosteroids have no place in the routine therapy of chronic urticaria, although they may be useful for urticarial vasculitis or the urticarial lesions of serum sickness. High doses are required to benefit patients with chronic urticaria, and these doses cannot be maintained for the many years that numerous patients with chronic urticaria would require them. After the patient with chronic urticaria has experienced the relief provided by 50 mg of oral daily prednisone, he or she will not be satisfied with having a disease that recurs completely at lower doses. The patient may continue to change physicians, seeking one who will prescribe the higher doses. Inevitably, such patients may have many complications from long-term high-dose corticosteroid therapy. Prednisone should be considered only for short-term management of severe urticarial flares or serious angioedema. Other second-line therapies include montelukast, thyroxine, nifedipine, colchicine, and sulfasalazine (Table 6–6).

Table 6–4 Comparison of the physical urticarias

Urticaria	Relative frequency	Precipitant	Time of onset	Duration	Local symptoms	Systemic symptoms	Tests	Mechanism	Treatment
Symptomatic dermatographism	Most frequent	Stroking skin	Minutes	2–3 hours	Irregular pruritic attacks	None	Scratch skin	Passive transfer, IgE, histamine, possible role of adenosine triphosphate, substance P, possible direct pharmacologic mechanism	Continual antihistamines
Delayed dermatographism	Rare	Stroking skin	30 minutes to 8 hours	<48 hours	Burning, deep swelling	None	Scratch skin, observe early and late	Unknown	Avoidance of precipitants
Pressure urticaria	Frequent	Pressure	3–12 hours	8–24 hours	Diffuse, tender swelling	Flu-like symptoms	Apply weight	Unknown	Avoidance of precipitants; if severe, low doses of corticosteroids given for systemic effects
Solar urticaria	Frequent	Various wavelengths of light	2–5 minutes	15 minutes to 3 hours	Pruritic wheals	Wheezing, dizziness, syncope	Phototest	Passive transfer, reverse passive transfer, IgE, possible histamine	Avoidance of precipitants; antihistamines, sunscreens, antimalarials
Familial cold urticaria	Rare	Change in skin temperature	30 minutes to 3 hours	<48 hours	Burning wheals	Tremor; headache; arthralgia; fever	Expose skin to cold air	Unknown	Avoidance of precipitants
Essential acquired cold urticaria	Frequent	Cold contact	2–5 minutes	1–2 hours	Pruritic wheals	Wheezing, syncope, drowning	Apply ice-filled copper beaker to arm, immerse	Passive transfer, reverse passive transfer, IgE (IgM), histamine, vasculitis can be induced	Cyproheptadine hydrochloride, other antihistamines; desensitization; avoidance of precipitants
Heat urticaria	Rare	Heat contact	2–5 minutes (rarely delayed)	1 hour	Pruritic wheals	None	Apply hot water-filled cylinder to arm	Possibly histamine; possibly complement	Antihistamines; desensitization; avoidance of precipitants
Cholinergic urticaria	Very frequent	General overheating of body	2–20 minutes	30 minutes to 1 hour	Papular, pruritic wheals	Syncope; diarrhea; vomiting, salivation; headaches	Bathe in hot water; exercise until perspiring, inject methacholine chloride	Passive transfer; possible immunoglobulin; product of sweat gland stimulation; histamine, reduced protease	Application of cold water or ice to skin; hydroxyzine regimen; refractory period; anticholinergics
Aquagenic urticaria	Rare	Water contact	Several minutes	30–45 minutes	Papular, pruritic wheals	None reported	Apply water compresses to skin	Unknown	Avoidance of precipitants; antihistamines
Vibratory angioedema	Very rare	Vibrating against skin	2–5 minutes	1 hour	Angioedema	None reported	Apply vibration to forearm	Unknown	Avoidance of precipitants; application of inert oil

From Jorizzo JL, Smith EG. The physical urticarias. Arch Dermatol 1982; 118: 194–201, with permission.

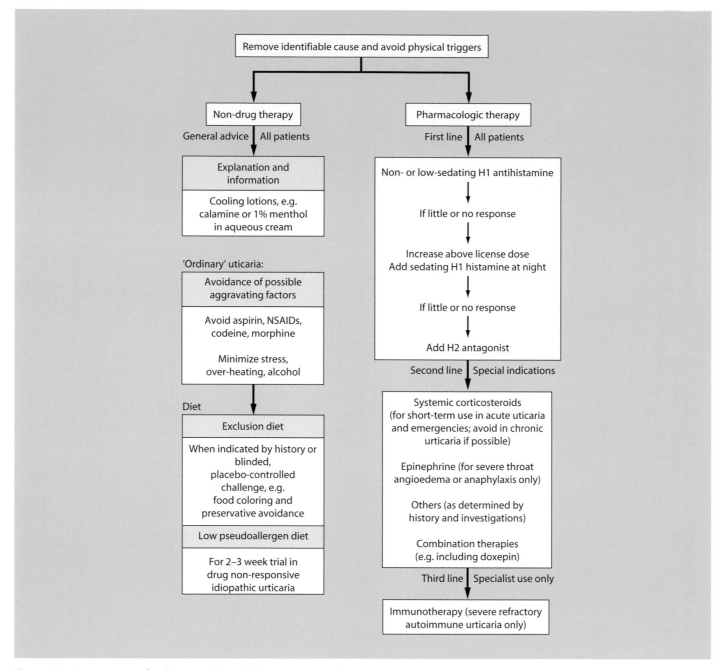

Figure 6–4 Management of ordinary and physical chronic urticarias. (From Bolognia JL, Jorizzo JL, Rapini RP, eds. Dermatology 2e, Vol 1; page 273; With permission from Clive EH Grattan and Anne Kobza Black 2008. © Mosby. Elsevier Inc.)

Table 6–5 Antihistamines for chronic urticaria

Class	Examples	Chemical family	Half-life (hours)	Daily adult dose*
Classic (sedating)	Chlorpheniramine (1)	Alkylamine	25	4 mg tid (up to 12 mg at night)
	Hydroxyzine (1)	Piperazine	20	10–25 mg tid (up to 75 mg at night)
	Diphenhydramine (2)	Ethanolamine	4	10–25 mg at night
	Doxepin** (1)	Tricyclic antidepressant	17	10–50 mg at night
Second-generation	Acrivastine (1)	Alkylamine	2–4	8 mg tid
	Cetirizine*** (1)	Piperazine	7–11	10 mg once daily
	Loratadine (1)	Piperidine	8–11	10 mg once daily
	Mizolastine (1)	Piperidine	13	10 mg once daily
Newer second-generation	Desloratadine (1)	Piperidine	19–35	5 mg once daily
	Fexofenadine (1)	Piperidine	17	180 mg once daily
	Levocetirizine (1)	Piperazine	7–10	5 mg once daily
H_2 antagonists†	Cimetidine (1)		2	400 mg bid
	Ranitidine (2)		2–3	150 mg bid

A short-acting classic antihistamine may be added at night to a daily second-generation antihistamine with or without the addition of an H_2 antagonist for maximal antihistamine blockade. Key to evidence-based support: (1) prospective controlled trial; (2) retrospective study or large case series; (3) small case series or individual case reports.
*Current prescribing manuals should be consulted for details on doses in children.
**Possesses potent H, and H_2 antihistaminic properties.
***The active metabolite of hydroxyzine.
†Used in combination with H_1 antagonists.
From Bolognia JL, Jorizzo JL, Rapini RP. Dermatology, 2nd edn. Volume 1. Mosby, Elsevier Inc.

Table 6–6 Second-line medications for chronic or physical urticaria

Generic name	Drug class	Route	Dose	Special indication/associated diseases
Prednisone (2)	Corticosteroid	Oral	0.5 mg/kg qd	Severe exacerbations (days only)
Epinephrine (2)	Sympathomimetic	sc, im (self-administered)	300–500 µg	Angioedema of throat/anaphylaxis
Montelukast (3)	Leukotriene receptor antagonist	Oral	10 mg qd	Aspirin-sensitive urticaria
Thyroxine (2)	Thyroid hormone	Oral	50–150 µg qd	Autoimmune thyroid disease
Nifedipine (1)	Calcium antagonist	Oral	10–40 mg modified-release qd	Hypertension
Colchicine (3)	Neutrophil inhibitor	Oral	0.6–1.8 mg qd	Neutrophilic infiltrates in lesional biopsy specimens
Sulfasalazine (3)	Aminosalicylates	Oral	2–4 g qd	Delayed pressure urticaria

Current prescribing manuals should be consulted for details on dose, drug interactions, and contraindications for individual patients. The stated doses represent guidelines only. Key to evidence-based support: (1) prospective controlled trial; (2) retrospective study or large case series; (3) small case series or individual case reports.
From Bolognia JL, Jorizzo JL, Rapini RP. Dermatology, 2nd edn. Volume 1. Mosby, Elsevier Inc.

Newer data showing the presence of autoantibodies in many patients with chronic idiopathic urticaria have led to trials of immunosuppressive therapies, including cyclosporine (3–5 mg/kg/day), intravenous immunoglobulin (2 g/kg in total over 5 days), and plasmapheresis. Phototherapy with psoralens and ultraviolet A light (PUVA) has also been reported to be beneficial. Ultimately the cost and potential morbidities of these therapies and their inability to deliver the desired long-term remissions limit their value in patients with chronic idiopathic urticaria.

Patients with chronic idiopathic urticaria require a physician with an emotionally supportive attitude who provides a realistic explanation of what to expect. The patient must be told that even maximal antihistamine therapy will not eliminate erythema, but rather will only control the urtication and pruritus.

SUGGESTED READINGS

Brown NA, Carter JD. Urticarial vasculitis. Curr Rheumatol Rep 2007; 9: 312–319.

Grattan CE, Sabroe RA, Greaves MW. Chronic urticaria. J Am Acad Dermatol 2002; 46: 645–657.

Guldbakke KK, Khachemoune A. Etiology, classification, and treatment of urticaria. Cutis 2007; 79: 41–49.

Kaplan AP. Diagnostic test for urticaria and angioedema. Clin Allergy Immunol 2000; 15: 111–126.

Lee EE, Maibach HI. Treatment of urticaria. An evidence-based evaluation of antihistamines. Am J Clin Dermatol 2001; 2: 27–32.

Simons FE. Advances in H1-antihistamines. N Engl J Med 2004; 351: 2203–2217.

Zuberbier T, Maurer M. Urticaria: current opinions about etiology, diagnosis and therapy. Acta Dermatol Venereol 2007; 87: 196–205.

B. Asher Louden
and Joseph L. Jorizzo

Chapter | **7** |

Erythema Multiforme, Stevens–Johnson Syndrome, and Toxic Epidermal Necrolysis

Erythema multiforme (EM) is an acute, self-limited mucocutaneous syndrome characterized by erythematous papules and targetoid lesions. As the name implies, EM may be extremely variable with regard to the spectrum of cutaneous lesions present, the associated systemic signs and symptoms, the etiology, and the tendency for episodes to recur. Infectious agents, specifically herpes simplex virus (HSV), are now widely believed to precipitate EM in a majority of cases. Since von Hebra's early coining of the term erythema multiforme, the concept of this disease has been confused such that there is little agreement among clinicians as to the exact boundaries of the syndrome. There is little disagreement, however, that the relatively benign syndrome of classic, often acral, target lesions (as described by von Hebra) should be called EM minor, henceforth referred to here solely as EM.

Stevens–Johnson syndrome (SJS) and toxic epidermal necrolysis (TEN) are mucocutaneous illnesses with significant associated morbidity and mortality that form a separate severe SJS–TEN spectrum. Epidermal necrosis and involvement of two or more mucosal surfaces are characteristic of SJS and TEN. Targetoid lesions can be observed as well, but are seen more frequently in milder forms of SJS, or at least earlier in disease progression. Drugs are the causative agent in a majority of SJS–TEN cases, with sulfonamides, nonsteroidal anti-inflammatory drugs (NSAIDs), and anticonvulsants being most frequently implicated. There is some overlap in etiology, however, with drugs occasionally inciting episodes of EM and infectious agents leading to SJS–TEN.

All three defined entities – EM and the spectrum from SJS to TEN – display similar histopathologic characteristics when targetoid lesions are sampled. Nikolsky-positive areas show more advanced changes, as will be discussed. The distinction between these can only be drawn clinically. Histologic findings are most useful in distinguishing these diseases from other differential diagnoses.

Treatments for the conditions vary greatly from one end of the spectrum to the other. Identification of the causative agent, whenever possible, is of the utmost importance. Given the paucity of evidenced-based treatments, especially for SJS–TEN, current approaches are based largely on case series and circumstantial evidence alone.

PATHOGENESIS

An immune-mediated pathogenesis has long been suspected for EM and SJS–TEN. Current concepts center on host immune response to various specific antigenic stimuli, such as HSV infection, drugs, and, presumably, the antigens associated with other causes. In the majority of EM patients, cutaneous lesions result from cytotoxic reactions against HSV antigens expressed in epidermal keratinocytes. In most patients with SJS–TEN, a cytotoxic reaction results from immunoreactivity against keratinocytes expressing drug-related antigens. This mechanism supports the theory that these patients are felt to be immunogenetically predisposed to developing their disease. Although similar in theory, there are many differences between the two reaction patterns.

Multiple etiologic agents have been implicated as causes of EM (Table 7–1). The best-documented causes include the infections induced by recurrent HSV and *Mycoplasma*. Reactions to many drugs have also been postulated as causes of EM. Interestingly, drug reactions and mycoplasmal infections most often produce SJS. The drugs most frequently associated with SJS–TEN spectrum diseases include sulfa drugs, NSAIDs, anticonvulsants, penicillins, allopurinol, and tetracyclines. Other associations with EM include mononucleosis, other viral infections (e.g., mumps, poliomyelitis, milker's nodule, and vaccinia), granuloma inguinale, psittacosis, histoplasmosis, syphilis, streptococcal infection, radiation therapy of tumors, sarcoidosis, pregnancy, carcinomas, reticuloses, leukemias, systemic lupus erythematosus, and other collagen–vascular diseases. A significant percentage of cases remain idiopathic.

As stated previously, HSV types 1 and 2 trigger the overwhelming majority of EM. Varicella zoster virus has not been shown to elicit a similar cutaneous reaction. Modern molecular biologic techniques have demonstrated fragments of HSV DNA in the cutaneous lesions of EM in more than 80% of cases. Most often, these strands encode a viral DNA polymerase.

Viral elements can reach distant body sites via hematogenous routes, by way of either immune complexes or mononuclear cells. Increased expression of adhesion mole-

Table 7–1 Possible causes of EM or SJS–TEN

Infectious agents
  Herpes simplex
  Mycoplasma pneumoniae
  Epstein–Barr virus
  Mumps
  Polio
  Calymmatobacterium
  Streptococcus
  Vaccinia
  Yersinia
  Tuberculosis
  Treponema pallidum
  Chlamydia
  Deep mycoses (e.g., histoplasmosis)

Medications
  Sulfonamides
  NSAIDs
  Carbamazepine
  Phenytoin
  Allopurinol
  Barbiturates
  Penicillins
  Tetracyclines
  Phenylbutazone

Other conditions
  Irradiation of tumors
  Immunizations
  Connective tissue disease (e.g., systemic lupus erythematosus)
  Sarcoidosis
  Inflammatory bowel disease
  Pregnancy

cules permits trafficking from the blood to endothelial cells and on to keratinocytes. Ultraviolet light, a known trigger of EM, is one suspected physical agent upregulating this pathway.

CD8+ T lymphocytes predominate in the sparse epidermal inflammatory infiltrate. After an appropriate stimulus, an apoptotic reaction, or chain reaction, ensues. As in SJS–TEN, CD4+ cells make up a majority of the dermal infiltrate. The dermal inflammatory reaction is frequently greater in EM than in SJS–TEN. This is in stark contrast to the degree of epidermal necrosis, which is much greater in SJS–TEN.

HLA-DQ3 has been shown to be linked with EM. Other HLA antigens have also been investigated. HLA-B12 is increased in frequency in patients with TEN, HLA-B*5801 appears to be associated with allopurinol-induced SJS/TEN, HLA*38 is increased in TEN due to lamotrigine, and HLA-B*73 appears to be increased in patients with oxicam-induced TEN. It is likely that additional studies will identify other antigens associated with SJS–TEN, which may differ for induction by specific drugs. In a recent study from Japan, HLA-A*0206 was strongly associated with SJS–TEN, whereas HLA-A*1101 was less frequent in TEN and HLA-B*5901 exhibited a high odds ratio for SJS–TEN with ocular complications.

The large extent of epidermal necrosis in TEN, despite the minimal number of inflammatory cells present, has long puzzled investigators. Recent evidence implicates an interaction of the death receptor Fas (CD95) and Fas ligand (FasL) on epidermal keratinocytes. Interaction of Fas and FasL induces signaling which rapidly leads to apoptosis. In normal skin, FasL is expressed intracellularly in low levels. Lesional skin from TEN patients has been shown to express higher levels of lytically active cell surface FasL. These greater levels of exposed FasL could explain the massive amount of epidermal necrosis seen. Antibodies present in pooled human intravenous immunoglobulins (IVIg) may block Fas-mediated keratinocyte death. Use of IVIg for treatment of TEN rests on this theory. Perforin/granzyme pathways have also been suggested as having a role in the pathogenesis of TEN.

CLINICAL MANIFESTATIONS

Erythema Multiforme

Typically, EM begins with nonspecific prodromal symptoms such as malaise, fever, and sore throat. The cutaneous eruption occurs as a primarily acral, symmetric eruption of asymptomatic to burning or pruritic erythematous macules. These lesions evolve into the characteristic dusky to purpuric, possibly vesiculobullous, target lesions (Fig. 7–1). Individual lesions last from 1 to 2 weeks, but may be replaced by succeeding waves of lesions. The entire episode may last 4–6 weeks. Erythematous macules, papules, and urticarial lesions may be associated with the more diagnostic target lesions. Sites of trauma (Koebner's isomorphic phenomenon), especially physical trauma or sun-exposed sites, may be favored.

Stevens–Johnson Syndrome

SJS is more likely to be characterized by generalized – especially truncal – lesions. Individual lesions are less typically targetoid and are more likely to be confluent areas of erythema

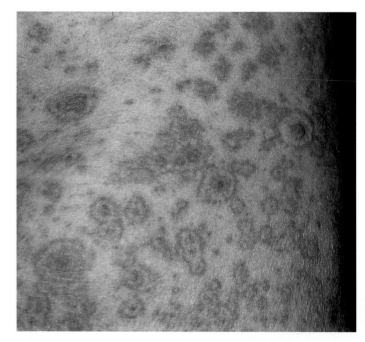

Figure 7–1 Erythema multiforme with typical target lesions.

with some purpura or urticarial lesions (Fig. 7–2). Large bullae may be seen, at times giving the impression of subclinical TEN (see following discussion). The proximal nailfold may be affected, and nail matrix dystrophy may result. Mucosal lesions are seen more commonly than in EM: they are present in almost all patients. These lesions present as superficial erosions anywhere in the oral cavity (Fig. 7–3), on the vaginal mucosa, or on the conjunctivae (Fig. 7–4). The penile corona (Fig. 7–5) or the esophagus may also be affected. Mucosal complications may include keratitis, conjunctival scarring, uveitis, scleral perforation, urethral stricture, and esophageal stricture. Patients often experience high fevers, arthralgias, arthritis, and myalgias; they may even experience hepatitis, bronchopulmonary disease, glomerulonephritis, or acute renal tubular necrosis. Rarely, severe prostration or even death may occur.

Toxic Epidermal Necrolysis

The term toxic epidermal necrolysis was coined by Lyell in the mid-1950s to refer to a severe illness characterized by a generalized scalded appearance of the skin and by life-threatening serum sickness-like features. Subsequently, the staphylococcal scalded skin syndrome was identified as a distinct entity occurring primarily in children, with the scalded appearance resulting from an exfoliative toxin produced by group 2 phage type 71 staphylococci. TEN is thought by many investigators to represent the most severe end of the SJS–TEN spectrum. Patients usually report prodromal features similar to those observed in EM and SJS. These are rapidly followed by a generalized macular erythema that progresses to confluent erythema with skin tenderness and vesiculation. Targetoid lesions may also occur (Fig. 7–6). Large, flaccid bullae with a positive Nikolsky sign (spread of the blister under pressure to adjacent skin) follow shortly afterwards (Fig. 7–7). The mucosal involve-

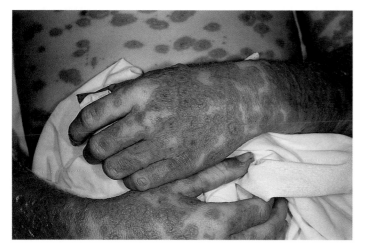

Figure 7–2 Stevens–Johnson syndrome. Targetoid lesions as well as multiple bullae were early manifestations in this adolescent. (Reprinted with permission from Color atlas of dermatology, 2nd edn. Philadelphia: WB Saunders, 2000.)

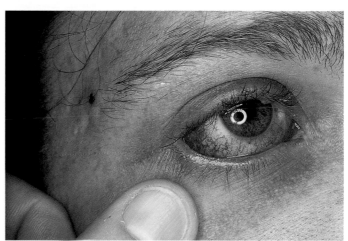

Figure 7–4 Stevens–Johnson syndrome: conjunctivitis.

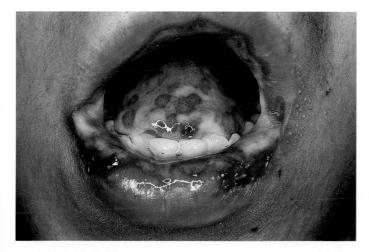

Figure 7–3 Erosive glossitis and erosive lesions on the lips in this patient with erythema multiforme and involvement of multiple mucosal surfaces.

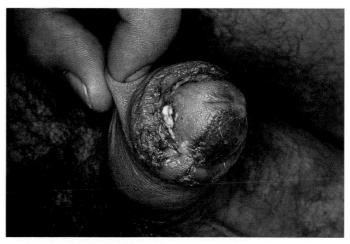

Figure 7–5 Stevens–Johnson syndrome with involvement of mucosal surfaces.

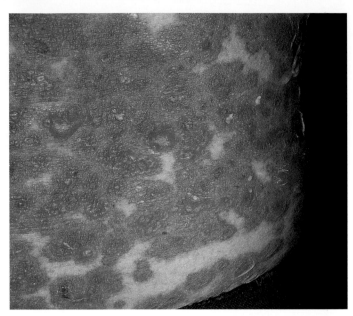

Figure 7–6 Toxic epidermal necrolysis presumed to be due to corticosteroid therapy. This patient began with painful lesions that rapidly developed into widespread epidermal loss. Among his earliest lesions were targetoid lesions, some with blisters.

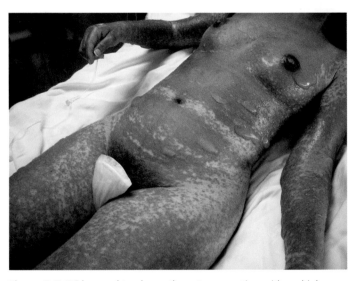

Figure 7–7 Widespread tender erythematous eruption with multiple bullae in a patient with toxic epidermal necrolysis.

ment is similar to that of SJS. The nails may be lost. Gastrointestinal, pulmonary, and renal involvement may be severe. Recovery may be slow, but it may be complete without cutaneous or mucosal scarring if excellent care is administered early in the disease course, usually in an intensive care or burn unit setting. Mucosal, cutaneous, and nail scarring may result if secondary infection occurs. The mortality rate approaches 30%. The most common cause of TEN is hypersensitivity to a systemically administered medication such as those mentioned above. A number of cases remain idiopathic.

Differential Diagnosis

The differential diagnosis of EM and SJS–TEN must be divided into two categories: a differential list for the cutaneous erup-

tion and one for the mucosal lesions, which may at times occur alone. Other chronic erosive mucosal diseases include pemphigus vulgaris (with the diagnostic histopathologic findings showing acantholysis, and with diagnostic direct and indirect immunopathologic examinations), paraneoplastic pemphigus (with a diagnostic immunopathologic examination), herpetic gingivostomatitis (with diagnostic histopathologic findings of multinucleated giant cells, a diagnostic culture, and/or the use of polymerase chain reaction), recurrent aphthous stomatitis (with the morphology and time course of the lesions suggesting the diagnosis), cicatricial pemphigoid (with suggestive histopathologic findings of dermoepidermal junction blister and confirmatory direct immunofluorescence), and erosive lichen planus (with a diagnostic histopathologic examination). The oral lesions of EM are acute in onset, last about 2 weeks, and histopathologically show focal epidermal necrosis, a dermoepidermal junction zone blister, and a perivascular lymphocytic infiltrate.

The differential diagnosis of the cutaneous lesions of EM is extensive, particularly if the typical target lesions are not noticed. Patients with typical EM with target lesions may have other cutaneous lesions that are clinicopathologically similar to those of simple erythema, urticaria, annular erythemas, viral exanthemas, secondary syphilis, toxic shock or mucocutaneous lymph node syndrome, or the following vasculitides: cutaneous small-vessel (leukocytoclastic) vasculitis, pustular vasculitis (disseminated gonococcemia or meningococcemia, or lesions of Behçet's or bowel bypass syndromes), or vasculitis associated with collagen–vascular diseases. Rowell's syndrome, characterized by EM-like lesions in a patient with lupus erythematosus, is also in the differential diagnosis. It is not known whether Rowell's syndrome represents a distinct entity or the coexistence of two distinct disorders. Detection of the classic target lesions and typical histopathologic features facilitate confirmation of the diagnosis.

In typical cases the explosive presentation and dramatic physical findings leave little confusion about the diagnosis of TEN. However, other blistering conditions, including drug-induced linear IgA bullous dermatosis, paraneoplastic pemphigus and pemphigus vulgaris, may closely resemble TEN. SJS–TEN spectrum has been subclassified as SJS when there is <10% body surface area with separation of the epidermis from the dermis, TEN when there is >30% separation, and overlap SJS–TEN when the separation is >10% but <30%. The staphylococcal scalded skin syndrome is excluded by histopathologic confirmation of a more superficial blister than that seen in TEN. This can be performed rapidly via microscopy on specimens prepared using frozen sections. Early TEN can be confused with morbilliform drug eruptions, physical and/or chemical injury, and toxic erythroderma.

Histopathologic Findings

Although the classic target lesions of EM do have a reproducible, typical histopathologic appearance, the clinician must be aware that individual vascular-based cutaneous lesions evolve over several days, and that the histopathologic findings in an individual lesion will vary, depending on when in a lesion's lifespan it is biopsied. Also, if the clinician samples a lesion with the clinical characteristics of erythema or urticaria rather than with those of a target lesion, the histopathologic appearance may mimic that of those conditions. Biopsy specimens should be taken from the periphery of target lesions, not from the center, to have the best chance of showing keratinocyte changes.

Typical lesions show endothelial swelling, a superficial perivascular mononuclear cell infiltrate, and papillary dermal edema. The epidermal changes, when combined with these nonspecific dermal changes, allow the diagnosis to be made. The focal necrosis of keratinocytes and spongiosis associated with vacuolar alterations of basal epidermal cells that may progress to a dermoepidermal junction zone blister are characteristic. The basement membrane remains intact and the lesions do not produce scarring. Extravasation of erythrocytes does occur in the dermis, but leukocytoclasia (infiltration of neutrophils with a breaking-up of their nuclei) and fibrinoid necrosis of blood vessel walls never occur. Oral lesions show similar histopathologic changes.

Direct immunofluorescence microscopy from lesions of EM is not diagnostic; however, a biopsy for immunofluorescence microscopy should usually be performed (especially for mucosal lesions) to exclude autoimmune bullous diseases such as paraneoplastic pemphigus, linear IgA bullous dermatosis, and pemphigus vulgaris. In early lesions of EM, immunoreactants such as C_3 and IgM may be detected in a granular pattern in the dermal blood vessels. These findings are not specific and are not of real value in confirming a diagnosis of EM.

The histopathologic appearance of lesions of TEN is identical to that of EM with extreme epidermal necrosis. The extent of epidermal necrosis may only be evident clinically, depending on the evolution of the sampled lesion. Most patients with SJS–TEN should a have biopsy for routine processing and immunofluorescence microscopy. The cutaneous basement membrane remains at the base of the blister in TEN. Therefore, if secondary infection is prevented, it is believed that scarring will not occur; however, clinically, results vary widely. Scarring may occur on mucosal surfaces, the scalp, the fingernails, and the skin, probably as a result of secondary infection.

Evaluation

A cost-effective yet adequate evaluation of the patient with EM or SJS–TEN must address both confirmation of the diagnosis and exclusion of significant underlying disease as a cause. There are no specific laboratory abnormalities associated with EM; therefore, the diagnosis is based on clinical parameters, with histopathologic confirmation as reviewed previously. Patients with EM may have leukocytosis, an elevated erythrocyte sedimentation rate, elevated liver function test results, proteinuria, and occasionally hematuria.

In addition to the routine histopathologic examination, a more prompt bedside evaluation of oral mucosal blisters may involve a Tzanck preparation. The roof of the vesiculobullous lesion is removed with a number 15 blade, the blister fluid is removed, and the base is scraped firmly but without inducing bleeding. The material obtained in this manner is placed on a glass slide and stained with Wright, Giemsa, or other suitable stain. EM blisters show only mixed inflammatory cells, but the acantholytic cells of pemphigus vulgaris or the multinucleate giant cells of herpes simplex infections can be excluded.

A thorough history and physical examination should be a prerequisite for the laboratory evaluation of the underlying causes of SJS–TEN spectrum illnesses. A careful drug history is particularly important. Obviously, suspected drugs should not be readministered, owing to the risk of even more severe reactions. The signs and symptoms of infection must be sought. The history may suggest recent vaccination or hyposensitization as a precipitant.

A high index of suspicion for HSV infection is particularly relevant in recurrent EM. The diagnosis of herpes virus infection can be confirmed by Tzanck's preparation of an active vesicle, biopsy of a herpetic lesion, or culture of the virus from a herpetic lesion. Immunoperoxidase-labeled monoclonal antibodies and polymerase chain reaction are sensitive techniques that can substantiate the diagnosis of HSV infection. It is often difficult to distinguish the herpetic lesion from the EM lesion on mucosal surfaces. It can be difficult to confirm HSV infection owing to the time lag between HSV infection and onset of EM.

If other infections are suspected clinically, appropriate imaging and laboratory studies can be ordered for confirmation. A complete blood count, erythrocyte sedimentation rate, urinalysis, and liver function tests may be useful screening procedures in patients with EM and SJS–TEN spectrum illnesses. Specialized tests (e.g., sinus and dental X-rays for suspected infections in those sites; hepatitis B surface antigen; cultures for bacteria, fungi, and viral agents; syphilis serology; tuberculin skin testing; antinuclear antibody profile; rheumatoid factor; pregnancy test; and specialized procedures to diagnose other diseases or occult malignancies) can be ordered as suggested by the history, physical examination, and screening laboratory tests. The clinician should realize that as many as one-third to half of the cases of EM are idiopathic.

Treatment

There is no treatment that has been demonstrated in a double-blind study to shorten the course of EM. EM may be an uncomplicated, self-limited condition that requires no treatment. The underlying causes should be identified when possible, because subsequent exposure could lead to a more severe recurrence.

Recurrent EM that is caused by HSV infection may be prevented by reducing the frequency of herpes infections (e.g., by sunscreen use on the lips to reduce the frequency of sun-exacerbated herpes labialis). Oral acyclovir (as low as 200 mg twice daily), valacyclovir (500 mg daily), or famciclovir (250 mg twice daily) can be used for a number of years in low oral doses to significantly reduce the incidence of herpes infection recurrences. Although once-daily dosing improves compliance, twice-daily dosing might smooth blood levels, especially if patients are late with daily dosing.

Patients with SJS–TEN require supportive care. Obviously, an underlying drug allergy or infection must be diagnosed and corrected. Supportive care may include maintaining the patient's fluid balance, prescribing antihistamines for pruritus or NSAIDs for arthralgias and fever, and providing local care with compresses or whirlpool baths to soothe and debride bullous lesions. Mucosal lesions require careful attention. Ophthalmologic consultation should be obtained early to prevent corneal scarring from secondary bacterial infections. Oral care should include compresses and oral rinses. Urethral stricture must be prevented in male patients with penile coronal involvement. These patients should also be monitored to exclude urinary retention.

Systemic corticosteroid therapy is a controversial treatment in SJS–TEN. Unfortunately, a double-blind study has never been conducted to confirm the efficacy of this treatment. A retrospective study in children suggested that corticosteroid-related complications may outweigh the benefit of corticosteroid therapy in the pediatric age group. A recently published retrospective study in Europe, however, suggested a benefit for corticosteroids over supportive care alone in adults with SJS–TEN. A tapering course of prednisone may be used early in the treatment of selected patients with serum sickness-like illness (e.g., fever, myalgias, arthralgias, etc.) after an infectious cause has been excluded. High-dose intravenous corticosteroids are also an option, especially in severe cases. The mortality rate in SJS may approach 5–10%. Patients with drug-induced SJS–TEN should wear a bracelet carrying a warning of their allergy because a second exposure to the particular drug may result in even more severe illness. However, there are also patients who have been re-exposed to putative agents that caused their disease and have had no further reactions.

TEN is associated with a mortality rate approaching 30%. Reports of the successful use of high-dose intravenous immunoglobulin (IVIg) provide hope that this prognosis can be dramatically reduced. Therapy must be given early in the course of the disease over several days – usually 3 – in order to deliver a total of 3 g/kg. The use of IVIg is controversial owing to reports suggesting a lack of benefit; but close examination of such reports notes variable times from the onset for administration, and the use of doses lower than 3 g/kg. In addition, it is possible that responses differ from one preparation of IVIg to another, and most of the case series have variable numbers of patients with comorbid conditions that might affect the outcome.

Anecdotal use of cyclosporine during the acute (i.e., Nikolsky test-positive) period has been described. TNF-α inhibitors have also been suggested, but cautious use is recommended owing to the detrimental effects seen with thalidomide. Conceptually, therapies that affect Fas–FasL interaction should be given during the Nikolsky-positive phase of the illness. Supportive therapy is otherwise similar to that for SJS, with the added need to care for a patient with almost total loss of integument. This care usually requires an intensive care or burn unit. Maintenance of fluid and electrolyte balance and prevention of infection require constant vigilance. Artificial dressings (e.g., OP-Site, DuoDERM, Vigilon, or keratinocyte culture grafts) that are designed for the care of burned patients may be life-saving.

SUGGESTED READINGS

Brice S, Krzemien D, Weston W, Huff J. Detection of herpes simplex virus DNA in cutaneous lesions of erythema multiforme. J Invest Dermatol 1989; 93: 183–187.

Chan HL, Stern RS, Arndt KA, et al. The incidence of erythema multiforme, Stevens–Johnson syndrome, and toxic epidermal necrolysis: a population based study with particular reference to reactions caused by drugs among outpatients. Arch Dermatol 1990; 126: 43–47.

Fernandez AP, Kerdel FA. The use of intravenous immune globulin in dermatology. Dermatol Ther 2007; 20: 288–305.

Lonjou C, Borot N, Sekula P, et al., and the RegiSCAR study group. A European study of HLA-B in Stevens–Johnson syndrome and toxic epidermal necrolysis related to five high-risk drugs. Pharmacogenet Genomics 2008; 18: 99–107.

Pereira F, Mudgil A, Rosmarin D. Toxic epidermal necrolysis. J Am Acad Dermatol 2007; 56: 181–200.

Roujeau JC. Steven's–Johnson syndrome and toxic epidermal necrolysis are severity variants of the same disease, which differs from erythema multiforme. J Dermatol 1997; 24: 726–729.

Schneck J, Stat D, Fagot J, et al. Effects of treatments on the mortality of Stevens–Johnson syndrome and toxic epidermal necrolysis: a retrospective study on patients included in the prospective EuroSCAR Study. J Am Acad Dermatol 2008; 58: 33–40.

Viard I, Welvei P, Ballani R, et al. Inhibition of toxic epidermal necrolysis by blockade of CD95 with human intravenous immune globulin. Science 1998; 282: 490–493.

Weston WL, Brice SL, Jester JD, et al. Herpes simplex virus in childhood erythema multiforme. Pediatrics 1992; 89: 32–34.

Wolkentein PE, Ronjeain JC, Revuz J. Drug-induced toxic epidermal necrolysis. Clin Dermatol 1998; 16: 399–408.

Chapter | 8 |

Manisha J. Patel,
Joseph L. Jorizzo, and
Jeffrey P. Callen

Erythema Nodosum and Other Panniculitides

Panniculitis refers to inflammation within the subcutaneous fat. The exact nature of the infiltrate may depend on when the biopsy is taken in relation to the age of the lesion undergoing biopsy. The panniculitides have been divided into four categories based on histopathologic criteria: (1) septal; (2) lobular; (3) mixed septal and lobular; and (4) panniculitis with vasculitis. Table 8–1 presents one of the currently accepted classifications for the panniculitides.

ERYTHEMA NODOSUM

Erythema nodosum is a relatively common dermatosis characterized by the occurrence of tender, nonulcerative nodules on the legs, resulting from primarily acute inflammation in the subcutaneous fat (i.e., panniculitis). It is a reactive process that is usually self-limited, lasting 3–6 weeks. The lesions are often symmetrical. The anterior tibial surface is the most common site of involvement. Patients may have accompanying serum sickness-like signs and symptoms, such as fever, malaise, arthralgias, and arthritis. Mainly younger patients (age range 20–40 years), primarily females, are affected. Up to one-third of affected patients may experience a recurrence.

Erythema nodosum was first described in the English literature by Robert Willan in 1807. Patients with erythema nodosum often present to primary care physicians; therefore, it is particularly important that physicians understand this cutaneous entity.

Pathogenesis

Although the pathogenesis of erythema nodosum remains unknown, several lines of evidence support a circulating immune complex-mediated pathogenesis. Clinically, patients classically have serum sickness-like signs and symptoms, such as fever, malaise, arthralgias, arthritis, and myalgias, often associated with circulating immune complex-mediated disease. The histopathologic detection of a primarily neutrophilic, vessel-based, septal panniculitis is also consistent with this hypothesis. Nonspecific in vitro assay results (e.g., C1q binding assay) have been positive in a significant percentage of patients with erythema nodosum, especially those with sarcoidosis or streptococcal pharyngitis. In addition, immunoreactants (e.g., IgG and C3) have been demonstrated in subcutaneous septal blood vessels in early lesions from some patients with erythema nodosum; this observation provides only nonspecific support for a circulating immune complex-mediated pathogenesis. These findings, and the occurrence of erythema nodosum in patients with diseases with strong circulating immune complex associations, such as inflammatory bowel disease, Behçet's syndrome, and bowel bypass syndrome, will no doubt prompt future investigators to apply modern immunoblotting and immunoperoxidase techniques to the identification of specific antigens in the circulating immune complexes and in septal blood vessels, respectively, to assess the role of specific immune complexes in disease pathogenesis.

Erythema nodosum has been associated with a host of underlying conditions (Table 8–2). Perhaps the associated diseases contribute antigens to circulating immune complexes that are then deposited in septal blood vessels in the subcutaneous fat, producing the lesions of erythema nodosum.

An important etiologic category for erythema nodosum is bacterial infection. Streptococcal infection is a major cause of erythema nodosum. The onset of erythema nodosum may follow acute streptococcal infection by 2–3 weeks. Other bacterial causes of erythema nodosum include tuberculosis, leprosy, brucellosis, lymphogranuloma venereum, leptospirosis, and yersinial infection. Chlamydial infections have also been associated with erythema nodosum. Tuberculosis was one of the leading causes of erythema nodosum earlier in the 20th century. Erythema nodosum occurs during primary exposure to the tuberculosis bacilli, possibly even before skin test conversion. Rather than occurring early in the course of leprosy, erythema nodosum leprosum occurs as a reactional form of leprosy, usually in patients whose disease is towards the lepromatous end of the leprosy spectrum. The lesions of erythema nodosum leprosum may be atypical in location and clinical appearance.

Erythema nodosum also occurs following primary exposure to deep fungal organisms. This is especially true for coccidioidomycosis (i.e., San Joaquin Valley fever) and for histoplasmosis. Erythema nodosum may be seen less commonly with other deep fungal infections, such as blastomycosis and

Table 8–1 A proposed classification of the panniculitides

I. Septal panniculitis
A. Erythema nodosum
B. Villanova's disease or subacute nodular migratory panniculitis
II. Lobular panniculitis
A. Weber–Christian disease or relapsing febrile nodular nonsuppurative panniculitis (idiopathic lobular panniculitis)
B. Rothman–Makai syndrome or lipogranulomatosis subcutanea
C. Subcutaneous fat necrosis of the newborn
D. Posterior panniculitis
E. Enzymatic panniculitis
1. Pancreatic
2. α_1-Antitrypsin deficiency
F. Physical or factitious panniculitis
G. Cytophagic panniculitis
H. Lipodystrophy syndromes
I. Connective tissue panniculitis (scleroderma or myositis)
III. Mixed panniculitis (e.g., lupus profundus or lupus erythematosus panniculitis)
IV. Panniculitis with vasculitis
A. Small-vessel vasculitis (postcapillary venule), leukocytoclastic vasculitis
B. Medium-sized vessel vasculitis (arterioles or small arteries)
1. Polyarteritis nodosa
2. Erythema induratum (nodular vasculitis)

Table 8–2 Evaluation of the patient with erythema nodosum

I. History
A. Drugs (e.g., oral contraceptives or antibiotics)
B. Exposure to infectious agents
C. Symptoms of an infection
D. Symptoms of bowel disease
II. Physical examination
III. Laboratory studies
A. Skin test for tuberculosis
B. Throat culture
C. Anti-DNase B titer (for *Streptococcus*)
D. Pregnancy test
IV. Radiographic examination
A. Chest X-ray

sporotrichosis, and it has been attributed even to underlying severe dermatophytosis.

Viral infections may also be a cause of erythema nodosum. Although herpes simplex virus and hepatitis B and C infections are the principal viral culprits, milker's nodule, measles, human immunodeficiency virus (HIV), and other viruses have occasionally been implicated.

Erythema nodosum may be a manifestation of parasitosis, such as a hookworm infestation. Other infections or infestations that are less commonly associated with erythema nodosum include toxoplasmosis and secondary syphilis.

Sarcoidosis is an important cause of erythema nodosum. Erythema nodosum lesions occur with serum sickness-like signs and symptoms and pulmonary hilar adenopathy in what is called Löfgren's syndrome. This represents stage I pulmonary sarcoidosis. These patients may have a more benign form of sarcoidosis that usually resolves; only a few patients who present with Löfgren's syndrome later develop the other systemic pulmonary manifestations of sarcoidosis.

Drug hypersensitivity is another major etiologic group to be considered in the evaluation of patients with erythema nodosum. The most common drugs that cause erythema nodosum are the oral contraceptives. All too frequently, these agents are overlooked as a cause as the physician embarks on a costly evaluation and drug regimen modification approach to evaluate the patient with erythema nodosum. Sulfonamides and related agents have also been implicated. Although drug allergy is difficult to prove in patients with erythema nodosum, the following medications have been implicated: trimethoprim–sulfamethoxazole, salicylates, selective serotonin reuptake inhibitors (SSRIs), aromatase inhibitors (used in the treatment of hormone receptor-positive breast cancer), ciprofloxacin, phenacetin, and (historically) iodides and bromides.

Various underlying diseases have also been associated with erythema nodosum. Patients with inflammatory bowel diseases such as ulcerative colitis and Crohn's disease and with infectious colitis such as that from *Yersinia enterocolitica* infection may develop erythema nodosum. The onset of the cutaneous disease and of serum sickness-like signs and symptoms often correlates with increasing bowel disease and high levels of circulating immune complexes. Patients with Behçet's disease and bowel bypass syndrome may have erythema nodosum-like lesions, perhaps by a similar mechanism. Patients with a malignancy, especially of the lymphoreticular system, may have erythema nodosum. Erythema nodosum may also occur during pregnancy. A significant percentage (>50%) of patients have idiopathic erythema nodosum.

Clinical Manifestations

The lesions of erythema nodosum usually begin suddenly as painful, red, round nodules (Fig. 8–1) that range from 1 to 5 cm in size. They are most commonly located bilaterally on extensor surfaces. The shins are the classic site of involvement. The lesions typically evolve over a 3-week period through a bruise-like cycle of discoloration. Other sites of reported involvement include the arms, trunk, and face. The lesions of erythema nodosum do not ulcerate, which is an important differential point from the findings in other panniculitides. Arthralgias, arthritis, fever, and malaise may be associated serum sickness-like features. The lesions may resolve with a mild post-erythemal desquamation. Up to one-third of patients

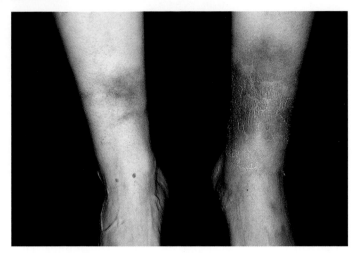

Figure 8–1 Erythema nodosum. This patient has typical erythematous, tender nodules on the lower extremities.

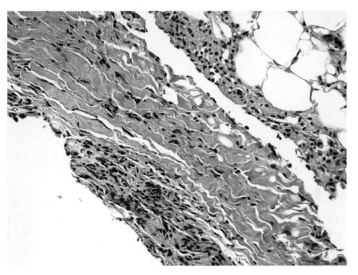

Figure 8–2 Histology of erythema nodosum (×20). This section shows a mostly septal panniculitis composed of lymphocytes and histiocytes, as well as septal fibrosis. (Courtesy of Gary Goldenberg, MD.)

may experience recurrent bouts of erythema nodosum, with each average episode lasting 2–4 weeks.

Differential Diagnosis

Usually, clinicians are able to establish that the lesions of erythema nodosum are a panniculitis based on the clinical examination. Therefore, the approach to the differential diagnosis involves excluding other forms of panniculitis. Examples of other types are panniculitis that is the result of pancreatic disease (this may be suppurative); lupus panniculitis; and nodular vasculitis (this may be suppurative and chronic and located on the posterior leg). Superficial migratory thrombophlebitis may be confused with panniculitis, despite occurring as a result of the inflammation of larger veins, because the inflammation from the phlebitis spreads to involve the surrounding fat. The lesions of thrombophlebitis tend to be arranged in a linear fashion along the veins and last from 1 to 7 days, instead of several weeks as do the lesions of erythema nodosum. Erythema induratum, now termed nodular vasculitis, is a more chronic form of panniculitis. It may produce suppurative, scarring lesions that affect primarily the calves. Disseminated bacterial, fungal, or tuberculous infections may rarely mimic erythema nodosum (infectious panniculitis). Other forms of panniculitis, such as those associated with lupus erythematosus or pancreatitis, can usually be distinguished on clinicopathologic grounds. A recent case has been reported of a patient with classic clinical features of nephrogenic systemic fibrosis whose specimen demonstrated unique histologic features of septal panniculitis with lymphocytic aggregates and Miescher's radial granulomas mimicking erythema nodosum. Cellulitis rarely causes confusion. Panniculitis that is caused by subcutaneous injections, other exogenous factors (e.g., cold exposure), or factitious disease must also be considered.

Histopathologic Findings

Because erythema nodosum is a panniculitis, a punch biopsy specimen is inadequate for interpretation. The deepest punch biopsy will sample only superficial subcutaneous fat, and so a small but deep incisional biopsy is required. The histopathologic findings of erythema nodosum are focused on the septal areas of the panniculus. Acute lesions show a primarily neutrophilic perivascular reaction. Endothelial swelling of blood vessel walls is commonly seen. Necrosis of the fat is not observed. Older lesions show a more mononuclear cellular reaction. There are variable numbers of giant cells, usually of foreign body type, as well as a few eosinophils and histiocytes. Miescher's radial granulomas can be seen, which are composed of small nodules of spindle to oval histiocytes arranged around a minute slit. In early lesions the fibrous septa are widened with edema and fibrinoid change, and in older lesions fibrosis can be found (Fig. 8–2). In acute or chronic erythema nodosum the centers of the fat lobules remain clear, and the inflammation is focused on the peripheral septal areas.

Evaluation

Evaluation of the patient with erythema nodosum should proceed in two directions. First, the diagnosis must be confirmed as erythema nodosum, and then underlying disease must be excluded (see Table 8–2). The diagnosis is usually made on clinical grounds. If the diagnosis is not certain, a biopsy may be required. A portion of the biopsy specimen may be cultured for bacteria, fungi, and acid-fast bacilli.

Patients with erythema nodosum often have a significant elevation of the Westergren erythrocyte sedimentation rate, peripheral leukocytosis, and elevated γ-globulin levels because acute-phase reactants are associated with the serum sickness-like illness. A thorough history and review of systems and a physical examination to look for the causes reviewed previously are essential. A chest radiograph should also be a mandatory part of the evaluation of the patient with erythema nodosum because of the possibility of detecting early changes of tuberculosis, sarcoidosis, or deep fungal infection. A purified protein derivative tuberculin test for tuberculosis can also be performed. The possibility of current or recent streptococcal infection can be assessed by a throat culture, and anti-DNase B titer. A complete blood count and urinalysis should be performed. In women of childbearing age, a pregnancy test can be performed.

Further evaluation can be performed in a cost-effective manner if it is guided by the history, physical examination, and laboratory screening test results. For example, the patient with gastrointestinal symptoms should be evaluated more completely for inflammatory bowel disease, and possibly for yersinial enterocolitis. Geography is also a relevant factor because tuberculosis and yersinial infections are less common in the United States, and coccidioidomycosis and histoplasmosis are important etiologic considerations in the southwestern United States and Ohio River Valley, respectively. The use of oral contraceptives should not be ignored in a complete drug history, because dermatologists often are consulted by patients with erythema nodosum who have undergone expensive laboratory evaluation and changes in medications but who are still taking their oral contraceptives. Discontinuation of the oral contraceptive is often followed by a prompt clinical remission.

Treatment

If an underlying cause for the erythema nodosum is found, this should be addressed as a key to treatment. Most patients also require symptomatic treatment. Nonsteroidal anti-inflammatory drugs (NSAIDs), in particular aspirin and indomethacin, are useful, because they relieve fever and arthralgias and also may alleviate the pain from the cutaneous lesions. Potassium iodide (SSKI) is an important treatment for patients with more resistant disease. It can be given as an oral solution in daily doses of up to 900 mg for 3–4 weeks (0.3 mL equals 300 mg). This therapy is relatively safe, except for occasional gastrointestinal upset or cutaneous eruptions; however, it is contraindicated in patients with hyperthyroidism. Systemic corticosteroid therapy is occasionally required. In patients treated with systemic corticosteroids, cautious exclusion of infections that might be worsened by this treatment (e.g., tuberculosis or a deep fungal infection) is required.

LOBULAR PANNICULITIDES

Idiopathic, chronic, lobular panniculitis is characterized by multiple recurrent subcutaneous nodules with accompanying fever. There is controversy regarding the designation of this entity. Other clinical features that commonly occur are arthralgias and myalgias. Some patients also have recurrent abdominal pain. In addition to the cutaneous lesions, any area of the body containing fat can be affected by what has been called Weber–Christian disease.

The laboratory abnormalities associated with Weber–Christian disease include an elevated erythrocyte sedimentation rate, anemia, leukopenia or leukocytosis, depression of complement components, and evidence of circulating immune complexes.

There is no specific therapy for this type of panniculitis. Reports have centered on the use of anti-inflammatory agents, including aspirin, NSAIDs, oral corticosteroids, antimalarials, and immunosuppressants, including cyclophosphamide and cyclosporine. In addition, colchicine, dapsone, and potassium iodide may be effective in some individual patients.

Panniculitis Associated with α₁-Antitrypsin Deficiency

Several groups of patients with a lobular or septal panniculitis have been found to have a deficiency of α_1-antitrypsin. There are differences in the clinical and histopathologic manifestations, but little difference in the associated conditions present in the two groups with or without α_1-antitrypsin deficiency. Specifically, the patients with α_1-antitrypsin deficiency are more likely to have ulceration and drainage. Recognition of these patients may be important on several grounds. First, debridement of the lesion should be avoided. Second, in patients believed to have factitious panniculitis, α_1-antitrypsin deficiency should be considered. Third, these patients should be evaluated for pulmonary disease and should be advised to avoid smoking. Fourth, therapy with α_1-proteinase inhibitor concentrate may be helpful.

Lipoatrophic Panniculitis

Several conditions that have been described in children often result in lipoatrophy following an inflammatory reaction. There is a range of diseases that perhaps includes Rothman–Makai syndrome (lipogranulomatosis subcutanea), lipoatrophic panniculitis, lipophagic panniculitis of childhood, and localized lipoatrophy (atrophic connective tissue disease panniculitis). These children tend to have multiple erythematous lesions, most commonly on the extremities, which resolve with subcutaneous atrophy. The patients are often febrile. They may have associated autoimmune phenomena, such as juvenile chronic arthritis, Hashimoto's thyroiditis, or diabetes mellitus. There is no known effective therapy, but some patients have responded to oral glucocorticosteroids, oral antimalarials, or oral dapsone.

Histiocytic Cytophagic Panniculitis

Histiocytic cytophagic panniculitis was described by Winkelman as a chronic histiocytic disease of the subcutaneous fat, with accompanying inflammatory panniculitis, fever, serositis, and reticuloendotheliomegaly. The process has also been linked to neoplastic processes such as lymphoma and malignant histiocytoses. Hemorrhagic complications, perhaps caused by thrombocytopenia, have occurred. Thorough oncologic evaluation is required. Aggressive therapy with cytotoxic agents and/or radiation therapy are offered early in this process.

Factitious Panniculitis

Factitious panniculitis due to external trauma caused by the injection of foreign substances is not uncommon and should be considered in any patient with panniculitis and unusual clinical or histopathologic features. In traumatic lesions an organizing hematoma is often demonstrated histologically, whereas with injection of a foreign material, refractile bodies or a 'Swiss cheese' effect is encountered. Occasionally, spectro-scopic and/or chromatographic techniques are necessary to identify the causative injected material. The treatment involves behavior modification and psychotherapy techniques.

SUGGESTED READINGS

Craig AJ, Cualing H, Thomas G, et al. Cytophagic histocytic panniculitis – a syndrome associated with benign and malignant panniculitis: case comparison and review of the literature. J Am Acad Dermatol 1998; 39: 721–736.

Krasowska D, Szymanek M, Schwartz RA, Myslinski W. Cutaneous effects of the most commonly used antidepressant medication, the selective serotonin reuptake inhibitors. J Am Acad Dermatol 2007; 56: 848–853.

Mana J, Marcoval J. Erythema nodosum. Clin Dermatol 2007; 25: 288–294.

Picco P, Galtorno M, Vignola S, et al. Clinical and biological characteristics of immunopathological disease-related erythema nodosum in children. Scand J Rheumatol 1999; 28: 27–32.

Prestes CA, Winkelmann RK, Su WPD. Septal granulomatous panniculitis: comparison of the pathology of erythema nodosum migrans (migratory panniculitis) and chronic erythema nodosum. J Am Acad Dermatol 1990; 22: 477–483.

Requena L, Sanchez Yus E. Erythema nodosum. Semin Cutan Med Surg 2007; 26: 114–125.

Requena L, Sanchez Yus E. Panniculitis. Part I. Mostly septal panniculitis. J Am Acad Dermatol 2001; 45: 163–183.

Requena L, Sanchez Yus E. Panniculitis. Part II. Mostly lobular panniculitis. J Am Acad Dermatol 2001; 45: 325–361.

Wood AM, Stockley RA. Alpha one antitrypsin deficiency: from gene to treatment. Respiration 2007; 74: 481–492.

Chapter | 9 | *Gil Yosipovitch*

Pruritus

Pruritus is a complex symptom that is very similar to pain and affects all humans in the course of their lives. Chronic pruritus is defined as an itch which lasts more than 6 weeks. It has a significant impact on patients' quality of life, very similar to chronic pain. It is the primary symptom in a diverse range of inflammatory skin diseases, such as atopic eczema, psoriasis, dry skin and chronic urticaria (Table 9–1). It can occur without any primary skin eruption associated with underlying systemic diseases (Table 9–2), and can be the presenting symptom of lymphoma, hepatic diseases such as biliary cirrhosis, and hepatitis C viral infection. It can occur in relation to primary damage to nerve fibers, such as post-herpetic neuropathy, as well as in afferent nerves in the central nervous system as in multiple sclerosis. Pruritus is a common symptom in psychiatric diseases such as obsessive compulsive disorders, and in delusions of parasitosis.

SKIN SIGNS OF CHRONIC PRURITUS

There are common skin lesions that develop in pruritus as a result of repetitive scratching and rubbing the skin. These lesions are not considered a primary skin eruption. They include excoriations – prurigo nodules – which are excoriated papules that lead to nodule formation. These are usually distributed on the extensor side of the limbs and upper back. Lichenification is a thickened plaque with marked accentuation of the skin creases which develops as a result of continuous rubbing and scratching in areas that the patient can easily scratch and rub, such as the nape of the neck, below the elbow, the ankle, the buttocks, and the genitalia. Changes in skin pigmentation – both hyper- and hypopigmentation – in darker skin can occur because of repeated scratching.

The Butterfly Sign

The middle of the back which cannot be reached may show normal skin or relative hypopigmentation, in contrast to the hyperpigmentation of the areas subjected to persistent scratching, thereby resulting in a butterfly pattern.

Shiny Finger Nails

The finger nails may be shiny because of prolonged rubbing. Excoriated lesions resulting from repetitive scratching as well as eczematous lesions can become infected, particularly in patients with atopic dermatitis.

COMMON COMPLICATIONS IN PATIENTS WITH GENERALIZED PRURITUS

Patients with chronic pruritus often have difficulty sleeping, agitation, depression, and decreased sexual desire and sexual function suggestive of a significant impairment of quality of life.

DIAGNOSIS

When no diagnosis of a primarily dermatological disorder can be made, a history, review of systems, physical examination, and screening laboratory examination are needed.

A detailed history is important. One should investigate whether the patient suffers from generalized or localized itching. A localized itch may be associated with a burning sensation and pain in peripheral neuropathy, such as damage to cervical nerves in brachioradial pruritus. Careful history also includes a drug history, as drugs such as opiates, aspirin, penicillin, and antimalarials can induce itch without a cutaneous eruption. A simple question, such as whether pruritus occurs in other family members, can indicate the possibility of scabies and prevent unnecessary investigation. Recent travel to endemic areas of parasitic infection and gastrointestinal complaints may be suggestive of parasitic infection. A positive review of systems, especially in relation to general health, such as weight loss, night sweats and tremor, could point to a systemic cause.

Some pruritic states have specific clinical patterns. Despite severe pruritus, chronic urticaria does not usually show secondary skin lesions associated with scratching. Patients with cholestatic itch initially present with itch in an acral distribu-

Table 9–1 Common skin diseases and infectious skin diseases that cause pruritus

Atopic eczema
Psoriasis
Contact dermatitis
Urticaria
Dry skin
Elderly idiopathic itch
Seborrheic dermatitis
Lichen planus
Cutaneous T-cell lymphoma
Scars and post burns
Pityriasis rosea
Bullous pemphigoid (including the pre-bullous phase)
Dermatitis herpetiformis
Pregnancy-associated cutaneous eruptions
Superficial fungal diseases
Folliculitis
Scabies
HIV
Varicella
Onchocerciasis

Table 9–2 Systemic diseases that cause itch

End-stage chronic renal disease

Cholestasis
  Primary biliary cirrhosis
  Hepatitis C viral infection
  Cholestasis of pregnancy

Hematopoietic
  Hodgkin's lymphoma
  Non-Hodgkin's lymphoma
  Mastocytosis
  Multiple myeloma
  Polycythemia vera
  Iron deficiency anemia
  Myeloid and lymphocytic leukemias
  Myelodysplastic disorders

Solid malignant tumors (paraneoplastic manifestation)

Endocrine
  Hyperthyroidism
  Hypothyroidism
  Mastocytosis
  Anorexia nervosa

Drugs (such as opioids, hydroxyethyl starch, chloroquine)

Collagen diseases
  Dermatomyositis
  Scleroderma
  Sjögren's syndrome

Itch in post-transplant patients

Peripheral neuropathy
  Post-herpetic neuralgia
  Brachioradial pruritus
  Notalgia paresthetica

Central nervous system neuropathy
  Multiple sclerosis
  Brain tumors
  Cerebrovascular events

Psychogenic itch
  Delusional state of parasitophobia
  Obsessive compulsive disorder
  Depression

tion in the palms and soles, whereas patients with other chronic types of itch rarely do so. Neuropathic itch in disease entities such as post-herpetic neuralgia and brachioradial pruritus involves itch in the relevant nerve distributions.

EXAMINATION

A thorough physical examination with particular attention to lymph nodes (lymphoreticular malignancy), and organomegaly of liver and spleen (lymphoreticular malignancy and paraneoplastic manifestations), is essential. Fine tremor may suggest underlying hyperthyroidism. Examination of the genital area, finger webs, the ulnar border of palms, wrists, elbows, axilla and nipples is carried out to exclude scabies.

INVESTIGATIONS

Based on the initial findings, further laboratory evaluation and imaging studies may be necessary. Although the appropriate tests will vary with the individual circumstances, one suggested approach is to obtain the studies indicated in Table 9–3. Most patients with pruritus will not need further tests. A detailed history and examination will reveal the cause. Investigations in patients with pruritus with an eruption include a skin biopsy and appropriate laboratory investigations. Figure 9–1 provides an algorithm for the diagnosis and investigation of pruritus.

PATHOPHYSIOLOGY OF GENERALIZED PRURITUS

In many cases, pruritus originates in the upper layers of the skin, although damage to nerve fibers along the peripheral and central nervous system can induce itch. There are histamine and nonhistaminergic C nerve fibers that transmit itch. These C nerve fibers represent only 5–10% of the C nerve fibers and have slow conduction velocity.

There are many mediators involved in pruritus, both peripheral and central. Important mediators include histamine, proteinases, substance P, nerve growth factor, prostaglandins and interleukins, and central mediators including opiates. For the most part, 'itch factors,' or pruritogens, in the various systemic diseases in which itching occurs have not yet been identified.

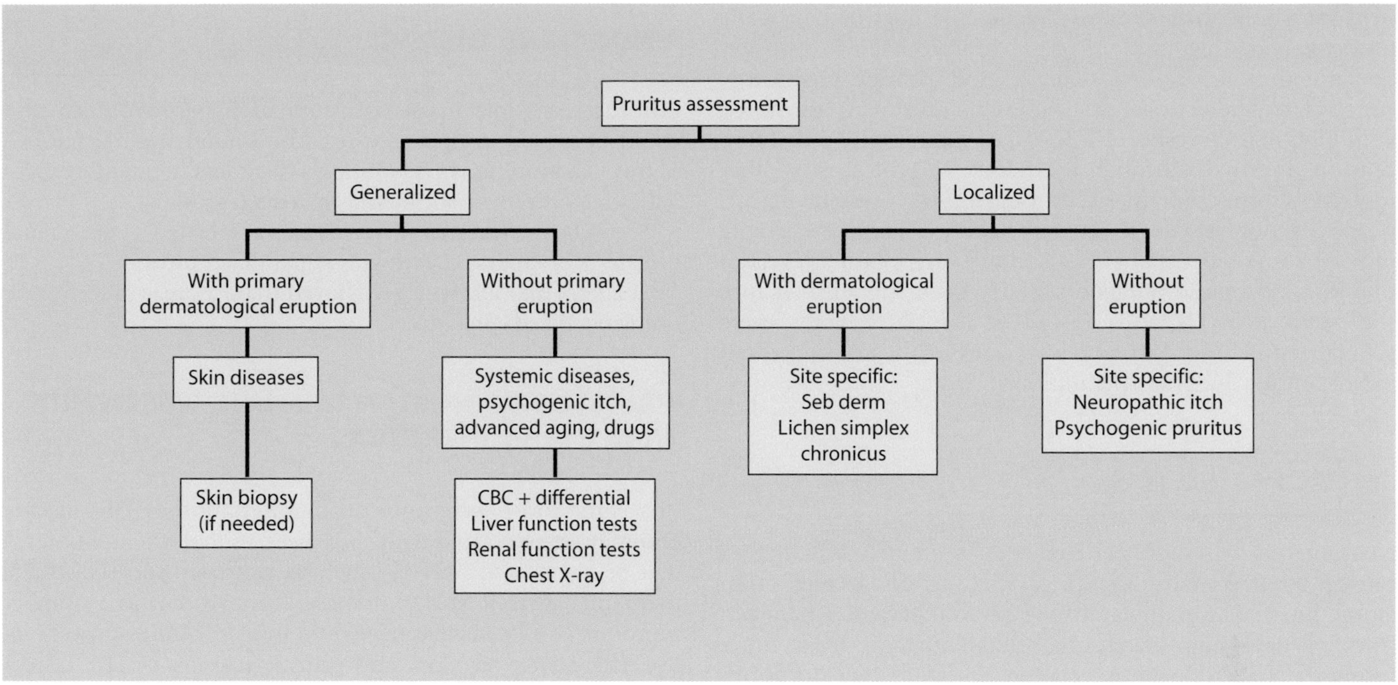

Figure 9–1 An algorithm for the diagnosis and investigation of pruritus. (Adapted from Yosipovitch G, Dawn AG, Greaves MW. Pathophysiology and clinical aspects of pruritus. In: Goldsmith KS, Wolff K, Gilchrest B, et al., eds. Fitzpatrick's dermatology in general medicine, 7th edn. New York: McGraw Hill, 2008; 902–911.)

Table 9–3 Initial laboratory studies in patients with generalized pruritus

I. Complete blood count and differential

II. Chemistry profile
   A. Hepatic enzymes
   B. Urea nitrogen and creatinine levels

III. Thyroid function (e.g., thyroid-stimulating hormone)

IV. Chest radiography

V. Optional
   A. Stool examination for parasites
   B. HIV testing
   C. Abdominal and chest imaging
   D. Skin biopsy for routine and immunofluorescence microscopy

It has recently been suggested that generalized pruritus is induced by an imbalance between the μ and the κ opioid systems. Activation of μ opioid receptors stimulates itch perception, whereas κ opioid receptor stimulation inhibits μ-receptor effects both centrally and peripherally.

END-STAGE RENAL FAILURE (ESRF) PRURITUS

Pruritus is a frequently disabling and distressing symptom of ESRF. It affects more than 50% of patients, especially those on dialysis, and has a significant impact on sleep and mental and physical function. In the International Dialysis Outcomes and Practice Patterns study, which evaluated more than 18 000 patients on hemodialysis, pruritus was associated with a 17% higher mortality risk, an effect that was no longer significant after adjustment for measures of sleep quality. This observation suggests that sleep disturbances may have an important role in the greater mortality risk associated with ESRF pruritus. The pathophysiology of ESRF pruritus is poorly understood. Current data point toward a role for the immune system and opioidergic systems. Early hypotheses of the pathogenesis of the pruritus caused by renal failure related the pruritus to secondary hyperparathyroidism, but other factors such as calcium and phosphate levels may have a role in itch. Subtotal parathyroidectomy was occasionally associated with the control of ESRF pruritus. It has been postulated that ESRF itch is associated with a proinflammatory state with elevated C reactive protein and T-helper type 1 cells. In concordance with this theory, immunomodulators such as ultraviolet light (UVB), thalidomide, and topical immunomodulators such as tacrolimus reduced pruritus. The pruritus can be so intense that excoriations lead to cutaneous nodules (prurigo nodularis). The most prevalent body site is the back, but the arms, head, and abdomen are also commonly affected. The symptom tends to be more severe at night.

PRURITUS OF CHOLESTASIS

Cholestatic pruritus is highly distressing. It often begins in an acral distribution but later becomes generalized. Clinicians are familiar with the causes of cholestasis, including intrahepatic (e.g., hepatitis of all causes), extrahepatic (e.g., bile duct stricture, cholelithiasis, or malignant bile duct or pancreatic tumors), and drug induced (e.g., chlorpromazine, testosterone, norethindrone, phenothiazines, tolbutamide, erythromycin estolate, and estrogens). Cholestatic pruritus is associated with high plasma levels of bile salts. Whether bile salts cause pruritus directly or through the release of proteases or other molecules from epidermal cells, hepatocytes, or tissue macrophages is not yet clear. Therapy with cholestyramine may provide some relief. Patients also have high plasma levels of opioids, and opioid antagonists have been shown to reduce cholestatic itch. Hepatitis C can be associated with severe generalized itching, and in severe cases itch is considered an indication for liver transplantation.

NEUROPATHIC ITCH

Neuropathic itch has been defined as an itch initiated or caused by a primary lesion or dysfunction at any point along the afferent pathway of the nervous system. Characteristics of neuropathic itch that differentiate it from other forms of itch include the associations with other sensory symptoms in a dermatomal distribution and the presence of other neural damages, including motor damage or autonomic damage.

Neuropathic itch can coincide with pain, as is seen in 30–40% of patients with post-herpetic neuralgia. Characteristic sensory complaints associated with neuropathic itch are burning, paresthesia, tingling, and stinging. Localized itching can follow dermatomes at the level of C5–C8, such as the dorsolateral aspect of the arms in brachioradial pruritus, and unilateral itch midback in dermatomes at the level of T2–T6 in notalgia paresthetica.

LYMPHOMAS, LEUKEMIA, AND HEMATOLOGIC DISEASE

Pruritus is an important sign that may have prognostic significance in several of the malignant lymphomas. It could be the presenting symptom of lymphoma. Widespread cutaneous T-cell lymphoma and erythrodermic forms, including Sézary syndrome (T-cell leukemia), cause an intractable severe itch that is difficult to treat. Thirty percent of patients with Hodgkin's lymphoma experience generalized pruritus at some time during the course of their disease. The pruritus of Hodgkin's lymphoma is usually related to the disease's activity. Pruritus from any cause is often experienced more intensely at night. Pruritus is an infrequent accompanying symptom of multiple myeloma. The mechanism of pruritus in these conditions remains unknown.

Approximately 50% of patients with polycythemia rubra vera develop pruritus that usually occurs after exposure to water (bath itch). This short-lasting pruritus is most probably mediated by increased histamine release from mast cells. Iron deficiency is associated with pruritus. This is reversible with iron supplementation. The mechanism of pruritus in iron deficiency is unknown.

ENDOCRINE DISEASE

Pruritus is an important symptom of hyperthyroidism and could be a presenting symptom. The underlying mechanism of this itch is unknown. Hypothyroidism less frequently causes itch related to the associated asteatosis (dry skin).

Secondary hyperparathyroidism associated with renal disease is often associated with generalized pruritus.

Diabetes mellitus is now believed to be a cause of localized, not generalized, pruritus.

PRURITUS OF HUMAN IMMUNODEFICIENCY VIRUS (HIV) INFECTION

Itch is the most common skin manifestation of HIV disease and may be associated with skin diseases that are more prevalent or aggravated by HIV, such as psoriasis and seborrheic dermatitis, as well as skin dryness. It may occur as a primary symptom of HIV, such as in eosinophilic folliculitis, insect bite hypersensitivity reaction, and pruritic papules of HIV. These papular pruritic eruptions cause severe itch. The majority of these patients with pruritus have advanced disease with CD4 counts below 50 cell/mm^3.

PREGNANCY

Pregnant women may experience generalized pruritus as a result of cholestasis, which is common in pregnancy; in addition, several dermatoses of pregnancy which are extremely itchy have been described, such as polymorphic eruption of pregnancy and pemphigoid (herpes) gestationis (see Chapter 35).

TREATMENT OF PRURITUS

There are no specific antipruritic drugs that benefit all forms of pruritus. Treatment depends on identifying and removing the cause, whether systemic or cutaneous. If treatment of the cause is not possible there are a number of preventive and therapeutic treatment options. Treatments are divided into topical and systemic.

Topical treatments to relieve itch are particularly helpful for pruritus resulting from skin inflammation. These include emollients and moisturizers, especially when the skin is dry, such as in old age, atopic eczema, and ESRF itch. Although they are capable of relieving pruritus due to inflammatory skin disease, corticosteroids are not intrinsically antipruritic. Topical immunomodulators such as tacrolimus or pimecrolimus have a role in itch associated with eczema.

Coolants and counterirritants such as menthol, which activate nerve fibers for cold, inhibit C nerve fibers that transmit warmth and itch. Other topical agents include local anesthetics such as pramoxine and topical capsaicin, which have a role in the treatment of localized itch, in particular that associated with neuropathic itch.

Systemic corticosteroids are not indicated, except when the diagnosis of a specific steroid-responsive disease (such as bullous pemphigoid) has been established.

Systemic antipruritic treatments include drugs that are used for neuropathic pain, such as gabapentin, pregabalin, and selective serotonin reuptake inhibitors such as mirtazapine and paroxetine. As mentioned, opioids have a role in systemic generalized itch. Therefore, opiate antagonists such as naltrexone have been used for the treatment of pruritus, in particular itch associated with cholestasis, but owing to their significant side effects they are not commonly used. There are currently new κ agonists in development that seem a promising avenue for treating severe pruritus. Butorphanol is a κ agonist and μ antagonist that is a commercially available analgesic and has fewer side effects than the μ antagonists. It has been reported to be effective for different types of severe generalized pruritus.

Antihistamines are only antipruritic if the pruritus is caused by histamine, as in urticaria. They only benefit nonhistamine-mediated itch through their sedating tranquilizing properties. First-generation H_1 antihistamines such as hydroxyzine have marked sedative and anticholinergic actions and are useful in severe chronic urticaria, enabling patients with chronic itch to sleep. Second-generation antihistamines such as loratadine, desloratadine, cetirizine, and levocetirizine are suitable in the daytime for relief of pruritus due to urticaria. The role of these nonsedating antihistamines in other pruritic disorders is limited. Thalidomide was found to have a role in treating chronic itch, but because of the high cost and monitoring requirements is rarely used.

Phototherapy has been used for more than a decade to treat different types of itch. UVB therapy, both broadband and narrowband, seems to be the most effective. The treatment is safe and can be repeated as necessary. It is beneficial for itch associated with atopic dermatitis, psoriasis, and chronic renal failure. Remissions may last for as long as 18 months.

Several studies have shown that behavioral modification therapy reduces the intensity and perception of itch. Other possible behavioral interventions include stress reduction and biofeedback. These treatments are especially effective in chronic pruritus associated with psychogenic cofactors.

SUGGESTED READINGS

Summey BT Jr, Yosipovitch G. Pharmacologic advances in the systemic treatment of itch. Dermatol Ther 2005; 18: 328–332.

Yosipovitch G, Greaves MW, Schmelz M. Itch. Lancet 2003; 361: 690–694.

Yosipovitch G, Greaves M, Fleischer A, McGlone F, eds. Itch: basic mechanisms and therapy. New York: Marcel Dekker, 2004.

Yosipovitch G, Dawn AG, Greaves MW. Pathophysiology and clinical aspects of pruritus. In: Goldsmith KS, Wolff K, Gilchrest B, et al., eds. Fitzpatrick's dermatology in general medicine, 7th edn. New York: McGraw Hill, 2008; 902–911.

Yosipovitch G, Dawn AG, Greaves MW. Cutaneous neurophysiology. In: Bolognia JL, Jorizzo JL, Rapini RP, et al., eds. Dermatology, 2nd edn. London: Mosby, 2008; 81–90.

Aaron M. Loyd
and Joseph L. Jorizzo

Chapter | **10** |

Erythroderma

Erythroderma, also called exfoliative dermatitis, is a clinical final common pathway for a number of underlying cutaneous diseases. Erythroderma can be viewed as representing an acute or chronic 'cutaneous failure' analogous to renal failure. Dermatoses as varied as eczemas, psoriasis, drug eruptions, and cutaneous T-cell lymphoma (mycosis fungoides) can cause the clinicopathologic picture of erythroderma. The entire cutaneous organ is inflamed. Dermal inflammation, seen as perivascular infiltration and mild edema, is accompanied by a psoriasis-like thickening of the epidermis. This combination of dermal and epidermal change is nonspecific histopathologically and is often termed psoriasiform dermatitis. This final common pathway histopathologically is reminiscent of the nonspecific glomerulonephritis often seen in patients with chronic renal failure. Regardless of cause, erythroderma is a serious and sometimes fatal condition often requiring hospitalization. This chapter will focus on adult erythroderma, as the differential diagnosis of pediatric erythroderma includes genodermatoses and is beyond the scope of this discussion.

CAUSE AND PATHOGENESIS

Varied dermatological and internal disorders may underlie erythroderma, although up to one-third of cases remain idiopathic after extensive evaluation (Table 10–1). Most frequently encountered are primary dermatological disorders that have generalized. This group encompasses one-third to half of erythrodermic patients.

Of the primary dermatoses, psoriasis and atopic dermatitis are the most common. It should be emphasized that these two diseases are distinct clinicopathologic entities. Atopic dermatitis is an eczematous disease characterized histopathologically by exocytosis (epidermal migration) of mononuclear cells with resultant spongiosis (intercellular epidermal edema). Psoriasis is a papulosquamous disease characterized by rapid epidermal turnover and exocytosis of neutrophils into epidermal microabscesses.

Other eczematous diseases also may result in erythroderma. Allergic contact dermatitis is a delayed hypersensitivity reaction with the epidermis as a target organ. Seborrheic dermatitis, nummular dermatitis, and photoallergic reactions are examples of other eczematous diseases that can underlie erythroderma.

Other papulosquamous diseases that sometimes resemble psoriasis and can cause erythroderma are pityriasis rubra pilaris and Reiter's syndrome. Rarer dermatoses, such as pemphigus foliaceus (an autoimmune bullous disease that occurs spontaneously or that is sometimes induced by drugs such as penicillamine or captopril) and various ichthyoses (genodermatoses characterized by fish-like scaling), also can produce erythroderma.

Drug eruptions from various oral medications can produce erythroderma. About 10% of all erythrodermas are believed to be the result of drug hypersensitivity. Common medications associated with this reaction pattern include sulfa drugs (e.g., trimethoprim–sulfamethoxazole), allopurinol, chlorpromazine, gold salts, penicillin, barbiturates, and phenytoin. It is likely that there is a genetic predisposition for the development of drug hypersensitivity syndrome (also known as drug reaction with eosinophilia and systemic symptoms) from phenytoin and other related compounds. A recent epidemiologic study of chronic dermatitis suggested that calcium channel blockers may be involved as a causative feature, but this report did not address whether erythroderma was part of the group studied.

The significant incidence of underlying malignancy seen in patients with erythroderma should also be of concern to the evaluating physician. Sézary syndrome is a form of cutaneous T-cell lymphoma characterized by circulating malignant helper T cells (Sézary cells) and erythroderma. Patients with other lymphoreticular malignancies, such as Hodgkin's disease and B-cell lymphomas, and solid tumors from the lung or gastrointestinal tract, also occasionally present with erythroderma.

Erythroderma may also herald other severe systemic diseases, including acquired immunodeficiency syndrome and graft-versus-host disease.

As is apparent from the varied list of underlying diseases, there is most likely no single pathogenesis for erythroderma. From an immunological perspective, erythroderma may be caused by diseases of presumed type II (circulating antibody directed against a peripheral target, e.g., pemphigus foliaceus), and type IV (delayed hypersensitivity, e.g., allergic contact dermatitis) mechanisms and by diseases of unknown cause

Table 10–1 Some causes of erythroderma

I. Pre-existing dermatosis
A. Eczema/dermatitis
1. Atopic dermatitis
2. Contact dermatitis
3. Stasis dermatitis
4. Seborrheic dermatitis
B. Psoriasis
C. Pityriasis rubra pilaris
D. Ichthyosis
E. Pemphigus foliaceus
II. Drug reaction
III. Malignancy
A. Cutaneous T-cell lymphoma
B. Other lymphomas and leukemias
C. Other malignancy
D. Acquired immunodeficiency syndrome (AIDS)
IV. Idiopathic

as a result of the large arteriovenous shunting that occurs in the inflamed skin.

HISTOPATHOLOGIC FINDINGS

The histopathologic appearance of the skin in erythroderma is usually nonspecific. If the process is subacute, the stratum corneum often shows parakeratosis (retention of nuclei in corneocytes), and the epidermis shows eczema-like spongiosis. Mononuclear cells migrate into the epidermis (exocytosis). A psoriasis-like thickening of the entire epidermis is seen. Dermal changes include edema, vasodilation, and a primarily mononuclear cell infiltrate. Eosinophils also may be seen. Occasionally, diagnostic changes can be found. In patients with Sézary syndrome, the mononuclear cells may have primarily atypical-appearing cerebriform nuclei (Sézary cells). In pemphigus foliaceus, acantholysis is seen in the upper epidermis. In extensive scabies, biopsy often reveals the infectious cause.

The lymph node changes seen in the lymphadenopathy of erythroderma are called dermatopathic lymphadenopathy. The lymph node architecture is well preserved. Lymph follicles are enlarged, with large germinal centers. The paracortical areas are dramatically enlarged. Even in patients with cutaneous T-cell lymphoma (Sézary syndrome or mycosis fungoides), a biopsy of the lymph nodes early in the course of the disease may show only dermatopathic lymphadenopathy.

EVALUATION

An overview of the evaluation of the patient with erythroderma is provided in Table 10–2. In all patients, a thorough cutaneous examination must be undertaken. Technically, erythroderma is defined as involving 100% of the cutaneous surface, although management of the patient with 90% body surface area erythema is similar to that for erythroderma. In such patients, residual areas diagnostic of an underlying dermatosis (e.g., psoriasis, or a form of eczema) might be identifiable at the interface between normal and abnormal skin. Pityriasis rubra pilaris, with areas of erythema and 'islands of sparing,' may be considered more highly in the differential diagnosis in these situations. A positive Nikolsky sign (the creation of a superficial blister by rubbing the skin) may be obtained in a few patients with erythroderma who have pemphigus foliaceus. Infiltrated plaques that suggest cutaneous T-cell lymphoma may be identified. It is particularly important to repeat the cutaneous examination frequently during treatment, because clues to a visible underlying cutaneous condition may be unmasked with clinical improvement.

The patient should be assessed thoroughly for significant lymphadenopathy. Unless the diagnosis is absolutely clear (e.g., in a patient with longstanding atopic dermatitis that has gradually evolved into erythroderma, or in a patient with longstanding psoriasis that shows a similar evolution), a lymph node biopsy to search for lymphoma should be considered.

The patient with erythroderma also warrants a careful complete history and physical examination and, sometimes, monitoring in hospital. These patients lose their capacity

(e.g., psoriasis) and malignant diseases (e.g., cutaneous T-cell lymphoma). The factors within each disease that trigger the entire cutaneous surface to become inflamed and to develop a nonspecific 'chronic cutaneous failure' pattern clinicopathologically remain speculative.

CLINICAL MANIFESTATIONS

The entire cutaneous surface is generally hot, red, scaly, and indurated. The qualities that separate eczematous eruptions (vesiculation and the distribution of the lesions) from psoriasis (well-marginated plaques with silvery scales) are largely lost. However, one should search for features of an underlying dermatosis, such as waxy palmar keratoderma in pityriasis rubra pilaris. Peripheral edema may be marked. The patient is usually shivering, owing to the loss of heat associated with the massive diversion of blood flow through the skin.

Pruritus leads to scratching, which often produces the secondary changes of excoriation, crusting, and lichenification (accentuation of skin markings as a result of rubbing). A diffuse, nonscarring alopecia may be present. Longstanding erythroderma is associated with the ridging and pitting of nails seen in proximal (i.e., nail matrix-related) nail dystrophies. The post-inflammatory hyperpigmentation may be generalized.

Almost all patients with erythroderma have associated generalized lymphadenopathy. Although lymphoma must be ruled out, the lymph node swelling is usually reactive, or dermatopathic. Hepatosplenomegaly may also be seen, and is not necessarily a sign of a poor prognosis. Signs of high-output cardiac failure must be sought in these patients, who are at risk

Table 10–2 Evaluation of the patient with erythroderma

I. History
Particular attention should be paid to history of pre-existing dermatoses; family history of skin disease; medication history; history of possible contactants, including work and hobby exposure; and a review of systems for clues to a possible occult malignancy and for symptoms of high-output cardiac failure, anemia, and hypothermia.

II. Physical examination
Particular attention should be paid to possible areas of normal skin (does the border suggest a possible underlying disease?), lymphadenopathy, signs of anemia or high-output cardiac failure, signs of underlying disease during resolution of the erythroderma (e.g., plaques of cutaneous T-cell lymphoma or of psoriasis), and signs of underlying malignancy.

III. Skin biopsy
Attention should be paid to nonspecific changes of erythroderma or specific findings of cutaneous T-cell lymphoma or pemphigus foliaceus.

IV. Lymph node biopsy (if indicated)
Dermatopathic findings and to exclude malignancy.

V. Laboratory studies
General tests are done, such as a complete blood count (e.g, eosinophilia, which possibly is more suggestive of a drug cause or anemia secondary to malabsorption of iron or a malignancy), erythrocyte sedimentation rate, serum chemistry screen, chest X-ray, stool guaiac test, urinalysis, electrocardiogram (may show a pattern of high-output failure or changes of volume overload), and Sézary cell preparation (false-positive test possible).

for thermoregulation. They lose heat to the environment and usually shiver. A fever can be masked in this setting. To maintain a normal body temperature, these patients experience an increase in metabolism that may result in progressive debilitation.

Patients with erythroderma have increased cutaneous blood flow, raised venous pressure with hypervolemia (but intravascular volume depletion and increased third-space fluid), and increased cardiac output. Although patients with a normal cardiac reserve may not be affected, those with cardiac disease and elderly patients may suffer serious, even fatal, effects.

Individuals with chronic erythroderma are often anemic. Although hemodilution may be a factor acutely, the anemia may be associated with iron and/or folate deficiency. Iron and folate may be lost from the rapidly dividing epidermal cells as a result of scaling, although malabsorption is the currently accepted hypothesis.

Patients with erythroderma experience increased thirst and oliguria acutely. These changes are attributed to water retention in the form of edema and to increases in water loss through the skin (intravascular volume depletion with increased third-space fluid).

Patients with erythroderma have been shown to have an associated protein-losing enteropathy with steatorrhea that responds to treatment of the skin alone. They also have a low serum albumin level. Although this may be in part dilutional, protein loss in the bowel and scaling probably play a significant role. Hepatic synthesis of albumin may be normal to increased.

The companion to a meticulous complete physical examination is a careful and complete history. The clinician should focus on the personal and family history that is suggestive of underlying dermatoses, elicit a complete medication history, and provide a list of exposures that might cause contact dermatitis. A review of systems oriented toward detecting clues of possible underlying malignancy is also crucial.

Patients over age 50 or those with a history suggesting a possible underlying malignancy should be investigated for occult carcinoma, and particularly for lymphoma. This evaluation should be guided by the findings from the history, physical examination, and screening laboratory tests. A chest X-ray should be performed. A test to determine the presence of blood in the stool should be performed. A lymph node biopsy to exclude lymphoma can be performed unless the cause of the erythroderma is known. A cutaneous biopsy, albeit usually nonspecific, must be performed to look for diagnostic features of cutaneous T-cell lymphoma, psoriasis, or, more rarely, pemphigus foliaceus. Immunohistochemical techniques may provide an efficient means of ruling out neoplastic erythroderma, as many 'idiopathic' erythrodermas are later diagnosed as lymphoma.

Routine laboratory abnormalities are not specific for erythroderma. Patients with Sézary syndrome may have a high percentage of Sézary cells in their circulation. Caution must be exercised, because patients with erythroderma not associated with a lymphoproliferative disorder may have in their circulation activated T cells, which are often difficult to distinguish from Sézary cells. Gene-rearrangement analysis may be useful in selected patients. Laboratory monitoring of anemia and albumin and electrolyte levels is part of following the patient's systemic response to the cutaneous disease.

COURSE AND TREATMENT

Erythroderma should be considered a serious condition that may require short-term management in hospital. Occasionally, it may be fatal. The drug-induced form of erythroderma usually resolves completely within several weeks after discontinuation of the offending medication. Erythroderma induced by allergic contact dermatitis also has an excellent prognosis if the offending antigen is identified and eliminated. Patch testing, however, cannot be performed during the acute stage of the illness.

Erythroderma associated with psoriasis or atopic dermatitis may convert from erythroderma to simple extensive involvement with those diseases, facilitating clinical diagnosis. Erythroderma associated with occult malignancy often responds to treatment of the malignancy; however, the prognosis is related to that of the malignancy. In general, patients with a malignancy and erythroderma do poorly. Finally, patients with idiopathic erythroderma often seem to experience a chronic course.

Deaths in patients with erythroderma may be the result of a malignancy, cardiovascular compromise, and infection (e.g., septicemia or pneumonitis), or as a complication of therapy. Underlying systemic diseases, such as malignancy, must be diagnosed and treated appropriately.

Acute supportive care in hospital requires careful attention to hydration, serum protein levels, electrolyte balance, circulatory status, and temperature regulation. The patient's room should be kept comfortably warm.

Topical corticosteroid therapy should be a mainstay of treatment. Intermediate-strength corticosteroids should be applied frequently to a clean, dry cutaneous surface. Wet-wrap occlusion may be used. Stubborn cases of erythroderma may benefit from combined tar ointment and ultraviolet light treatments, similar to the Goeckerman regimen used to treat psoriasis.

Whirlpool or hydrosound treatments once daily are invaluable in debriding excess scale and reducing the bacterial colonization on the inflamed cutaneous surface. Wet compresses can also be used for this purpose. Occlusive plastic (i.e., 'sauna') suits favored by some physicians can cause problems because their mechanism of enhancing topical corticosteroid penetration into the skin is hydration from sweating. Perspiration can be irritating to inflamed skin, and the suit may promote bacterial overgrowth.

Systemic antibiotics are required for patients with true cutaneous or systemic infection, and sometimes these are administered to patients with heavy cutaneous bacterial colonization with *Staphylococcus aureus*. Systemic corticosteroid therapy often is initiated to treat erythroderma; however, several words of caution are required. Short-term tapering courses of prednisone or other systemic corticosteroids may be associated with severe rebound flares of the disease after tapering. Patients with psoriatic erythroderma should not be given systemic corticosteroid therapy because of the risk of rebound with severe pustular psoriasis on tapering. Patients with idiopathic erythroderma may have a prolonged course leading to unacceptable side effects if high-dose systemic corticosteroid therapy is continued long term. Ultraviolet light therapy (narrowband UVB or PUVA) and systemic therapy with methotrexate, mycophenolate, azathioprine, and, for limited periods, cyclosporine are indicated for many patients. Anti-TNF-α and other biologic agents are also often helpful.

SUGGESTED READINGS

Callen JP, Bernardi DM, Clark RA, Weber DA. Adult-onset recalcitrant eczema: a marker of noncutaneous lymphoma or leukemia. J Am Acad Dermatol 2000; 43: 207–210.

Fierro MT, Novelli M, Quaglino P, et al. Heterogeneity of circulating CD4+ memory T-cell subsets in erythrodermic patients: CD27 analysis can help to distinguish cutaneous T-cell lymphomas from inflammatory erythroderma. Dermatology 2008; 216: 213–221.

Kanthraj GR, Srinivas CR, Devi PN, et al. Quantitative estimation and recommendation for supplementation of protein loss through scaling in exfoliative dermatitis. Int J Dermatol 1999; 38: 91–95.

Levine N. Exfoliative erythroderma: skin biopsy is required to determine the cause of this pruritic eruption. Geriatrics 2000; 55: 25.

Morar N, Dlova N, Gupta AK, et al. Erythroderma: a comparison between HIV positive and negative patients. Int J Dermatol 1999; 38: 895–900.

Pruszkowski A, Bodemer C, Fraitag S, et al. Neonatal and infantile erythrodermas: a retrospective study of 51 patients. Arch Dermatol 2000; 136: 875–880.

Rothe MJ, Bialy TL, Grant-Kels JM. Erythroderma. Dermatol Clin 2000; 18: 405–415.

Seghal V, Srivastave G, Sardana K. Erythroderma/exfoliative dermatitis: a synopsis. Int J Dermatol 2004; 43: 39–47.

Purpura

The clinical finding of purpura is associated not only with some of the most rapidly life-threatening illnesses known, but also with some of the most common and benign conditions of daily life. Although the evaluation of a patient with purpura can occasionally be complicated, in many cases a good history and physical examination in conjunction with some simple tests may be all that is required.

Purpura is a generic term for visible hemorrhage in the skin and mucous membranes. More specific terms describe particular types of purpura, and subtyping purpura is essential for an efficient diagnosis. The term petechia generally implies an area of hemorrhage 4 mm or less in diameter (Fig. 11–1). If the condition is severe, petechiae may become confluent in areas, forming ecchymoses, but the predominant and the newest lesions will be petechial. An ecchymosis is a deep reddish-blue, purplish, or blue-black macule, usually at least 1–1.5 cm in its greatest dimension. As used in this chapter, the terms petechiae and ecchymoses are also restricted to lesions which never have a blanchable component, implying a noninflammatory etiology of simple hemorrhage for such lesions. A contusion is a major trauma-induced lesion that may be purpuric, and frequently has trauma-related soft-tissue swelling and tenderness. The traditional term palpable purpura is best applied to a lesion which is partially but not completely blanchable, implying a component of early inflammation, and is often palpable. Retiform purpura is a term which describes hemorrhage which may be inflammatory or noninflammatory, but is characterized by a distinctive shape, with branching or reticulate patterning of the whole lesion or of its edges. Noninflammatory retiform purpura most characteristically is due to microvascular occlusive disease in the skin.

PATHOGENESIS

Cutaneous hemorrhage may result from intravascular, vascular, and extravascular causes, and many differential diagnoses use this approach. It may be more helpful to approach the bedside diagnosis of purpura from a morphological perspective, using the distinctive morphology of purpura to decide between three possible broad pathogenic mechanisms: simple hemorrhage, inflammatory hemorrhage (vessel-directed inflammation), or occlusive hemorrhage with minimal inflammation. This differential applies to lesions of purpura which are primary, meaning that the mechanism of the lesion is also the sole cause of the hemorrhage. Clinical judgment is needed to distinguish purpura which is secondary, for example secondary to scratching, and into an area of inflammation such as cellulitis or stasis dermatitis.

Simple Hemorrhage

Simple hemorrhage can be divided into two differentials, petechial and ecchymotic.

Petechial Simple Hemorrhage

Thrombocytopenia or platelet dysfunction

Platelet counts above 50 000/mm^3 are usually not accompanied by purpura unless an abnormality of platelet function exists or there is a separate injury. Therefore, thrombocytopenia that might result in hemorrhage occurs at platelet counts of 50 000/mm^3 or less, and typically is not seen until the platelet count is 10 000/mm^3 or below. A variety of disorders can at times produce this degree of thrombocytopenia (Table 11–1). Although severe thrombocytopenia may result in ecchymotic hemorrhage, usually the predominant morphology in any given patient is petechial. Conversely, platelet function defects may result in petechial hemorrhage and must be considered in this differential, but seem more often to lead to scattered minor trauma-related ecchymoses. Although thrombocytopenic hemorrhage may occur anywhere, typically it is increased in dependent areas or at sites of minor trauma.

Intravascular pressure spikes

Petechial hemorrhage may also result from strong or repetitive localized increases in intravascular pressure. For example, straining during childbirth may produce petechial hemorrhage above the clavicles, solely from the vigorous Valsalva-like pressure effects. This can also occur with vigorous repetitive coughing or retching. In children, vigorous crying may produce a similar supraclavicular distribution of petechial hemorrhage. Ligature placement or strangulation may also produce distinctive patterns of petechial hemorrhage.

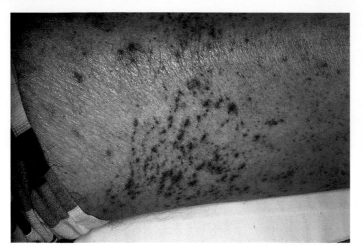

Figure 11–1 Small petechiae in an individual with thrombocytopenia.

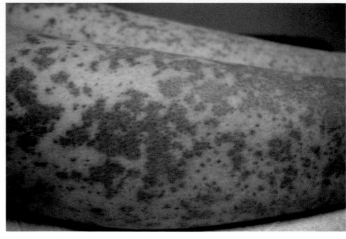

Figure 11–2 Typical lesions of palpable purpura in a patient with cutaneous small-vessel vasculitis.

Minimally inflammatory microvascular syndromes

There are a variety of minimally inflammatory syndromes affecting the very smallest dermal vessels which may result in petechial hemorrhage, most included within the syndromes of chronic pigmented purpuras. The most likely to mimic simple petechial hemorrhage is Schamberg's purpura, which typically affects elderly men. This disease typically localizes to the legs, and produces multiple noninflammatory petechiae. These are often clustered in groups, and may over time leave a 'cayenne pepper' background pigmentation, leading to easy diagnosis. However, early in the course of disease, if the lesions are not clustered, they may mimic the dependent distribution of thrombocytopenic hemorrhage. The syndrome of Waldenström's benign hypergammaglobulinemic purpura may also produce dependently distributed petechial hemorrhage, which clinically and often histologically is noninflammatory. However, platelet numbers and function are normal, and hemorrhage typically occurs episodically in this syndrome, most often accompanied by burning at the site of new lesions.

Platelet function is also important. Intravascular hemorrhage associated with normal platelet counts may result from congenital or hereditary platelet function defects. More commonly encountered are acquired platelet function defects, especially those caused by drugs or metabolic abnormalities, such as severe renal or hepatic impairment. Another type of acquired platelet function defect occurs in patients with monoclonal gammopathies in which there may be interference with normal platelet function by the protein. Finally, patients with myeloproliferative disease and thrombocytosis in the range of $1\,000\,000/mm^3$ will often have platelet dysfunction, and such patients may have problems with both hemorrhage and thrombosis.

Coagulation cascade problems in hemostasis

The ability to form a normal platelet plug is the most important factor for normal hemostasis in the small vessels that supply the skin. The coagulation cascade system becomes important as the diameter of the vessel increases, and increasing forces of pressure and flow require reinforcement of the platelet plug by fibrin clots. This explains why patients with hemophilia or other procoagulant deficiencies of the coagulation cascade system usually do not present with spontaneous petechial hemorrhage. Instead, they present with relatively minor trauma-related injury of larger vessels in skin, fat, joint, or muscle, with the development of an overlying ecchymosis.

Other intravascular causes of hemorrhage

Petechiae may develop in nondependent areas as a result of abrupt increases in capillary and postcapillary venule pressure. Forceful and repetitive Valsalva-like maneuvers, such as paroxysmal vomiting, violent coughing, or straining during childbirth, can cause petechial hemorrhage in supraclavicular areas even in patients whose platelet number and function are normal.

The Gardner–Diamond syndrome, or psychogenic purpura, is sometimes included in discussions of intravascular causes of hemorrhage. Whether this syndrome results from more than factitious disease remains controversial.

Vascular Causes

Vascular causes of hemorrhage include both inflammatory and noninflammatory disorders.

Inflammatory causes

Inflammatory hemorrhage should include only those disorders in which vessel-directed inflammation is evident. Perivascular inflammation that is not vessel directed should not be considered vasculitis, and it does not result in palpable purpura, the hallmark lesion of inflammatory hemorrhage. Lesions of palpable purpura are characterized by a port-wine color, incomplete blanching on pressure or diascopy, and palpability (Fig. 11–2). Such lesions, when due to immune complex deposition, usually develop first in dependent areas, which in a bedridden patient may be the back and buttocks. An important cause of palpable purpura is small-vessel leukocytoclastic vasculitis, which has a variety of causes, including idiopathic,

Table 11–1 Partial differential diagnosis for purpura

I. Petechial (nonpalpable)
  A. Hemostatically relevant thrombocytopenia (platelet count <50 000/mm^3, usually <10 000/mm^3)
    1. Idiopathic thrombocytopenic purpura
    2. Thrombotic thrombocytopenic purpura (some cases)
    3. Disseminated intravascular coagulation
    4. Drug-related thrombocytopenia
      a. Peripheral destruction: quinidine, quinine
      b. Marrow: idiosyncratic or dose related
    5. Marrow infiltration, fibrosis, or failure
  B. Abnormal platelet function
    1. Congenital or hereditary platelet function defects
    2. Acquired platelet function defects (e.g., aspirin, renal or hepatic insufficiency, monoclonal gammopathy)
    3. Thrombocytosis in myeloproliferative disease (>1 000 000/mm^3)
  C. Elevated intravascular pressure (Valsalva maneuver-like causes)
  D. Chronic pigmented purpura (occasionally palpable, caused by minimal small-vessel inflammation)

II. Ecchymotic
  A. Procoagulant defect (often localized to sites of minor trauma)
    1. Hemophilia
    2. Anticoagulants
    3. Disseminated intravascular coagulation
    4. Vitamin K deficiency
    5. Hepatic insufficiency with poor procoagulant synthesis
  B. Poor dermal support of vessels (usually localized to sites of minor trauma)
    1. Actinic (senile) purpura
    2. Corticosteroid therapy, topical or systemic
    3. Scurvy
    4. Systemic amyloidosis (light chain related)
    5. Ehlers–Danlos syndrome, primarily types I, IV, VI, VIII, and X
    6. Pseudoxanthoma elasticum
  C. Abnormal platelet function (see above)
  D. Other
    1. Benign hypergammaglobulinemic purpura of Waldenström (as a result of mild vessel inflammation, usually causes macular hemorrhage, but can produce palpable purpura)

III. Palpable purpura
  A. Classic palpable purpura
    1. Small-vessel leukocytoclastic vasculitis syndromes
      a. Post-infectious, drug-induced, or idiopathic IgG, IgM immune complex vasculitis
      b. Post-infectious, drug-induced, or idiopathic IgA-predominant vasculitis (Henoch–Schönlein purpura)
      c. Mixed cryoglobulinemia
      d. Associated with lupus, rheumatoid arthritis, Sjögren's syndrome
      e. Small-vessel lesions of Wegener's, Churg–Strauss, or lymphomatoid granulomatosis
    2. Pityriasis lichenoides et varioliformis acuta (PLEVA) syndrome
    3. Erythema multiforme (some variants)
  B. Target lesions
    1. Erythema multiforme
  C. Inflammatory retiform purpura (usually vasculitic, both retiform morphology and prominent early erythema)
    1. IgA-predominant small-vessel leukocytoclastic vasculitis (some)
    2. Syndromes of small- and medium-vessel leukocytoclastic vasculitis, such as rheumatic vasculitis, polyarteritis, and Wegener's granulomatosis (occasionally)
    3. Some early lesions of warfarin- or heparin-induced necrosis demonstrate erythema, but this tends to be at the margin of large, confluent areas of necrosis

IV. Noninflammatory retiform purpura (occlusion syndromes, usually retiform morphology without early erythema)
  A. Disorders of platelet plugging: myeloproliferative thrombocytosis, heparin necrosis, rarely thrombotic thrombocytopenic purpura, paroxysmal nocturnal hemoglobinuria
  B. Disorders of cold-related cryogelling or agglutination
  C. Disorders of vessel invasive organisms: ecthyma gangrenosum, aspergillus and other opportunistic fungi, disseminated strongyloidiasis
  D. Disorders of local or systemic control of coagulation: inherited or acquired severe protein C or S deficiency (acquired includes some sepsis/disseminated intravascular coagulation, coumadin necrosis, some antiphospholipid antibody syndromes), some atrophie blanche
  E. Disorders of embolization: cholesterol or oxalate emboli, atrial myxoma, crystalglobulins
  F. Miscellaneous disorders: cutaneous calciphylaxis, Degos' disease, sickle cell ulcerations

post-infectious, and drug-related; Henoch–Schönlein purpura; mixed cryoglobulinemia; connective tissue disease, such as systemic lupus erythematosus and rheumatoid arthritis; and Wegener's granulomatosis or the allergic granulomatosis of Churg–Strauss syndrome, with or without granulomatous changes. However, the physical findings of palpable purpura may occasionally result from disorders in which vessel-directed inflammation is caused by a predominantly mononuclear cell infiltrate, as in urticarial vasculitis, Sjögren's syndrome-related vasculitis, hypocomplementemic vasculitis, erythema multiforme, and the pityriasis lichenoides group (especially PLEVA [pityriasis lichenoides et varioliformis acuta] syndrome).

The finding of palpable purpura indicates only inflammatory hemorrhage, and a biopsy of an early lesion (less than 24–48 hours old) is necessary to demonstrate the composition of the initial inflammatory infiltrate and the presence of relevant immune complexes. This has important clinical implications because a patient with cutaneous small-vessel vasculitis may have associated visceral or renal involvement, whereas a patient with palpable purpura as a result of erythema multiforme is instead at risk for the development of mucosal injury, which can be severe.

Mild inflammatory conditions that may result in purpura, and occasionally in palpable purpura, include the syndromes of chronic pigmented purpura and benign hypergammaglobulinemic purpura of Waldenström. Chronic pigmented purpura includes several subsets, but patients with this problem usually have areas of recurring hemorrhage, often petechial, with surrounding erythema and brown hyperpigmentation as a result of hemosiderin deposition in the dermis (Fig. 11–3). Because petechial hemorrhage is common in this syndrome, often the patient or the physician is concerned that there is a serious underlying disorder, such as leukemia. However, chronic pigmented purpura is not associated with internal disease.

Waldenström's hypergammaglobulinemic purpura is usually characterized by macular hemorrhage in either dependent areas or areas covered by restrictive clothing. This condition may be idiopathic or may occur in association with Sjögren's syndrome, sarcoidosis, or other diseases having a polyclonal gammopathy. These lesions may be associated with a burning sensation and may show little or no inflammation on biopsy. This disorder is best characterized by the presence of an IgG (not IgM) rheumatoid factor, which is demonstrable using analytic ultracentrifugation of serum or plasma. Unfortunately, because this technology is no longer widely used, only those cases with a typical clinical picture and a polyclonal hypergammaglobulinemia will tend to be included in this diagnosis.

Noninflammatory causes

Bland occlusion syndromes typically present as noninflammatory (and usually retiform) palpable purpura. In these syndromes, fibrin clot, cryoglobulin gel, or other material occludes multiple vessels, and this initial occlusion is followed by propagation of a thrombus within the retiform (livedoid) network of superficial dermal venules (Figs 11–4 and 11–5). The list of causes is extensive; these are categorized in Table 11–1. It is important to recognize this subset of purpura as distinct from inflammatory hemorrhage because, although the therapy differs according to the syndrome, all are treated differently from the syndromes of inflammatory hemorrhage.

Occasionally, lesions of inflammatory retiform purpura will occur. Usually, these result from vasculitides that affect both medium-sized and small vessels, such as Wegener's granulomatosis, lupus or rheumatoid vasculitis, and some types of polyarteritis nodosa. However, when such a clinical picture is caused by small-vessel involvement alone, it strongly suggests an IgA-predominant leukocytoclastic vasculitis. Many such patients have multisystem disease, and prolonged or recurrent courses and ulcerations may be more likely in adults. In this setting, the early lesions tend to be classic palpable purpura, with a strong tendency towards the linking of lesions in a livedoid pattern, creating some confluent areas of epidermal or dermal necrosis.

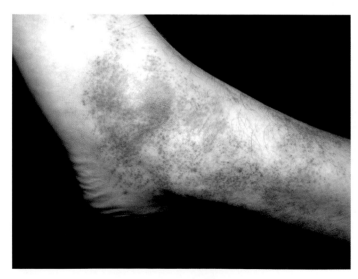

Figure 11–3 Clustered petechial hemorrhage with background hyperpigmentation typical of chronic pigmented purpura.

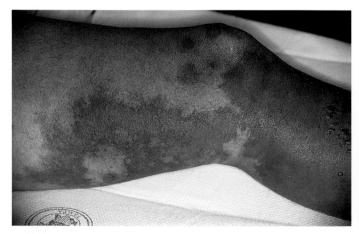

Figure 11–4 Noninflammatory retiform purpura in a patient with disseminated intravascular coagulation, Gram-negative sepsis, and diffuse small-dermal-vessel thrombosis and perivascular hemorrhage. These lesions demonstrate little or no erythema (blanching component). (Courtesy of Dr Neil A. Fenske, Tampa, FL.)

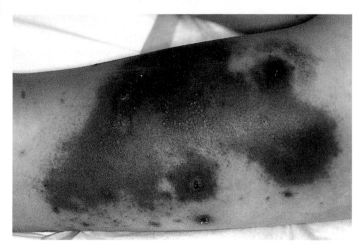

Figure 11–5 Purpura fulminans following a varicella infection. Note the retiform extensions at the margins of palpable purpura. Little or no erythema is present.

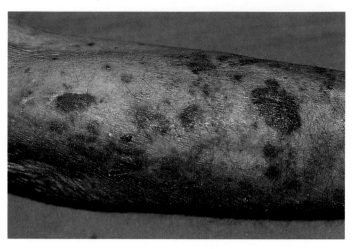

Figure 11–6 Ecchymosis as a result of corticosteroid application. Also, note the cutaneous atrophy produced by topical steroids. (Courtesy of Dr Neil A. Fenske, Tampa, FL.)

Noninflammatory vascular hemorrhage can occasionally occur as a result of defects in the vascular wall, but such hemorrhage is typically ecchymotic and nonpalpable. The purpura resulting from vessel infiltration in light chain-related systemic amyloidosis is a good example. Because the collagen and elastin content of very small blood vessels is minimal, cutaneous hemorrhage in association with the Ehlers–Danlos syndrome or pseudoxanthoma elasticum is usually not the result of a vessel wall abnormality, but rather of poor vessel wall support by the surrounding connective tissue. The Kasabach–Merritt syndrome, usually seen in infants, occurs when the abnormal vasculature of a giant cutaneous or visceral hemangioma induces platelet consumption and thrombosis; a clinical picture mimicking disseminated intravascular coagulation may result.

Extravascular Causes

Extravascular causes of hemorrhage may include either major trauma or minor trauma to the skin. Major trauma results in hemorrhage even in normal skin, is associated with remembered injury, significant tissue swelling, tenderness, or obvious abrasions, and is seldom a diagnostic problem. Purpura related to minor trauma may occur in the absence of obvious tissue swelling and often without the patient's recollection of trauma. Such hemorrhage is usually the result of poor support of the small blood vessels by surrounding abnormal connective tissue. The areas of skin most likely to be traumatized include the extensor surface of the forearms, the anterior lower legs, and the dorsum of the hands. Purpura that is caused in part by external trauma tends to be distributed in a geometric pattern, e.g., linearly on the forearm in a scraping injury, or linearly across a periarticular flexural crease. Perhaps the most common type of minor trauma-related purpura is actinic purpura. Most senile purpura should in reality be classified as actinic or solar, because it occurs only in chronically sunexposed areas with actinic degeneration of the connective tissue. Corticosteroid excess (endogenous or iatrogenic) is another common cause of poor connective tissue support (Fig. 11–6).

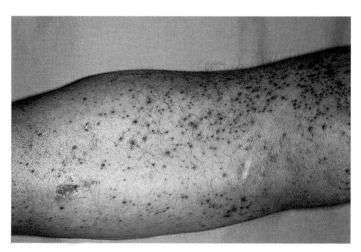

Figure 11–7 Perifollicular purpura in a patient with vitamin C deficiency. (Courtesy of Dr Kenneth E. Greer, Charlottesville, VA.)

The presence of perifollicular hemorrhage should suggest the diagnosis of scurvy and requires a nutrition-directed history to exclude scurvy as a cause (Fig. 11–7). The reason for the initial perifollicular localization of vitamin C deficiency is not known. The hemorrhage is probably caused by a collagen defect, because ascorbic acid is a necessary factor for the formation of normal collagen. Light chain-related systemic amyloidosis is a rare but important cause of dramatic minor trauma-related hemorrhage, owing to infiltration of vessel walls and replacement of normal connective tissue by infiltration. Waxy-appearing papules and plaques, or purpura easily induced by light stroking or pinching of the skin, strongly suggest the diagnosis of light chain-related systemic amyloidosis. Cutaneous hemorrhage as a result of Ehlers–Danlos syndrome and pseudoxanthoma elasticum is usually caused by the poor tissue support the vessels receive in involved areas.

The autoerythrocyte sensitization (Gardner–Diamond) syndrome is most likely factitious in its pathogenesis. The disorder occurs primarily in young women who often have significant emotional problems, and is manifested by the rapid

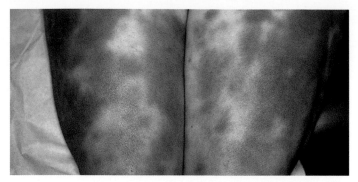

Figure 11–8 Multiple bruises in a patient with Gardner–Diamond syndrome.

development of unexplained noninflammatory purpura (Fig. 11–8). Laboratory studies of immune function and coagulation are within normal limits. It is said that the injection of autologous erythrocytes will reproduce the lesions. Manipulation of injection sites by the patient has been demonstrated in some individuals with this diagnosis. These patients are extremely difficult to treat.

CLINICAL MANIFESTATIONS

Purpuric Lesion

The first task in unraveling the cause of purpura is to prove that the lesion is purpuric. The color of the lesion should be the result of hemoglobin, i.e., bright red for fully oxygenated; reddish-blue, blue-black, or purple for less-saturated hemoglobin; and blue-black to black for hemorrhage associated with hemorrhagic tissue necrosis. The brown pigmentation of hemosiderin (resulting from the breakdown of hemoglobin) can be impossible to distinguish from melanin pigment, and it is therefore less reliable in establishing past hemorrhage.

Diascopy

Next, at least some of this color must be proved to reside extravascularly. This is done by diascopy, applying direct pressure to a lesion. This is generally done best by using the thicker glass of a pocket hand lens rather than the currently available fragile glass slides. This direct pressure compresses the dermal vessels in the area, and any blood within the vessels should flow away from the area. Blood in the dermis or clotted within the vessels cannot move. A critical assessment is whether a color appropriate for hemorrhage remains within the area being compressed.

Three types of lesion can yield misleading information on diascopy. A tangled mat of small vessels may develop kinks or occluded sections while compressed, thereby trapping blood within vessel segments. A lesion may be too firm, or may develop over soft areas of the skin and simply be pushed into the skin without sufficient compression. For example, cherry (senile) angiomas may be firm, or if they overlie a prominent panniculus (such as on the abdomen) they may be impossible to compress. Finally, any cutaneous eruption may become

hemorrhagic when sufficiently traumatized or if it develops in an area of high hydrostatic pressure, e.g., a pruritic area traumatized by scratching, or an active dermatitis occurring near the ankle in an ambulatory patient. By contrast, the presence of symmetrical hemorrhage, especially in dependent areas, or hemorrhage in lesions that the patient cannot easily scratch, and the absence of excoriations suggests that the hemorrhage is primary rather than secondary.

Inflammation

Having established a lesion as primary purpura, the next task to assess is the degree of inflammation. At the bedside, this is determined by gauging the percentage of color that is blanchable, which represents erythema and correlates with the degree of inflammation, and by noting the residual color that does not blanch and hence represents hemorrhage. Nonpalpable petechiae and simple ecchymoses typically show little or no color change on diascopy, and these represent lesions of simple hemorrhage. Many lesions of palpable purpura contain elements of both inflammation (erythema) and hemorrhage (purpura), depending on the pathogenesis of the vessel injury and the age of the lesion. Typical lesions of small-vessel leukocytoclastic vasculitis most commonly present as port-wine papules 5–10 mm in diameter (classic palpable purpura), but a subset of vasculitides may present as inflammatory retiform purpura. When due to immune complex deposition, these lesions are concentrated in dependent areas (areas of the highest hydrostatic pressure), whereas clinically identical lesions associated with antineutrophil cytoplasmic antibody (ANCA)-positive syndromes (e.g., Wegener's, microscopic polyarteritis) are much more like to occur in a random pattern of distribution. Such vasculitic lesions initially have a prominent component of erythema, which becomes less intense and finally disappears as the individual lesion evolves, leaving hemorrhage, vesicles, or ulceration in its place.

Other forms of inflammatory hemorrhage exist. For example, the lesion most characteristic of erythema multiforme is a target lesion consisting of a central region of intense inflammation with epidermal necrosis or vesicle formation, often associated with an element of purpura. This central area is surrounded by an area of flesh-colored to slightly pale skin, representing relative ischemia, and then by a zone of erythema, thought to represent reactive hyperemia. Erythema multiforme is often idiopathic; the known causes are most frequently medications (including 'health foods,' vitamins, and other nonprescription items) and herpes simplex infections, especially in recurrent cases.

Bland Occlusion

A third variant of palpable purpura is that which begins as a simple occlusion or thrombosis, usually of multiple dermal vessels, in the absence of significant early inflammation. Such lesions are often palpable but not erythematous, and tend to develop in a livedoid or retiform pattern. Hemorrhage occurs in a perivascular distribution during the early ischemic phase of a lesion as endothelial junctions break down. Inflammation is usually absent initially, but may ultimately develop as a response to ischemic necrosis. Such bland occlusion occurs in a variety of clinical settings, including some types of disseminated intravascular coagulation, or with monoclonal cryoglobulinemia.

HISTORY AND PHYSICAL FINDINGS

Because purpura has many different causes, the associated history and physical findings vary greatly. For instance, arthralgias, arthritis, fever, and visceral lesions may accompany cutaneous small-vessel vasculitis. Monoclonal cryoglobulinemia results from benign or malignant lymphoproliferative disease, which may have other manifestations. Hepatitis C infection is now recognized as the most common cause of what was formerly termed essential cryoglobulinemia. Syndromes of disseminated intravascular coagulation usually occur in association with sepsis, malignancy, or other serious underlying disorders. Although many clinicians now seem to use the term purpura fulminans to imply extensive purpuric lesions of any type, the term was originally coined to describe the findings in patients whose dermatologic lesions resulted from extensive noninflammatory thrombosis, presenting clinically as noninflammatory retiform purpura.

HISTOPATHOLOGIC FINDINGS

Both petechiae and ecchymoses show simple extravasation of red blood cells into the dermis on biopsy, the difference being the total volume of extravasation. Patients with inflammatory hemorrhage may show leukocytoclastic vasculitis, characterized by the presence of at least some neutrophils in and around vessel walls, the presence of perivascular nuclear dust (representing degenerated neutrophil nuclei), and fibrinoid necrosis of the vessel wall. This is the histologic correlate of most forms of necrotizing vasculitis. Other types of inflammatory hemorrhage, such as erythema multiforme, may have relatively few neutrophils in an infiltrate composed largely of mononuclear cells. Syndromes of bland occlusion or thrombus typically include multiple dermal vessels occluded by pink to hyaline material with intermingled red cells, perivascular extravasation of red cells, and often little to no inflammation in early lesions.

Understanding the differences in lesional evolution between these processes is essential in the correct interpretation of clinical and biopsy findings. The earliest lesions of leukocytoclastic vasculitis might have much more erythema than hemorrhage, with early signs of neutrophil-rich inflammation, and significant remaining components of the immune complexes that triggered the lesion. A later stage of the lesion might have comparable degrees of purpura and erythema, a full-blown fibrinoid necrosis on biopsy, but total destruction or removal of the inciting immune complexes in the vessel wall. A resolving lesion would have little or no erythema and a nonspecific inflammatory infiltrate.

By contrast, bland occlusion syndromes typically begin with little inflammation, prominent hemorrhage, and propagation of a clot within vessels; significant necrosis may develop later, followed by a wound-healing response of nonspecific inflammation. Ulcers from any cause may have features of secondary leukocytoclastic vasculitis at their margins. Choosing an appropriate lesion to biopsy is essential for a proper diagnosis. Fundamental to this appropriate selection is recognizing the distinct clinical evolution of lesions that result from different pathogenic processes.

DIFFERENTIAL DIAGNOSIS

The differential diagnosis of purpura is extensive, sometimes confusing, and usually challenging. Table 11–1 lists a partial differential diagnosis that uses morphologic features to separate groups by their likely pathogenesis.

EVALUATION

The history provides much useful information in the assessment of purpuric syndromes, e.g., a family history of a bleeding or thrombotic disorder, the use of drugs that might affect platelet function or coagulation, the presence of underlying metabolic disease that might affect clotting parameters, or a constellation of symptoms that might suggest a particular disease or syndrome.

The bedside correlation of morphology with pathogenesis allows a much more thoughtful and focused approach to aspects of the history and physical examination relevant to the pathogenesis of hemorrhage. This is important in both choosing and interpreting appropriate tests. Abnormal values are not always indicative of important disease, or they can be misleading. For example, a prolonged partial thromboplastin time (PTT) usually implies a coagulation factor deficiency and would correlate with a tendency to develop ecchymotic hemorrhage. The finding of lupus anticoagulant can also prolong the PTT, but if it causes disease will result not in simple ecchymosis but instead in noninflammatory palpable purpura as a result of dermal vessel thrombosis.

A complete blood cell count and differential can be used to assess the number and morphology of platelets, to screen for schistocytes (which suggest a microangiopathic anemia, as may be seen in disseminated intravascular coagulation), and to explore the likelihood of myeloproliferative disease. A bleeding time is a useful screen of abnormal platelet function, but a history is usually adequate for diagnosing the most frequent cause of platelet dysfunction, i.e., aspirin use. Reasonable screens for defects in the coagulation cascade system include the PTT and the prothrombin time. More specialized clotting studies, such as protein C and protein S levels, are important in cases of bland occlusion syndromes. Screens for the antiphospholipid antibody syndrome might include a PTT or dilute Russell viper venom test to look for lupus anticoagulant activity, occasionally a Venereal Disease Research Laboratory (VDRL) test to look for false positives, and anticardiolipin or antiphospholipid antibody tests. Most studies suggest that elevated IgG anticardiolipin antibodies are more likely to be predictive of or explain thrombosis, but IgM antibodies can occasionally be responsible for thrombotic disease. Unfortunately, IgG or IgM anticardiolipin antibodies have a high rate of false positivity in predicting thrombosis, and may be negative in patients whose thrombosis is due to lupus anticoagulant/antiphospholipid disease. Serum and plasma tubes drawn and spun down at body temperature are essential for excluding cryoglobulin- or cryofibrinogen-related disease. When the clinical picture is appropriate, an antinuclear antibody titer, SS-A and SS-B levels, rheumatoid factor titer, serum protein electrophoresis, or immunoelectrophoresis might be indicated. A biopsy of an appropriate lesion early in its evolution is important for the proper diagnosis of palpable purpura, and immunofluorescence studies for immune complexes are useful if leukocytoclastic vasculitis is suspected. Urinalysis to look for blood, cells, or crystals and testing the stool for occult blood are important to exclude associated or underlying disease, especially in vasculitic syndromes.

TREATMENT

Treatment in purpuric syndromes is directed at the specific cause of the hemorrhage, so the correct diagnosis is critical to proper care. The treatment of cutaneous vasculitis is discussed in Chapter 4.

SUGGESTED READINGS

Braverman IM. The angiitides. In: Braverman IM, ed. Skin signs of systemic disease, 3rd edn. Philadelphia: WB Saunders, 1998; 278–334.

Lee PH, Gallo RC. The vascular purpuras. In: Lichtman MA, Beutler E, Kipps TJ, et al., eds. Williams' hematology, 7th edn. New York: McGraw-Hill, 2006; 1857–1866.

Piette WW. The differential diagnosis of purpura from a morphologic perspective. Adv Dermatol 1994; 9: 3–24.

Piette WW. Purpura: mechanisms and differential diagnosis. In: Bolognia JL, Jorizzo JL, Rapini RP, eds. Dermatology, 2nd edn. London: Mosby, 2008; 321–330.

Piette WW. Cutaneous manifestations of microvascular occlusion. In: Bolognia JL, Jorizzo JL, Rapini RP, eds. Dermatology, 2nd edn. London: Mosby, 2008; 331–345.

Piette WW, Stone MS. A cutaneous sign of IgA-associated small dermal vessel leukocytoclastic vasculitis in adults (Henoch–Schönlein purpura). Arch Dermatol 1989; 125: 53–56.

Robson KJ, Piette WW. The presentation and differential diagnosis of cutaneous vascular occlusion syndromes. Adv Dermatol 1999; 15: 153–182.

Spicer TE. Purpura fulminans. Am J Med 1976; 61: 566–571.

Weinstein S, Piette WW. Cutaneous manifestations of antiphospholipid antibody syndrome. Hematol Oncol Clin North Am 2008; 22: 67–77.

Chapter | **12** |

Anneli R. Bowen and John J. Zone

Bullous Diseases

Immunobullous diseases can precipitate extreme stress to multiple organ systems. Severe cases can have extensive mucocutaneous involvement, and have the potential for secondary infection and fluid loss. These diseases are also associated with a variety of systemic disorders, both directly and indirectly. Furthermore, the requirement for systemic corticosteroid and immunosuppressive therapy may produce myriad systemic complications.

Comprehension of the biology of keratinocyte interactions with other keratinocytes and with the extracellular matrix is essential for understanding the autoimmune blistering diseases. Keratinocytes attach to each other by desmosomes, whereas they attach to the underlying basement membrane by hemidesmosomes (Fig. 12–1). Desmosomes consist of an intracellular cytoplasmic plaque made up of the molecules desmoplakin, plakophilin and plakoglobin. This cytoplasmic plaque interacts with the intracellular scaffolding of tonofilaments and anchors the keratin intermediate filaments to the hemidesmosome. The extracellular portion of the desmosome is comprised of desmogleins and desmocollins, which project onto the cell surface of the keratinocyte and contact desmosomal proteins of neighboring keratinocytes. Disruption of desmosomal interactions leads to acantholysis.

Hemidesmosomes attach basal keratinocytes to the underlying basement membrane. Together with the basement membrane zone (BMZ), hemidesmosomes form the dermoepidermal junction. Proteins that comprise the hemidesmosome are the bullous pemphigoid antigens 1 (BP230) and 2 (BP180), plectin and α6β4 integrin. BPAG1 is a 230 kDa intracellular molecule, whereas the 180 kDa BPAG2 is an anchoring filament that spans the keratinocyte extracellular membrane, extending into the BMZ. Disruption of hemidesmosomal interactions is implicated in bullous pemphigoid, pemphigoid (herpes) gestationis (discussed in Chapter 35), and linear IgA bullous dermatosis. The BMZ is divided into the lamina lucida and lamina densa, named according to their transmission electron microscopic appearance. Anchoring filaments extend from the hemidesmosome through the lamina lucida to the lamina densa, where they interact with collagen IV and laminin V. The papillary dermis attaches to the BMZ by anchoring fibrils, which either extend from the lamina densa down to dermal anchoring plaques, or loop back up to reattach to the

lamina densa. Anchoring fibrils are composed of collagen VII. The blistering in epidermolysis bullosa acquisita is thought to be due to disruption of molecular interactions in this region. Important structural proteins in the dermis include types I and II collagen and elastin.

PEMPHIGUS

Pemphigus is characterized by detachment of adhesions between keratinocytes (acantholysis). This process results in vesicles, bullae, and subsequent erosions of both cutaneous and mucosal surfaces. Affected skin in pemphigus vulgaris reveals flaccid blisters that generally develop on noninflamed skin, are readily broken, and progress to large, weeping, denuded areas (Fig. 12–2). Oropharyngeal erosions are common and may be the presenting sign (Fig. 12–3). The pemphigus group of diseases is divided into pemphigus vulgaris (with its variant pemphigus vegetans), pemphigus foliaceus (with its variants pemphigus erythematosus and fogo selvagem), IgA pemphigus, and paraneoplastic pemphigus.

Pathogenesis

The pathogenetic process in pemphigus is that of an organ-specific autoimmune disease. Lesional skin and usually serum demonstrate the presence of an IgG class autoantibody directed against desmoglein antigens present in normal squamous epithelium. The exact mechanism for this loss of self-tolerance is unknown, but CD4+ T cells recognize distinct epitopes of the extracellular portions of desmoglein 1 and 3, and preferentially produce T-helper type 2 (Th2) cytokines. Auto-antibody production in pemphigus vulgaris and pemphigus foliaceus is polyclonal, and most antibodies in active disease are of IgG_4 subclass. Patients in remission who have persistent pemphigus antibodies in their serum have mainly IgG_1 subtype.

Several lines of evidence support the critical role of antibodies to desmogleins in the clinical acantholytic process. First, the antibody is consistently present in lesional skin and the patient's serum. The serum autoantibody titers correlate with

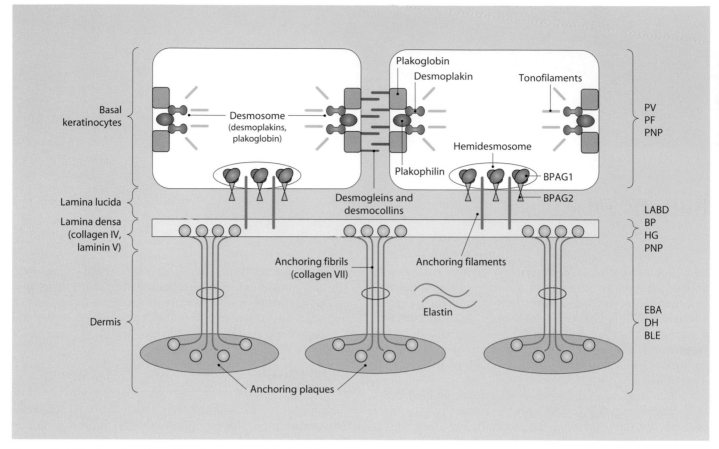

Figure 12–1 The dermal–epidermal junction consists of the basal keratinocytes, the basement membrane and the papillary dermis with their structural and attachment molecules. Diseases are listed on the right by the location of their target antigen(s). PV = pemphigus vulgaris, PF = pemphigus foliaceus, PNP = paraneoplastic pemphigus, LABD = linear IgA bullous dermatosis, BP = bullous pemphigoid, HG = herpes gestationis, EBA = epidermolysis bullosa acquisita, DH = dermatitis herpetiformis, BLE = bullous lupus erythematosus. BPAG1 and 2 = bullous pemphigoid antigens 1 and 2.

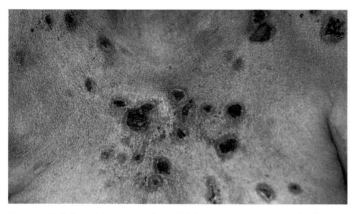

Figure 12–2 Pemphigus vulgaris. Multiple erosions on the trunk of this patient were preceded by blisters.

disease activity and there is a therapeutic response to plasmapheresis. Passive transfer of pemphigus from mothers to neonates occurs. Pemphigus antibody produces acantholysis when added to normal human skin in organ culture, and results in detachment when added to epidermal cell cultures. Further convincing evidence of the pathogenetic role of pemphigus antibody has been provided by the demonstration that IgG fraction purified from the serum of patients with pemphigus can induce a disease in neonatal mice that reproduces the clinical, histologic, and immunologic features of human pemphigus.

There are two alternative hypotheses to explain the autoantibody-mediated acantholysis: the desmoglein compensation hypothesis and the intracellular signaling hypothesis. In the desmoglein compensation hypothesis, binding of IgG to desmoglein molecules structurally disrupts epidermal cell adhesion. Desmoglein 1 expression is very low in mucosa, but it is expressed throughout the skin and increases in the more superficial layers. Desmoglein 3, by contrast, is expressed in all levels of mucosa, but only in and near the basal layer of the skin. Therefore, pemphigus foliaceus with Dsg 1 antibodies leads to superficial blistering in the skin, but no oral involvement. Pemphigus vulgaris with only Dsg 3 antibodies (mucosal-dominant pemphigus vulgaris) leads to oral erosions but minimal skin blisters. Amagai has proposed the 'desmoglein compensation theory' as an explanation of this phenomenon, suggesting that Dsg 1 in the skin can 'compensate' for the loss of Dsg 3 adhesion in this form of the disease. Finally, there can be no desmoglein compensation in pemphigus with both Dsg 1 and 3 antibodies (mucocutaneous pemphigus vulgaris), so acantholysis results in both skin and mucosa. Complement

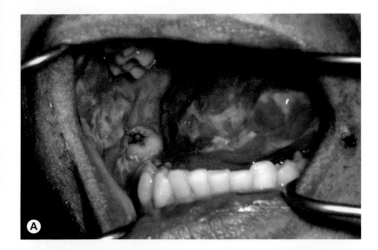

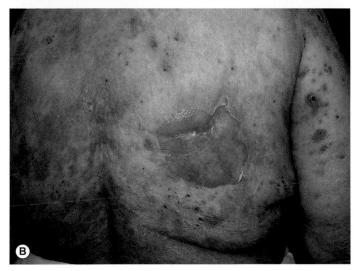

Figure 12–3 (A) Oral erosions of pemphigus are often the earliest lesions, as in this patient. (Courtesy of Mark Bernstein, MD, Louisville, KY.) (B) Pemphigus foliaceus in this elderly woman was initially misdiagnosed as impetigo

activation is not thought to play a role in acantholysis. The second hypothesis involves binding of IgG to the desmoglein cell surface antigen. This triggers transmembrane signaling and a series of intracellular pathways that lead to separation of the epidermal cells. These pathways are complex, but the validity of the process has been documented in vitro.

Although the stimulus for pemphigus antibody formation is unknown, the endemic nature of pemphigus foliaceus in Brazil suggests the involvement of an environmental factor, possibly an infectious agent. Most of the cases in Brazil occur in populations residing near rivers, and an insect vector for a microorganism has been proposed. Whether pemphigus in other geographic areas is precipitated by similar events is unknown. D-Penicillamine may produce pemphigus (predominantly pemphigus foliaceus) in patients being treated for rheumatoid arthritis, Wilson's disease, scleroderma, or other penicillamine-responsive disorders. Consequently, it is likely that a variety of stimuli may give rise to epidermal antigen intolerance.

There is a strong association of pemphigus vulgaris with the HLA class II alleles HLA DRB*0402, DRB*0401 and DQB1*0503. These HLA alleles may restrict autoreactive responses to desmoglein 3.

Classification

There are two histopathologically distinct forms of pemphigus. Pemphigus vulgaris is the most severe type and is characterized histopathologically by suprabasilar cleft formation, whereas pemphigus foliaceus is less severe and is distinguished by blister formation within or just beneath the granular layer. In pemphigus vulgaris and, to a lesser extent, pemphigus foliaceus, the blister may extend into surrounding nonblistered skin by applying shearing pressure to perilesional tissue (Nikolsky's sign).

Pemphigus vulgaris is the most common form of pemphigus and is generally seen in the fourth to sixth decades of life. It has, however, been described both in children and in the elderly. Prior to the use of corticosteroids, 50% of patients with the disease died within the first 12 months, most frequently from secondary cachexia, sepsis, and/or electrolyte imbalance. Now, with the broad utilization of immunosuppressants, the mortality is 5%.

Pemphigus vegetans is a rare variant of pemphigus vulgaris. Proliferative and verrucous lesions with surrounding pustules gradually develop from denuded bullae on intertriginous cutaneous surfaces. Such lesions were more common in the era before corticosteroid use and may represent a host response to the blistering process. Spontaneous remission is somewhat more likely in the vegetans form. Histopathologically one sees epidermal proliferation with hyperkeratosis, papillomatosis, and acantholysis with intraepidermal abscesses containing eosinophils.

Pemphigus foliaceus is generally less severe than pemphigus vulgaris. The superficial vesicles rupture easily, producing shallow erosions and crusting that clinically resemble impetigo. Clinical blistering may be totally absent. Lesions occur on the chest, back, and scalp, and may produce a seborrhea-like scaling with eventual spread to acral areas after a prolonged period. Clinically visible mucosal lesions are absent, even in advanced cases. Autoantibodies in pemphigus foliaceus are directed predominantly against desmoglein 1. Pemphigus herpetiformis is a morphologic variant of pemphigus vulgaris or pemphigus foliaceus that occurs as grouped vesicles.

Fogo selvagem is an endemic form of pemphigus foliaceus seen in Brazil. It occurs predominantly in children and young adults from poor rural areas. It is characterized by desquamation, erythroderma, and an intense burning in the sun-exposed skin, giving rise to the term fogo selvagem ('wild fire' in Portuguese). Histopathologically and immunopathologically it is indistinguishable from pemphigus foliaceus. Unlike other pemphigus variants, this condition can be seen in multiple members of a single family. There is an increased frequency of HLA-DRB1 haplotypes, DRB1*0404, 1402, 1406, and 1401. An environmental 'second hit' is suspected but not identified. Because of the clustering of cases near rivers, *Simulium* black flies have been suggested as a possible vector. IgM-anti-Dsg 1 is found in a majority of fogo selvagem patients in their native environment, but is uncommon in patients with other pemphigus phenotypes and in fogo selvagem patients who move to more urban settings, further supporting a recurrent environmental antigenic exposure in the pathogenesis of this disease.

Pemphigus erythematosus (Senear–Usher syndrome) represents a localized variant of pemphigus foliaceus characterized by erythematous lupus-like malar dermatitis. Patients frequently manifest an abnormal antinuclear antibody test as well as the presence of pemphigus antibody. Direct immunofluorescence microscopy may show immunoglobulin and complement components along the basement membrane, as well as characteristic intercellular pemphigus antibody deposition. This disorder is believed to represent the coexistence of lupus erythematosus and pemphigus foliaceus.

IgA pemphigus comprises a recently characterized group of IgA-mediated immunobullous diseases. This entity presents as vesicopustules with neutrophils and acantholysis, most commonly affecting the axillae and groin. Oral involvement is rare. IgA pemphigus is subdivided into two histologic types: the subcorneal pustular dermatosis type with blister formation subcorneally, and the intraepidermal neutrophilic type where blisters form throughout the epidermis. The IgA pemphigus antibodies in the subcorneal pustular dermatosis type recognize desmocollin 1, whereas rare IgA pemphigus sera recognize desmoglein 1 and 3. The antigen in the intraepidermal neutrophilic form remains uncharacterized. Only 50% of patients have circulating autoantibody on indirect immunofluorescence. The subcorneal pustular dermatosis form is clinically indistinguishable from Snedden–Wilkinson disease and must be differentiated by immunofluorescence studies. Rarely, either form of IgA pemphigus may exhibit concomitant expression of IgG autoantibodies – so-called IgA/IgG pemphigus.

Penicillamine and angiotensin-converting enzyme (ACE) inhibitor therapy have been associated with a variety of autoimmune disorders, including pemphigus vulgaris and pemphigus foliaceus. Pemphigus foliaceus accounts for 70% of the penicillamine-induced cases, and pemphigus vulgaris composes the remainder. The development of pemphigus may occur with a wide range of dosages and is often a late complication of therapy. After discontinuation of penicillamine therapy approximately half the patients resolve in 4 months, whereas the other half require suppressive corticosteroid therapy over a longer period. Autoantibodies from drug-induced patients have the same antigenic specificity on a molecular level as do those from idiopathic forms of pemphigus.

Pemphigus has occurred in association with thymoma and myasthenia gravis. Pemphigus vulgaris, pemphigus foliaceus, and pemphigus erythematosus have all been noted associations. There is little, if any, concordance between the clinical activities of the coexistent disorders. The concurrence is believed to involve an underlying failure of thymic-dependent lymphocytes in suppressing autoimmune disease.

The description of paraneoplastic pemphigus (PNP) as a distinct disorder by Anhalt et al. focuses this issue in a small subgroup of patients who had a clear-cut association of pemphigus with a tumor. The patients are clinically heterogeneous and somewhat atypical. Clinical descriptions partially resemble Stevens–Johnson syndrome, with target lesions and painful oral lesions seen on occasion. Some patients have been described as having a papulosquamous eruption, whereas others have tense bullae. The most common associations, in descending order, are non-Hodgkin's lymphoma, chronic lymphocytic leukemia, Castleman's disease, and solid tumors including carcinomas, sarcomas, and melanoma. Histologically, suprabasilar acantholysis has been described in some cases, whereas keratinocyte necrosis, basal cell vacuolization, interface inflammation, and even basement membrane blisters have been described in others.

The immunofluorescent pattern in paraneoplastic pemphigus is one of intercellular IgG deposition, which may be patchy and focal, and basement membrane zone IgG and complement deposition. Circulating autoantibodies bind to different tissue sources than standard pemphigus antibodies, including urinary bladder, respiratory epithelium, and desmosomal areas of myocardium and skeletal muscle. Indirect immunofluorescence to rat bladder is the most specific diagnostic tool. PNP sera react to a unique complex of antigens which includes the plakin protein family, including desmoplakin, bullous pemphigoid antigen 1 (BPAG1), envoplakin and periplakin, and desmogleins 1 and 3. Patients with paraneoplastic pemphigus may have antibodies to one or all of these antigens, or may start with few and with time develop antibodies to other paraneoplastic pemphigus antigens. This observed progression may represent epitope spreading.

Unique to paraneoplastic pemphigus is a large proportion of patients who develop bronchiolitis obliterans, a lethal pulmonary condition characterized by severe hypoxia, a relatively clear chest X-ray, and an association in at least one patient with IgG deposition in bronchial epithelium intracellular spaces. Because desmoplakins are present in bronchial epithelium it is possible that this pulmonary finding is autoimmune mediated. In summary, it appears that this is an unusual mucocutaneous disorder with myriad clinicopathologic findings, some of which are not a part of any of the forms of pemphigus.

Other sporadic and poorly understood associations with pemphigus include pernicious anemia, red blood cell aplasia, rheumatoid arthritis, and lymphomatoid granulomatosis.

Differential Diagnosis

The differential diagnosis of blistering disorders of the skin ranges from a wide variety of banal dermatoses to more serious and progressive disorders such as pemphigus, bullous pemphigoid (Fig. 12–4), and epidermolysis bullosa acquisita. These disorders require clinical, histopathologic, and immunopathologic evaluation for definite diagnosis. When the etiology of blistering disorders cannot be recognized, biopsy is warranted. Subsequent decisions are made on the basis of these findings. Histopathologic characteristics of potential blistering disorders that will not be discussed here in detail are listed in Table 12–1.

Many patients with oral ulcerations of pemphigus are misdiagnosed as having aphthous stomatitis. After months to years, however, such patients typically progress to have extramucosal involvement.

Acantholysis is the hallmark of immunologically mediated pemphigus, but it may also be seen in Grover's disease (transient acantholytic dermatosis), Darier's disease (keratosis follicularis), and Hailey–Hailey disease (benign familial pemphigus). In Grover's disease there is involvement of the trunk

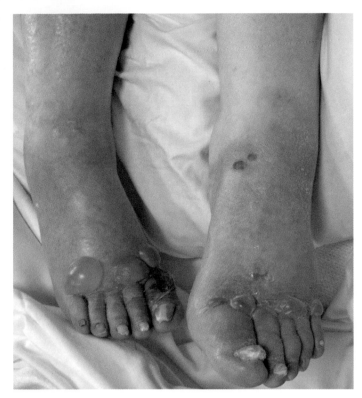

Figure 12–4 Tense bullae are representative of bullous pemphigoid.

Table 12–1 Blistering dermatoses

1. Subcorneal vesicles
  a. Bullous impetigo
  b. Staphylococcal scalded skin syndrome
  c. Miliaria
  d. Subcorneal pustular dermatosis
  e. Candidiasis

2. Spongiotic blisters
  a. Eczematous disorders, including allergic contact dermatitis, stasis dermatitis, irritant dermatitis, fungal dermatitis, etc.
  b. Incontinentia pigmenti

3. Ballooning degeneration of epidermal cells
  a. Herpes simplex
  b. Herpes zoster and varicella

with pruritic papulovesicles, but no oral involvement. It is frequently precipitated by sun exposure or heat and lasts for weeks to months, although chronic cases are not uncommon.

Darier's disease is an autosomal dominant disorder characterized by yellowish-brown crusted papules on the scalp, intertriginous areas, and seborrheic areas of the face and trunk. The disease is slowly progressive and seldom overtly bullous. Lesions are frequently perifollicular. Although acantholysis is suprabasilar, as in pemphigus vulgaris, characteristic dyskeratotic changes (corps ronds and grains) occur within the epidermis.

Hailey–Hailey disease (benign familial pemphigus) is an autosomal dominant disorder characterized by multiple grouped erythematous vesicles in intertriginous areas. Mucosal surfaces are usually spared. There is extensive loss of intercellular bridges, with partial coherence of cells throughout all levels of the epidermis.

The clinical pattern of these acantholytic disorders is usually distinctive from that of pemphigus. If confusion exists, direct immunofluorescence of perilesional skin is negative for IgG deposition in these disorders, whereas pemphigus patients demonstrate characteristic intercellular IgG deposition in stratified squamous epithelial tissues.

Patient Evaluation

Close examination of all mucous membranes is indicated. Oral involvement is the rule in pemphigus vulgaris, but esophageal as well as vulvar involvement may occur. Significant esophageal symptoms and even stricture may develop. Consequently, esophageal symptoms mandate endoscopy and possible biopsy. Patients presenting with blistering skin disorders that cannot be easily explained (e.g., friction blisters and contact dermatitis) require biopsy. If there is histopathologic acantholysis, biopsy of perilesional skin for direct immunofluorescence should be performed. Indirect immunofluorescence microscopy demonstrating pemphigus antibodies in the serum further confirms the diagnosis, and antibody titers typically correlate with disease activity. Disappearance of antibody from the serum frequently precedes remission.

Chest X-ray to rule out an associated thymoma and a search for clinical symptoms of myasthenia gravis is part of good clinical care, but a low yield of positive findings is to be expected. Culture of potentially infected lesions and close attention to protein loss and malnutrition are necessary in severe cases. Chest X-ray, tuberculosis skin test, complete blood count (CBC), and blood glucose determination should be undertaken prior to initiating corticosteroid or immunosuppressive therapy.

Treatment

Initial therapy of pemphigus involves complete suppression of blistering with oral prednisone (usually 1–2 mg/kg daily). Initial control with 3–4 mg/kg daily has been suggested, but in the authors' estimation is associated with unnecessarily severe side effects. Because therapy may need to be continued for years, corticosteroid side effects become a major clinical problem. Corticosteroid sparing may be accomplished by the addition of an immunosuppressive agent, as discussed below. Immunosuppression is continued in sufficient doses to suppress blistering until serum antibody titers become negative, at which time tapering of therapy should be attempted. Follow-up biopsy for direct immunofluorescence once clinical manifestations have cleared for >6 months on treatment can predict the likelihood of remission once medications are stopped. Ratnam and Pang showed that three-quarters of patients with negative direct immunofluorescence at this stage remain in remission, and those with negative direct immunofluorescence who do recur have mild disease. In contrast, all patients with a positive follow-up direct immunofluorescence tend to relapse within 3 months of discontinuing therapy.

Systemic methotrexate (oral, intravenous, or intramuscular) can be used in dosages of 20–50 mg per week, but may aggravate oral ulcers. Cyclophosphamide is effective in oral dosages of 1–3 mg/kg/day, and oral azathioprine may be used in dosages of 1–3 mg/kg/day. Mycophenolate mofetil is effective alone or in combination with steroids in doses of 1–3 g/day. Close attention should be paid to a variety of potential side effects, including leukopenia, hepatotoxicity, teratogenesis, sterility, oral ulcers, and cystitis, depending on the specific agent used. Patients with excessive toxicity from oral corticosteroids or cyclophosphamide may have reduced side effects with monthly pulse doses.

Plasmapheresis may be useful in pemphigus patients poorly controlled on conventional therapy. Six-liter exchanges on three separate occasions over a 3-week period are necessary to lower the antibody titer significantly. Immunosuppressants such as cyclophosphamide are then necessary to maintain the improvement and prevent the rebound of antibody levels that usually follows plasmapheresis.

Intravenous immunoglobulin (IVIg) therapy is emerging as a promising new treatment for many immune-mediated diseases. It works rapidly, and selectively lowers serum levels of pemphigus antibody. The clinical response in individual patients is variable. The concurrent administration of an immunosuppressive agent to prevent the synthesis of new antibody improves the efficacy. The dose is usually 2 g/kg/cycle, administered over 2–5 days. It is traditionally given in monthly cycles, but the optimal frequency of cycles is unknown. Caution needs to be taken to avoid fluid overload in elderly patients, and venous thrombosis may occur with administration.

Rituximab is a murine–human chimeric monoclonal antibody to CD20, an antigen present on B cells but not plasma cells. It is approved for use in B-cell lymphoma and is being used off-label for pemphigus and pemphigoid. Administration in a dose of 375 mg/m² once weekly for 4 weeks rapidly reduces the peripheral B-cell count to zero and sustains this level for 6–12 months. Clinical improvement occurs within days to weeks, indicating that mechanisms other than B-cell depletion may be active. Pemphigus antibodies decrease in response to therapy and complete remission may occur. The risk of fatal infection is increased, and at present it is recommended that it be reserved for severe disease unresponsive to conventional therapy.

Because of its neutrophil-mediated pathogenesis, the drug of choice for IgA pemphigus is dapsone. Doses of 100 mg/day are usually sufficient. For patients unable to tolerate dapsone, etretinate is an alternative, providing immunosuppression by interfering with neutrophil and monocyte chemotaxis.

BULLOUS PEMPHIGOID

Bullous pemphigoid (BP) is the most common subepidermal blistering disorder. It is characterized by subepidermal vesicles and bullae that, unlike the lesions of pemphigus vulgaris, do not rupture easily and rarely produce large areas of denuded skin. Oropharyngeal lesions occur commonly, and may be the only manifestation of the disease (mucous membrane pemphigoid). Cutaneous blisters generally arise from erythema-

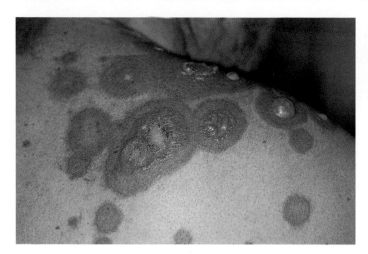

Figure 12–5 Multiple tense bullae arising on an urticarial base in a patient with bullous pemphigoid. (Reprinted with permission from Callen JP, Greer KE, Paller A, Swinyer L, eds. Color atlas of dermatology: A morphological approach, 2nd edn. Philadelphia: WB Saunders, 2000.)

tous or urticarial plaques (Fig. 12–5). BP is often self-limited, and in contrast to pemphigus vulgaris the mortality is low even in the absence of corticosteroid therapy. However, BP is a potentially serious disease because it typically occurs in older individuals whose compromised status predisposes them to infection and the complications of corticosteroid therapy. BP is characterized by deposition of IgG antibodies that react with basement membrane antigens in the lamina lucida, stimulating loss of dermoepidermal adherence.

Pathogenesis

Although the specific mechanisms responsible for blister formation in BP are not as well established as those in pemphigus, there is good evidence that IgG antibodies directed against antigens of the hemidesmosome of stratified squamous epithelium are pivotal. Perilesional skin and frequently serum from BP patients demonstrate the presence of IgG autoantibody directed against two distinct hemidesmosomal antigens: a 230 kDa glycoprotein bullous pemphigoid antigen 1 (BPAG1 or BP230) that reacts with circulating antibodies in 50–70% of cases, and the 180 kDa bullous pemphigoid antigen 2 (BPAG2 or BP180) with extracellular collagen-like domains that is reactive in 30–50% of cases. The BP antigens are normal components of the basement membrane zone, but, as is the case in pemphigus, patients become intolerant to these antigens. The HLA DQB1*0301 allele may be important in initial antigen processing. Autoreactive T lymphocytes producing Th1 and particularly Th2 cytokines are critically involved in the initiation of production of pathogenic autoantibodies in BP.

Antibodies to BPAG2, also known as collagen XVII, bind to a noncollagenous region of the molecule outside the cell membrane in the lamina lucida. Several points support the pathogenic role of anti-BPAG2 antibodies in bullous pemphigoid. Passive transfer experiments in mice have resulted in blister formation when rabbit-derived antibodies to murine BPAG2 are injected. Secondly, sensitive ELISA testing shows that BP180 antibody titers correlate with disease severity. Finally, IgG antibodies to BPAG2 in the related condition pemphigoid gestationis can cross the placenta and cause blisters in the fetuses of mothers with this disease. Passive transfer experiments in mice have produced inflammation and subepidermal blistering. Because BPAG1 is an intracytoplasmic molecule it has been suggested that anti-BPAG1 antibodies may develop secondarily after initial skin injury by anti-BPAG2 antibodies.

BPAG2 IgG antibodies are thought to cause blistering by complement and neutrophil activation. Several pieces of information support a role for complement in the pathogenesis of BP lesions. Complement deposits have been detected in vivo in the lamina lucida, and the complement membrane attack complex has been identified in involved skin. The stimulus for leukocyte attachment is activated complement components released by immune complex activation. Neutrophils are recruited by C5a-dependent pathways. Their pathogenicity is inferred by the finding that mice deficient in gelatinase-B (a neutrophil enzyme) were protected from blistering in passive transfer experiments. When neutrophils from normal mice were injected into the gelatinase-deficient mice they developed blisters.

Degranulation of mast cells mediated by either complement-derived anaphylatoxins, eosinophil activation, or a direct effect of IgG antibody is responsible for the release of chemotactic factors, proteolytic enzymes, and vasoactive amines which subsequently mediate dermoepidermal separation. IgE is emerging as an important pathogenic factor in BP. IgE antibodies against BPAG1 and BPAG2 have been detected in a high percentage of BP patients, with anti-BPAG1 IgE levels correlating with local eosinophil recruitment. SCID mice injected with an IgE-producing hybridoma directed toward the shed ectodomain of BPAG2 developed histologically evident subepidermal blisters in human skin grafts. Finally, IgE anti-BPAG2 is related to disease activity and severity.

Several reports have indicated that patients with BP may develop further blistering on exposure to ultraviolet light. The mechanism for this may be related to ultraviolet light activation of mast cells.

Classification

The term BP is generally reserved for patients demonstrating a chronic, vesiculobullous eruption involving predominantly nonmucosal surfaces. The distribution is usually widespread, with sites of predilection including the lower abdomen, inner thighs, groin, axilla, and flexural aspects of the arms and legs. BP antigen may vary in the amount distributed regionally, accounting for this classic distribution. However, 15–30% of patients demonstrate tense bullae limited to the pretibial area. Such cases are immunopathologically and histologically identical to BP, and no definite reason for the localized nature has been established. BP has been described in prepubertal children, but it is most common in the seventh and eighth decades of life. In the pre-corticosteroid era many cases resolved without treatment, although occasional patients developed aggressive and severe disease.

Some patients' biopsy specimens demonstrate a heavy inflammatory infiltrate around dermal blood vessels, with an admixture of neutrophils, eosinophils, and mononuclear cells.

The prominence of the eosinophil infiltration serves to differentiate this disorder from dermatitis herpetiformis histopathologically. The second histopathologic type is characterized by a sparse inflammatory infiltrate of mononuclear cells around superficial dermal blood vessels in the presence of prominent vesiculation in the basement membrane zone. Immunopathologic diagnosis is essential to separate this from other immunobullous diseases.

The term cicatricial pemphigoid is reserved for those forms of the disease characterized by blistering and scarring. Classically this is a disease of the elderly, involving erosions of mucosal surfaces, especially the conjunctiva (Fig. 12–6), but also including the nasopharynx, oropharynx, esophagus, larynx, urethra, and anal mucosa. The morbidity and mortality of the disorder are related to the scarring produced by the recurrent lesions. Associated skin lesions occur in a minority of cases. Eye involvement may result in conjunctival symblepharon with obliteration of the conjunctival sulcus. Subsequent scarring of the cornea may produce blindness. The gingivae are commonly involved, and the disease may present only as 'desquamative gingivitis.' Esophageal lesions begin as smooth-bordered erosions, but stricture may occur and require repeated dilatation. Direct immunofluorescence microscopy of mucous membrane tissue reveals IgG and/or IgA anti-BMZ antibody in more than 80% of cases. Immunofluorescent-negative cases may represent a technical problem with obtaining adequate tissue from mucosal surfaces such as the eye. However, it is important to obtain positive direct immunofluorescence results, even if multiple biopsies are required, in order to separate the disorder from pemphigus, lichen planus, and cicatrizing conjunctivitis secondary to irritants and allergens. Indirect immunofluorescence studies reveal circulating anti-BMZ antibodies of IgG or IgA class in less than 50% of cases. Antibodies in cicatricial pemphigoid recognize several BMZ molecules, including BPAG1 and 2, laminin V, α6β4 integrin, and type VII collagen. The scarring nature of this disease may be explained by the fact that the BPAG2 antibodies in cicatricial pemphigoid recognize the distal extracellular

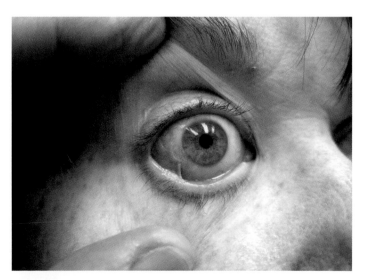

Figure 12–6 Scarring ocular disease in a patient with cicatricial pemphigoid.

domain (carboxy terminus) of this molecule, which ends in the lamina densa, in contrast to classic bullous pemphigoid patients where the more proximal NC16A domain of BPAG2 is targeted.

A specific localized scarring variant of cicatricial pemphigoid has been termed the Brunsting–Perry type. In this variant, scarring and blister formation occur on the head and neck without concomitant oral involvement. The pathogenesis of cicatricial pemphigoid is believed to be similar to that of BP, although the reason for localized disease and scarring is not understood.

There have been numerous evaluations of the association between BP and internal malignancy. BP has been reported in association with malignancies of the lymphoreticular system, skin, lung, breast, pancreas, kidney, and gastrointestinal tract. However, rarely have concurrent onset or a parallel course been documented. Ahmed and coworkers, as well as Stone and Schroeter, were able to find no increased rate of malignancy in their BP patients, but a study by Chorzelski et al. did claim a 10% association. Most authors have concluded that there is no increased incidence of malignancy in BP patients compared to age-matched controls. Thus, BP is best considered not to be a cutaneous marker of internal malignancy. However, recent evaluation of a subset of 35 cicatricial pemphigoid patients who had IgG serum antibodies directed against laminin V found that 10 patients had an associated malignancy.

This finding gives further credence to the need to characterize individual patients' antigen-binding profiles. Testing for specific antigen binding is only available in research laboratories at present, but indirect immunofluorescence on basement membrane split skin is a standard technique in immunopathology laboratories, and can suggest the presence of antibodies to laminin V on the basis of the uncommon dermal binding pattern.

BP has been reported in association with a wide variety of other disorders, including psoriasis, diabetes mellitus, lupus erythematosus, pernicious anemia, thyroiditis, polymyositis, and rheumatoid arthritis. It seems unlikely that any of these associations is important in pathogenesis, but the reasons for the associations remain unclear. In a case–control study in 1984 Chuang and associates found 20% of bullous pemphigoid patients had diabetes, compared to 2.5% of controls. This association remained significant even after correcting for age differences. The association with rheumatoid arthritis seems to be significant, and it has been hypothesized that the two disorders may share similar pathogenetic mechanisms.

Lichen planus pemphigoides has been described on many occasions. It is characterized by the typical outbreak of lichen planus followed by a bullous eruption with the histological and immunopathological findings of bullous pemphigoid. It is unclear whether these patients have coexistent lichen planus and bullous pemphigoid, or whether this is a distinct entity in which the inflammatory process of lichen planus stimulates an immune response to BP antigens.

Differential Diagnosis

The initial diagnostic approach to blistering disorders is reviewed under the differential diagnosis of pemphigus. If biopsy suggests that the blister is subepidermal, direct immunofluorescence microscopy of perilesional tissue is indicated. BP characteristically demonstrates linear deposition of IgG along the basement membrane. Some cases of pemphigoid have also been described as having IgG and IgA along the basement membrane, making the separation from linear IgA bullous dermatosis somewhat arbitrary.

Dermatitis herpetiformis is differentiated by its clinical appearance (see later discussion), as well as by the characteristic deposition of granular IgA in perilesional tissue. Linear IgA bullous dermatosis shows characteristic deposition of IgA along the basement membrane as the predominant and usually the only immunoglobulin. Linear IgA disease is sensitive to sulfone therapy.

Erythema multiforme may also show a subepidermal blister. Characteristic involvement of the palms and soles with target lesions (minor type) or involvement of mucous membranes and skin (major type) in an acute fashion is characteristic of erythema multiforme. Biopsy of erythema multiforme reveals individually necrotic keratinocytes, and direct immunofluorescence fails to reveal anti-BMZ antibody. Occasional patients with erythema multiforme may have immunoglobulins in superficial dermal blood vessels.

Bullous lupus erythematosus usually occurs in patients who fulfill the American Rheumatism Association (ARA) criteria for systemic lupus erythematosus. In addition, the disorder shows granular deposition of immunoglobulin along the BMZ. Such deposition may be sufficiently intense to give a band-like pattern that can be confused with BP. However, patients with bullous lupus erythematosus histopathologically demonstrate a neutrophilic infiltrate similar to that of dermatitis herpetiformis.

Bullous forms of lichen planus exist that are distinguished by an intense mononuclear infiltrate adjacent to the BMZ, absence of anti-BMZ antibodies, and characteristic epidermal changes of lichen planus, which allow differentiation.

Epidermolysis bullosa of the junctional and dystrophic types may show a blister at the dermoepidermal junction. Such cases are characterized by onset of blistering early in childhood, absence of the inflammatory infiltrate, and negative direct immunofluorescence. The scarring, progressive nature of these disorders is easily distinguishable clinically.

Porphyria cutanea tarda also shows pauci-inflammatory subepidermal blistering, which occurs in sun-exposed areas. Histologically, the dermal papillae irregularly extend into the bulla cavity. Direct immunofluorescence microscopy may be positive, further confusing this differentiation. The diagnosis of porphyria cutanea tarda is ultimately made on the basis of elevated 24-hour uroporphyrins. Pseudoporphyria related to the use of NSAIDs may give a clinical, pathologic and immunopathologic pattern identical to that of porphyria cutanea tarda, but the 24-hour uroporphyrin level is normal. Epidermolysis bullosa acquisita is discussed in detail later.

The mucous membrane lesions of cicatricial pemphigoid must be differentiated from those of oral lichen planus, erythema multiforme, aphthous stomatitis, Behçet's syndrome, and pemphigus. The differentiation from oral lichen planus and erythema multiforme can usually be made histopathologically. Aphthous stomatitis lesions tend to be small and punched out. Behçet's syndrome need only be considered if other components of the syndrome, including genital ulceration, pustular dermatosis, and iritis, are present. None of these disorders demonstrates anti-BMZ antibodies.

Patient Evaluation

Close examination of all mucosal and cutaneous surfaces is necessary. Esophageal involvement may produce stricture, and patients with esophageal complaints should be considered for endoscopy and possible biopsy. In the presence of symptoms and/or signs found by the general physical examination that suggest the possibility of internal malignancy, those findings should be evaluated. However, no detailed evaluation to rule out the possibility of malignancy is otherwise necessary. Potentially infected lesions should be cultured. Evaluation of the patient's general status, including CBC, chemistry profile, and urinalysis, is advisable because many patients will have associated complicating clinical problems attendant upon their age. Chest X-ray and tuberculosis skin testing should be undertaken prior to starting corticosteroid and/or immunosuppressive therapy.

Initial study attempts to correlate the titers of BP antibody with disease activity were unsuccessful. However, it had been observed that the disappearance of antibody from the serum usually heralded the onset of spontaneous remission. Recently an association between disease activity and antibody titers has been seen when antibody levels to the BPAG2 antigen are followed specifically by highly sensitive ELISA assays.

Treatment

The majority of patients with BP have a complete clinical remission following effective therapy. The mainstay of therapy for BP is parenteral corticosteroids. Oral prednisone, 40–60 mg daily, is generally adequate for initial treatment, and may be the only treatment necessary. With this agent, individual blisters generally resolve within 2–3 weeks and new blister formation ceases. A major complication of treatment is related to corticosteroid side effects, including increased susceptibility to infection, potential gastrointestinal bleeding, onset of diabetes mellitus, and the possible development of psychiatric symptoms. These problems may well be severe, in view of the elderly age group afflicted. Consequently, close attention to complications is necessary. Oral therapy with bisphosphonates is indicated to prevent steroid-induced osteoporosis if steroids are to be used for more than a few days. Some reports suggest a beneficial effect of the combination of tetracycline and niacinamide as initial therapy in mild cases.

Azathioprine, 1–3 mg/kg/day, is an especially effective agent when used to spare corticosteroid dosage in patients with BP. The onset of effect is slow; thus, after 4–6 weeks of treatment with azathioprine, corticosteroid doses can be gradually tapered. Cyclophosphamide and mycophenolate mofetil are effective and may be used in the manner described for pemphigus.

As with pemphigus, IVIg appears to be effective, especially in recalcitrant disease. Doses similar to those used in pemphi-

gus vulgaris have been effective in some patients, but definitive studies on its efficacy in pemphigoid are lacking.

Mucous membrane pemphigoid, if localized, may be treated with topical corticosteroid preparations, but usually requires systemic corticosteroid therapy. Dapsone may be helpful in controlling the oral lesions, but is often ineffective in preventing progressive ocular disease. Therapy with dapsone should be given in doses similar to those described for dermatitis herpetiformis (see later section on dermatitis herpetiformis). Eye involvement in cicatricial pemphigoid is particularly serious and warrants aggressive therapy. If initial response to oral corticosteroid therapy is not forthcoming, aggressive treatment with cyclophosphamide is indicated. However, ophthalmic involvement may be resistant to all therapies.

Localized BP of the extremities as well as some mucosal disease may be successfully treated with intradermal injections of small amounts of triamcinolone acetonide (2.5 mg/mL) used in combination with potent topical corticosteroids.

EPIDERMOLYSIS BULLOSA ACQUISITA

Epidermolysis bullosa acquisita (EBA) is a rare acquired bullous disease that generally occurs in adults and is distinguished by the involvement of extensor surfaces with blisters that heal slowly, leaving atrophic scars. Blisters appear mechanically induced and may lead to secondary milia formation (Fig. 12–7). Immunoglobulin and complement are deposited in a dense, linear pattern along the BMZ, as seen on direct immunofluorescence microscopy, and circulating IgG anti-BMZ antibody is present in about 50% of patients. Serologic studies demonstrate that this anti-BMZ antibody reacts with a 290 kDa antigen that is type VII collagen, the same antigen as for bullous systemic lupus erythematosus.

Pathogenesis

Histopathologically, EBA is characterized by a subepidermal blister with or without a neutrophilic inflammatory infiltrate. There is dense deposition of IgG and frequently complement components along the basement membrane. The majority of cases have a circulating IgG antibody which reacts on indirect immunofluorescence with the dermal side of salt-split skin (skin which has been separated in the lower lamina lucida by incubation with 1 M sodium chloride). This is in contrast to BP sera, which react with the epidermal side or both epidermal and dermal sides of such preparations. Blister formation has been reported to occur either below the lamina lucida or below the lamina densa. On immunoelectron microscopy the immune deposits of EBA are localized to the anchoring fibrils of the sublamina densa region. Lapiere and colleagues have identified the BMZ protein that is antigenic in the sublamina densa region as the noncollagenous (NC-1) domain of type VII collagen. Specifically, antibodies to the fibronectin-like repeats within collagen VII seem to be preferentially formed and probably interfere with collagen VII–laminin V interaction. Passive transfer experiments of IgG anti-collagen VII autoantibody have produced an EBA-like clinical picture in mice.

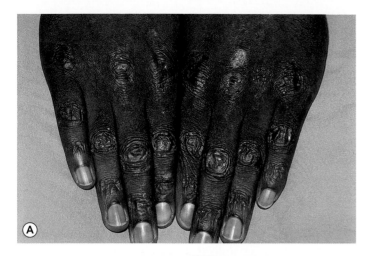

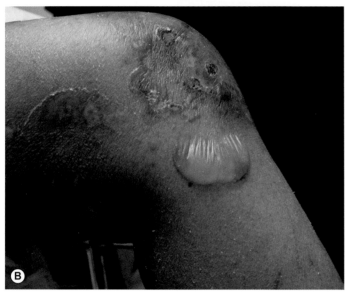

Figure 12–7 (A) Epidermolysis bullosa acquisita. Scars and milia are present in this patient who had multiple traumatically induced blisters on the dorsal hands. (B) Epidermolysis bullosa acquisita in a patient with systemic lupus erythematosus.

Preparations of EBA patients' anti-BMZ antibodies show both complement-activating and noncomplement-activating subclasses. However, the presence of complement-fixing antibodies does not correlate with the inflammatory or non-inflammatory clinical subtypes. Additionally, when the complement-fixing ability of EBA patients' serum is measured, it is absent to weak; therefore, it is unlikely that complement plays a major role in blister formation. Nevertheless, an organ culture system utilizing EBA antibody, tissue injury, and BMZ separation can be produced. Eventually, antibody deposition and the inflammatory process may produce sufficient damage to the anchoring fibrils such that minor trauma will produce a loss of dermoepidermal adhesion in the absence of the inflammatory process.

Classification

EBA is a sharply defined entity on the basis of its immuno-pathologic findings. However, there is a spectrum of clinical

and histopathologic manifestations of EBA. Blisters may arise on an inflammatory or a noninflammatory base. Milia may or may not be present. The inflammatory variant is frequently associated with nail dystrophy.

EBA has been reported to be associated with a variety of disorders, including rheumatoid arthritis, multiple myeloma, chronic thyroiditis, diabetes mellitus, lymphoma, amyloidosis, inflammatory bowel disease, and cryoglobulinemia. Many of these may be chance occurrences. The strongest associations appear to be with diabetes mellitus and Crohn's disease. The mechanism for these associations is unclear.

The distinction between EBA and bullous lupus erythematosus is complex. Cases with the clinical criteria for systemic lupus erythematosus and immunopathologic findings of EBA may well represent a subset of lupus patients in whom the immune dysregulation of lupus results in the production of antibodies to type VII collagen.

Differential Diagnosis

The differential diagnosis of subepidermal blistering disease is described under BP. However, EBA may be impossible to separate from BP on the basis of clinical findings alone. If circulating antibody is present, indirect immunofluorescence utilizing BMZ split skin as described above should be utilized. In the absence of circulating antibody, immunoelectron microscopy is the only reliable way to separate BP from EBA. In this situation EBA will demonstrate deposition of IgG in the sublamina densa area of the anchoring fibrils, whereas BP IgG deposition will be in the lamina lucida.

The classic clinical and histopathologic presentation of EBA closely resembles that of porphyria cutanea tarda, but EBA patients have normal uroporphyrins. Differentiation of EBA from other forms of epidermolysis bullosa includes the adult onset, as well as a negative family history of EBA. The inflammatory variant may also closely mimic drug-induced bullous erythema multiforme, which, however, lacks the characteristic findings of EBA on direct immunofluorescence.

Patient Evaluation

The evaluation of patients with EBA is essentially the same as that for patients with BP. However, because EBA can cause scarring on mucosal surfaces, a multidisciplinary approach involving gastroenterology, otolaryngology, ophthalmology, dentistry and speech therapy may be required to deal with these complications. Correlation of antibody titer with disease activity has not been well evaluated.

Treatment

The treatment of EBA is similar to that for BP. However, EBA tends to be progressive and unrelenting, and is much more resistant to treatment with systemic corticosteroids than is BP. In a review by Engineer, small series and case reports were summarized showing promising results with cyclosporine, colchicine, and IVIg.

DERMATITIS HERPETIFORMIS

Dermatitis herpetiformis (DH), or Duhring's disease, is characterized by involvement of extensor surfaces with grouped, pruritic, erythematous papulovesicles (Fig. 12–8). Biopsy demonstrates a blister at the basement membrane with accumulation of neutrophils in the dermal papillary tips. Perilesional skin demonstrates the pathognomonic deposition of granular IgA in dermal papillary tips. More than 90% of patients with DH have the HLA-DQ2 genotype, compared to 20% of controls. This offers a unique background on which gluten sensitivity and the subsequent IgA immune response develop. Virtually all DH patients have gluten-sensitive enteropathy on small bowel biopsy, but gastrointestinal symptoms occur in only about 25% of cases. The skin disease as well as the associated gluten-sensitive enteropathy improves with dietary restriction of gluten.

Pathogenesis

The skin disease as well as the intestinal lesions responds to a strict gluten-free diet, although it may take 3–6 months for the clinical improvement. IgA also clears from the skin with prolonged gluten restriction. This indicates a central role for gluten ingestion and IgA in the pathogenesis.

The HLA-DQ2 antigen is found in 90% of celiac disease and DH patients and only 20% of controls. It is believed that this genetic background is essential to presentation of the gluten antigen to the mucosal immune system. The intestinal lesion is then produced by an intestinal inflammatory infiltrate of mononuclear cells. However, it is unknown how gluten triggers IgA binding to skin, and how IgA triggers neutrophil infiltration and the inflammatory cascade. An antigen to which the IgA antibodies bind in the skin has been identified as epidermal transglutaminase (TG3).

The proposed pathogenesis of DH and celiac disease is an immune response to gliadin antigen, a digestion product of gluten which is present in rye, barley, and wheat. Glutamine residues within gliadin are absorbed into the lamina propria of the small intestine and deamidated by tissue transglutaminase (TG2). Deamidated gliadin then binds to the groove on dendritic antigen-presenting cells and the antigen is presented to T-helper cells. Plasma cells then produce IgA antibodies to multiple antigens, including gliadin, tissue transglutaminase, and epidermal transglutaminase. Natural killer lymphocytes cause villous atrophy. Circulating IgA antibodies to TG2 and TG3 result from this process and are an index of the severity of the intestinal inflammatory response. These antibodies decrease with adherence to gluten restriction.

The cutaneous lesions are probably produced by the IgA present in dermal papillae in combination with the epidermal transglutaminase (TG3) antigen. The intestinal inflammatory process is important for the activation of neutrophils, which infiltrate into the dermal papillae where the IgA immune complexes reside. Degranulation of neutrophils releases neutrophilic enzymes, which induce degradation of the lamina lucida and a basement membrane blister.

Clinical Features

Thyroid disorders have been reported in many cases of DH. These disorders include hyperthyroidism, hypothyroidism, thyroid nodules, and asymptomatic goiter. Thyroid peroxidase antibodies are seen in 40% of patients with DH. The abnormal findings are especially prominent in females, and some thyroid abnormality may occur in as many as 40% of female DH patients.

Lymphoma is known to occur with increased prevalence in patients with gluten-sensitive enteropathy. There are many case reports of abdominal lymphoma in patients with DH, but the only controlled study of this phenomenon was performed by Leonard and suggested a slight increase in the incidence of lymphoma (4%) in patients with DH. It was suggested that this incidence may be reduced by a gluten-free diet, although at present there are insufficient data to support this conclusion. An extremely large study would be necessary to evaluate the statistical validity of the association between DH and lymphoma. Consequently, it is best to assume that the incidence is approximately that of celiac disease, and appropriate evaluation should be performed if signs of lymphoma develop.

Differential Diagnosis

The differential diagnoses are those of subepidermal blistering disease, reviewed under the heading of bullous pemphigoid. The main clinical differentiation is with linear IgA disease. Direct immunofluorescence is essential to distinguish between linear IgA disease and dermatitis herpetiformis. Also helpful in differentiating the two is the fact that DH is closely associated with HLA-B8-DR3, whereas linear IgA disease has no HLA associations and does not respond to a gluten-free diet.

Patient Evaluation

Immunofluorescence is essential in diagnosis. Noninflamed perilesional skin harbors the greatest amount of IgA and is

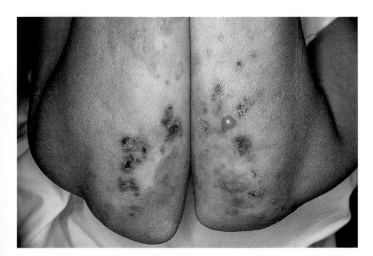

Figure 12–8 Grouped vesicles and bullae on the elbows of this patient with dermatitis herpetiformis. (Reprinted with permission from Callen JP, Greer KE, Paller A, Swinyer L, eds. Color atlas of dermatology: A morphological approach, 2nd edn. Philadelphia: WB Saunders, 2000.)

therefore the preferred biopsy site for direct immunofluorescence when DH is suspected. IgA anti-tissue transglutaminase antibodies are found in the serum of DH patients as well as those with celiac disease, and are an indication of gluten sensitivity. However, serum antibody tests should not be used for diagnosis in the absence of direct immunofluorescence.

Close clinical examination for thyroid nodules and thyromegaly is indicated as a baseline and at return visits. Detailed history of bowel symptoms, including bloating after eating, recurrent abdominal pain, diarrhea, and steatorrhea, is indicated. Patients who do not have obvious signs of gluten-sensitive enteropathy may frequently note improvement in these minimal symptoms when a gluten-free diet is instituted.

A CBC, chemistry profile, and urinalysis are necessary as baseline studies in all patients with DH. This approach not only screens for the malabsorption problems discussed previously, but also represents a baseline for subsequent abnormalities that may be induced by dapsone therapy. Serum thyroxine and thyrotropin hormone levels are evaluated as a baseline in view of the high incidence of thyroid abnormalities. Glucose-6-phosphate dehydrogenase levels should be checked as a baseline in patients who are black or of southern Mediterranean origin, as catastrophic hemolysis may result from the administration of dapsone in deficient patients. Evaluation for associated malabsorption is reviewed in Chapter 25.

Treatment

Dapsone is the drug of choice in the therapy of DH. Treatment with dapsone will adequately suppress (but not cure) the disease. Dapsone treatment requires continued monitoring and may be associated with significant side effects. Dapsone is available in 25 mg and 100 mg tablets. Initial treatment with 25 mg of dapsone by mouth daily usually improves symptoms within 24–48 hours in adults. Correspondingly smaller doses should be used in children. When it is taken daily, dapsone levels reach a steady state within 7 days. Maintenance therapy is then adjusted on a weekly basis to maintain adequate suppression of symptoms; the average maintenance dose is 100 mg daily (range 1–3 mg/kg/day). Occasional new lesions (two or three per week) are to be expected and are not an indication for altering daily dosage. Minor fluctuations in disease severity do occur and are probably related to oral gluten intake. Application of potent topical corticosteroid gel may be helpful in relieving symptoms of individual lesions. Hemolysis is the most common side effect of treatment. Dapsone is a strong oxidizer and produces a dose-related oxidant stress on normal aging red blood cells. Initial reduction of hemoglobin by 2–3 g is common, but subsequent partial compensation by reticulocytosis is the rule. Methemoglobinemia is seldom a severe problem, but it may be tolerated poorly in patients with cardiopulmonary decompensation. Other dose-related side effects are rare with doses <200 mg daily. These include toxic hepatitis, cholestatic jaundice, psychosis, and both motor and sensory neuropathy. Hypoalbuminemia may occur after chronic use. Carcinogenicity of dapsone has been reported in mice and rats, but has not been documented in humans. Rarely, infectious mononucleosis syndrome with fever and lymphadenopathy occurs.

Treatment with a gluten-free diet is successful in more than 90% of cases if the diet is adhered to for a minimum of 3–12 months. In such cases, initial suppression of symptoms with dapsone is usually necessary. When gluten restriction allows a decrease in dapsone requirement, the patient can gradually taper the dosage. Complete control of skin disease on a gluten-free diet obviates the need for hematologic follow-up. It also serves to treat the cause rather than the symptoms of the disease. Disadvantages of a gluten-free diet include the inconvenience of the diet, which some patients may find unappetizing. It must be stressed that the patient should actively participate in the decision to start a gluten-free diet, as individual patients vary in their willingness to take medications or adhere to diets over a prolonged period.

After initial baseline information is collected, a CBC should be checked weekly for 1 month, monthly for 6 months, and semiannually thereafter. Chemistry profile should be checked at 6 months and then annually to monitor for possible hepatotoxicity, changes in renal function, and hypoalbuminemia. IgA tissue transglutaminase antibodies can be monitored as an index of adherence to gluten restriction and improvement of the small intestinal inflammatory process.

LINEAR IgA BULLOUS DERMATOSIS

Linear IgA bullous dermatosis (LABD) is a chronic bullous disorder characterized by erosions and tense blisters, often on an erythematous base (Fig. 12–9). As many as 80% of patients with LABD have oral involvement. It is also known as linear IgA disease, IgA pemphigoid, and linear dermatitis herpetiformis. The distinction between LABD, bullous pemphigoid, and DH was made in 1979 by Chorzelski et al. based on direct immunofluorescence findings which demonstrated linear depositions of IgA along the BMZ in LABD.

Classification

Chronic bullous disease of childhood (CBDC) and LABD share the same histology and immunofluorescence findings. Although they have different clinical presentations, they are considered by most experts to be the same disease.

CBDC occurs in children, with a peak incidence at 4.5 years, and tends to remit by age 13. The characteristic distribution is the lower abdomen and perineum, although the extremities can be involved. Blisters occur in the so-called 'cluster of jewels' configuration, because new lesions appear at the periphery of old ones. Mucosal involvement is reported in 64% of cases.

LABD shows a slight female preponderance, with peak incidence at 60–65 years. Its clinical picture often resembles DH, with pruritic papules and vesicles on the extremities; however, larger vesicles and bullae similar to those of BP may occur. These may be linear or 'sausage shaped.' In about 60% of patients LABD may remit over several years.

LABD is unique in that it may be induced by drugs, and may remit after withdrawal of the offending drug. Vancomycin

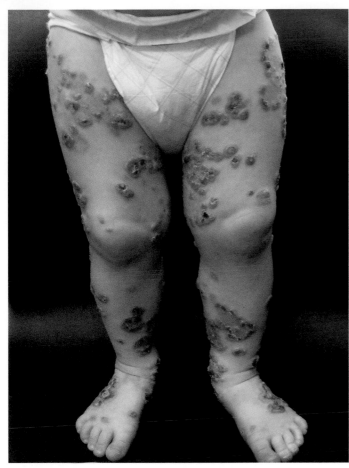

Figure 12–9 Grouped bullae representative of linear IgA bullous dermatosis in this child.

is the most common association, but others include amiodarone, ampicillin, captopril, childhood vaccinations, diclofenac, interferon-γ, interleukin-2, iodine, lithium, penicillin G, phenytoin, piroxicam, rifampin, somatostatin, and trimethoprim–sulfamethoxazole. The pathogenesis of this reaction is not understood.

Pathogenesis

In 1990 Zone et al. identified a 97 kDa protein antigen recognized in adult and childhood sera from LABD patients. This protein is identical to the extracellular portion of collagen XVII (BPAG2, BP180). This protein represents a proteolytic fragment of the shed ectodomain of BPAG2. The mechanism by which IgA basement membrane antibodies cause blistering is yet to be elucidated.

Some patients show linear IgA and linear IgG along the basement membrane, and this is thought to represent an immunologic overlap of LABD and bullous pemphigoid. These patients should be treated according to the predominant antibody pattern.

Numerous case reports link LABD to Hodgkin's disease and other B-cell lymphomas. Transitional cell cancer of the bladder and esophageal cancer have also been reported in association with LABD. Because IgA is among the antibodies deposited at the basement membrane in systemic lupus erythematosus (SLE), it is not clear whether the association between LABD and SLE is a true one. There is a real association between ulcerative colitis and LABD: in fact, one study showed ulcerative colitis present in five of 70 patients with LABD. Other disease associations include multiple sclerosis, dermatomyositis, Crohn's disease, hydatidiform mole, and rheumatoid arthritis.

Multiple drugs have been reported to induce LABD. The reaction usually occurs within days to weeks of ingestion. The most common medication is vancomycin, although penicillins, cephalosporins, ACE inhibitors, and NSAIDs have been reported. Several other medications have been described to produce LABD on rare occasions. A detailed medication history is indicated for all patients with LABD. Most cases resolve in 2–6 weeks after discontinuation of the offending drug.

Differential Diagnosis

The differential diagnosis of LABD is similar to that of the other immunobullous diseases discussed in this chapter. An important differentiation is between LABD and DH, and the key to this distinction is the direct immunofluorescence findings in LABD of linear IgA along the basement membrane. Based on histology alone, without clinical history and examination, LABD can be difficult to distinguish from the bullous eruption of systemic lupus erythematosus. Bullous lupus tends to affect patients already carrying the diagnosis of lupus, or who have other stigmata associated with the disease.

Patient Evaluation

Direct immunofluorescence is the cornerstone to making the diagnosis of LABD. Perilesional skin will show linear deposition of IgA (usually IgA$_1$ subclass, but occasionally IgA$_2$) along the basement membrane. Indirect immunofluorescence is positive in about 60–70% of cases. BMZ split skin is a somewhat more sensitive substrate for indirect immunofluorescence. Not surprisingly, most of the antibodies in LABD bind to the epidermal side of BMZ split skin, similar to the situation seen in bullous pemphigoid, with which LABD shares a major pathogenic antigen, BPAG2.

Treatment

As with other IgA and neutrophil-mediated diseases, the mainstay of treatment for LABD is dapsone. Dosage and management are similar to those used in dermatitis herpetiformis (DH), and the reader is referred to the discussion of this drug in that section of the chapter. As with DH, patients intolerant of dapsone may be controlled with sulfapyridine. There is evidence for the use of colchicine, combination tetracycline and nicotinamide, as well as IVIg in recalcitrant cases. Prednisone and immunosuppressive therapy as described for pemphigus and bullous pemphigoid is successful in resistant cases. LABD is rarely associated with gluten sensitivity, and a gluten-free diet is not indicated unless celiac disease can be documented.

SUGGESTED READINGS

Anhalt GJ, Kim SC, Stanley JR, et al. Paraneoplastic pemphigus. An autoimmune mucocutaneous disease associated with neoplasia. N Engl J Med 1990; 323: 1729–1735.

Bystryn JC, Rudolph JL. IVIg treatment of pemphigus: how it works and how to use it. J Invest Dermatol 2005; 125: 1093–1098.

Egan CA, Lazarova Z, Darling TN, et al. Anti-epiligrin cicatricial pemphigoid: clinical findings, immunopathogenesis, and significant associations. Medicine (Baltimore) 2003; 82: 177–186.

Egan CA, Zone JJ. Linear IgA bullous dermatosis. Int J Dermatol 1999; 38: 818–827.

Green PH, Cellier C. Celiac disease. N Engl J Med 2007; 357: 1731–1743.

Hertl M, Veldman C. Pemphigus – paradigm of autoantibody-mediated autoimmunity. Skin Pharmacol Appl Skin Physiol 2001; 14: 408–418.

Joly P, Mouquet H, Roujeau JC, et al. A single cycle of rituximab for the treatment of severe pemphigus. N Engl J Med 2007; 357: 545–552.

Liu Z, Diaz LA. Bullous pemphigoid: end of the century overview. J Dermatol 2001; 28: 647–650.

Murrell DF, Dick S, Ahmed AR, et al. Consensus statement on definitions of disease, end points, and therapeutic response for pemphigus. J Am Acad Dermatol 2008; 58: 1043–1046.

Rocha-Alvarez R, Ortega-Loayza AG, Friedman H, et al. Endemic pemphigus vulgaris. Arch Dermatol 2007; 143: 895–899.

Sardy M, Karpati S, Merkl B, et al. Epidermal transglutaminase (TGase 3) is the autoantigen of dermatitis herpetiformis. J Exp Med 2002; 195: 747–757.

Stanley JR, Amagai M. Pemphigus, bullous impetigo, and the staphylococcal scalded-skin syndrome. N Engl J Med 2006; 355: 1800–1810.

Woodley DT, Remington J, Chen M, et al. Autoimmunity to type VII collagen: epidermolysis bullosa acquisita. Clin Rev Allergy Immunol 2007; 33: 78–84.

Chapter | **13** | *Edward W. Cowen and Jeffrey P. Callen*

Skin Signs of Internal Malignancy

The skin often reflects internal processes, and patients' awareness of this leads them to consider malignancy as a potential cause for many cutaneous abnormalities. Indeed, there are many skin conditions that have been linked to internal malignancy in a specific and/or nonspecific manner. This chapter considers those cutaneous disorders that have been linked to internal malignancy, the precise manner in which the cutaneous disease and the neoplasm are related, and the evaluation necessary for the patient with a cutaneous sign of internal malignancy.

Curth previously suggested criteria by which to gauge the potential relationship of two disorders, in this case a cutaneous finding and neoplasia (Table 13–1). The disorders may occur concurrently or follow a parallel course; there may be a specific tumor site or cell type associated with the cutaneous disease; there may be a statistical association between the two processes; or there may be a genetic association between the two disorders. In this chapter, we examine these factors to determine whether a 'true' association exists for three categories of skin disease: (1) proliferative and inflammatory dermatoses; (2) hormone-secreting tumors; and (3) inherited syndromes.

PROLIFERATIVE AND INFLAMMATORY DERMATOSES

Acanthosis Nigricans

The characteristic clinical feature of acanthosis nigricans (AN) is hyperpigmented, velvety thickening of the skin on intertriginous surfaces. The eruption usually affects the axillary vault (Fig. 13–1), the neck, inguinal crease, nipples, and umbilicus, but may also involve areas of trauma, such as the elbows, knees, and knuckles. Frequently, the oral mucosa has a papillomatous thickening. In rare instances, the eruption can become generalized (Fig. 13–2). Verrucous or papillary lesions may accompany the typical lesions of AN. Patients may develop multiple seborrheic keratoses simultaneously.

AN can occur in many clinical scenarios, including obesity and insulin resistance, and as a manifestation of a number of heritable diseases (e.g., Crouzon's syndrome, congenital lipodystrophy). Once other associations have been excluded, the possibility of an underlying neoplasm must be strongly considered. In general, patients with malignant AN are older adults with a history of associated weight loss.

AN most often occurs simultaneously with the underlying malignancy; however, patients in whom the dermatosis preceded or followed the malignancy have also been reported. Approximately 90% of the tumors associated with AN arise within the abdominal cavity, particularly the gastrointestinal and genitourinary tracts. Adenocarcinoma of the stomach is the most commonly described cancer associated with malignant AN. However, malignancies outside the abdomen and non-adenocarcinomas have been reported. The course of malignant AN parallels the course of the tumor. The prognosis of malignant AN is poor, owing to the aggressive nature of the tumors with which it is associated. Malignant AN is a prototypic dermatological condition associated with malignancy, fulfilling all of Curth's 'postulates' except a genetic association.

Acrochordons (Skin Tags)

Skin tags are extremely common cutaneous lesions believed to be of little or no significance. Multiple acrochordons have been proposed as a marker of colonic adenomatous polyps. However, more recent studies have not supported an association between acrochordons and colonic polyps or colon cancer. Acrochordons are also a feature of the triad of skin manifestations associated with Birt–Hogg–Dube syndrome (along with fibrofolliculomas and trichodiscomas). However, because of the frequency of acrochordons in the general population, detection of a fibrofolliculoma or trichodiscoma is a more valuable marker for identification of this cancer-related genodermatosis.

Bazex Syndrome

Acrokeratosis paraneoplastica, or Bazex syndrome, is by definition always associated with an underlying malignancy. Acrokeratosis paraneoplastica develops progressively through three stages. The initial cutaneous signs consist of erythematous, violaceous, poorly defined macules with a fine adherent scale that occur over the acral areas of the body, including the fingers, toes, ears, and nose. A paronychial reaction is also

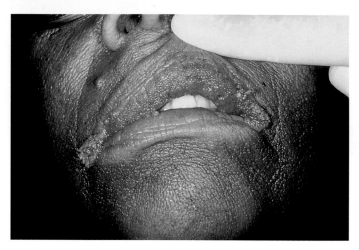

Figure 13–1 Mucosal surfaces may be involved in acanthosis nigricans, as demonstrated by this woman with adenocarcinoma of the stomach. (Courtesy of Dr Mark Holzberg, Atlanta, GA.)

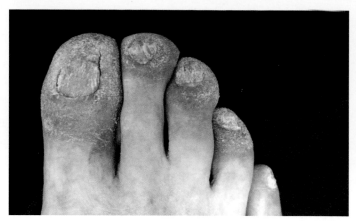

Figure 13–3 Acrokeratosis paraneoplastica. This patient developed an acral violaceous erythema almost simultaneously with a squamous cell carcinoma of his tonsillar pillar.

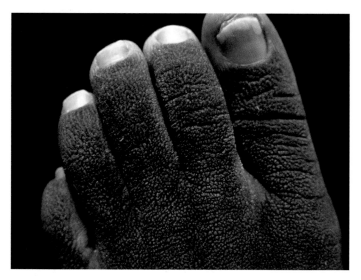

Figure 13–2 Acanthosis nigricans, generalized in a patient who also had erythema gyratum repens.

Table 13–1 Criteria used to associate dermatoses and neoplasia
Concurrent onset
Parallel course
Uniform neoplasm (site or cell type)
Statistical association
Genetic association

common. In the second stage, skin lesions begin to generalize and keratoderma develops. In the third stage, the eruption generalizes but still maintains its violaceous nature and predilection for acral involvement (Fig. 13–3). The three stages of the cutaneous disease parallel the growth and spread of the underlying tumor. Bazex syndrome is more common in men, and the underlying tumors are most often squamous cell carcinomas of the upper aerodigestive tract. As with acanthosis nigricans, the course of cutaneous involvement typically parallels the course of the tumor, thereby fulfilling the criteria to consider it a marker of internal malignancy.

Bowen's Disease

Bowen's disease is a form of squamous cell carcinoma in situ of the skin. Invasion of this neoplastic process can occur late in the course of the disease. Sun exposure and arsenic ingestion have been implicated in the etiology of Bowen's disease. The lesion of Bowen's disease is an erythematous plaque with scale and, occasionally, erosion. Prior to biopsy it is often treated as eczema or as psoriasis, which reveals the true nature of the process.

The frequency of malignancy in patients with Bowen's disease was first reported in 1959 to be as high as 80%; subsequently, however, the same authors revised their figures downward. Later, it was suggested that those patients with lesions on 'nonexposed' surfaces had a much greater propensity for the presence of an underlying malignancy. Data from Denmark do not show an increased risk for malignancy in patients with Bowen's disease or other cutaneous malignancies. No specific type of neoplasm has been strongly associated with Bowen's disease, and no parallel disease course. Thus, at present this entity should not be considered to be a marker of internal malignancy, and patients should not undergo an evaluation beyond the standard history and physical examination and appropriate age-related testing.

Bullous Dermatoses

Several of the bullous dermatoses have been reported to be associated with malignancies. Although the association of malignancy with bullous pemphigoid may be related primarily to the increased incidence of both bullous pemphigoid and malignancy in elderly patients, certain subsets of bullous pemphigoid appear to be associated with an increased risk of malignancy, in particular those patients with negative immunofluorescence results, those who have linear IgA disease, and those who have prominent mucosal lesions. Egan and colleagues reported solid organ malignancies in 10 of 35 patients with anti-epiligrin cicatricial pemphigoid (AECP). In eight cases the cancer was discovered within 14 months of the diagnosis of AECP. AECP is an uncommon, severe, and often scarring mucosal variant of pemphigoid associated with an IgG antibody directed against laminin 5. In contrast, two recent reviews of mucous membrane pemphigoid associated with antibodies to the β4α6 integrin subunits did not identify an increased risk of cancer. Furthermore, a wide variety of neoplasms have been associated with pemphigoid, and there does not appear to be a specific course relating the pemphigoid to the malignancy. Thus, at present the data do not support a relationship between bullous pemphigoid and malignancy, with the possible exception of certain pemphigoid subsets, particularly AECP.

Epidermolysis bullosa acquisita (EBA) has very rarely been associated with malignancy, most commonly of hematologic origin. However, several such reports describe patients with features of both EBA and cicatricial pemphigoid.

The pemphigus group of disorders is most commonly associated with thymoma and lymphoproliferative malignancies. Patients with thymomas also often develop myasthenia gravis. The pemphigus course does not coincide with that of the neoplasm. However, careful review of chest X-ray findings may be prudent to ensure a possible thymoma is not missed. In the early 1990s, Anhalt and coworkers reported an entity that they termed 'paraneoplastic pemphigus' (PNP). Patients with PNP develop severe mucosal erosions and ulcerations, polymorphic cutaneous lesions that may resemble erythema multiforme, and antibodies targeting a number of proteins, particularly envoplakin and periplakin (Fig. 13–4). However, several cases of lichenoid paraneoplastic pemphigus in patients treated with rituximab have been reported in which autoantibody detection was delayed or antibodies were not identified. The term

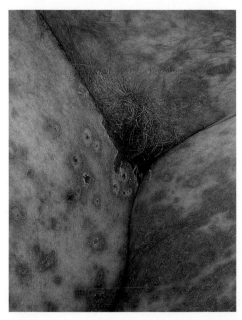

Figure 13–4 Paraneoplastic pemphigus. Multiple erythematous papules and vesicles in the groin of this patient. (Reprinted with permission from Callen JP, Greer KE, Paller A, Swinyer L. Color atlas of dermatology: A morphological approach, 2nd edn. Philadelphia: WB Saunders, 2000.)

paraneoplastic autoimmune multiorgan syndrome (PAMS) has been proposed in order to reflect the multiorgan system involvement now appreciated with PNP. Patients often also develop disease involving their bronchi and may die of respiratory failure (see Chapter 12 for further discussion of PNP/PAMS). The prognosis is poor, with very few survivors.

Intestinal lymphoma has been reported in association with dermatitis herpetiformis. This relationship appears to be caused by the presence of gluten-sensitive enteropathy in patients with this disease. In those patients whose condition is complicated by intestinal lymphoma, the removal of the tumor does not appear to affect the course of the cutaneous disease.

Porphyria cutanea tarda (PCT) has been associated with hepatic tumors, in particular primary hepatoma. This association is most likely a coincidental phenomenon, as hepatitis C virus infection is a risk factor for both PCT and hepatic carcinoma. The exact frequency of hepatic tumors in patients with PCT is not known; however, there are reports of concurrent onset and a parallel disease course. Careful evaluation of the liver, including hepatitis C antibody testing, is advised in all patients with PCT.

Dermatomyositis and Other Collagen–Vascular Disorders

As discussed in Chapter 2, dermatomyositis (DM) is clearly associated with malignancy; however, only rarely do patients with dermatomyositis have a concurrent onset and a parallel course of their tumors. The malignancy work-up of the patient with a new diagnosis of dermatomyositis should include an age-appropriate evaluation. Women should be carefully evaluated for malignancy of the breast and gynecologic system. Ethnicity should also be considered: nasopharyngeal carcinoma was the most common malignancy in a study of DM in Taiwan. All patients should have a chest X-ray and probably a CT scan of the chest and abdomen, as well as a stool hematest. Repeat examination should probably be performed annually for at least the first 3 years following the diagnosis of DM. At all times, unexplained symptoms or signs should be thoroughly evaluated.

Malignancies appear to be a coincidental occurrence in patients with lupus erythematosus. Several reports of lymphoreticular malignancies in patients with systemic lupus erythematosus probably reflect a complication of immunosuppressive therapy. Myeloma and paraproteinemias have been reported in patients with chronic cutaneous lupus erythematosus, but the frequency and significance of these findings are not clear.

Scleroderma may rarely be linked to malignancy, most frequently reported in women with longstanding diffuse involvement. Sites of fibrotic internal organ involvement appear to pose the greatest risk, particularly the lung and esophagus. There does not appear to be an association between the profile of scleroderma-related autoantibodies and the risk of internal malignancy.

The coexistence of cutaneous small-vessel vasculitis and malignant neoplasms has been noted and recently reported as paraneoplastic vasculitis. Cutaneous small-vessel vasculitis is a common finding, as are cutaneous and systemic polyarteritis nodosa. Most of the tumors reported with vasculitis are of the lymphoreticular system (particularly hairy cell leukemia), but sporadic cases associated with solid tumors have also been described. Occasionally the cutaneous disease is the initial finding in these patients, and a parallel course may also occur. The patient with cutaneous vasculitis probably does not require a specific evaluation for malignancy.

Eruptive Angiomas, Telangiectasias, and Seborrheic Keratoses

Reports linking the sudden appearance of angiomas or telangiectasias with internal malignancies have been published in the dermatological literature. Angiomatous lesions are common in the adult population and are seen as small, cherry-colored papules. It is not clear whether, when there is a rapid onset of the lesions, the physician should be concerned about a potential malignancy. The situation in regard to telangiectasias is similarly unclear.

The sudden appearance or growth of multiple seborrheic keratoses is known as the sign of Leser–Trélat (see Fig. 13–1). Numerous reports have linked this condition to various malignancies. Many of these patients also have AN, and the sign of Leser–Trélat is similarly associated with intra-abdominal adenocarcinoma, albeit to a lesser extent than malignant AN. Recent population studies have not demonstrated a link between multiple seborrheic keratoses and internal malignancy. However, a patient has been described who had demonstrable epidermal growth factor receptors on the seborrheic keratosis, with evidence that a melanoma produced this factor. In this patient, when the melanoma was excised, the keratoses regressed. Although all the criteria for an association with malignancy are not fulfilled, it seems reasonable to carefully evaluate patients with a sudden onset or growth of multiple seborrheic keratoses, including evaluation for other epidermal features associated with internal malignancy, such as AN and tripe palms. The work-up should include a history and physical examination, and imaging studies of the gastrointestinal and genitourinary systems.

Erythroderma

Erythroderma (exfoliative dermatitis) is a cutaneous reaction characterized by general erythema, edema, and scaling (see Chapter 10). The reaction may be accompanied by fever, lymphadenopathy, organomegaly, and/or leukocytosis. Malignancy was reported to be present in roughly 10–15% of patients. In most instances the malignancy is in the lymphoreticular system, but several reports of solid tumors have also been published. The course of the cutaneous disease often follows that of the tumor, and the discovery of the malignant process has often been linked to the diagnosis of the cutaneous disorder. Therefore, in all patients with erythroderma the possibility of an underlying neoplasm must be considered.

Figurate Erythemas

There are multiple figurate erythemas, but the only one that truly appears to be related to malignancy is erythema gyratum repens. In this eruption, erythematous lesions form gyrate or serpiginous bands that rapidly spread across the cutaneous surface (Fig. 13–5), producing a 'wood-grained' appearance. Nearly all patients with erythema gyratum repens have an associated malignancy, which is often discovered concurrently. The course also frequently parallels that of the neoplasm. There is no specific type or site for the malignant process. The presence of erythema gyratum repens mandates an extensive internal evaluation for malignancy.

Hypertrichosis Lanuginosa (Malignant Down)

Hypertrichosis is the excessive growth of hair without signs of virilization (Fig. 13–6). The sudden development of fine downy hair has been linked to the presence of an underlying neoplasm in all patients thus far reported. The malignancies are of varied sites and cell types, and are often discovered at the time of the diagnosis of hypertrichosis lanuginosa. Glossitis has also accompanied the malignancy-associated down, but

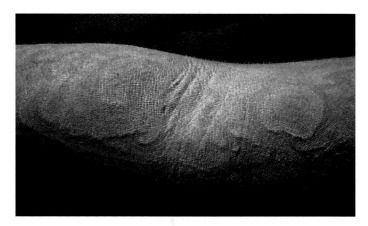

Figure 13–5 Erythema gyratum repens. Multiple bands of erythema in a dark-skinned individual.

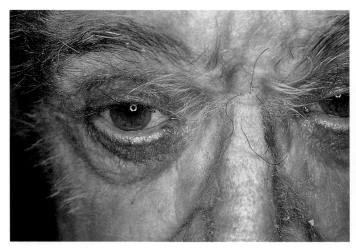

Figure 13–6 Hypertrichosis lanuginosa. This man developed fine lanugo hairs at the same time as he was discovered to have a squamous cell carcinoma of the lung.

it is believed to be a manifestation of vitamin deficiency rather than a related finding. Patients with this type of hair growth who do not have another clear explanation for their condition, such as a medication or endocrinopathy, should be evaluated for the possibility of an internal malignancy.

Acquired Ichthyosis

Acquired ichthyosis resembles ichthyosis vulgaris, and is characterized by rhomboidal scales with margins that are lifted off the surface of the skin. Acquired ichthyosis has been associated with malignancy, particularly lymphoreticular disorders. It was also associated with other paraneoplastic conditions, such as AN or the sign of Leser–Trélat. However, several other conditions have been associated with acquired ichthyosis, including hypothyroidism and sarcoidosis. Although there is a possible relationship with neoplastic diseases, the diagnosis of the malignancy is almost always known at the time of recognition of the ichthyosis.

Keratoacanthoma

Keratoacanthoma is a rapidly growing epidermal neoplasm that may be locally invasive but otherwise exhibits a benign course. In association with sebaceous neoplasms, keratoacanthomas are one of the cardinal features of the Muir–Torre syndrome, a variant of hereditary nonpolyposis colorectal cancer (HNPCC) Lynch syndrome II. Additional sporadic cases describing an association between multiple keratoacanthomas and internal malignancy have been described. However, because patients with keratoacanthoma tend to be elderly, this association may be an age-related phenomenon.

Migratory Thrombophlebitis (Trousseau Syndrome)

Although superficial thrombophlebitis is a relatively common medical condition, migratory thrombophlebitis is associated with a significant risk of underlying malignancy, most frequently of the pancreas, lung, and prostate. The veins of the neck, chest, abdomen, and lower extremities are involved either sequentially or simultaneously. The hypercoagulable state associated with cancer is probably multifactorial in origin, and may be induced by inflammatory cytokines, acute-phase reactants, circulating tissue factor, and cancer microparticles. Patients with migratory thrombophlebitis without a known underlying cause should have a thorough evaluation, including a CT scan of the abdomen.

Multicentric Reticulohistiocytosis

Multicentric reticulohistiocytosis is a rare disorder characterized by polyarthritis and nodular cutaneous lesions. The cutaneous lesions are small flesh-colored to violaceous nodules on the scalp, ears, face, extremities, trunk, and mucous membranes. The arthritis involves the joints of the hand and is destructive, eventually resulting in severe deformities of the fingers (Fig. 13–7). Roughly one-quarter of patients have an associated internal malignancy, usually a carcinoma. The exact

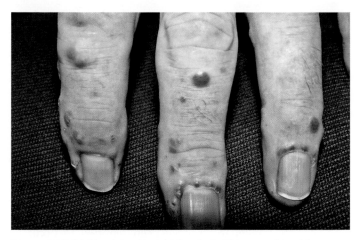

Figure 13–7 Multicentric reticulohistiocytosis. This man did not have a malignancy, but the lesions would be identical.

relationship – specifically the manner in which the disorder is associated with cancer – is not clear.

Mycosis Fungoides (Cutaneous T-Cell Lymphoma)

Cutaneous T-cell lymphoma (CTCL) is often a chronic disease characterized by poikiloderma or erythematous patches, plaques, or tumors (see Chapter 19). The disease is characterized histopathologically by epidermotrophic malignant T cells. Second primary malignancies have been reported to occur in patients with CTCL more frequently than would be predicted. Recent data from the Surveillance, Epidemiology, and End Results (SEER) program identified a significantly elevated risk for Hodgkin's disease and non-Hodgkin's lymphoma. New signs or symptoms in patients with CTCL must be carefully and thoroughly evaluated.

Necrobiotic Xanthogranuloma

The term necrobiotic xanthogranuloma with paraproteinemia was coined by Winkelmann to describe the destructive cutaneous lesions associated with the histopathologic finding of an inflammatory granuloma with xanthomatosis and panniculitis, and an associated paraproteinemia. Clinically, the lesions are yellow to red papules, nodules, or plaques that enlarge and become ulcerative. They have a predilection for periorbital skin. By definition, these lesions are associated with paraproteinemia and, infrequently, with myeloma.

Paget's Disease of the Breast and Extramammary Paget's Disease

Paget's disease of the breast is characterized by an erythematous, eczematous plaque surrounding the nipple and areola. This condition occurs in conjunction with a ductal adenocarcinoma of the breast, which has frequently metastasized to the axillary lymph nodes. Paget's disease is believed to be caused by an upward migration of malignant cells, and hence it is not truly a paraneoplastic sign but rather a specific malignant infiltrate.

Extramammary Paget's disease is the same clinicopathologic lesion as that found in Paget's disease of the breast, but occurs on a nonmammary surface, most often on the genital, axillary, or perianal skin (Fig. 13–8). Roughly 30–50% of patients with this condition have an underlying neoplasm, which generally occurs in areas underlying the area of involvement, such as the genitourinary or gastrointestinal tract. In patients with extramammary Paget's disease an evaluation of the areas contiguous to the disease should be undertaken.

Pityriasis Rotunda

Pityriasis rotunda is an unusual, round, noninflammatory lesion that occurs on the trunk and results in hyperpigmentation. Various malignancies have been reported to occur in conjunction with pityriasis rotunda. The condition has also been reported with numerous other potential etiologic agents. In a recent study from South Africa, pityriasis rotunda was reported in 10 patients, seven of whom had hepatocellular carcinoma. The relationship of this cutaneous condition to malignancy when present is not known. To date, there have not been patients whose pityriasis rotunda has followed the course of their neoplasm. Despite the lack of confirmatory data, it seems prudent to at least consider cancer in anyone with this rare cutaneous disease.

Punctate Keratoses and Arsenical Keratoses of the Palms and Soles

Punctate keratoses are discrete, flesh-colored, hyperkeratotic papules that occur on the palms and soles, most commonly in African-Americans. The lesions often have a central plug or a depressed, crater-like center. They are often numerous, but remain distinct from one another. Symptoms are uncommon.

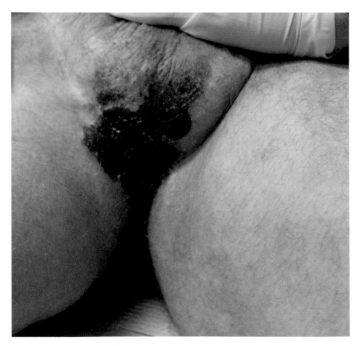

Figure 13–8 Extramammary Paget's disease. Chronic, scaly erythematous plaque in the groin. This patient did not have an underlying neoplasm.

Arsenical keratoses, albeit histopathologically distinct, may be clinically indistinguishable from punctate keratoses. Although the relationship between punctate keratoses and malignancy is controversial at best, chronic arsenic exposure in contaminated drinking water has been associated with bladder and lung carcinoma in addition to nonmelanoma skin cancer.

Pyoderma Gangrenosum and Other 'Neutrophilic' Dermatoses

Cases of various malignancies have been reported infrequently in patients with classic pyoderma gangrenosum. Patients with atypical bullous pyoderma gangrenosum in particular may have myeloid leukemia or be in a pre-leukemic state. Similarly, many patients with Sweet's syndrome (acute febrile neutrophilic dermatosis) have been reported to have myeloid leukemia (Fig. 13–9). Paraneoplastic neutrophilic lesions on the face may simulate erysipelas. In patients with malignancy-associated neutrophilic dermatoses the discovery of the leukemia often occurs simultaneously with the recognition of the cutaneous abnormality. The cutaneous lesions disappear when the leukemia is in remission, and may recur when the leukemia relapses. It seems reasonable to evaluate all patients with atypical pyoderma gangrenosum or Sweet's syndrome with careful hematologic studies, including a bone marrow examination in selected patients.

Pachydermoperiostosis

Acquired pachydermoperiostosis manifests as thickening of the skin, hypertrophic osteoarthropathy, and clubbing of the nails. The condition may result in a coarse facial appearance resembling acromegaly. In addition, the skin of the distal extremities is frequently involved. The palms and soles may also become hyperkeratotic. Clubbing may occur without the other features of the syndrome, but has the same malignancy implications.

These disorders are most frequently associated with lung neoplasia. However, the changes are not exclusively paraneo-

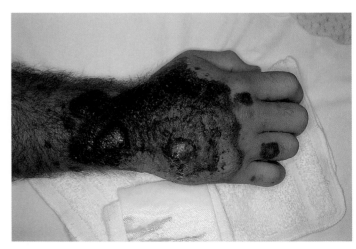

Figure 13–9 Sweet's syndrome (acute febrile neutrophilic dermatosis) in a patient with acute myelogenous leukemia. At the time that this picture was taken he was severely thrombocytopenic, hence the massive hemorrhage.

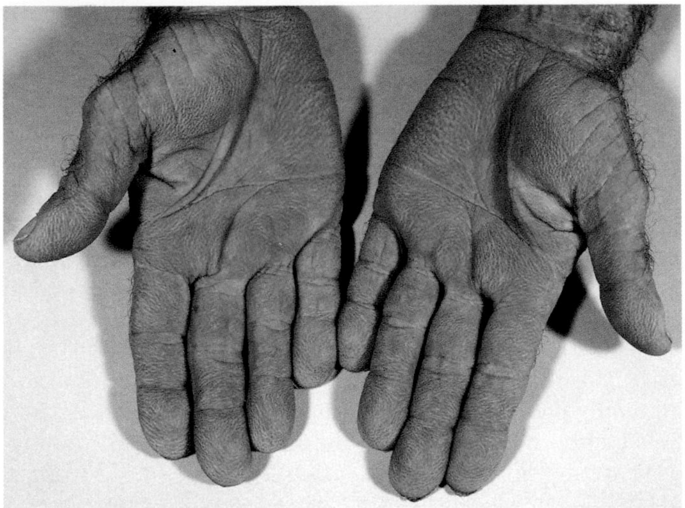

Figure 13–10 Tripe palms: rugose changes on the palms of both hands. (Courtesy of Jon Dyer, MD, Columbia, MO.)

plastic and may also occur in the setting of benign pulmonary and cardiac disease. The incidence of malignancy in patients with pachydermoperiostosis is unknown. Also, it is not clear whether tumor therapy affects the course of the skin or nail disease. Thus, clubbing with or without pachydermoperiostosis should be considered to be a sign of cardiopulmonary disease, and the possibility of lung cancer should be considered.

Tripe Palms

Tripe palms is a cutaneous paraneoplastic syndrome characterized by a thickened, moss-like, velvety texture of the palms (Fig. 13–10). The appearance of the palmar surface is similar to the intertriginous changes found in AN. Some patients with tripe palms also manifest AN, but the majority do not. Often, a malignancy is found concurrently with the recognition of the cutaneous disease. Most of the cancers are found in the stomach and lungs. In the absence of AN, tripe palms is most often associated with a lung cancer. It is not known whether the cutaneous disease course parallels that of the malignancy.

Vitiligo

Vitiligo or a vitiligo-like leukoderma has been reported in conjunction with malignant melanoma. Furthermore, a recent report linked vitiligo in older individuals (over 40 years) with various malignant neoplasms. This association has not been confirmed. In the authors' view, the onset of vitiligo in an adult warrants a full skin examination, including a Wood's light examination.

HORMONE-SECRETING SYNDROMES

Carcinoid Syndrome

Carcinoid syndrome is produced by tumors that secrete 5-hydroxytryptamine (5HT) and other vasoactive amines. The tumors are most common in the gastrointestinal tract, but they

also occur in the lungs or ovaries. Clinically, flushing, diarrhea, abdominal pain, wheezing, and occasionally shortness of breath occur. Tumors from the gastrointestinal tract do not produce symptoms until they metastasize to the liver, because under normal circumstances the liver is able to detoxify the amines responsible for the production of symptoms. Tumors in other locations are capable of producing symptoms prior to metastasis. The diagnosis of carcinoid syndrome is made by finding elevated levels of 5-hydroxyindoleacetic acid (or other metabolites or vasoactive amines) in the urine. Removal of the tumor results in a cessation of symptoms.

Ectopic Adrenocorticotropic Syndrome

Certain tumors are capable of amine precursor uptake and decarboxylation and are therefore known as APUDomas. These tumors usually originate in the lungs (bronchial adenoma or oat cell carcinoma), gastrointestinal tract (carcinoid), or glandular tissues. Ectopic adrenocorticotropic hormone (ACTH)-producing tumors result in many of the typical signs and symptoms of Cushing's syndrome, with the exception of obesity. Intense hyperpigmentation is rare in Cushing's disease, but is common in patients with ectopic production of ACTH. The most common tumor that produces this syndrome is oat cell carcinoma of the lung.

Necrolytic Migratory Erythema (Glucagonoma Syndrome)

Necrolytic migratory erythema is an eruption strongly associated with glucagon-producing pancreatic neoplasms (see Chapter 21). The characteristic cutaneous eruption begins in the groin area as irregular erythematous patches studded with superficial flaccid erosions, vesicles, and bullae. The erythema and bullous lesions may coalesce into circinate and/or polycyclic psoriasiform plaques. The eruption may be confused with seborrheic dermatitis, intertrigo, or candidiasis. Erythematous lesions at the corners of the mouth (angular cheilitis) and glossitis also develop. Other findings include new-onset diabetes mellitus, anemia, weight loss, and diarrhea. The clinical and histological similarity of necrolytic migratory erythema to acrodermatitis enteropathica and vitamin B deficiencies suggests that necrolytic migratory erythema may be a skin manifestation of nutritional deficiency induced by excessive glucagon secretion by the pancreatic tumor. In fact, iatrogenic necrolytic migratory erythema has been induced by the administration of glucagon to treat persistent hypoglycemia. Although removal of the glucagonoma results in resolution of skin symptoms, more than 50% of patients have hepatic metastases at the time of diagnosis, so the prognosis is generally poor.

INHERITED SYNDROMES ASSOCIATED WITH INTERNAL CANCER

Birt–Hogg–Dube Syndrome (OMIM #135150)

Birt–Hogg–Dube syndrome was first described in 1977 as a triad of fibrofolliculoma, trichodiscoma, and acrochordon.

Subsequent to this description, Birt–Hogg–Dube syndrome was linked to a risk of spontaneous pneumothorax and renal cell cancer. Mutations in the BHD gene, FLCN, on chromosome 17p11.2, were identified in 2002, but the function of the folliculin protein remains unclear. Characteristic fibrofolliculoma facial lesions begin in the third decade as small white to skin-colored flat papules, and may range from few scattered lesions to near-confluent involvement of the face and neck (Fig. 13–11). Affected individuals may develop multiple renal neoplasms of variable histology simultaneously in both kidneys, including unusual oncocytic–chromophobe hybrid tumors.

Cowden's Disease (OMIM #158350)

Cowden's disease, Bannayan–Ruvalcaba–Riley syndrome, and Lhermitte–Duclos disease share overlapping clinical features, including macrocephaly, hamartomatous gastrointestinal polyps, and lipomas, and are collectively referred to as PTEN hamartoma tumor syndromes. The most characteristic findings of Cowden's disease are trichilemmomas located around the nose and central face, multiple keratotic papules on the face, neck, ears, and hands, and multiple papules on the oral mucosa that coalesce to form a cobblestone appearance. Systemic

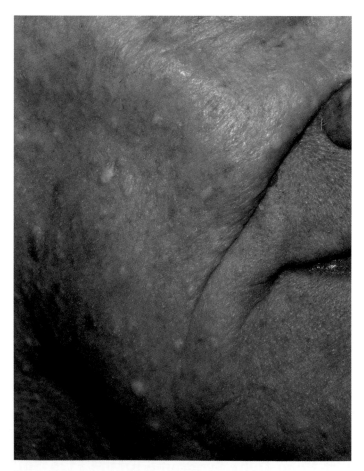

Figure 13–11 Birt–Hogg–Dube syndrome. Multiple white fibrofolliculomas on the face.

manifestations include polyposis of the gastrointestinal tract, tumors of the thyroid gland, ovarian cysts, and fibrocystic disease of the breast. All of the hamartoma tumor syndromes are associated with germline mutations in the PTEN gene (10q23.3) and an increased risk of malignancy in several organ systems. Women are at very high risk of breast cancer, often bilateral, but men with Cowden's disease are at risk of breast malignancy as well. The overall prevalence of malignant tumors may be as high as 40–50%, specifically adenocarcinoma of the breast (20%), adenocarcinoma of the thyroid (7%), squamous cell carcinoma of the skin (4%), and cancers of the colon, prostate, uterus, cervix, bladder, or blood (<1% each). A careful evaluation of patients with this syndrome and all family members for underlying malignancies is necessary. Some authorities have even gone so far as to suggest prophylactic mastectomy in women with this disease.

Gardner's Syndrome (OMIM #175100)

Gardner's syndrome is a variant of familial adenomatosis polyposis. Patients with Gardner's syndrome develop epidermoid cysts, fibromas, lipomas, and desmoid tumors. Multiple osteomas may develop. Bilateral congenital hypertrophy of the retinal pigment epithelium is an early ocular finding. Epidermoid cysts appear in early childhood on the face, trunk, and scalp, and may precede the identification of colonic polyposis by many years. Concern for malignant transformation of the polyps often leads to prophylactic total colectomy in childhood. Patients are also at risk of neoplasia of other organ systems, particularly central nervous system malignancy (Turcot's syndrome).

Hereditary Leiomyomatosis and Renal Cell Cancer (OMIM #150800)

Hereditary leiomyomatosis and renal cell cancer is an autosomal dominant cancer syndrome characterized by cutaneous leiomyomas, uterine leiomyomas (fibroids), and renal cell cancer. Germline mutations in fumarate hydratase (FH), a Krebs' cycle enzyme, predispose to this syndrome. Cutaneous leiomyomas are ovoid pink nodules that often cluster together. They are frequently described as painful or sensitive to touch (Fig. 13–12). Uterine fibroids are nearly universal in women with FH mutations, leading in most cases to hysterectomy. The penetrance of renal cell cancer in affected individuals is lower than that of cutaneous and uterine leiomyomas. However, FH mutation-related renal cell cancer typically follows an aggressive clinical course, and regular screening is necessary for early detection of these tumors.

Multiple Endocrine Neoplasia (OMIM #131100 (Type 1); #171400 (2A); #162300 (2b))

The multiple endocrine neoplasias (MEN) are discrete dominantly inherited genetic disorders associated with a very high prevalence of benign and malignant endocrine neoplasms.

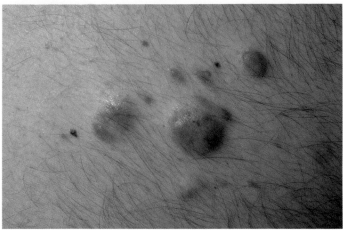

Figure 13–12 Hereditary leiomyomatosis and renal cell cancer. Cluster of painful red nodular leiomyomas on the upper back.

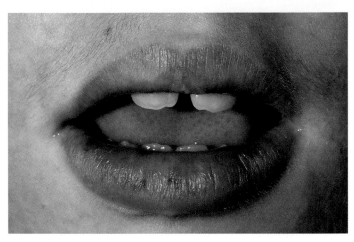

Figure 13–14 Peutz–Jeghers syndrome. Multiple lentiginous macules on the lips.

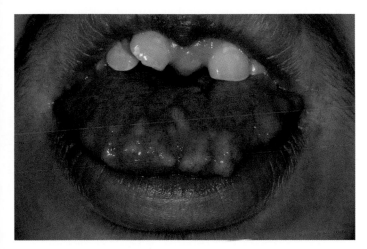

Figure 13–13 MEN 2b. Thickened lips and multiple neuromas of the tongue in a young man with metastatic medullary thyroid carcinoma.

MEN type 1 is associated with parathyroid adenoma in nearly all patients, as well as pituitary tumors, and a variety of pancreatic neoplasms. Multiple facial angiofibromas are common in MEN 1. Collagenomas, café-au-lait macules, gingival papules, and lipomas are less frequent cutaneous findings. Patients with MEN 2a develop parathyroid adenoma, pheochromocytoma, and medullary thyroid carcinoma. The only cutaneous manifestation of MEN 2a is lichen amyloidosis. MEN 2b is associated with mucosal and intestinal neuromatosis, pheochromocytoma, and medullary thyroid carcinoma. Affected individuals present with a marfanoid habitus and coarse facial features, the latter due to neuronal infiltration of the eyelids, lips, and tongue (Fig. 13–13).

Muir–Torre Syndrome (OMIM #158320)

Muir–Torre syndrome is a variant of hereditary nonpolyposis colorectal cancer (HNPCC) Lynch syndrome II with multiple sebaceous tumors, including adenomas, adenocarcinomas, and epitheliomas. It is associated with deleterious mutations in DNA mismatch repair genes, including MLH1 and MSH2. The presence of multiple sebaceous tumors or keratoacanthomas, or early onset of these skin lesions, should prompt a careful personal and family history evaluation for similar skin lesions and internal malignancy. If suggestive features are identified, testing for mutations in the mismatch repair genes is warranted. Although the visceral tumors in patients with Muir–Torre syndrome appear to behave in a more benign fashion than similar sporadic tumors, 60% will develop metastatic disease. In addition, 50% of patients with Muir–Torre syndrome present with an internal malignancy before manifesting skin lesions. Therefore, careful screening of other at-risk family members is important.

Peutz–Jeghers Syndrome (OMIM #175200)

Mucocutaneous pigmented macules (Fig. 13–14) and hamartomatous polyps of the gastrointestinal tract are characteristic of Peutz–Jeghers syndrome. Lentigines tend to cluster around the lips, on the oral mucosa, and on acral areas of the body. This disorder is inherited in an autosomal dominant pattern, but spontaneous mutations account for 50% of the cases. Peutz–Jeghers syndrome is associated with germline mutations in the LKB1 gene (19p13.3) which encodes a multifunctional serine–threonine kinase. Affected individuals may present in adolescence with anemia, bloody stools, or intermittent abdominal pain due to intussusception from intestinal polyps. Increased aromatase activity resulting from calcifying Sertoli cell testicular tumors may induce gynecomastia as another presenting sign of the syndrome in boys. Patients are at an increased risk of both intestinal and extraintestinal malignancies, including breast, pancreatic, ovarian, testicular, and cervical cancer, mandating yearly cancer screening beginning at age 10.

Table 13–2 Paraneoplastic disorders

Disorders that fit Curth's criteria

Acanthosis nigricans and possibly the sign of Leser–Trélat
Bazex syndrome
Carcinoid syndrome
Ectopic ACTH syndrome
Erythema gyratum repens
Glucagonoma syndrome
Hypertrichosis lanuginosa
Neutrophilic dermatoses
Paget's disease
Paraneoplastic pemphigus

Disorders associated statistically with cancer

Arsenical keratoses
Bowen's disease
Dermatomyositis
Exfoliative dermatitis
Extramammary Paget's disease
Generalized pruritus without a primary cutaneous eruption
Mycosis fungoides
Pityriasis rotunda
Porphyria cutanea tarda

Dermatoses possibly associated with cancer

Acquired ichthyosis
Anti-epiligrin cicatricial pemphigoid
Multicentric reticulohistiocytosis
Necrobiotic xanthogranuloma
Classic pyoderma gangrenosum
Polymyositis
Tripe palms
Vasculitis
Vitiligo

ACTH = adrenocorticotropic hormone.

von Recklinghausen's Disease (OMIM #162200)

von Recklinghausen's disease (neurofibromatosis) is an autosomal dominant disorder that is discussed elsewhere (see Chapter 36). Approximately 2–5% of the patients with this syndrome will develop a malignancy, many of which represent a malignant degeneration of the neurofibroma. However, these patients may also develop astrocytomas, glioblastomas, meningiomas, and bilateral pheochromocytomas. If the patient with neurofibromatosis develops symptoms of headache, backache, or hypertension, the potential for internal malignancy must be considered, and appropriate tests should be ordered.

CONCLUSIONS

The cutaneous disorders associated with malignancy are reviewed in Table 13–2. They are classified as: (1) those that fit Curth's postulates and thus warrant specific investigation; (2) those that are statistically related to internal malignancy but do not require extensive malignancy investigations; and (3) those with only a possible association with cancer. Further work is needed to delineate the exact relationship of these cutaneous disorders with their potentially associated internal neoplasms. Epidemiologic studies that involve statisticians in the experimental design are needed to further evaluate many of the syndromes that may be malignancy-related.

SUGGESTED READINGS

Anhalt GJ. Paraneoplastic pemphigus. Adv Dermatol 1997; 12: 77–96.

Brenner S, Tamir E, Maharshak N, Shapira J. Cutaneous manifestations of internal malignancies. Clin Dermatol 2001; 19: 290–297.

Callen JP, ed. Skin signs of internal malignancy. Semin Dermatol 1984; 3: 265–359.

Curth HO. Skin lesions and internal carcinoma. In: Andrade R, Gumport SL, Popkin GL, Reed TD, eds. Cancer of the skin. Philadelphia: WB Saunders, 1976; 1308–1343.

Egan CA, Lazarova Z, Darling TN, et al. Anti-epiligrin cicatricial pemphigoid and relative risk for cancer. Lancet 2001; 357: 1850–1851.

Moore RL, Dever TS. Epidermal manifestations of internal malignancy. Dermatol Clin 2008; 26: 17–29.

Nguyen VT, Ndoye A, Bassler KD, et al. Classification, clinical manifestations, and immunopathological mechanisms of the epithelial variant of paraneoplastic autoimmune multiorgan syndrome: a reappraisal of paraneoplastic pemphigus. Arch Dermatol 2001; 137: 193–206.

Ponti G, Ponz de Leon M. Muir–Torre syndrome. Lancet Oncol 2005; 6: 980–987.

Thiers BH, Callen JP, Cannick L. Dermatologic manifestations of internal malignancy. In: Rigel DS, Friedman RJ, Dzubow LM, et al., eds. Cancer of the skin. Philadelphia: Elsevier, 2005; 371–384.

Wooton M. Systemic sclerosis and malignancy: a review of the literature. South Med J 2008; 101: 59–62.

Chapter | **14** | *Warren W. Piette*

Metastatic Disease

The skin is an uncommon site of metastasis. Recognition of cutaneous metastases is important, however, as skin metastases may be the first sign of malignancy, may represent the most accessible site to obtain histologic confirmation of tumor origin in a patient suspected of having a malignancy, or may affect therapeutic decisions as the first sign of extranodal metastatic disease in a patient with known malignancy.

EPIDEMIOLOGY

Studies published before 1970 found a frequency range of 0.7–4.4% for cutaneous metastases in cancer patients. Brownstein and Helwig found that sarcomas with cutaneous metastases represented only 3% of all such metastases in men and 2% in women. A 1987 study by Spencer and Helm found a 9% incidence of cutaneous metastases at autopsy in 7518 patients with carcinoma (including melanoma), sarcoma and bone marrow and lymphopoietic malignancies, with a 6.6% incidence of cutaneous spread by leukemia or lymphoma.

In a 1990 study, Lookingbill et al. found just under a 5% incidence of cutaneous metastases in 7316 patients with carcinoma (excluding melanoma). The incidence of cutaneous metastases at the time of cancer diagnosis was 1%, and in only 0.6% was the skin metastasis the first sign of internal cancer. In a 1993 follow-up study of carcinoma, 10.4% of 4020 patients with metastatic carcinoma (including melanoma) had cutaneous metastases. In 7.6% of these cases (6.4% if melanoma is excluded) skin metastasis was the first sign of extranodal disease. The tumor types in the 427 patients with cutaneous metastases in the 1993 study are shown in Table 14–1, including the difference in incidence of tumor types between men and women. Solitary cutaneous metastases of carcinomas are most frequently associated with lung cancers (53% of lung patients with cutaneous metastases) or an unknown primary (35%). A retrospective analysis spanning 1990 to 2005 of patients with biopsy-proven skin metastases and correlative clinical data and most with known stage IV cancer, found that skin metastasis was the presenting sign in 12% (6 of 50). In 45% of biopsies from these patients, the lesions were not suspected of being skin metastases because of unusual clinical presentations. Metastases from small cell car-cinomas and sarcomas were histologically misinterpreted as primary skin tumors. A study from 2007 of 1287 patients with internal malignancy found a 27.4% rate of metastasis, with cutaneous metastases found in only 1.2% of all patients, most frequently nodules localized on the anterior chest. In only one case was cutaneous metastasis the presenting sign.

Melanoma and cancers of the breast and upper respiratory tract have the highest tendency to metastasize to skin: more than 10% of metastases by these tumor types are to skin. In contrast, lung and colorectal cancers have a very low tendency to metastasize to skin. Despite this, they are still common causes of cutaneous metastases simply because they are such common cancers.

PATHOGENESIS

The exact mechanisms leading to invasion and metastasis of tumors are not known, but a number of factors have some theoretic and experimental support. There is evidence that some metastases are produced from a specialized minor sub-population of cells; that some metastases are clonal in origin; and that tumor cells are usually less genetically stable than nonmetastatic tumor cells. This evidence suggests that most cells in a tumor are not important in terms of metastasis because they lack the particular factors needed to establish distant metastases.

In order to metastasize, tumor cells must successfully complete multiple critical steps in sequence. For a carcinoma, this might begin with invasion through an epithelial basement membrane into the extracellular environment. Very quickly, the tumor must solicit invasion of new vessels or vessel progenitors into the tumor itself. Next, one or more cells must cross the differently composed basement membrane of the vessel, intercalate between the endothelial cells themselves, and invade the circulation, a process termed intravasation. Once in the circulation, they must survive for some indefinite period in a suspended state. Normally, loss of adhesion in epithelial cells triggers a process known as anoikis, leading to apoptotic cell death. Avoiding apoptosis is obviously critical to surviving in the circulation long enough to accomplish the next steps in metastasis, which include adhesion to a distant

Table 14–1 Cutaneous involvement by carcinoma (including melanoma)* (Lookingbill et al. 1993)

Distribution in men (n = 127)		Distribution in women (n = 300)	
Primary site	*Rounded (%)*	*Primary site*	*Rounded (%)*
Melanoma	32%	Breast	71%
Lung (13/19 adenocarcinoma, 2/19 oat cell carcinoma)	12%	Melanoma	12%
Colon/rectum	11%	Ovary, unknown primary, oral cavity, lung**	5–2%
Oral cavity	9%	Colon/rectum, endometrium, bladder, uterine cervix, stomach, bile duct, pancreas, endocrine**	<2%
Unknown primary	9%		
Larynx	6%		
Kidney, upper digestive tract, breast, nasal sinuses, bladder, esophagus**	5–2%		
Endocrine, stomach, pancreas, liver**	<2%		

*Carcinoma accounts for the overwhelming majority of cutaneous metastastes (see text).
**Listed in descending order of frequency.

capillary bed, and extravasation between the endothelial cells and across the vessel membrane. Tumor extravasation probably mirrors many aspects of normal leukocyte trafficking, adhesion, and extravasation. Tumor cells must next invade a different extracellular environment, proliferate, and re-establish a vascular supply. Studies suggest that a large number of cells may enter the circulation, and that many may even successfully exit the circulation, but most fail to proliferate in a foreign extracellular environment, making colonization of the target organ the most challenging phase of metastasis. Many advances in cancer therapy may result from a better understanding of tumor immunology and of the molecular mechanisms for each of these critical steps in metastasis. The relative role of tumor cell properties and host defense mechanisms in the metastatic process is unknown.

CLINICAL MANIFESTATIONS

Site

Tumor may spread to the skin by direct extension from an underlying malignancy, through lymphatic conduits to the skin, by metastasis or embolization through lymphatic or blood vessels, or rarely through direct implantation of tumor during surgery (oral cavity, laryngeal, kidney, colorectal, breast, ovarian), or following thoracocentesis and percutaneous needle biopsies of pleura, prostate, liver, kidney, pancreas, and thyroid.

The generalization that most cutaneous metastatic deposits overlie the primary tumor is only partially accurate. For example, breast and oral cavity cancers preferentially involve the anterior chest and face, respectively, whereas lung and kidney carcinomas may metastasize to any region of the skin.

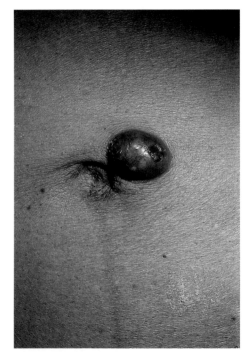

Figure 14–1 Sister Mary Joseph's nodule. Metastatic adenocarcinoma of the stomach to an area near the umbilicus.

The scalp, face, and neck are the most common cutaneous metastatic sites for breast, lung, and oral cavity cancers. The chest is most often involved by breast or lung carcinoma. Metastases to the back and extremities are unusual. Intra-abdominal, pelvic, and breast malignancies sometimes metastasize to the umbilicus, giving rise to the so-called Sister Mary Joseph's nodule, named after the nurse who first described this phenomenon (Fig. 14–1).

Appearance

Cutaneous metastases most commonly manifest as single or clusters of flesh-colored or slightly erythematous nodules. Although ulceration may occur, it is unknown in metastatic carcinoma (Fig. 14–2). Depending on the type of cancer, its vascularity, and any associated pigment production, lesions may also be violaceous, pink, brown, black, or white. Most cutaneous metastases occur as multiple nodules.

Certain patterns of cutaneous metastasis are noteworthy, and most of these occur more often as a manifestation of breast carcinoma than of any other tumor (Table 14–2). Nodules in the scalp may cause circumscribed hair loss termed alopecia neoplastica, which may be cicatricial (Fig. 14–3). Lymphatic obstruction may result in superficial nonpitting dermal edema with depressions at the site of hair follicles, resulting in an orange-peel or peau d'orange appearance. Massive lymphatic obstruction by inflammatory breast cancer may appear as carcinoma erysipelatoides, a condition resembling erysipelas wherein the chest wall skin manifests warmth, erythema, edema, and tenderness. Sometimes confused with

mastitis, this condition can be differentiated because the sudden onset, fever, chills, and elevated white blood cell count seen in mastitis are not present in metastatic carcinoma. Inflammatory carcinoma may also be seen in association with metastases from the pancreas, parotid, tonsils, stomach, lung, colon, rectum, and pelvis (Fig. 14–4). The first sign of colorectal adenocarcinoma may be inflammatory carcinoma of the inguinal region, supraclavicular area, or head and neck. Breast

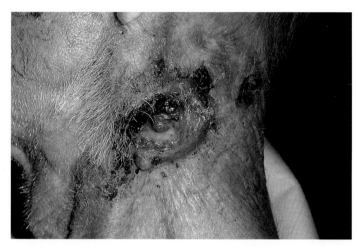

Figure 14–2 A large, nodular lesion, representative of metastatic disease from the larynx.

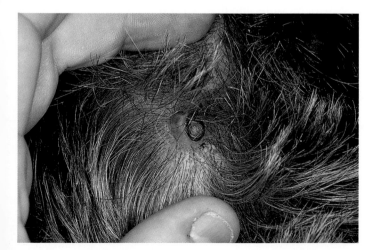

Figure 14–3 This nodule in the scalp represents metastatic renal cell carcinoma.

Table 14–2 Cutaneous presentations of breast carcinoma
Nodules: most breast cancer metastases, whether local or distant, are nodular, with just under 10% of nodules showing ulceration. Some may mimic cylindromas or pilar cysts.
Inflammatory: up to 10% of breast cancer metastases, more common in women with pendulous breasts. Erythematous patch or plaque with an active spreading border resembling erysipelas. Occasionally may mimic erythema annulare. Clinical appearance of inflammation is caused by capillary congestion from tumor cells, and there is minimal to no inflammatory infiltrate on biopsy.
Bullous, lymphangiomatous, or zosteriform pattern: breast, rarely lung, cervical, gastric, or ovarian carcinoma.
Sclerotic syndromes: **Cicatricial**: alopecia in scalp shows scarring alopecia, typically painless, nonpruritic, pink to red, and smooth-surfaced. This is more likely to represent hematogenous, rather than lymphatic, spread. Scalp plaques may also resemble discoid lupus, lichen planopilaris, pseudopelade, or morpheaform basal cell carcinoma. **Morphea-like (eburneum carcinoma)**: breast, rarely stomach, lung, mixed tumor, lacrimal gland. **Carcinoma telangiectasia**: pinpoint telangiectases or telangiectatic papules, which may overlie sclerotic plaques, or may present as violaceous papulovesicles resembling lymphangioma circumscriptum. **Carcinoma en cuirasse**: fibrosis affecting trunk, causing encased (en cuirasse) appearance. Usually begins as scattered firm papulonodules, which coalesce into a noninflammatory sclerodermoid plaque. **Eburneum carcinoma or carcine eburnée** is used to describe less extensive sclerodermoid change, and cancer cells may be sparse and difficult to identify histologically.
Paget's disease: sharply demarcated plaque of patch or erythema and scaling on nipple or areola. Almost always associated with underlying cancer. **Extramammary Paget's disease** can resemble Paget's clinically and histologically. May occur in the axilla, external ear canal, eyelid, or anogenital region, and may at times be verrucous. There are three types: one unassociated with cancer, one associated with an adjacent apocrine or eccrine gland carcinoma, and one associated with visceral cancer, usually gastrointestinal or genitourinary.
Breast carcinoma of the inframammary crease: exophytic nodule clinically suggestive of a primary cutaneous squamous or basal cell carcinoma, intertrigo, or callus. More likely to occur in women with pendulous breasts.
Metastatic mammary carcinoma of the eyelid: painless eyelid swelling with induration or nodularity. Described in at least 13 patients. In 8, lesion had prominent histiocytoid lesions microscopically.

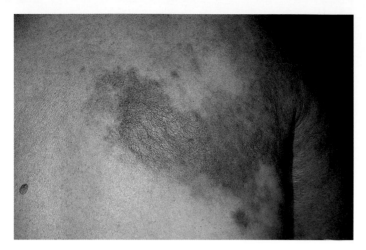

Figure 14–4 Metastatic carcinoma with a cellulitic appearance on the back as a result of carcinoma of the breast. This patient also had dermatomyositis.

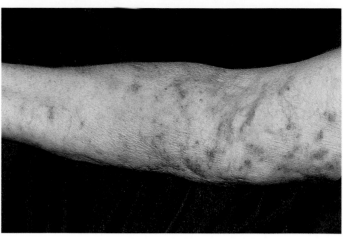

Figure 14–5 Stewart–Treves syndrome. Reoccurrence of breast carcinoma in an arm with lymphedema following an axillary node dissection.

cancer may also present on the anterior chest wall as a nodular sclerotic plaque termed carcinoma telangiectasia, which is characterized by broad sclerotic plaques containing multiple overlying telangiectasias and telangiectatic papules. A variant called carcinoma en cuirasse, also the result of lymphatic obstruction from breast cancer, manifests as intensely sclerotic plaques that may be studded with nodules. Another sclerotic variant of metastatic breast cancer called eburneum carcinoma appears as morphea-like plaques in which sparsely distributed cancer cells may be difficult to identify.

Colorectal adenocarcinoma, in addition to presenting as inflammatory carcinoma, may also appear as a sessile or pedunculated nodule on the buttocks, grouped vascular nodules on groin or scrotal skin, a facial tumor, scalp cyst, persistent cutaneous fistulation after surgery, or may mimic hidradenitis suppurativa.

The characteristic pattern and appearance of metastatic lesions may be altered when such lesions arise in areas of previously damaged skin. For example, if metastases develop in an area of skin previously injured by radiation therapy directed at the primary tumor, the cutaneous metastases are much more likely to show early erosion or ulceration and may be associated with radiation therapy-related hyperpigmentation, telangiectases, or atrophy. Metastatic lesions in such a location may be difficult to differentiate from a primary carcinoma because neoplasms such as basal cell and squamous cell carcinomas, sarcoma, and atypical fibroxanthoma may arise de novo in areas of radiation dermatitis and, occasionally, from other types of chronic injury, such as burn scars or chronic cutaneous ulcers.

Special Types

Cutaneous angiosarcomas usually present in elderly individuals as ill-defined dark red to dark blue nodules and plaques, often located on the scalp or face. This subset of angiosarcoma is thought to arise in the skin. Typically, its extent at the time of diagnosis is well beyond clinically apparent margins, due

both to direct invasion and to more distant cutaneous metastasis. Also, angiosarcoma or lymphangiosarcoma may arise in vessels of chronic cavernous hemangiomas (rarely in port-wine stains) or in areas of chronic lymphedema, such as those that may develop in the upper extremities following mastectomy and axillary node dissection (Stewart–Treves syndrome) (Fig. 14–5). Although probably beginning at a single site, these types of tumors often remain undetected until multiple local metastases have developed.

Metastatic renal cell carcinoma accounts for some particularly interesting phenomena. Although renal cell carcinoma accounts for only about 2% of neoplasms, it may account for up to 10% of cutaneous metastases. As previously mentioned, it metastasizes to the scalp more frequently than do most other tumors. Moreover, there is a high incidence of metastasis occurring late – often 3 or more years after apparent complete removal of the primary tumor. Renal cell carcinoma and thyroid carcinoma are the two types of internal malignancy most likely to have frankly vascular cutaneous metastases, which may be easily compressible, may rapidly refill on the release of pressure, and may even pulsate spontaneously, especially if situated over a bony surface, such as on the scalp or forehead. At least one case of renal cell carcinoma mimicking Kaposi's sarcoma clinically and histologically has been described.

Cutaneous carcinomas rarely occur in children, probably because carcinoma itself is rare in this age group. Leukemia is the second most common cause of skin metastases in children, neuroblastoma metastases being the most common. Neuroblastoma is the most common solid malignant tumor of childhood, and cutaneous metastases are frequent in infants with this disease, becoming much less frequent with increasing age (32% of neonatal patients, but only 3% of patients of all ages). The lesions are usually bluish nodules, sometimes termed 'blueberry muffin' (a term also used for some lesions of ectopic hematopoiesis seen in early childhood). A characteristic feature is blanching induced by palpation or stroking of lesions. This blanching usually lasts 30–60 minutes and is

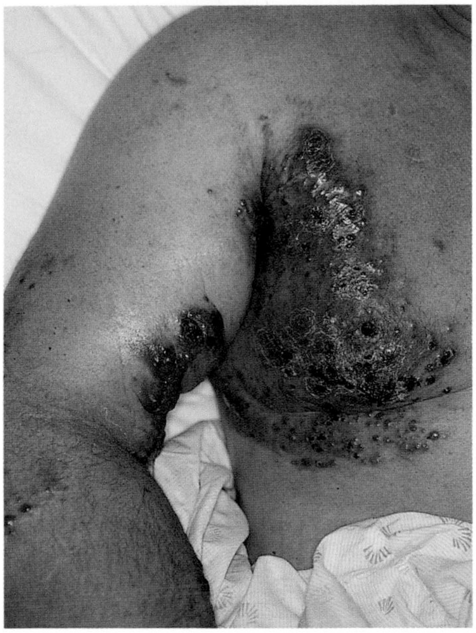

Figure 14–6 Multiple pigmented nodules from metastatic melanoma.

followed by a 2-hour refractory period. Two other frequent manifestations of neuroblastoma include periorbital ecchymoses ('raccoon eyes') and heterochromia iridis, a variation in the color of the iris.

Melanoma is usually cutaneous in origin, and it often develops multiple metastatic cutaneous or visceral lesions (Fig. 14–6). Kaposi's sarcoma is another tumor that is cutaneous in origin and frequently has multiple cutaneous – and occasionally visceral – lesions. Evidence suggests that these multiple lesions represent a multifocal origin of the tumor rather than multiple metastatic lesions, due to transformation by herpes virus. Primary cutaneous tumors, such as Merkel cell tumors, atypical fibroxanthomas, malignant fibrohistiocytomas of the skin, dermatofibrosarcoma protuberans, sebaceous carcinomas, melanomas, squamous cell carcinomas, and even basal cell carcinomas, may occasionally develop noncutaneous metastatic lesions. In this setting, it is important to recognize the cutaneous lesions as the primary malignancy rather than as a manifestation of a noncutaneous primary tumor.

DIFFERENTIAL DIAGNOSIS

Because of the multiple clinical presentations of cutaneous metastases, the differential diagnosis can include a wide range of changes in the skin induced by inflammation, infection, benign neoplasia, and primary malignant cutaneous tumors, as noted previously and in Table 14–2. A biopsy specimen should be obtained from any patient presenting with the recent finding of one or more growing nodules, particularly if inflammation is absent. In other settings, the physician must maintain a high index of suspicion that a localized eruption might be caused by cutaneous metastases, particularly in a patient with unexplained systemic findings.

HISTOPATHOLOGIC FINDINGS

Cutaneous metastases usually resemble the primary tumor histologically; however, metastases may demonstrate less differentiation. Histologic features of a cutaneous metastasis may allow identification of such primary tumors as small cell carcinoma of the lung, clear cell carcinoma of the kidney, carcinoid, and teratoma; however, in most instances definitive identification is impossible. For example, renal cell carcinoma may show characteristic tubular arrangements of glycogen-rich clear cells within a highly vascular stroma, but in many cases a definite diagnosis remains elusive. Clear cells may also originate from the lung, liver, ovary, endometrium, cervix, and vagina. In one series, nearly 50% of malignant cutaneous clear cell metastases were histologically misdiagnosed as benign lesions.

Immunohistochemical studies are important in refining the histologic differential diagnosis of many cutaneous tumors. Some data suggest that detection of p63 (an oncogene belonging to the p53 gene family) may be helpful in distinguishing primary and metastatic skin tumors. The least differentiated keratinocytes of the epidermis and epidermal appendages, and the myoepithelial cells of sweat glands express p63, as do most tumors that arise from these cells. Albeit not absolute, most benign and malignant primary skin tumors express p63, whereas most noncutaneous metastatic disease does not. This may be especially helpful in assessing adenocarcinomas of unknown origin. Other antigens useful in making this histologic differential diagnosis are B72.3, calreticulin, and CK5/6. Metastatic renal cell carcinoma may be confused with cutaneous adnexal neoplasms, and in this setting CD10 positivity appears to favor renal cell carcinoma over skin primaries of eccrine or apocrine origin, but is much less helpful in primary cutaneous sebaceous carcinoma.

The principal sites of primary squamous cell carcinoma include the lung, oral cavity, esophagus, larynx, and cervix. When the cutaneous squamous cell carcinoma is excluded, well-differentiated variants usually pose no histologic diagnostic problem. However, poorly differentiated squamous cell carcinomas may resemble lymphomas or anaplastic tumors.

Electron microscopy and histochemical techniques occasionally assist in identifying likely primary sites. The greatest challenge lies in the clinical and histologic evaluation of the patient with metastatic disease and an unknown primary tumor. The clinical and histologic evaluation of patients with cutaneous disease as the first sign of malignancy is discussed in the next section.

EVALUATION AND PROGNOSIS

Metastases from an unknown primary site are found in about 4% of all cancer patients. Despite this low incidence, the incidence of unknown primary tumors (UPTs) is higher than ovarian cancer, non-Hodgkin's lymphoma, or rectal carcinoma. Patients with UPTs are characterized by a history of disease of less than 3 months, rapid progression, and a random pattern of metastasis. For example, in UPT patients with a supraclavicular lymph node presentation, the primary tumors found at necropsy were as likely to be located below as above the diaphragm. Regardless of the cell of origin, UPTs seem to share a partial or complete loss of chromosome 1p.

The clinical course is usually rapidly progressive and fatal. The primary site becomes obvious in only 25% of patients during their lifetime, but is identifiable in 70% at autopsy. This means that in 30% of patients with metastatic disease not limited to the skin, no primary tumor is ever identified, even after death. The most common origin of UPTs are lung (30%) and pancreas (20%), followed by large bowel, kidneys, and breast.

Patients and relatives often become anxious when a primary site of cancer cannot be identified, usually because of concerns that the physician's care is substandard, or that knowledge of the primary site might greatly improve the chances for effective therapy. As a result, patients are often subjected to a battery of investigations that yield distressingly little valuable clinical information. Instead, the work-up should be focused on reasonable investigations of likely primary sites based on the presentation, and especially on distinguishing treatable subsets of UPTs. In most patients the clinical evaluation should be brief and focused, with a careful history and complete physical examination, hematologic and biochemical profiles, chest radiography, and chest computed tomography (CT). Mammography is indicated in women with clinical features suggestive of metastatic breast cancer; some include it in the panel for any patient with UPT. CT of the abdomen and pelvis may identify a primary site in 10–40% of patients, especially pancreas, kidney, hepatobiliary tract, and ovary, with pancreatic carcinoma most commonly found.

In UPTs, light microscopy allows classification into four pathologic subgroups: adenocarcinoma 50–60%, poorly differentiated adenocarcinoma 30–40%, squamous cell carcinoma 5–8%, and poorly differentiated neoplasm 2–5%. In the two groups with poorly differentiated histology, immunohistochemical analysis may be helpful. Commonly used antibodies to define tumor lineage include common leukocyte antigen (lymphoma), cytokeratin (carcinoma), S-100 protein (melanoma), and vimentin (mesenchymal tumors). Relatively specific immunohistochemical tests used to diagnose metastatic adenocarcinomas of unknown primary origin include prostate-specific antigen, thyroglobulin, estrogen and progesterone receptor proteins, thyroid transcription factor-I, and surfactant apoproteins. Of these, prostate-specific antigen and thyroglobulin are the most specific. Blood β-HCG or α-fetoprotein may be useful in young men with poorly differentiated carcinoma. Other specific tumors can be identified by neuron-specific enolase (neuroendocrine carcinoma), and possibly β-HCG (germ cell tumors).

After immunohistochemical evaluation, 30–70% of undifferentiated neoplasms appear to be non-Hodgkin's lymphomas, whereas in 10–20% a diagnosis of melanoma or sarcoma is apparent.

THERAPY

Patient subsets with specific treatment implications have now been described, and account for approximately 40% of all patients with UPTs. Local therapies are useful for focal metastases of head and neck squamous cell cancer or melanoma. Patients with squamous cell carcinoma in cervical lymph node metastasis often have an occult head or neck tumor, and even if the tumor primary cannot be found, may have an important response to surgery or radiotherapy. In patients with inguinal lymph nodes containing squamous cell carcinoma, the primary tumor should be sought in the perineal or anorectal area. This subgroup may have a reasonable response to lymph node excision and radiotherapy. Palliative hormone therapy is indicated for breast, endometrial, or prostatic cancer. Even if a primary cannot be identified, men with prostate-specific antigen elevated in serum or present in the tumor should be treated for metastatic prostate cancer, and women with estrogen receptor-positive UPTs should receive a trial of hormonal therapy as in breast cancer. Chemotherapy for metastatic germ cell tumors, trophoblastic tumors, Hodgkin's disease, or non-Hodgkin's lymphoma may be curative, so efforts at identification and treatment of these subgroups are critically important. Chemotherapy may achieve a significant and clinically relevant response in patients with breast, ovarian, oat cell lung, head and neck squamous cell, or transitional urothelial cancer.

Some patients with metastatic cancer with no identifiable primary, and who do not appear to fit into any of the above therapeutic groups, may respond to chemotherapy. Recent studies of empiric taxane-containing therapies have produced higher response rates than previous regimens, and have probably extended survival.

SUGGESTED READINGS

Bahrami S, Malone JC, Lear S, Martin AW. CD10 expression in cutaneous adnexa neoplasms and a potential role for differentiating cutaneous metastatic renal cell carcinoma. Arch Pathol Lab Med 2006; 130: 1315–1319.

Brownstein MH, Helwig EB. Patterns of cutaneous metastasis. Arch Dermatol 1972; 105: 862–868.

Brownstein MH, Helwig EB. Spread of tumors to the skin. Arch Dermatol 1973; 107: 80–86.

Gu U, Kilic A, Gonul M, et al. Spectrum of cutaneous metatases in 1287 cases of internal malignancies: a study from Turkey. Acta Dermatol Venereol 2007; 87: 160–162.

Hainsworth JD. Management of patients with cancer of unknown primary site. Oncology (Huntington) 2000; 14: 563–574.

Hammar SP. Metastatic adenocarcinoma of unknown primary origin. Hum Pathol 1998; 29: 1393–1402.

Ivan D, Nash JW, Prieto VG, et al. Use of p63 expression in distinguishing primary and metastatic cutaneous adnexal neoplasms from metastatic adenocarcinoma to skin. J Cutan Pathol 2007; 34: 474–480.

Kanitakis J, Chouvet B. Expression of p63 in cutaneous metatases. Am J Clin Pathol 2007; 128; 753–758.

Lookingbill DP, Spangler N, Sexton FM. Skin involvement as the presenting sign of internal carcinoma. J Am Acad Dermatol 1990; 22: 19–26.

Lookingbill DP, Spangler N, Helm KF. Cutaneous metastases in patients with metastatic carcinoma: a retrospective study of 4020 patients. J Am Acad Dermatol 1993; 29: 228–236.

Maher-Wiese VL, Wenner NP, Grant-Kels JM. Metastatic cutaneous lesions in children and adolescents with a case report of metastatic neuroblastoma. J Am Acad Dermatol 1992; 26: 620–628.

McClatchey AI. Modeling metastasis in the mouse. Oncogene 1999; 18: 5334–5339.

Resnik KS, DiLeonardo M, Gibbons G. Clinically occult cutaneous metastases. J Am Acad Dermatol 2006; 55: 1044–1047.

Rolz-Cruz G, Kim CC. Tumor invasion of the skin. Dermatol Clin 2008; 26: 89–102.

Sariya D, Ruth K, Adams-McDonnell R, et al. Clinicopathologic correlation of cutaneous metastases: experience from a cancer center. Arch Dermatol 2007; 143: 613–620.

Schwartz RA. Cutaneous metastatic disease. J Am Acad Dermatol 1995; 33: 161–182.

Spencer PS, Helm TN. Skin metastases in cancer patients. Cutis 1987; 39: 119–121.

Cutaneous Manifestations of Leukemias, Myelodysplastic and Myeloproliferative Syndromes, and Systemic Lymphomas

Specific or nonspecific lesions of the skin may occur in many hematopoietic malignancies or destructive reactive processes. Specific lesions are those in which there are tumor cells in the skin; nonspecific lesions, which are more common, do not have tumor cells but must be considered to be a cutaneous reaction to the malignancy. Specific cutaneous lesions are expected in primary cutaneous T- and B-cell lymphomas (Chapter 19), and in the cutaneous histiocytoses (Chapter 17). This chapter will focus on the cutaneous syndromes associated with leukemias, systemic lymphomas, and myeloproliferative and myelodysplastic syndromes.

PATHOGENESIS

The specific cutaneous lesions of leukemia or lymphoma result from direct infiltration of the epidermis, dermis, or subcutaneous fat by malignant cells. Depending on the degree and depth of infiltration, specific cutaneous lesions can present as papules, plaques, nodules, or ulcers. Early cutaneous involvement may result from specific tissue-homing patterns of the malignant cell. Late cutaneous involvement is seldom due to selective tissue trafficking, but rather to a complication of a large tumor cell burden. Nonspecific lesions do not contain obvious tumor cells, but are associated with the malignancy. This association may be direct and well understood, such as cutaneous infection or hemorrhage caused by tumor-related cytopenias, or may be less direct and poorly understood paraneoplastic changes, such as acquired ichthyosis, exfoliative dermatitis, or generalized pruritus.

CLINICAL MANIFESTATIONS

Specific Lesions

Specific cutaneous lesions occur much less frequently and develop much later in the course of most leukemias and systemic lymphomas than in primary cutaneous lymphomas. As might be expected from the predominance of T-cell malignancies in primary cutaneous lymphomas, patients with natural killer (NK)/T-cell-derived neoplasms are more likely to develop specific cutaneous lesions of systemic lymphomas, presumably because of an increased tendency of some of these cells to home to skin. However, this is offset by the much lower incidence and prevalence of systemic T-cell lymphomas compared to systemic B-cell lymphomas and non-T-cell leukemias.

Specific cutaneous lesions in leukemias and lymphomas usually present as flesh-colored, erythematous, or distinctive plum-colored papules or nodules that often have a rubbery consistency on palpation (Fig. 15–1). Specific lesions range in size from a few millimeters to several centimeters in diameter, and are randomly distributed. Ulceration of cutaneous nodules is not common but can occur; cutaneous ulceration may also result from necrosis of involved lymph nodes with secondary overlying cutaneous necrosis.

Specific leukemic or lymphomatous infiltrates may localize in sites of dermal inflammation. This inflammation could result from processes as varied as surgical, thermal, or traumatic injury; intramuscular injections; and herpes simplex or herpes zoster lesions.

Leukemia

Early cutaneous involvement occurs more frequently in acute myelomonocytic and monocytic leukemia than in other leukemias and most systemic lymphomas. Infiltrated, hyperplastic, and friable gingival tissue strongly favors the diagnosis of acute myelomonocytic or monocytic leukemia, and biopsy specimens of such tissue should confirm the diagnosis. Oral involvement can occur rarely with other types of acute leukemia and, even more rarely, with chronic leukemias and lymphomas.

The syndrome of aleukemic leukemia cutis is the earliest cutaneous presentation possible. In this syndrome, lesions containing blast cells develop in the skin in the absence of peripheral blood and, occasionally, bone marrow evidence of leukemia. Such lesions may be present several months before diagnosis, but the full leukemic syndrome ultimately develops.

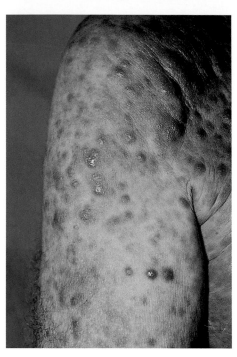

Figure 15–1 Multiple erythematous to violaceous nodules in a man with lymphoblastic lymphoma.

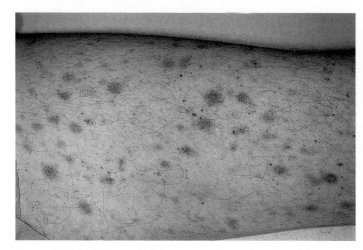

Figure 15–2 Multiple small violaceous papules and small nodules in a man with a blast cell crisis of acute myelogenous leukemia.

Aleukemic leukemia cutis has been reported predominantly with acute myelomonocytic leukemia, much less often with acute monocytic leukemia, and rarely preceding acute lymphoblastic leukemia/lymphoma.

Granulocytic sarcoma is a rare tumor of malignant myeloid cells, which may present in the skin. It may precede the development of acute myelogenous leukemia (one form of aleukemic leukemia cutis), it may accompany acute myelogenous leukemia, or it may develop in myelodysplastic syndromes or chronic myelogenous leukemia at the time of leukemic transformation. Lesions are typically flesh-colored or erythematous papules or nodules in a child or young adult. Chloroma is an alternative name for granulocytic sarcoma when the solid mass of blast cells in the skin shows a diagnostic yellowish-green coloration following cutting of the lesion during pathologic examination. The greenish discoloration is attributed to the presence of high concentrations of myeloperoxidase in the myeloblasts.

Acute promyelocytic leukemia rarely involves sites other than blood and bone marrow, but skin is the most commonly affected extramedullary site, accounting for half the cases. The cutaneous presentations are clinically similar to those of acute myelogenous leukemia or granulocytic sarcoma. As noted previously, leukemia cutis may localize to sites of burns, trauma, injections, herpes, scars, or Hickman catheter use. Acute promyelocytic leukemia may be particularly prone to occur at sites of vascular puncture with blood draws or catheters, with a review suggesting that most reported cases of promyelocytic sarcoma occurred at puncture sites for venepuncture, central venous catheters, or bone marrow aspiration.

The term chronic myelogenous leukemia is now considered to encompass four syndromes. Classic chronic myelogenous

leukemia has also been called chronic granulocytic leukemia and chronic myeloid leukemia, and is by far the most common subset. It is usually Philadelphia chromosome positive and presents with anemia, elevation of mature neutrophils and other granulated leukocytes, sometimes thrombocytosis, and frequently splenomegaly. This disease typically ends in an accelerated phase often evolving to acute leukemia, usually myelocytic but occasionally lymphocytic. Chronic myelogenous leukemia spares the skin until an accelerated blast phase or blast crisis develops, at which time multiple flesh-colored or erythematous papules and nodules may rapidly develop (Fig. 15–2). An unusual manifestation of chronic myelogenous leukemia is a tender, edematous, purpuric area of induration on the lower leg that resembles stasis dermatitis but which is due to a perivascular and periappendigeal myeloid infiltration of the dermis. The three much less common subsets of chronic myelogenous leukemia include chronic myelomonocytic leukemia, juvenile myelomonocytic leukemia, and chronic neutrophilic leukemia. These are generally much more aggressive diseases when untreated, and much less treatment responsive than classic myelogenous leukemia. These are less likely than chronic myelogenous leukemia to have specific skin infiltrates, but are perhaps more likely to develop nonspecific lesions, either paraneoplastic (as in Sweet's syndrome) or cytopenic (infections or hemorrhage) manifestations of malignant disease.

Both Chediak–Higashi syndrome and Griscelli syndrome have autosomal recessive inheritance of pigmentary, hematologic, immunologic, and neurologic abnormalities. Dysfunction of lysosomes and melanosomes is common to both. Both are now known to have defects in the secretion of perforin-containing granules, essential for lymphocyte cytotoxicity; this may explain some of the nonphagocytic immune defects. Both may also have an 'accelerated phase,' with blood and systemic features similar to those of familial lymphohistiocytosis, and this may also be a consequence of perforin-related immune deficiency (see Chapter 17).

Chronic lymphocytic leukemia (CLL) is overwhelmingly B-cell derived in most countries where it is common (<2% T-cell). In predominantly Asian countries where it is much less common, CLL may be T cell in origin in up to 18% of patients. In B-cell CLL, lesions due to primary infiltration of skin are rare, but small malignant B cells may frequently infiltrate infectious or inflammatory cutaneous lesions in patients with CLL. Chronic T-cell leukemia has recently been combined with T-cell prolymphocytic leukemia, but together these account for less than 5% of CLL in western countries. About a third of patients have cutaneous involvement, usually manifesting as localized or extensive erythema or erythematosus papules or plaques. The more extensive the erythema, the more important it is to distinguish from Sézary syndrome (Chapter 19). Some (but not all) T-cell CLL and prolymphocytic leukemias are HTLV-1 associated; HTLV-1 linkage is much more likely in areas of endemic HTLV-1 infection.

Malignant cell infiltration of facial skin can be so extensive that a leonine facies results, mimicking that seen occasionally with primary cutaneous lymphomas (usually T-cell). Chronic lymphocytic leukemia is the most common cause of this rare complication of leukemia or systemic lymphoma. Mikulicz's syndrome is most commonly associated with Sjögren's syndrome, and less often sarcoidosis or lupus erythematosus; very rarely it may be secondary to infiltration by leukemia or non-Hodgkin's lymphoma. The lymphocytic infiltration of the lacrimal, orbital, and salivary glands that characterizes Mikulicz's syndrome, whether benign or malignant, produces the same clinical findings of xerostomia and reduced lacrimation.

Hairy cell leukemia, or leukemic reticuloendotheliosis, is associated with mucocutaneous manifestations in roughly 20% of patients. These findings are often related to disease-associated thrombocytopenia, with some patients developing spontaneous purpura or epistaxis. Macular and papular lesions are also reported in patients with hairy cell leukemia, but the character of the infiltrate in such lesions is not well described. Specific infiltration of the lips by hairy cell leukemia can produce macrocheilia, mimicking the Melkersson–Rosenthal syndrome.

Several leukemia/lymphoma syndromes are discussed under the systemic lymphoma category in order to consolidate the discussion of lymphoma classification.

Myeloproliferative Syndromes, Myelodysplastic Disease, and Extramedullary Hematopoiesis

Extramedullary hematopoiesis is a physiologic process in early to mid-stage human embryologic development, but normally ends well before birth. Postnatal cutaneous extramedullary hematopoiesis is a very rare cutaneous syndrome seen most commonly in neonates following certain congenital infections (especially toxoplasma, rubella, cytomegalovirus, and herpes virus) or with severe anemia (Rh or ABO incompatibility, twin transfusion syndrome, or severe inherited or congenital anemias). In infants, lesions are frequently blue to blue-red papules or nodules, giving rise to the term 'blueberry muffin baby.' Even more rare in adults, it is most frequently associated with idiopathic myelofibrosis (estimated prevalence 0.4%), and less frequently with chronic myeloid leukemia, pachydermoperiostosis, and pilomatricomas. Cutaneous lesions are

pink, red, or violaceous in color and may resemble hemangiomas, but more typically are papules, plaques or nodules on the trunk. Some lesions develop ulcerations, bullae, or perilesional hemorrhage. Splenectomy may slightly increase the likelihood of cutaneous extramedullary hematopoiesis in marrow replacement syndromes. Because the spleen is the usual site of early and often massive extramedullary hematopoiesis when bone marrow is replaced by tumor or fibrosis, it is possible that the removal of this organ might predispose these patients to cutaneous hematopoiesis.

Specific cutaneous lesions of myeloproliferative syndromes and myelodysplastic diseases usually develop only in the setting of transformation to acute leukemia, or blast crisis of chronic myelogenous leukemia. Specific cutaneous lesions are less common in these syndromes than are the nonspecific lesions due to cytopenias or to Sweet's syndrome.

Systemic Lymphomas

Immunophenotyping and gene rearrangement studies have dramatically altered perceptions regarding the cutaneous presentation of lymphomas. The reports of true histiocytic (monocyte–macrophage) lymphomas continue to decrease as improved methods of identifying cell lineages are applied to what are initially indeterminate large cell-containing lesions (Chapter 17). Most such cases appear to be either B- or T-cell lymphomas. Additionally, until recently most studies supported the view that B-cell malignancies seldom present as cutaneous lesions in the absence of extracutaneous disease. With phenotyping, it is now clear that some B-cell lymphomas in fact may be skin limited indefinitely, although they can be difficult or impossible to distinguish from lymphocytoma cutis or other pseudolymphomas on cellular morphology alone. Primary cutaneous T- and B-cell lymphomas (Chapter 19) must be distinguished from systemic T- and B-cell lymphomas with cutaneous involvement. This is especially important in those systemic lymphomas that may present with cutaneous disease and relatively occult systemic disease, because the prognosis and therapeutic approach are usually dramatically different between the two, even when the histologic appearance is similar or identical.

Although there are reports of Hodgkin's disease presenting as a skin-limited disorder, specific cutaneous lesions of Hodgkin's disease are rare at any stage. When specific lymphomatous infiltrates of Hodgkin's disease occur in the skin, they develop late in the course of the disease and are thought to result from retrograde flow of lymphoma cells from obstructed infiltrated lymph nodes. Another setting for specific cutaneous involvement of Hodgkin's disease occurs when massive nodal enlargement results in the necrosis of overlying skin.

Human T-cell leukemia virus is an important etiologic agent for a subset of systemic cutaneous lymphomas, and is discussed later. Human immunodeficiency virus (HIV) infection with acquired immune deficiency syndrome (AIDS) is associated with a large increase in the incidence of non-Hodgkin's lymphoma. In this setting the disease runs an aggressive course, with constitutional symptoms and early extensive multisystem involvement. Hodgkin's and T-cell lymphomas are rare in patients with AIDS. The B-cell predominance is attributed in part to Epstein–Barr virus, which is now recognized as an important agent for lymphoma induction in many immunodeficiency states. Extranodal cutaneous involvement occurs roughly as often in HIV-associated non-Hodgkin's lymphoma (<10%) as in non-Hodgkin's lymphoma overall.

A number of T-cell leukemias and systemic lymphomas frequently result in early or extensive cutaneous disease. Several of these, with a propensity for leukemic presentations, have already been discussed, including: precursor T-lymphoblastic leukemia/lymphoma, T-cell chronic lymphocytic leukemia/prolymphocytic leukemia, adult T-cell leukemia/lymphoma, and NK/NK-like T-cell leukemia/lymphoma.

Most of the systemic T-cell lymphomas with prominent cutaneous involvement would fit into three categories in the WHO classification: peripheral T-cell lymphoma, unspecified (includes nasal and nasal-type NK/T-cell group, most angiocentric lymphomas); subcutaneous panniculitis-like T-cell lymphoma; and CD30+ anaplastic large cell lymphoma. Intravascular T-cell lymphoma will be discussed below with its B-cell counterpart.

Peripheral T-cell lymphoma is more common in Asia than in western countries, and the incidence of the angiocentric lymphoma subset is much higher (32%) than in western countries (<10%), primarily because of the inclusion of the nasal-type NK/T-cell lymphoma in this category. This neoplasm is highly associated with Epstein–Barr virus in Asia, but not in western countries. Despite the common occurrence of HTLV-1-related lymphoma in endemic areas of Japan, the incidence of this viral-related syndrome is very rare in Korea and other Asian countries outside Japan. A comparison of two series of peripheral T-cell lymphomas from different parts of the world is included in Table 15–1, and allows comparisons of these tumors by western and eastern regions, by survival, and by incidence of skin involvement.

The CD30+ anaplastic large cell systemic lymphoma differs from the primary cutaneous syndrome in that it is anaplastic large cell kinase (ALK)-1 positive, and frequently positive for the t(2,5) translocation, both of which are uniformly negative in the cutaneous form. Leukemic and nodal involvement is expected in the systemic variety, and the rate of disease progression demands much more aggressive therapy than for the cutaneous form. CD30– anaplastic large cell lymphoma is an aggressive lymphoma syndrome whether it presents as systemic or an apparent primary cutaneous disease.

NK cell and NK-like T-cell leukemia/lymphoma is a predominantly extranodal syndrome derived from large granular lymphocytes. The azurophilic Giemsa granules contain cytolytic proteins, including perforin. These cells are CD56+, and cutaneous presentations are common. One study suggests that patients with blastic NK-cell lymphoma/leukemia tend to present at an older age (56 vs 46 years) and to have a somewhat better prognosis, though both groups represent aggressive disease (median survival 15 vs 25 months with skin disease). The remarkable propensity of some CD56+ NK lymphomas to present with widespread nodules of tumor with minimal apparent systemic disease initially may be explained by work suggesting that at least some of these malignancies might be better termed plasmacytoid dendritic cell leukemia/lymphoma (CD4 and CD56 positive without other lineage-specific markers) with a homing pattern similar to that of Langerhans' dendritic cell disease. These plasmacytoid dendritic cells seem to be an important component of the innate immunity system. A subset of NK and NK-like T-cell lymphomas is included in classifications of primary cutaneous T-cell lymphomas as nasal or nasal-type lymphomas (lethal midline granuloma, polymorphic reticulosis), and may be associated with Epstein–Barr virus. Although many of these lymphomas are angiocentric, this is not a uniform finding. Although this is a rare syndrome, it is not uncommon for these patients to present with cutaneous nodules and leukemia without nasal localization. Others have

Table 15–1 Comparison of peripheral T-cell lymphomas from western and eastern countries by REAL (Revised European–American Lymphoma) classification subsets

Subset of peripheral T-cell lymphoma	Percent of total in European study (n = 174) 1*	Percent of total in Asian study (n = 78) 2*	Median survival in months		Percent of subset with skin involvement	
			1*	2*	1*	2*
Peripheral T-cell, unspecified	54%	40%	22	18	12%	16%
Angiocentric	8%	32%	25	51	7%	4%
Anaplastic large cell	17%	17%	65	NR	20%	38.5%
Angioimmunoblastic	13%	6%	20	4	18%	20%
Intestinal	7%	2%	4	–	0%	0%
Panniculitic	–	2%	–	–	–	50% (n = 2)

1* López-Guillermo A et al., 1998.
2* Kim K et al., 2002.
NR = median survival not reached at time of study; therefore best survival of group.

presented with subcutaneous panniculitic lesions and hemophagocytosis. In some patients the large cells have been CD30 positive. Given the variety of clinical and pathologic presentations, the aggressive course, and the usually poor prognosis of this disease, staining for CD56 antigen should be considered in large cell leukemias or lymphomas with early cutaneous involvement. The angiocentric subsets of NK and NK-like T-cell lymphomas should also be distinguished from lymphomatoid granulomatosis and other angiocentric or angiodestructive lymphomas. Lymphomatoid granulomatosis is an angiocentric B-cell neoplasm rich in reactive T cells. It is typically a multisystem disease, with early skin and lung involvement more suggestive of granulomatous vasculitides than of lymphoma. Occasional patients with lymphomatoid granulomatosis have disease which appears to be skin limited, and may not require aggressive systemic therapy.

Adult T-cell leukemia/lymphoma is endemic to southwest Japan and the Caribbean region, but sporadic cases have increased, partly due to sharing of contaminated syringes by intravenous drug abusers, and can be seen worldwide. There are multiple subsets of this disease, distinguished in part by rate of progression and ranging from very aggressive disease to relatively indolent syndromes. Lymphadenopathy, leukocytosis, hypercalcemia, lytic bone lesions, hepatomegaly, and skin involvement are common features. Skin involvement can mimic that of mycosis fungoides or Sézary syndrome (including the development of Pautrier's microabscesses), but more typical lesions are localized erythema, erythematosus plaques, or larger nodules or tumor masses. Malignant cells typically are CD4+ (as are those in mycosis fungoides/Sézary syndrome), but usually have more pronounced nuclear irregularity with lobulation ('flower cells'), which distinguishes these cells from those of classic cutaneous T-cell lymphoma. Likewise, HTLV-1 positivity is expected in this syndrome, but is extremely rare in other T-cell lymphomas, including the primary cutaneous lymphomas.

Angioimmunoblastic lymphoma, previously known as angioimmunoblastic lymphadenopathy with dysproteinemia or immunoblastic lymphadenopathy, is associated with polyclonal B-cell activation. It usually starts with the rapid onset of generalized lymphadenopathy with fever, malaise, and weight loss in older individuals. Hepatosplenomegaly is frequently present. Polyclonal hypergammaglobulinemia, anemia, a positive direct Coombs' test, leukocytosis, eosinophilia, thrombocytopenia, and hypoalbuminemia are frequent laboratory findings. Cutaneous manifestations are common. Generalized pruritus or excessive sweating occurs in up to one-third of patients, and up to 40% have some type of cutaneous eruption. Generalized macular or papular erythema is the most common, but purpura, urticaria or urticarial lesions, nodular and ulcerative lesions, scleromyxedema-like lesions, and erythroderma have also been described. An association with eczema craquelé-like dermatitis, transient acantholytic dermatitis, dermatitis herpetiformis-like bullous skin lesions, and Kaposi's sarcoma has also been reported. This syndrome is now considered a moderately aggressive T-cell lymphoma, which may transform into a more aggressive and obvious lymphoma pattern such as immunoblastic sarcoma.

Many of the B-cell leukemias and systemic lymphomas have already been discussed, including precursor B-lymphoblastic leukemia/lymphoma, chronic B-cell lymphocytic leukemia (small lymphocytic B-cell lymphoma is the nodal lymphoma counterpart, with earlier node involvement and later leukemic phase), and lymphomatoid granulomatosis. Follicle-center cell lymphoma and marginal zone lymphoma have counterparts in the primary cutaneous B-cell lymphomas (Chapter 19), as well as systemic lymphoma syndromes with occasional mid- to late-course cutaneous involvement. These two B-cell categories are the most common nodal lymphomas. Mantle cell lymphoma is a less common but aggressive form of B-cell lymphoma with some tendency for skin involvement in the later stages. Diffuse large B-cell lymphoma includes a number of somewhat aggressive systemic lymphomas, intravascular B-cell lymphomas, and entities which many experts feel warrant separate consideration, including the primary cutaneous syndromes of primary cutaneous follicle-center cell lymphoma and diffuse large B-cell lymphoma of the leg (Chapter 19). Intravascular B-cell lymphoma, previously known as malignant angioendotheliomatosis, is a rare but distinct lymphoma that is almost completely confined within vascular lumina. Although central and peripheral nervous system involvement is the most common presentation, cutaneous involvement is a close second and is obviously much easier to sample. A high index of suspicion is important in making this diagnosis, because patients usually present with nonspecific central nervous system abnormalities and frequently have fever, malaise, weight loss, and evidence of antinuclear antibody, rheumatoid factor, or anti-red cell autoantibodies, suggesting a rheumatologic disorder. The cutaneous lesions most often consist of multiple red to violaceous papules, plaques, or nodules, and these may occasionally ulcerate. Cutaneous presentations include isolated instances of widely distributed macular hyperpigmentation and a T-cell type, mimicking squamous cell carcinoma of the foreskin. A biopsy specimen will show distended vessels in the dermis and occasionally in the subcutis, and will contain discohesive, cytologically atypical lymphocytes. Immunophenotyping reveals an overwhelming predominance of B-cell lymphoma, but intravascular T-cell lymphoma is reported.

Nonspecific Lesions

A number of nonspecific cutaneous lesions may occur in association with leukemia, myeloproliferative and myelodysplastic syndromes, and lymphoma. Some nonspecific cutaneous manifestations are so common that they are seldom helpful in the diagnosis, but they can be difficult therapeutic problems. Other types of nonspecific involvement may be so uncommon in other settings, or so distinctive in appearance, that not only is a specific diagnosis of leukemia or lymphoma suggested, but also sometimes even the exact type of lymphoma or leukemia can be inferred (Table 15–2). For example, acute neutrophilic febrile dermatosis (Sweet's syndrome) is a distinctive syndrome characterized by painful edematous papules or plaques, usually in association with fever, arthralgias, and neutrophilic leukocytosis. An association with malignancy has been reported in 10–15% of cases, though reporting bias of cancer-associated cases is likely to have inflated this percentage somewhat. Reported malignancies are usually hematopoietic, usually acute myelogenous leukemia, or less often myeloproliferative

Table 15–2 Nonspecific mucocutaneous lesions associated with lymphomas and leukemias

Caused by cytopenias
Pallor
Purpura, especially petechial
Gingival hemorrhage
Oral ulcerations with neutropenia
Infections, especially opportunistic

Pathogenesis not known	Most characteristic association
Acute febrile neutrophilic dermatosis (Sweet's syndrome)	Acute myelogenous leukemia. GSF and GCSF treatment for cytopenias may also induce Sweet's-like lesions or lesional histology
Atypical pyoderma gangrenosum	Acute myelogenous leukemia (also plasma cell dyscrasia)
Generalized pruritus	Hodgkin's disease (occasionally other lymphomas; pruritus common with cutaneous T-cell lymphomas)
Vasculitis	Occasionally with leukemias and lymphomas, especially hairy cell
Exfoliative erythroderma	Cutaneous T-cell lymphoma, rare in B-cell lymphoma
Acquired ichthyosis	Hodgkin's disease, occasionally, lymphocytic lymphoma, Kaposi's sarcoma
Vesicular disease	Possible associations of linear IgA disease with hematologic malignancies Paraneoplastic pemphigus highly associated with mostly malignant lymphoproliferative disease or with thymoma
Xanthomas	Plasma cell dyscrasias, leukemia with café-au-lait spots: juvenile chronic granulocytic leukemia

or myelodysplastic syndromes. Sweet's syndrome may also arise in the course of therapy, either as histologic Sweet's-like lesions in the skin following the use of granulocyte colony-stimulating factor (GCSF) for treatment-related leukopenia, or as a result of cell differentiation in ALL-*trans*-retinoic acid (ATRA) treatment of acute promyelocytic leukemia. Sweet's syndrome must be differentiated from ATRA syndrome of promyelocytic leukemia. ATRA syndrome is manifested by fever, weight loss, respiratory distress, interstitial pulmonary infiltrates, pleural and pericardial effusions, episodic hypotension, and acute renal failure; skin lesions are not reported.

Pyoderma gangrenosum, a distinctive ulcerating disorder, is also associated with hematopoietic disorders, especially acute myelogenous leukemia, myelodysplastic syndromes, multiple myeloma, or monoclonal gammopathy, and occasionally myeloproliferative disease. Overlap clinical presentations between classic Sweet's syndrome lesions and pyoderma gangrenosum ulcers have been reported using the following terms: atypical Sweet's syndrome, bullous Sweet's syndrome, bullous pyoderma gangrenosum, superficial pyoderma gangrenosum, and neutrophilic dermatosis of the dorsal hands. These hybrid clinical lesions seldom arise in nonmalignancy-associated Sweet's syndrome. Persistent unexplained anemia may be the best hematologic indicator of an underlying marrow dyscrasia in patients with Sweet's syndrome without obvious signs or symptoms of malignancy.

Paraneoplastic pemphigus is almost invariably linked to immunoproliferative or lymphoproliferative disease, including lymphomas, lymphocytic leukemia, Castleman's disease, and thymoma. Severe mucosal involvement is a hallmark of this disease, along with pemphigoid-like bullous disease, and erythema multiforme-like lesions. Pulmonary disease is often present in patients with paraneoplastic pemphigus and portends a poor prognosis. Many of the patients have a history of prior lymphoma, and in these patients it has been postulated that there may be a small nidus of cells that produce the auto-antibodies responsible for the clinical manifestations. Few therapies have been effective, but the recent introduction of rituximab has been of benefit for many of these patients.

Nonspecific lesions that favor the diagnosis of acute leukemia or myelodysplasia may result from marrow failure caused by replacement of normal marrow by abnormal blasts. The resulting anemias will produce skin pallor; a marked thrombocytopenia may produce cutaneous hemorrhage (especially petechiae); and severe neutropenia may be suspected when certain opportunistic infections, such as disseminated candidiasis, disseminated aspergillosis, or mucormycosis, develop. Conversely, erythrocytosis accounts for the plethora and ruddy cyanosis seen in polycythemia rubra vera.

Xanthomas (or xanthogranuloma) and multiple café-au-lait macules (as seen in neurofibromatosis) have been associated with the development of leukemia: of 24 reported patients, all were children, most were boys, and all but one developed juvenile chronic granulocytic (myelomonocytic) leukemia.

Because leukemias and lymphomas are frequently treated with intensive chemotherapeutic regimens, such patients have a high incidence of chemotherapy-related cutaneous syndromes, some of which are listed in Table 15–3.

DIFFERENTIAL DIAGNOSIS

Skin findings can suggest the presence of a hematopoietic disorder, but the diagnosis of leukemia, lymphoma, or other disorder ultimately depends on firm histologic evidence, often combined with specialized cell marker studies when skin lesions contain malignant cells.

Pseudolymphoma of the skin is a term applied to a group of dermatoses that, on the basis of clinical and/or histologic findings, are difficult to distinguish from leukemia or lymphoma involving the skin (Fig. 15–3). Such dermatoses include

Table 15–3 Chemotherapy-related mucocutaneous findings

Alopecia, anagen effluvium and telogen effluvium

Hyperpigmentation, generalized, localized, and patterned

Nail dystrophies and dyspigmentations

Inflammation or necrosis with extravasation

Radiation or phototoxic recall or enhancement reactions

Acral erythema

Xerosis

Stomatitis, due to chemotherapy or to neutropenia

Photosensitivity

Angioedema, urticaria

Cutaneous eruption of lymphocyte recovery

Neutrophilic eccrine hidradenitis

Flushing reaction

Kaposi's sarcoma (increased in lymphoma, also increased with immunosuppression)

Epidermal growth factor receptor inhibitors (gefitinib, cetuximab, erlotinib, panitumumab)

Papulopustular eruption most frequent, usually in seborrheic areas

Abnormal growth of eyelashes, scalp, or facial hair

Xerosis

Paronychia, often with pyogenic granuloma

Telangiectasias

Anaphylactic infusion reaction with cetuximab: rare

Multikinase inhibitors

Imatinib
  Most common: edema, exanthem-like eruption
  Most severe: Stevens–Johnson, AGEP

Dasatinib
  Most common: localized or generalized eruptions in 35%, stomatitis/mucositis 16%, pruritus 11%

Nilotinib
  Most common: 'rashes' 20%, pruritus 15%, dry skin 12%

Sorafenib
  Most common: rash/scaling 66%, hand/foot skin reaction 62%, alopecia 53%, stomatitis/pharyngitis 35%, dry skin 23%, flushing 16%, edema 15%
  Seborrheic dermatitis-like eruption common

Sunitinib
  Most common: bullae, periorbital edema, symmetric acral erythemas
  Transient yellow skin discoloration may occur

Proteasome inhibitors

Bortezomib
  Erythematous nodules or plaques, upper body erythematous papular eruption – biopsy said to show necrotizing vasculitis

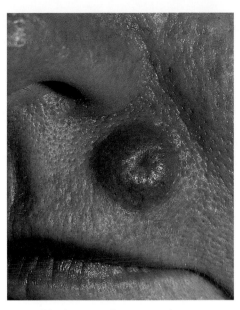

Figure 15–3 A nodular lesion on this patient's lip is representative of a benign lymphocytic infiltrate. (Courtesy of Dr Donald Hazelrigg, Evansville, IN.)

lymphocytic infiltration of Jessner, reticular erythematous mucinosis, arthropod bite reactions, nodular scabies, actinic reticuloid, drug-induced pseudolymphoma syndrome, and lymphocytoma cutis.

Drug-induced pseudolymphoma syndrome is usually the result of phenytoin administration, but can occur with related compounds, including barbiturates and carbamazepine. There is probably a genetic predisposition for the development of this syndrome. Generalized lymphadenopathy, hepatosplenomegaly, fever, arthralgias, and eosinophilia are typical findings; generalized pruritic erythematous macules or papules are the most common cutaneous manifestations. Rare instances of cutaneous nodule formation have been described. This syndrome is usually rapidly reversible following discontinuation of the offending drug, but rare progression to lymphoma has occurred.

Lymphocytoma cutis is known by a number of other names, including cutaneous lymphoid hyperplasia, cutaneous lymphoplasia, and Spiegler–Fendt sarcoid. The cutaneous lesions are usually asymptomatic violaceous or flesh-colored papules or nodules. They are most commonly located on the face, but they can occur anywhere in either a grouped or a random pattern, and may develop into large confluent plaques. On rare occasions, spontaneous ulceration of these lesions may occur. Changes in the size and extent of established lesions are frequent, and spontaneous regression, which may take years to occur, is common. Histologic examination of lesional specimens is important in the differentiation from lymphoma, as is the absence of visceral lesions. Some patients whose conditions were originally diagnosed as lymphocytoma cutis later develop lymphoma, but it is unclear whether these instances indicate a true transformation or merely reflect the difficulties in detecting small monoclonal populations of cells. Although it is unusual for lesions of lymphocytoma cutis to be lesions of systemic lymphoma, many such lesions are now considered to be indolent primary cutaneous B-cell lymphomas (Chapter 19).

HISTOPATHOLOGIC FINDINGS

Although the histopathologic findings of cutaneous lesions of non-T-cell lymphoma or leukemia depend on the specific type of malignancy, certain generalizations can be made. Most leukemias and non-Hodgkin's lymphomas that involve the skin histologically show a monomorphous infiltrate, which may be vasocentric or may extensively infiltrate or efface portions of the dermis and subcutaneous fat. A thin upper dermal zone immediately below the epidermis (Grenz zone) is usually spared, even in extensively infiltrated lesions of non-T-cell tumors. Many lymphomas may show nodular or follicular arrangements of lymphoma cells in involved lymph nodes, but despite this, the cutaneous lesions resulting from the infiltration of these lymphomas almost never show follicular or nodular patterns. Primary cutaneous B-cell lymphomas may have suggestive histologic findings, but in the absence of immunophenotypic evidence they can be impossible to distinguish from lymphocytoma cutis. In the absence of prominent cytologic atypia, the decision to proceed with phenotyping or gene-rearrangement studies is a matter of clinical judgment, which depends partly on the morphology and chronicity of the lesions, the clinical setting, and helpful but often nondiagnostic histologic criteria.

Diffuse and confluent masses of lymphocytes in the dermis are typical of lymphocytoma cutis. Although germinal centers are typical in lymphocytoma cutis and are extremely rare in secondary cutaneous lymphomas, primary cutaneous B-cell lymphomas often have features that suggest a germinal center morphology. Also, germinal centers may be part of a reactive process at the periphery of a lymphomatous infiltrate. For these reasons, the finding of germinal centers cannot be used to rule out malignancy absolutely.

The type of dense lymphocytic perivascular infiltrate typically seen in a cutaneous lesion of chronic lymphocytic leukemia and well-differentiated lymphocytic lymphoma can be seen in a number of nonmalignant settings (e.g., cutaneous lupus erythematosus, lymphocytic infiltrate of Jessner, polymorphous light eruption, and drug-induced pseudolymphoma). Such histologic findings can be properly interpreted only in conjunction with the clinical setting, the lesional morphology, and occasionally, additional special studies, including cell marker surveys.

A variety of granulomatous reactions mimicking sarcoidosis or extravascular granulomas of granulomatous vasculitides have been reported in the settings of lymphoma and leukemia. Although not specific, such lesions may suggest the correct diagnosis when the clinical findings are not consistent with those of sarcoidosis or granulomatous vasculitis.

EVALUATION

History and physical examination (with special emphasis on the skin and lymph nodes) remain the keystone for the proper diagnosis of hematopoietic neoplasms involving the skin. The type of cutaneous lesion (specific or nonspecific), the histologic appearance of specific lesions, the pace of the disease, and the hematologic findings are useful in establishing the need for further studies, which include bone marrow examination or lymph node biopsy, routine and scanning radiography, or a diligent search for an associated underlying infection. Improvements in cell identification by immunologic and molecular biologic techniques are also essential for increased precision in the diagnosis and classification of leukemias and lymphomas.

TREATMENT

The best treatment for both the specific and nonspecific eruptions of leukemia or lymphoma is the cure or control of the underlying systemic disease. When such control cannot be achieved by currently available chemotherapy, immunotherapy, or radiation therapy, or when responses are slow or incomplete, local therapy may be more important. Local radiation therapy can often induce regression or remission of specific (tumor-containing) cutaneous lesions. If radiation therapy is not effective or is not acceptable to the patient, or if previous treatment precludes further local radiation, the intralesional injection of triamcinolone acetonide at concentrations of 5–20 mg/mL may occasionally be helpful. Cutaneous and subcutaneous atrophy may rarely be severe following such injections, and the full effect of intralesional therapy may not be evident for 3–4 weeks afterwards.

A new approach to the treatment of malignant disorders has been signaled by the development of imatinib mesylate (ST1571, Gleevec), a tyrosine kinase inhibitor. Bcr-Abl is an oncogene kinase and the causative molecular abnormality of chronic myelogenous leukemia (CML). Inhibition of this kinase by imatinib mesylate appears to be dramatically effective in treatment trials of CML, with 88% complete hematologic response in interferon-resistant or -intolerant patients, and major responses in 21% of accelerated-phase CML and 13.5% of blast-phase CML. Additional tyrosine kinase inhibitors have been developed to treat imatinib resistance, either by restoring inhibition of Bcr-Abl or through inhibition independent of the Bcr-Abl kinase. Dasatinib and nilotinib are such agents, and have been studied primarily in imatinib-resistant CML. Sorafenib is a multikinase inhibitor released in the United States for treatment of renal carcinoma; sunitinib is a multitargeted tyrosine kinase inhibitor released for treatment of metastatic renal cell carcinoma and for imatinib-resistant gastrointestinal stromal tumor (GIST). A second group of targeted anticancer agents include the epidermal growth factor receptor inhibitors. This receptor is important as an activator of several other tyrosine kinase pathways, and inhibition of these pathways has been effective in treating many cancers, including colorectal, breast, pancreatic, and head and neck squamous cell carcinomas, and nonsmall cell lung cancers. Gefitinib and erlotinib are orally administered; cetuximab and panitumumab are administered intravenously. Cetuximab is usually combined with irinotecan, a topoisomerase I inhibitor. These new targeted therapies have been associated with new patterns of cutaneous toxicity, some of which are noted in Table 15–3. The revival of thalidomide and the development of lenalidomide are changing the therapeutic approach to multiple myeloma, and both appear to offer some promise in the treatment of myelodysplastic disease and some leukemias. In addition, there have been reports of the benefit of thalidomide for associated nonspecific lesions such as myelodysplastic-associated Sweet's syndrome. Lenalidomide induces a direct cytotoxic effect against hematopoietic clones affected by chromosome 5q deletions.

Therapy for nonspecific lesions, when treatment for systemic disease is inadequate, depends on the particular type of cutaneous involvement. Specific therapy for pruritus, erythroderma, vasculitis, bullous dermatoses, and the reactive dermatoses is discussed in the appropriate chapters of this book.

The possibility of a viral, fungal, or bacterial origin for the cutaneous lesions must always be considered. Therefore, an early biopsy of suspicious lesions for histologic examination and culture should be considered, especially in patients who are leukopenic or otherwise immunocompromised.

The major risk of treating lymphocytoma cutis would seem to be the risk of omission. Indolent B-cell lymphomas that are primary in the skin may have some risk of spreading extracutaneously, and such lymphomas can be difficult to separate from the pseudolymphoma group. Because many therapies are likely to alter histologic and immunologic studies on any recurring lymphocytic infiltrate, the extent of the work-up needed in each case should be considered before initiating therapy of an infiltrative lesion. Intralesional corticosteroid injections, cryotherapy, and low-dose radiation therapy are often helpful in treating symptomatic lesions of lymphocytoma cutis.

SUGGESTED READINGS

Bain BJ. Lymphomas and reactive lymphoid lesions in HIV infections. Blood Rev 1998; 12: 154–162.

Bangham CRM. HTLV-1 infections. J Clin Pathol 2000; 53: 581–586.

Burns MK, Kennard CD, Dubin HV. Nodular cutaneous B-cell lymphoma of the scalp in the acquired immunodeficiency syndrome. J Am Acad Dermatol 1991; 25: 933–936.

Cao W, Liu YJ. Innate immune functions of plasmacytoid dendritic cells. Curr Opin Immunol 2007; 19: 24–30.

Chang SE, Huh J, Choi JH, et al. Clinicopathological features of CD56+ nasal type T/natural killer cell lymphomas with lobular panniculitis. Br J Dermatol 2000; 142: 924–930.

Gamache-Ottou F, Feuillard J, Saas P. Plasmacytoid dendritic cell leukaemia/lymphoma: towards a well defined entity? Br J Haematol 2007; 136: 539–548.

Heidary N, Naik H, Burgin S. Chemotherapeutic agents and the skin: an update. J Am Acad Dermatol 2008; 58: 545–570.

Jabbour E, Cortes J, O'Brien S, et al. New targeted therapies for chronic myelogenous leukemia: opportunities to overcome imatinib resistance. Semin Hematol Oncol 2007; 44: S25–S31.

Kantarjian HM, Talpaz M. Imatinib mesylate: clinical results in Philadelphia chromosome-positive leukemias. Semin Oncol 2001; 28: 9–18.

Kim K, Kim WS, Jung CW, et al. Clinical features of peripheral T-cell lymphomas in 78 patients diagnosed according to the Revised European-American lymphoma (REAL) classification. Eur J Cancer 2002; 38: 75–81.

López-Guillermo A, Cid J, Salar A, et al. Peripheral T-cell lymphomas: Initial features, natural history, and prognostic factors in a series of 174 patients diagnosed according to the REAL Classification. Ann Oncol 1998; 9: 849–855.

Martel P, Laroche L, Courville P, et al. Cutaneous involvement in patients with angioimmunoblastic lymphadenopathy with dysproteinemia. A clinical, immunohistological, and molecular analysis. Arch Dermatol 2000; 136: 881–886.

McEvoy MT, Connolly SM. Linear IgA dermatosis: association with malignancy. J Am Acad Dermatol 1990; 22: 59–63.

Melchert M, Kale V, List A. The role of lenalidomide in the treatment of patients with chromosome 5q deletion and other myelodysplastic syndromes. Curr Opin Hematol 2007; 14: 123–129.

Ngu IWY, Sinclair EC, Greenaway S, Greenberg ML. Unusual presentation of granulocytic sarcoma in the breast: a case report and review of the literature. Diagn Cytopathol 2001; 24: 53–57.

Nguyen VT, Ndoye A, Bassler KD, et al. Classification, clinical manifestations, and immunologic mechanisms of the epithelial variant of paraneoplastic autoimmune multiorgan syndrome. A reappraisal of paraneoplastic pemphigus. Arch Dermatol 2001; 137: 193–206.

Ohno S, Yokoo T, Ohta M, et al. Aleukemic leukemia cutis. J Am Acad Dermatol 1990; 22: 374–377.

Piette WW, Trapp JF, O'Donnell MJ, et al. Acute neutrophilic dermatosis with myeloblastic infiltrate in a leukemia patient receiving ALL-trans-retinoic acid. J Am Acad Dermatol 1994; 30: 293–297.

Revenga R, Horndler C, Aguilar C, Paricio JF. Cutaneous extramedullary hematopoiesis. Int J Dermatol 2000; 39: 957–958.

Sanz MA, Larrea L, Sanz GF, et al. Cutaneous promyelocytic sarcoma at sites of vascular access and marrow aspiration. A characteristic localization of chloromas in acute promyelocytic leukemia? Haematologica 2000; 85: 758–762.

Schmuth M, Ramaker J, Trautmann C, et al. Cutaneous involvement in prelymphomatous angioimmunoblastic lymphadenopathy. J Am Acad Dermatol 1997; 36: 290–295.

Slater DN. Cutaneous CD56 natural killer and natural killer-like T-cell lymphoma. Br J Dermatol 2000; 142: 853–855.

Stroup RM, Sheibani K, Moncada A, et al. Angiotropic (intravascular) large cell lymphoma: a clinicopathologic study of seven cases with unique clinical presentations. Cancer 1990; 66: 1781–1788.

Susser WS, Whitaker-Worth DL, Grant-Kels JM. Mucocutaneous reactions to chemotherapy. J Am Acad Dermatol 1999; 40: 367–398.

Suzuki R, Nakamura S, Suzumiya J, et al., for NK-Cell Tumor Study Group. Blastic natural killer cell lymphoma/leukemia (CD56-positive blastic tumor). Prognostication and categorization according to anatomic sites of involvement. Cancer 2005; 104: 1022–1031.

Tallman MS, Andersen JW, Schiffer CA, et al. Clinical description of 44 patients with acute promyelocytic leukemia who developed the retinoic acid syndrome. Blood 2000; 95: 90–95.

Tamura K, Sawada H, Izumi Y, et al. Chronic lymphocytic leukemia (CLL) is rare, but the proportion of T-CLL is high in Japan. Eur J Haematol 2001; 67: 152–157.

Willard RJ, Turiansky GW, Genest GP, et al. Leukemia cutis in a patient with chronic neutrophilic leukemia. J Am Acad Dermatol 2001; 44: 365–369.

Chapter | **16** | *Warren W. Piette*

Dysproteinemias, Plasma Cell Disorders, and Amyloidosis

A wide variety of diseases associated with monoclonal immunoglobulin or light chain production may cause cutaneous lesions. In some instances these lesions are directly related to the monoclonal protein, as in many cases of cryoglobulinemia. In other instances the cutaneous lesions result from abnormalities in the metabolism of monoclonal proteins, as in light chain-related systemic amyloidosis. In still others, cutaneous lesions occur in diseases frequently associated with plasma cell dyscrasias.

Any discussion of monoclonal proteins must include monoclonal gammopathy of undetermined significance (MGUS). MGUS is defined as a serum monoclonal protein <30 g/L; <10% plasma cells in the bone marrow; and the absence of end-organ damage (hypercalcemia, renal insufficiency, anemia, and/or bone lesions [CRAB]). Although this disorder is uncommon in young individuals, its incidence increases with age, reaching 3% in those 50 years of age or older, and 5% in those over 70. The risk of progression to multiple myeloma or a related disorder is 1% per year. Three risk factors are useful in predicting the likelihood of progression (as measured at 20 years' follow-up): (1) an increase in serum free light chains; (2) an MGUS of nonimmunoglobulin G (IgG) origin; or (3) a serum M protein of 15 g/L or more. The risk of multiple myeloma at 20 years was 58% with all three risk factors, 37% with two risk factors, 21% with one risk factor, and 5% when no risk factors were present. Smoldering myeloma is a term used to describe an asymptomatic phase of myeloma characterized by a serum IgG or IgA monoclonal protein >30 g/L and/or >10% plasma cells in the bone marrow, but no evidence of myeloma-related end-organ damage. In this group, the cumulative probability of progression to active multiple myeloma or amyloidosis was 51% at 5 years, 66% at 10 years, and 73% at 15 years, with a median time to progression of 4.8 years.

This discussion of cutaneous disease associated with monoclonal protein disorders is divided into three parts, as follows: (1) disorders directly related to monoclonal proteins (cryoglobulinemia, hyperviscosity syndrome, or cold agglutinin disease); (2) disorders associated with monoclonal protein production (such as POEMS syndrome, normolipemic plane xanthomas, and scleromyxedema); and (3) disorders directly related to amyloid deposition.

DISORDERS DIRECTLY RELATED TO MONOCLONAL PROTEINS

Pathogenesis

Monoclonal proteins may cause disease directly by acting as cryoglobulins, by raising serum viscosity, or by acting as cold agglutinins. Cryoglobulins are immunoglobulins that precipitate on exposure to cold. They may be unstable in other settings, such as in the hyperosmotic environment found in the kidneys, or in microvascular areas with a slow blood flow. The most critical factor that determines the behavior of the cryoglobulin in vivo is the temperature at which it begins to precipitate. If that temperature approaches those found in the cutaneous microvasculature on cold exposure, cold-induced disease is usually significant. If it precipitates only at a temperature well below room temperature, the symptoms will not be cold related. Cryoglobulins are divided into three categories, depending on their composition. Type I cryoglobulins consist of a single monoclonal protein; type II are composed of a monoclonal immunoglobulin with anti-IgG (rheumatoid factor) activity that binds to polyclonal serum IgG; and type III cryoglobulins consist of polyclonal immunoglobulins, usually with anti-IgG activity, that bind to polyclonal serum IgG (a polyclonal rheumatoid factor). Roughly 5–10% of myeloma proteins and macroglobulins are cryoprecipitable. Types I and II cryoglobulinemia are often (but not always) associated with a lymphoproliferative disorder or plasma cell dyscrasia. Patients with type II cryoglobulinemia may have IgM, IgG, or IgA as their monoclonal rheumatoid factor. The possibility that rheumatoid factor may be an IgM or IgA is important because IgM or IgA monoclonal proteins may not be detected by routine serum protein electrophoresis when bound to polyclonal IgG.

The hyperviscosity syndrome results from a significant increase in whole blood viscosity. Such an increase may be related to an increase in the cellular elements in the blood, as in polycythemia vera or primary thrombocythemia. It may also result from a change in serum viscosity as a result of the presence of large amounts of monoclonal protein in the blood. If immunoglobulin related, the hyperviscosity syndrome is usually caused by a monoclonal IgM protein. Monoclonal IgG or IgA can cause the hyperviscosity syndrome, but only if the monoclonal antibody is present in the serum at higher concentrations, or if the patient's serum is prone to self-aggregation.

Cold agglutinin disease is actually a cold antibody-induced autoimmune hemolytic anemia. The antibody, usually IgM, binds to the red cell in the cold and initiates complement activation; it then elutes at body temperature while the complement activation proceeds to red cell lysis. The cold agglutinin also promotes temperature-dependent agglutination of red cells, leading to sludging or occlusion of the blood flow in the microvasculature exposed to cold temperatures.

Clinical Manifestations

Cryoglobulinemia

Type I cryoglobulins are usually IgM and therefore primarily intravascular; however, they can also be composed of IgG. They are likely to precipitate at temperatures easily attained in the cutaneous microvasculature. Both of these factors contribute to clinically important cold-induced disease. Such disease

may present as Raynaud's phenomenon, livedo reticularis, digital infarcts, peripheral gangrene, or purpura; the latter may be palpable (Fig. 16–1A,B), exhibit central necrosis, or have a livedoid or retiform component (Fig. 16–1C).

Cold sensitivity is more variable with types II and III cryoglobulins because these are usually bound to normal IgG. The classification of essential mixed cryoglobulinemia is now known to be composed primarily of patients with hepatitis C viral infection. Mixed cryoglobulins may be detected as cryoproteins or as rheumatoid factor in the laboratory; in the patient, they are more likely to cause disease as an immune complex than as a cryogelling protein. For this reason, mixed cryoglobulinemias tend to present with features of leukocytoclastic (necrotizing) vasculitis that affect both small and medium-sized vessels in the skin and elsewhere. Palpable purpura, digital infarcts, arthralgias and arthritis, and glomerulonephritis are the usual clinical features. Some patients with an underlying lymphoproliferative disease may develop angioedema with urticaria as a result of C1 esterase inhibitor depletion; the monoclonal protein in such patients may also behave as a cryoglobulin in the test tube. Finally, some cases of cold-induced urticaria are caused by a circulating cryoglobulin without evidence of any associated disease.

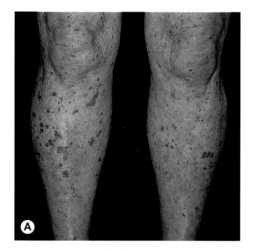

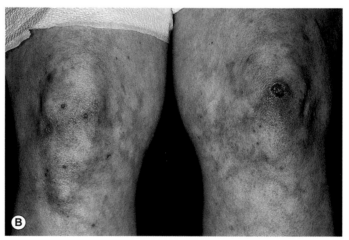

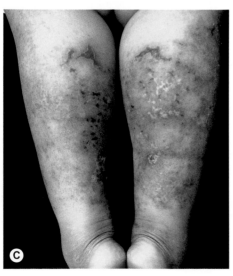

Figure 16–1 (A,B) Palpable purpura in a patient with cryoglobulinemia. (C) Retiform necrotic lesions in a patient with type I cryoglobulinemia.

Hyperviscosity Syndrome

Hyperviscosity syndrome may present as mucous membrane bleeding, retinopathy, neurologic disturbances, hypervolemia, or cardiac failure, and if caused by a cryoglobulin, Raynaud's phenomenon. Symptoms require a four- to fivefold increase in blood viscosity, seldom seen with <4 g/dL serum concentrations of IgM if the result of monoclonal proteins. Hyperviscosity alone may not fully explain the increased bleeding tendency in these patients. Additional factors in some patients are antibody activity against clotting factors, platelet dysfunction as a result of surface coating by immunoglobulin, and other poorly understood clotting defects.

Cold Agglutinin Disease

Cold agglutinin disease is characterized clinically by episodes of hemolytic anemia, hemoglobinuria, and cold-mediated vaso-occlusive phenomena. Patients may develop acrocyanosis, Raynaud-like phenomenon, or generalized livedo reticularis, but cutaneous ulcerations or necrosis are unusual. Jaundice or pallor may follow a severe episode of hemolysis. Cold agglutinin disease occurs in two forms: primary (idiopathic) and secondary. Patients with primary cold agglutinin disease may develop features diagnostic of, or similar to, Waldenström's macroglobulinemia, whereas secondary forms follow certain infections. Cold agglutinins can also be categorized by their red cell antigen affinity. The antibodies are usually directed against the I/i antigen system, and, rarely, against Pr group antigens. Anti-I antibodies occur primarily in association with idiopathic disease, *Mycoplasma* pneumonia, and some lymphomas; anti-i-specific antibodies are associated with infectious mononucleosis and some lymphomas. The cold agglutinins are monoclonal in primary and lymphoma-associated disease and polyclonal in post-infectious disease. The rare cases of IgA cold agglutinin disease are also characterized by red cell agglutination in the microvasculature, but hemolytic anemia does not develop because the cell-bound IgA does not fix complement.

Waldenström's Macroglobulinemia

This is a disease characterized by a serum monoclonal IgM spike and by malignant lymphoplasmacytoid proliferation, primarily in the bone marrow, liver, spleen, and lymph nodes. In some patients the IgM paraprotein may behave as a monoclonal (type I) cryoglobulin or a cold agglutinin. Urticarial vasculitis associated with an IgM monoclonal protein, bone pain with hyperostosis, and intermittent fever is known as Schnitzler's syndrome.

Cryofibrinogenemia

Cryofibrinogen is a plasma complex of fibrin, fibrinogen, and fibronectin that can precipitate on cooling and clot when combined with thrombin. Cryofibrinogenemia occurs as a primary disorder, or as an associated disorder in patients with neoplasia, acute infections, collagen vascular disorders, or thromboembolic disease. It was recently recognized that patients with cryofibrinogenemia often present with recurrent painful cutaneous ulcerations of the lower leg and foot. Purpura, often nonpalpable, may accompany the ulcers, which are usually small. The ulcerations heal with ivory stellate scars, resembling the cutaneous features of livedoid vasculopathy (Fig. 16–2).

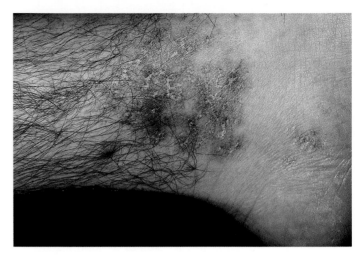

Figure 16–2 Purpuric nodules within a livedoid vasculopathy-like eruption in a patient with hepatitis C-related cryoglobulinemia.

Differential Diagnosis

The differential diagnosis for cryoglobulinemia or cold agglutinin disease depends on the disease's manifestations. In cases of mixed cryoglobulinemia presenting as leukocytoclastic vasculitis, the differential diagnosis primarily includes other necrotizing vasculitides. Hyperviscosity syndrome is usually caused by a clonal lymphoproliferative disorder, but it can result from other hematologic disorders, such as polycythemia vera. Raynaud's phenomenon may be idiopathic (Raynaud's disease), or may be secondary to an autoimmune connective tissue disease, including scleroderma, lupus erythematosus, rheumatoid arthritis, or Sjögren's syndrome. Other diseases may resemble Raynaud's phenomenon; in addition to those mentioned in this section, conditions such as ergotism, Buerger's disease, chilblains (pernio), and acrocyanosis should be considered. In patients presenting with lesions of dermal vessel occlusion (cold agglutinin disease or monoclonal cryoglobulinemia), disorders that must also be considered include cryofibrinogenemia, disseminated intravascular coagulation, thrombotic thrombocytopenic purpura, warfarin- or heparin-induced necrosis, and paroxysmal nocturnal hemoglobinuria (see Chapter 11).

Histopathologic Findings

Early cutaneous lesions of monoclonal cryoglobulinemia demonstrate intravascular amorphous eosinophilic material that is composed principally of precipitated cryoglobulin. There is often red blood cell extravasation into the dermis. Inflammation is usually minimal, is located perivascularly, is lymphohistiocytic, and appears to be a response to, rather than a cause of, necrosis, which results from vessel occlusion. By contrast, early cutaneous lesions of mixed cryoglobulinemia show histopathologic changes of leukocytoclastic (necrotizing) vasculitis, including neutrophilic infiltration of the vessel wall, nuclear fragments of dead neutrophils (nuclear dust), and fibrinoid necrosis of the vessel walls. Immunoreactant deposition in vessel walls can be seen on direct immunofluorescence microscopy, although this is a nonspecific finding. The exact histologic picture depends on the age of the lesions that undergo biopsy, although such information is seldom provided in reported studies and is generally ignored when analyzing data on histologic findings. Positive immunofluorescence microscopic findings are not expected in lesions more than 24–48 hours old, and the neutrophilic infiltrate may be largely replaced by a lymphohistiocytic infiltrate as the lesion evolves. Therefore, older lesions in patients with either intravascular gelling or leukocytoclastic vasculitis on biopsy may show similar nondiagnostic changes.

Cutaneous lesions that are the result of cryofibrinogenemia, cold agglutinin disease, or paroxysmal nocturnal hemoglobinuria should show histologic evidence of multiple dermal vessel thrombosis, usually in the absence of significant inflammatory infiltrate. The histologic findings are essentially identical to those seen in the cutaneous lesions of disseminated intravascular coagulation.

Evaluation

Although the detection and analysis of a serum or urine monoclonal immunoglobulin or Bence Jones protein (i.e. light chain) was classically accomplished via serum or urine protein electrophoresis, immunofixation techniques have proved to be significantly more sensitive. Recently, the serum free light chain assay has emerged as the most sensitive method for the detection of plasma cell dyscrasias characterized by overproduction of light chains. When a patient is suspected of having a cryoprotein-related disease, a simple screening procedure may be helpful. Blood is drawn for both serum and plasma sampling and kept at body temperature until the cellular elements have been removed. Following at least overnight refrigeration, each sample is then examined for evidence of a cryoprecipitate. A cryoglobulin should appear in both the serum and the plasma sample, whereas cryofibrinogen will appear in only the plasma fraction. Immunofixation of the precipitated cryoglobulin can then define its composition. Patients found to have type I or II cryoglobulins should be examined for an underlying plasma cell dyscrasia or lymphoproliferative disorder. Patients with type II or III cryoglobulins should be evaluated for hepatitis C viral infection; non-hepatitis-related disease may be secondary to an underlying connective tissue or autoimmune disease, or to other chronic infections or inflammatory diseases.

Confirmation of a presumptive diagnosis of cold agglutinin disease or paroxysmal nocturnal hemoglobinuria usually requires consultation with hematologists and hematopathologists. Vessel occlusion caused by cold agglutinins is rare, although cold agglutinins can be detected at low levels in many different acute and chronic diseases. If hyperviscosity syndrome is suspected, serum viscosity measurements are usually easily obtained from clinical laboratories, but whole blood viscosity measurements remain a specialized research procedure.

Treatment

The treatment of cryoglobulinemia depends on the clinical features. If clinically relevant cold sensitivity is present (usually associated with an IgM type I cryoglobulin), adequate clothing and avoidance of cold exposure are essential and may be all that is required. For those with more severe disease, treatment of the underlying plasma cell dyscrasia or lymphoproliferative disorder is indicated. In patients with type II or III cryoglobulinemia, in whom necrotizing vasculitis is the usual presenting finding, therapy will depend on the manifestations. Cutaneous lesions may respond to oral dapsone or colchicine therapy, whereas aggressive therapy with systemic corticosteroids in combination with immunosuppressive or cytotoxic agents may be required in severe systemic disease. In hepatitis C-related cryoglobulinemia, antiviral therapy may reduce the vasculitis but can occasionally induce flaring. Patients with specific underlying etiologic disorders may respond to effective treatment of that disorder. Plasmapheresis may provide temporary but rapid relief of symptoms in patients with high levels of circulating cryoglobulins, and it may be synergistic when combined with chemotherapy in appropriate cases. Intravenous γ-globulin therapy is occasionally successful in cryoglobulinemia and refractory vasculitis.

Cold agglutinin disease is best treated by keeping the patient (particularly the extremities) warm. Cytotoxic agents may be useful in some patients, but plasmapheresis is contraindicated because it may induce severe hemolytic anemia. Post-infectious cases of cold agglutinin disease are usually self-limiting.

For patients in whom simple measures do not address the clinical manifestations of cryofibrinogenemia, the use of an oral anabolic steroid such as stanozolol (4–8 mg/day) or danazol may prove beneficial, with rapid pain relief and ulcer healing observed in a number of patients. Stanozolol and danazol are androgenic steroids with fibrinolytic properties, but unfortunately stanozolol has recently been removed from the market in the United States. Other therapies for livedoid vasculopathy associated with cryofibrinogenemia include heparin, warfarin, streptokinase, plasmapheresis, immunosuppressive agents, and tissue plasminogen activator.

DISORDERS ASSOCIATED WITH MONOCLONAL PROTEIN PRODUCTION

Pathogenesis

This group of disorders is united by the frequent finding of an associated monoclonal gammopathy. Some diseases are almost always associated with a monoclonal gammopathy (e.g., POEMS syndrome, scleromyxedema), whereas others are frequently associated with a monoclonal gammopathy (e.g., normolipemic plane xanthoma). Many diseases have a greater than chance association with the presence of a serum or urine monoclonal protein, but this is not required for typical disease expression (e.g., scleredema). The known relationship between these diseases and the expression of monoclonal protein will be mentioned in the context of the individual diseases.

Clinical Manifestations

POEMS Syndrome

This was recognized as a distinct entity in Japan in 1968 and is also known as the Crow–Fukase or Takatsuki syndrome. This disease is reported primarily in Japan, but cases have now been described in the United States. POEMS is an acronym for polyneuropathy, organomegaly, endocrinopathy, M-protein, and skin changes. In the largest series to date (102 patients), men were affected twice as frequently as women, and patients were young to middle-aged adults with a mean age of 46 years (compared to mean age of myeloma presentation of 62 years). All patients had peripheral polyneuropathy (usually sensorimotor), 97% had elevated cerebrospinal fluid protein, and 62% had papilledema. Organomegaly was manifested as hepatomegaly in 82% of the patients, lymphadenopathy in 65%, and splenomegaly in 39%. The most common endocrine abnormalities were impotence (78%) and gynecomastia (68%) in men, and amenorrhea (68%) in women. Additional endocrine findings in this and other series include glucose intolerance (28–48%), hyperthyroidism (10–24%), and hyperprolactinemia, adrenal insufficiency or hypercalcemia (rare).

Most patients (75%) have had a serum or, rarely, a urine monoclonal spike. Of these spikes, approximately 55% are IgG_1 and 40% are IgA_1. Although in some of these patients the disease may ultimately progress to multiple myeloma, this does not always occur. Slightly more than half of patients with POEMS syndrome had bone lesions, and 85% of patients with bone lesions had osteosclerotic lesions, with or without osteolytic lesions; this is in contrast to a large series of patients with myeloma in whom osteosclerotic lesions comprised only 0.5–3.0% of bone lesions. Also, unlike the findings in osteolytic multiple myeloma, anemia, hypercalcemia, and renal insufficiency are uncommon, and extensive bone marrow infiltration by plasma cells is rare.

Cutaneous changes are common in this disorder, and reported changes include diffuse hyperpigmentation (93–98%); peripheral edema (92%); and sometimes anasarca, hypertrichosis (78–81%), a poorly characterized skin thickening (77–85%), and digital clubbing (56%). Cutaneous angiomas occur in 24–44% of patients and include cherry, verrucous, subcutaneous, or 'glomeruloid' angiomas (Fig. 16–3). The histopathological finding of a glomeruloid angioma is highly indicative of this syndrome. That circulating levels of vascular endothelial growth factor (VEGF) are markedly increased in these patients may provide some explanation for the vascular and circulatory changes in POEMS. This increase in VEGF may come from aggregating platelets overly rich in VEGF, which could provide very high local microcirculatory concentrations of VEGF. In patients with POEMS in association with multicentric Castleman's disease, viral interleukin (IL)-6 produced by human herpesvirus-8 could also lead to increased circulating levels of VEGF. Terry's nails, Raynaud's phenomenon, and sicca syndrome have also been described. Biopsy findings of the skin are often nonspecific, but include hyperpigmentation, dermal thickening caused by edema and an increase in collagen and proteoglycan, microvascular proliferation, and occasional large fibroblasts in the dermis.

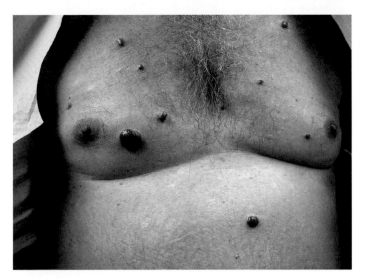

Figure 16–3 Multiple angiomas in this patient with POEMS syndrome.

Variable findings include ascites, pleural effusions, fever, polycythemia, leukocytosis, thrombocytosis, and an elevated erythrocyte sedimentation rate. POEMS syndrome may predispose to arterial and venous thromboses and stroke. Associations with Castleman's disease have been reported, as have presentations such as flushing, hypotension, and bronchial spasm, mimicking carcinoid. As awareness of this syndrome increases, it is likely that its recognition in the United States will increase, particularly in the group of patients with cryptogenic polyneuropathies or isolated osteosclerotic bone lesions. The AESOP (adenopathy and extensive skin patch overlying a plasmacytoma) syndrome describes a distinctive presentation of a slowly extending violaceous skin patch overlying a solitary plasmacytoma of bone, associated with enlarged regional lymph nodes. Of the four reported patients, all had neuropathy and two developed POEMS syndrome. Treatment of the plasmacytoma resulted in resolution of the syndrome in all but one of the patients. Of note, according to the current WHO–EORTC classification of cutaneous B-cell lymphomas with primary cutaneous manifestations, cases previously designated as primary cutaneous plasmacytomas are now classified as primary cutaneous marginal zone B-cell lymphomas.

Cutaneous Plasmacytomas

These are rare and may be solitary or multiple. Most of these cutaneous lesions are smooth, nontender, cutaneous or subcutaneous nodules, skin-colored to violaceous, and 1–5 cm in diameter, and they may be crusted or ulcerated. They are usually located on the trunk, extremities, or face. Cutaneous plasmacytomas indicate a large tumor cell burden in patients with multiple myeloma, and therefore they usually occur late in the course of the disease. Lesions may develop either as an extension from underlying bone or as distinct cutaneous metastases. All immunoglobulin classes have been associated with cutaneous plasmacytomas, but most are IgG- or IgA-producing cells. Although IgD myeloma is rare, patients with this disease have a higher incidence of extramedullary lesions, including cutaneous plasmacytomas (up to 18%). The IgD subset of myeloma usually develops in young men and has an aggressive course.

In a few instances a solitary cutaneous plasmacytoma may be an isolated finding, even with long-term follow-up. Because the number of plasma cells in such a lesion is small and the amount of immunoglobulin synthesized is directly related to cell numbers, such patients are unlikely to have a serum monoclonal antibody spike. Conversely, the presence of a monoclonal spike suggests extracutaneous disease.

Cutaneous and Systemic Plasmacytosis

Plasma cell-rich lesions have been described in cutaneous and systemic plasmacytosis as well as plasma cell orificial mucositis. Cutaneous and systemic plasmacytosis is a rare disorder reported almost exclusively in patients of Japanese descent, and is characterized by widespread reddish-brown macules (due to polyclonal plasma cell infiltration), polyclonal hypergammaglobulinemia, peripheral adenopathy (~60%), and sometimes infiltration of the lung, liver, spleen, or kidney. Although rare, these disorders present with so extensive an infiltration of plasma cells that, on biopsy, they may mimic cutaneous plasmacytomas.

Necrobiotic Xanthogranuloma with Paraproteinemia

This is a distinctive entity, typically presenting with yellowish periorbital plaques or nodules that tend to ulcerate and heal with scar formation. Lesions may also develop on the trunk or proximal limbs, especially in flexural areas (Fig. 16–4). The lesions often extend deeply into the dermis and subcutis and, on biopsy, show both Touton and foreign body giant cells, broad areas of altered collagen, and necrobiosis on a background of extensive granulomatous inflammation. Most patients have a monoclonal gammopathy (IgG, often κ), many have leukopenia, and although bone marrow plasmacytosis is common, multiple myeloma or other lymphoproliferative disorders are rare. In one series, hepatomegaly or splenomegaly was reported in 20 of 48 patients.

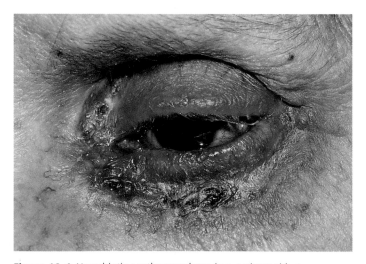

Figure 16–4 Necrobiotic xanthogranuloma in a patient with a paraproteinemia.

Other Xanthomatous Disease

Other xanthomatous disorders may occasionally indicate an underlying plasma cell disorder. Xanthoma disseminatum is a disorder that usually develops in patients 25 years old or younger and is associated with an increased incidence of monoclonal gammopathy or multiple myeloma in adults (see Table 17–2). Generalized plane xanthomatosis has also been associated with multiple myeloma. Lesions in this disorder are yellow to yellow-brown flat plaques, and, when generalized, they typically involve the head, eyelids, neck, and upper trunk. Rarely, patients with multiple myeloma have an anti-lipoprotein antibody as their monoclonal protein, and this may result in an abnormal lipid profile and, occasionally, in the development of xanthomas.

Benign Hypergammaglobulinemic Purpura of Waldenström

This is characterized by flat, petechial or small purpuric lesions on the lower extremities in association with polyclonal hypergammaglobulinemia. New lesions may develop in cycles and may be preceded by a burning sensation. Most patients have an IgG anti-IgG rheumatoid factor that is not demonstrated by current standard rheumatoid factor testing; it precipitates in the 12–15S range on analytic ultracentrifugation. Some of these IgG rheumatoid factors have been shown by specialized tests to be monoclonal, and this may relate to the small but increased incidence of multiple myeloma or lymphoproliferative disorders in some patients after several years of disease. Both primary and secondary forms of this disease have been described. At least half the patients with primary disease in one series who were followed for 5 years developed evidence of an associated disease, occasionally malignant but usually autoimmune. Such autoimmune diseases include keratoconjunctivitis sicca, Sjögren's syndrome, lupus erythematosus (particularly anti-Ro [SS-A]-positive disease), undifferentiated connective tissue disease, or sarcoidosis.

Scleromyxedema

This is a type of generalized lichen myxedematosus (also known as papular mucinosis) that presents with coalescent erythematous to yellow papules and plaques (Figs 16–5, 16–6). Usually located on the face, neck and forearms, these plaques may mimic the facial features of acromegaly or generalized myxedema. These patients may suffer from intense pruritus. They may also have esophageal dysmotility, myopathic changes, arthritis, neuropathy, or cardiac disease.

Patients with scleromyxedema frequently have an associated monoclonal gammopathy and may have a characteristic finding on serum protein electrophoresis of a 'slow γ-region' migrating protein (extreme migration toward the negative electrode). Evidence suggests that this unusual migration pattern is not caused by a response to a common antigen, because careful studies in some patients appear to show different idiotype characteristics from patient to patient. Some studies found that sera from these patients produced a mucin-stimulatory effect on fibroblasts in vitro, and one study suggested – but did not prove – that the abnormal protein was not the stimula-

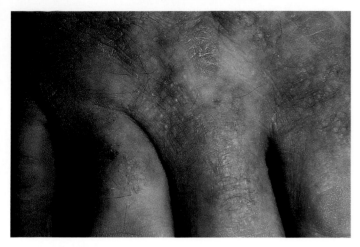

Figure 16–5 Multiple small papules in a linear array in a patient with papular mucinosis and paraproteinemia.

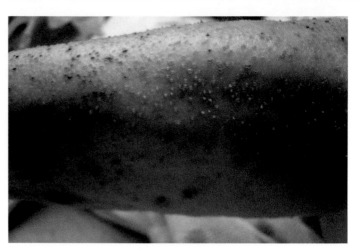

Figure 16–7 Multiple follicular keratotic lesions in this patient with myeloma.

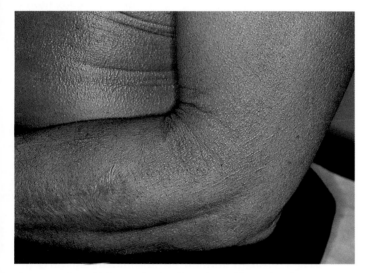

Figure 16–6 Multiple papules that have formed linear bands in a patient with lichen myxedematosus.

tory factor. Despite the frequent (albeit not obligatory) presence of monoclonal protein in this disease, associated lymphoproliferative malignancies have not been reported.

Other Disorders

Other cutaneous diseases may have a rare, but apparently real, association with monoclonal gammopathies due to plasma cell dyscrasias or lymphoproliferative diseases. Such diseases include scleredema adultorum, erythema elevatum diutinum, subcorneal pustular dermatosis, pyoderma gangrenosum, some forms of acquired angioedema (patients can develop a monoclonal protein with anti-C1 esterase activity, for example), and, more rarely, dermatomyositis, dermatitis herpetiformis, cutaneous T-cell lymphoma, and Kaposi's sarcoma. Although IgG paraprotein-associated disorders are usually the most common, some of these disorders (erythema elevatum diutinum, subcorneal pustular dermatosis, and pyoderma gangrenosum) appear to have a strong IgA association, which is

as yet unexplained. Dermatitis herpetiformis is frequently associated with polyclonal IgA gammopathy, but the increased incidence of malignancies in this disease is due to enteropathy-associated T-cell lymphoma, not myeloma. Spicule-like hyperkeratosis (follicular > nonfollicular) has been reported as a rare but distinctive cutaneous finding in patients with myeloma (Fig. 16–7), as has crystal-storing histiocytosis; the latter is also associated with lymphoproliferative disorders. Although skin involvement is rare in crystal-storing histiocytosis, the histologic findings are distinctive: macrophages with thin crystalloid structures in the cytoplasm, consisting of phagocytosed crystals of immunoglobulins. Additional rarely reported associations include possible increased sensitivity to developing halogenoderma, pityriasis rotunda, and linear IgA bullous dermatosis.

Treatment

The therapy of these disorders is aimed largely at controlling the underlying disease process when present. Multiple myeloma usually responds to thalidomide, lenalidomide, or bortezomib (a proteasome inhibitor), either alone or in combination with weekly systemic corticosteroids. Autologous hematopoietic stem cell transplantation is considered the standard of care for patients under the age of 60 after they have responded to medical therapy. POEMS syndrome may be treated with radiation therapy for isolated osteosclerotic lesions, or with regimens similar to those used for myeloma if warranted by systemic symptoms. Cutaneous plasmacytomas are treated with radiation and/or chemotherapy. Individual lesions show a partial response to intralesional injections of tumor necrosis factor (TNF)-α. Patients with Schnitzler's syndrome have been reported to respond to anakinra therapy. Therapy of xanthoma disseminatum is often ineffective, but cutaneous lesions may respond if systemic cytotoxic therapy is otherwise indicated. Individual lesions may respond to cryotherapy. The therapy of hypergammaglobulinemic purpura in the absence of a lymphoproliferative disorder is largely symptomatic, and the therapeutic agents used to treat vasculitis should be considered (see Chapter 4). Necrobiotic xanthogranuloma and scleromyxedema may respond to therapy with alkylating agents such as melphalan, but the benefits must outweigh the risks, including the long-term risk of leukemogenesis. Scleromyxedema occasionally responds to therapy with topical high-potency corticosteroids, topical dimethyl sulfoxide, systemic corticosteroids, oral isotretinoin, thalidomide, cytotoxic therapy, phototherapy, plasmapheresis, or extracorporeal photochemotherapy. Recently, autologous hematopoietic stem cell transplantation has been reported as successful in a number of patients with scleromyxedema, but the durability of the response is uncertain.

AMYLOIDOSIS

Amyloidosis is a general term used to describe a group of conditions characterized by the extracellular deposition of an abnormal protein that has a specific set of staining properties and a fibrillar ultrastructure. Cutaneous deposition of amyloid can occur in primary systemic amyloidosis (i.e., amyloidosis associated with plasma cell dyscrasia and light chain related), in secondary systemic amyloidosis caused by chronic inflammatory conditions, in patients undergoing chronic hemodialysis, in distinctive familial syndromes of amyloidosis, and in a variety of localized cutaneous amyloidoses.

Pathogenesis

The deposition of amyloid is still an incompletely understood process, but all disorders of amyloid deposition have in common the synthesis of amyloid fibrils from a precursor protein and the binding of a ring-shaped amyloid P component onto the amyloid fibril. Although most proteins in humans and other species are synthesized in an α-helical structure, amyloid proteins are among the few that are synthesized in a β-pleated sheet structure, which is much less biodegradable.

There are 18–20 known precursor proteins for amyloid, and at least seven known proteins that can serve as precursors for amyloid fibril deposition in the skin: (1) light chain monoclonal protein; (2) serum protein A; (3) β_2-microglobulin; (4) plasma transthyretin (prealbumin); (5) gelsolin; (6) cystatin C; and (7) keratin or keratin-related proteins. The pattern of amyloid deposition correlates with the precursor protein type, which in turn depends on the underlying syndrome. This means that the clinical pattern of disease may suggest the type of amyloid precursor involved, and hence the most likely sites for biopsy. Also, the pattern of cutaneous deposition may be predictive for the presence or absence of extracutaneous disease, and for the likely fibril source.

Clinical Manifestations (Table 16–1)

Light Chain-Related Systemic Amyloidoses

The age-adjusted incidence of light chain-related amyloidosis is between 5.1 and 12.8 per million person-years, accounting for 1300–3200 new cases annually in the United States. This

is roughly one-fifth the incidence of multiple myeloma, and about the same incidence as Hodgkin's disease or Ph1-positive chronic granulocytic leukemia. Men account for 60–65% of cases, and only 1% of patients are under the age of 20. Fatigue and weight loss are the most common presenting symptoms. Light-headedness is also common, and may be secondary to nephrotic syndrome with volume contraction, to cardiac amyloidosis with low stroke volume, or to autonomic neuropathy with orthostatic hypotension.

The light chain-derived systemic amyloidoses (amyloid light chain fibril, or AL) occur in the setting of primary systemic amyloidosis and an associated plasma cell dyscrasia. True myeloma-associated amyloidosis is uncommon. Even when patients with AL amyloidosis have >10% plasma cells in the bone marrow, lytic bone lesions, myeloma cast nephropathy, and anemia secondary to marrow replacement are rare. It is assumed that all AL fibril-type systemic amyloidoses are caused by a monoclonal protein. Blood or urine immunofixation studies for monoclonal immunoglobulin or light chain protein are positive in nearly 90% of cases, and both should be obtained if AL amyloidosis is suspected. Even in those instances in which no monoclonal abnormality can be detected, the problem is thought to be one of test sensitivity. More recently, the serum free light chain assay, which is nearly 100% sensitive, has improved diagnostic accuracy; in contrast to immunofixation, it is a quantitative assay. Subcutaneous fat aspiration is positive in 70–80% of patients with AL amyloidosis.

The reported incidence of cutaneous lesions in AL-derived systemic amyloidosis ranges from 10% to 40%. The most common lesions include purpura, papules, plaques, and nodules, but bullous eruptions (sometimes mimicking porphyria cutanea tarda or epidermolysis bullosa acquisita), scleroderma-like cutaneous infiltration, pigmentary changes, nail dystrophies, acral localized acquired cutis laxa, and alopecia have been reported. Purpura is most common (Figs 16–8, 16–9) and is usually attributed to amyloid infiltration of the dermal blood vessels and supporting tissue, resulting in problems with hemostasis following mild trauma. Rare causes of hemorrhage in AL amyloidosis include depletion of Factor X by adsorption to splenic amyloid deposits, and acquired von Willebrand syndrome, apparently secondary to the plasma cell dyscrasia. Deposition of AL amyloid is most prominent on the upper body. Stroking or pinching the skin usually induces purpura in lesions in these areas, and spontaneous periorbital hemorrhage is commonly seen following Valsalva-like maneuvers (coughing or vomiting) or a dependently positioned head. Papules and plaques are most often yellow to skin-colored, nonpruritic, and frequently hemorrhagic. A waxy or translucent character in such papules is strongly suggestive of AL-type amyloid deposition. Papular deposition of amyloid is most common on the central face, eyelids, lips, tongue, buccal mucosa, postauricular areas, neck, and intertriginous zones. Rarely, tissue infiltration by amyloid may present as proptosis, ophthalmoplegia, periarticular soft tissue enlargement, or skeletal muscle pseudohypertrophy. Infiltration of lacrimal or parotid glands may cause keratoconjunctivitis sicca or may mimic Sjögren's syndrome. Deposits of AL amyloid can involve almost any internal structure, but the most character-

Table 16–1 Characteristics of systemic amyloidoses

Feature	Light chain-related AL	Secondary/Reactive AA	Dialysis-associated A β-microglobulin	Heredofamilial ATTR & others
Underlying disease	Almost always associated with monoclonal protein	Usually associated with chronic infection or inflammatory disease	Usually occurs after long-term dialysis	Usually related to altered protein, most frequently transthyretin
Major clinical presentation	Cardiac, renal, gastrointestinal, carpal tunnel	Renal	Chronic arthralgias, destructive arthropathy, carpal tunnel syndrome	Dependent on family, but commonly neuropathic
Renal	Expected	Expected	Already on dialysis	
Hepatic	Usually	Usually	Uncommon	
Spleen	Often	Often	Uncommon	
Cardiac	Frequently impaired	Deposits common, but impairment very rare	Uncommon	
Periarticular	Occurs, carpal tunnel common	Rare	Expected, carpal tunnel common	
Neurologic	Common, often autonomic	Rare		
Macroglossia	12–15%	No	One case reported	
Cutaneous findings	Clinical lesions 10–40%, subclinical deposits frequent	Clinical lesions rare, subclinical deposits frequent	Clinical skin lesions rare, subclinical deposits occasional	Syndrome dependent: clinical lesions occur in several, subclinical deposits expected in some syndromes

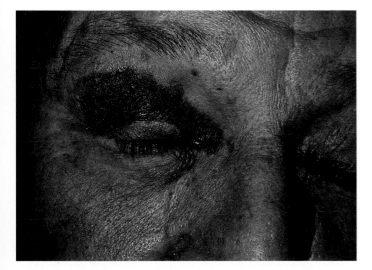

Figure 16–8 'Pinch purpura' in a patient with multiple myeloma. This represents amyloidosis of the skin.

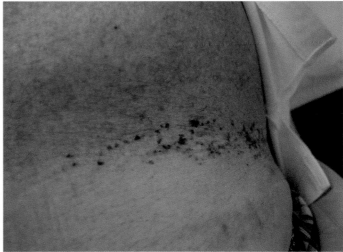

Figure 16–9 Widespread purpura due to amyloidosis occurring as a late manifestation of myeloma.

istic associated features include peripheral neuropathy, carpal tunnel syndrome, orthostatic hypotension as a result of autonomic neuropathy, macroglossia, congestive heart failure (secondary to a restrictive cardiomyopathy), and nephrotic syndrome.

In patients with AL amyloidosis and multiorgan dysfunction the prognosis is 1–2-year survival. Modest therapeutic efficacy of chronic alkylating therapy is supported by several studies, but patients may die before they have had sufficient time to respond. Some studies have shown benefit of high-dose chemotherapy with hematopoietic stem cell transplantation, but numbers are small and toxicity is high, especially if there is existing multiorgan dysfunction or cardiac disease.

Reactive or Secondary Amyloidosis

Acquired systemic amyloidosis of the amyloid A (AA) protein fibril type is usually seen in association with a chronic inflammatory process, such as rheumatoid arthritis, leprosy, tuberculosis, syphilis, chronic osteomyelitis, or chronic inflammatory bowel disease. It may also be associated with certain long-standing cutaneous disorders that may be the source of chronic inflammation, such as decubitus ulcers, stasis ulcers, thermal burns, neglected basal cell carcinomas, hidradenitis suppurativa, dystrophic epidermolysis bullosa, psoriasis and psoriatic arthritis, and reactive arthritis (previously referred to as Reiter's disease). In the United States, secondary amyloidosis is rare because chronic inflammation secondary to infection is rare. Amyloid fibrils in this setting are derived from chronically elevated serum protein A, an apolipoprotein. This protein increases with inflammation, during pregnancy, and with advancing age. Any organ may be involved, but significant hepatic, splenic, and renal infiltration is most typical. Also, unlike systemic AL fibril disease, cardiac infiltration in AA fibril disease almost never results in cardiac dysfunction.

Deposition of amyloid in the skin is common in AA amyloidosis and may be detected by subcutaneous fat aspiration or, less often, by blind skin biopsy. However, clinically apparent skin lesions are rare. Macular purpura is one of the few reported manifestations. The rarity of skin lesions in this syndrome distinguishes it from AL amyloidosis. The presence of cutaneous lesions in a patient with systemic amyloidosis strongly suggests AL rather than AA amyloidosis.

Hemodialysis-Related Amyloidosis

A more recently recognized category of systemic amyloidosis is termed hemodialysis-related amyloidosis and is dependent on β_2-microglobulin. This single polypeptide chain (length 100 amino acids) is normally present on all cell membranes, except erythrocytes and trophoblastic cells, and is the constant β-chain portion of the class I histocompatibility antigen molecule. The β_2-microglobulin molecule is constantly shed from cell membranes, and like many proteins it is freely filtered through the glomerulus and reabsorbed in the proximal tubule, where it is catabolized. In renal failure this major catabolic pathway is lost, and serum levels rise. The incidence of systemic amyloidosis in this condition depends partly on the length of time the patient has been undergoing dialysis, but most β_2-microglobulin-associated amyloidosis occurs in patients dialyzed for 8 or more years. The amyloid is deposited primarily in perineural and periarticular structures, joints, bones, skin, and subcutaneous tissue. Patients typically present with shoulder periarthritis, carpal tunnel syndrome, and flexor tenosynovitis of the hands. The incidence of carpal tunnel syndrome in this group ranges from 2% to 31%. Other major clinical manifestations of this deposition are chronic arthralgias and destructive arthropathy. Less frequent sites of involvement include the rectal mucosa, liver, spleen, kidney, prostate, and blood vessels. Macroglossia is rare. In one series, 16 of 16 skin biopsy specimens were negative for amyloid, but subcutaneous abdominal fat aspiration was positive in nine of 25 (36%) of these patients. Subcutaneous amyloid masses (amyloidomas) have been reported.

Familial Syndromes of Systemic Amyloidosis

A number of familial syndromes have the frequent deposition of amyloid in various organs in common. Familial Mediterranean fever, inherited in an autosomal recessive fashion, results in an AA fibril type of systemic amyloidosis that is secondary to the frequent inflammatory episodes characteristic of this disease. The remaining familial amyloidosis syndromes may differ considerably from kindred to kindred, but are usually inherited in an autosomal dominant fashion. The incidence of familial amyloidoses in referral centers is 10–20% of the number of AL amyloid cases seen. Several types share the features of peripheral polyneuropathy, autonomic nervous system dysfunction, and varying involvement of the heart, gastrointestinal tract, and eyes. Atrophic scars, ulcerations, or petechiae may occur in these patients, and patients with familial amyloidotic polyneuropathy may have cutaneous amyloid deposition noted in biopsy specimens. Plasma transthyretin protein (prealbumin) has been shown to be the amyloid precursor protein in several forms of familial amyloidosis, with more than 60 known amino acid substitutions that can lead to amyloid disease. Abnormal transthyretin can be identified by isoelectric focusing of serum that can separate wild-type from variant, or by DNA-based testing for a mutant transthyretin gene. Gelsolin (an actin-modulating protein) is now known to be the fibril source in hereditary gelsolin amyloidosis (AGel amyloidosis), and cutis laxa is a principal clinical manifestation of this disease, along with skin fragility and intracutaneous bleeding. In Iceland there is a hereditary cerebral hemorrhagic disease secondary to the deposition of amyloid fibrils derived from cystatin C, a proteinase inhibitor. In 12 of 12 patients with this disorder who were tested, prominent subclinical cutaneous deposition of cystatin C-derived amyloid was demonstrated by light microscopy of punch biopsy specimens. Patients with the Muckle–Wells syndrome, a familial disorder characterized by repeated febrile episodes, a painful urticarial eruption, and progressive deafness, develop an amyloid nephropathy due to amyloid A (AA) fibril deposition.

Skin-Limited Amyloidoses

A variety of primary cutaneous amyloidoses have been described, including lichen amyloidosis; macular amyloidosis; biphasic amyloidosis; and amyloidoses of the anosacral, bullous, poikiloderma-like, and dyschromic types. These syndromes are seen uncommonly in the United States, lichen amyloidosis being seen the most frequently. Patients with lichen amyloidosis develop pruritic, hyperkeratotic, skin-colored or hyperpigmented papules, particularly on the anterior lower extremities, although other areas may be involved. Those with macular amyloidosis have pruritic, oval, grayish-brown macules that may coalesce to rippled or reticular hyperpigmented patches on the lower extremities or back. Patients with both macular and papular lesions are sometimes classified as having biphasic amyloidosis, but macular, biphasic, and lichen amyloidoses probably represent a continuum of the same process. These cutaneous amyloidoses are thought to have a keratin protein as the amyloid fibril precursor and are considered an amyloid keratin protein (AK) type of amyloidosis. The biopsy specimens in these disorders show distinctive changes that aid in distinguishing them from systemic amyloidosis. Variants, such as poikilodermatous or vitiliginous amyloidoses, have been reported; these may develop early in life and may be associated with short stature or light sensitivity (e.g., amyloidosis cutis dyschromica). Familial syndromes of lichen amyloidosis have also been reported. Familial primary localized cutaneous amyloidosis is an autosomal dominant disorder associated with chronic pruritus and AK amyloid deposition in the dermis. This syndrome is associated with missense mutations in the oncostatin M-specific receptor β gene (OSMRβ). This mutation may offer new insight into pruritus mechanisms. Several reports now exist of a familial syndrome of multiple endocrine neoplasia (MEN) type 2a associated with lichen amyloidosis.

Localized amyloid AK deposition may occur around or within a number of cutaneous growths, including actinic keratoses, basal cell carcinomas, Bowen's disease (a form of in situ squamous cell carcinoma), and seborrheic keratoses. In these settings, the amyloid deposition is not clinically evident. Patients undergoing psoralen–ultraviolet A light (PUVA) treatment also may have subclinical cutaneous amyloid deposition, presumably of the AK type.

Although nodular (tumefactive) cutaneous amyloidosis is also considered to be a form of primary cutaneous amyloidosis, it is not the result of AK disease. Amyloid deposition in nodular cutaneous amyloidosis is thought to derive from a light chain precursor produced at the site by surrounding clonally restricted plasma cells. This type of amyloidosis presents as nodules on the face, extremities, trunk, or genitalia. These nodules are usually skin-colored and frequently have overlying epidermal atrophy or features resembling anetoderma. The mean age at diagnosis is 55 years, with a range of 20–87 years, and there is no gender predilection. Patients with nodular cutaneous amyloidosis require regular follow-up because some may develop systemic amyloidosis, presumably of the AL fibril type. Initial reports suggested a 50% progression rate to systemic amyloidosis, but more recent data suggest that the rate is less than 10%. Local light chain production and conversion to AL amyloid should not result in a detectable serum or urine monoclonal protein; its presence should suggest the need for further work-up and close follow-up.

Differential Diagnosis

The differential diagnosis for systemic amyloidoses depends on the syndrome, but AL amyloidosis should always be considered in the differential diagnosis of cephalad-distributed waxy papules or unexplained hemorrhage induced by mild trauma. Patients with the AA or familial syndromes of amyloid frequently have no specific cutaneous amyloid lesions. Lichen and macular amyloidosis may be confused with localized pigmentary disorders, lichen simplex chronicus, notalgia paresthetica, and prurigo nodularis.

Histopathologic Findings

Subcutaneous abdominal fat aspiration may be helpful in confirming a diagnosis of systemic amyloidosis in patients with AL, AA, or some familial amyloid syndromes. When performed and interpreted by an experienced group, the biopsies appear to be relatively sensitive, specific, and safe.

A biopsy of clinical lesions in AL-derived systemic amyloidosis should provide diagnostic evidence of amyloid deposition. Even in patients without clinical lesions, a biopsy of apparently normal skin may reveal cutaneous deposits of amyloid in up to 50% of individuals with systemic AL-type amyloidosis. Amyloid deposits are usually located in the superficial dermis and dermal vessels. Epidermal atrophy (or at least the loss of rete ridges) is an associated finding. Congo red staining with green birefringence under polarized light is the most specific stain for amyloid, although other stains, such as methyl violet, crystal violet, or thioflavine T, may be more sensitive.

Despite the rarity of clinical lesions in AA fibril-type (secondary) systemic amyloidosis, a biopsy of apparently normal skin may yield evidence of amyloid deposition. The pattern of amyloid deposition differs from that seen with the AL type. The deposits are usually deep in the dermis and subcutaneous fat, and are occasionally in a perivascular or periappendageal distribution. Amyloid deposition in hemodialysis-related amyloidosis and in several familial amyloid syndromes (dependent on transthyretin, gelsolin, or cystatin C) has been similar to that described for AA fibril-type amyloidosis. As discussed previously, subcutaneous fat pad aspiration is frequently positive in AL, AA, and perhaps other systemic amyloidoses, but this test requires experience to interpret and to avoid overstaining the tissue with Congo red.

Lichen amyloidosis and macular amyloidosis have a biopsy appearance unlike that of AL or AA amyloidosis. Amyloid is deposited in the papillary tips, with rete ridge elongation and sparing of dermal blood vessels. The changes in macular amyloidosis are sometimes minimal. Cutaneous tumor-associated amyloidosis is a pathologic curiosity; its recognition as an entity is important primarily to prevent its misinterpretation as evidence of a more serious amyloid disorder. The cutaneous deposits in nodular cutaneous amyloidosis are localized to the nodules. Extensive dermal and subcutaneous deposits within the lesions are typical, as is blood vessel wall infiltration. Plasma cells are usually prominent; giant cells and focal calcification may be seen.

Evaluation

The evaluation of a patient with biopsy-proven cutaneous amyloid deposition must be directed by the setting. The presence or absence of clinical lesions, the site sampled (lesional or nonlesional skin, subcutaneous fat), the presence of associated systemic findings, and the specific histologic features seen on the biopsy specimen are all important in determining the most appropriate evaluation for an individual patient. For example, the presence of waxy hemorrhagic facial papules with histologic features of epidermal atrophy, significant dermal amyloid deposition, and amyloid infiltration of vessel walls is nearly diagnostic of AL-type systemic amyloidosis. In such a case, a thorough search for an associated plasma cell dyscrasia, via immunofixation electrophoresis of serum and urine and the serum free light chain assay, is mandatory. By contrast, the presence of skin-colored pruritic papules on the lower extremity that, when sampled, show features of papillary tip amyloid deposition, sparing of vessels, and rete ridge elongation would be sufficient for the diagnosis of lichen amyloidosis and would obviate the need to search for a systemic cause.

Treatment

The therapy of amyloidosis, regardless of the type, is difficult, probably owing to the insolubility of this protein. The treatment of AL systemic amyloidosis is usually unsatisfactory, although some patients have had slowing of disease progression or even partial regression of amyloid deposition following chronic alkylating agent chemotherapy (usually melphalan) plus corticosteroids. Because AL systemic amyloidosis is a reflection of a plasma cell dyscrasia, recent and future advances in therapy will probably parallel those of myeloma, e.g., thalidomide, lenalidomide, bortezomib, hematopoietic stem cell transplants. The therapy of AA systemic amyloidosis is directed, when possible, towards treating or eliminating the underlying disorder leading to chronic inflammation. Colchicine can prevent or greatly diminish attacks and AA amyloid deposition in patients with familial Mediterranean fever. The treatment of lichen and macular amyloidosis is often unsatisfactory. Nonetheless, attempts should be made to control the pruritus, and occasional good results have been reported with the use of topical or intralesional corticosteroid therapy, corticosteroid-impregnated tape, topical pramoxine, topical retinoic acid, topical dimethyl sulfoxide, systemic etretinate, or dermabrasion.

SUGGESTED READINGS

Appiah YE, Onumah N, Wu H, et al. Multiple myeloma-associated amyloidosis and acral localized acquired cutis laxa. J Am Acad Dermatol 2008; 58: S32–S33.

Arita K, South AP, Hans-Filho G, et al. Oncostatin M receptor-beta mutations underlie familial primary localized cutaneous amyloidosis. Am J Hum Genet 2008: 82: 73–80.

Boom BW, Brand A, Bavinck JN, et al. Severe leukocytoclastic vasculitis of the skin in a patient with essential mixed cryoglobulinemia treated with high-dose γ-globulin intravenously. Arch Dermatol 1988; 124: 1550–1553.

Brouet JC, Clauvel JP, Danon F, et al. Biological and clinical significance of cryoglobulins. A report of eighty-six cases. Am J Med 1974; 57: 775–788.

Burnside NJ, Alberta L, Robinson-Bostom, Bostom A. Type III hyperlipoproteinemia with xanthomas and multiple myeloma. J Am Acad Dermatol 2005; 53: S281–S284.

Campistol JM, Solé M, Muñoz-Gomez J, et al. Systemic involvement of dialysis – amyloidosis. Am J Nephrol 1990; 10: 389–396.

Cohen SJ, Pittelkow MR, Su WPD. Cutaneous manifestations of cryoglobulinemia: clinical and histopathologic study of seventy-two patients. J Am Acad Dermatol 1991; 25: 21–27.

Colaco SM, Miller T, Ruben BS, et al. IgM-λ paraproteinemia with associated cutaneous lymphoplasmacytic infiltrate in a patient who meets diagnostic criteria for POEMS syndrome. J Am Acad Dermatol 2008; 58: 671–675.

Dispenzieri A. POEMS syndrome. Blood Rev 2007; 21: 285–299.

Drueke TB. Extraskeletal problems and amyloid. Kidney Int 1999; 56: S89–S93.

Falanga V, Kirsner RS, Eaglstein WH, et al. Stanozolol in treatment of leg ulcers due to cryofibrinogenemia. Lancet 1991; 338: 347–348.

Falk RH, Comenzo RL, Skinner M. Medical progress: the systemic amyloidoses. N Engl J Med 1997; 337: 898–909. Comments in N Engl J Med 1998; 338: 264–265.

Falk RH, Skinner M. The systemic amyloidoses: an overview. Adv Intern Med 2000; 45: 107–137.

Frankel AH, Singer DRJ, Winearls CG, et al. Type II essential mixed cryoglobulinaemia: presentation, treatment and outcome in 13 patients. Q J Med 1992; 82: 101–124.

Gabriel SE, Perry HO, Oleson GB, Bowles CA. Scleromyxedema: a scleroderma-like disorder with systemic manifestations. Medicine 1988; 67: 58–65.

Garcia T, Dafer R, Hocker S, et al. Recurrent strokes in two patients with POEMS syndrome and Castleman's disease. J Stroke Cerebrovasc Dis 2007; 16: 278–284.

Gertz MA, Lacy MQ, Dispenzieri A. Amyloidosis. Hematol Oncol Clin North Am 1999; 13: 1211–1233.

Green T, Grant J, Pye R, Marcus R. Multiple primary cutaneous plasmacytomas. Arch Dermatol 1992; 128: 962–965.

Grunewald K, Sepp N, Weyrer K, et al. Gene rearrangement studies in the diagnosis of primary systemic and nodular primary localized cutaneous amyloidosis. J Invest Dermatol 1991; 97: 693–696.

Hashiguchi T, Arimura K, Matsumuro K, et al. Highly concentrated vascular endothelial growth factor in platelets in Crow-Fukase syndrome. Muscle Nerve 2000; 23: 1051–1056.

Janier M, Bonvalet D, Blanc MF, et al. Chronic urticaria and macroglobulinemia (Schnitzler's syndrome): report of two cases. J Am Acad Dermatol 1989; 20: 206–211.

Kalajian AH, Waldman M, Knable AI. Nodular primary localized cutaneous amyloidosis after trauma: a case report and discussion of the rate of progression to systemic amyloidosis. J Am Acad Dermatol 2007; 57: S26–S29.

Kiuru-Enari S, Keski-Oja J, Haltia M. Cutis laxa in hereditary gelsolin amyloidosis. Br J Dermatol 2005; 152: 250–257.

Kois JM, Sexton FM, Lookingbill DP. Cutaneous manifestations of multiple myeloma. Arch Dermatol 1991; 127: 69–74.

Kos CA, Ward JE, Malek K, et al. Association of acquired von Willebrand syndrome with AL amyloidosis. Am J Hematol 2007; 82: 363–367.

Kyle RA, Rajkumar SV. Monoclonal gammopathy of undetermined significance and smouldering multiple myeloma: emphasis on risk factors for progression. Br J Haematol 2007; 139: 730–743.

Lee MR, Choi,HJ, Lee EB, Baek JH. POEMS syndrome complicated by extensive arterial thromboses. Clin Rheumatol 2007; 26: 1989–1992.

Leonard AL, Meehan SA, Ramsey D, et al. Cutaneous and systemic plasmacytosis. J Am Acad Dermatol 2007; 56: S38–S40.

Lipsker D, Rondeau M, Massard G, Grosshans E. The AESOP (adenopathy and extensive skin patch overlying a plasmacytoma) syndrome: report of 4 cases of a new syndrome revealing POEMS (polyneuropathy, organomegaly, endocrinopathy, monoclonal protein, and skin changes) syndrome at a curable stage. Medicine 2003; 82: 51–59.

List AF. Lenalidomide – the phoenix rises. N Engl J Med 2007; 357: 2183–2186.

McFadden N, Ree K, Søyland E, Larsen TE. Scleredema adultorum associated with a monoclonal gammopathy and generalized hyperpigmentation. Arch Dermatol 1987; 123: 629–632.

Mellqvist UH, Lenhoff S, Johnsen HE, et al. and the Nordic Myeloma Study Group. Cyclophosphamide plus dexamethasone is an efficient initial treatment before high-dose melphalan and autologous stem cell transplantation in patients with newly diagnosed multiple myeloma: results of a randomized comparison with vincristine, doxorubicin, and dexamethasone. Cancer 2008; 112: 129–135.

Mehregan DA, Winkelmann RK. Necrobiotic xanthogranuloma. Arch Dermatol 1992; 128: 94–100.

Myers BM, Miralles GD, Taylor CA, et al. POEMS syndrome with idiopathic flushing mimicking carcinoid syndrome. Am J Med 1991; 90: 646–648.

Patterson JW, Parsons JM, White RM, et al. Cutaneous involvement of multiple myeloma and extramedullary plasmacytoma. J Am Acad Dermatol 1988; 19: 879–890.

Pock L, Stuchlik D, Hercogova J. Crystal storing histiocytosis of the skin associated with multiple myeloma. Int J Dermatol 2006; 45: 1408–1411.

Rubinow A, Cohen AS. Skin involvement in generalized amyloidosis. Ann Intern Med 1978; 88: 781–785.

Terpos E, Sezer O, Croucher P, Dimopoulos MA. Myeloma bone disease and proteasome inhibition therapies. Blood 2007; 110: 1098–1104.

Touart DM, Sau P. Cutaneous deposition diseases. Part I. J Acad Dermatol 1998; 39: 149–171.

Wang WJ. Clinical features of cutaneous amyloidoses. Clin Dermatol 1990; 2: 13–19.

Wong CK. Treatment of cutaneous amyloidosis. Clin Dermatol 1990; 2: 108–111.

Yiannias JA, El-Azhary RA, Gibson LE. Erythema elevatum diutinum: a clinical and histopathologic study of 13 patients. J Am Acad Dermatol 1992; 26: 38–44.

Cutaneous Manifestations of Macrophage/Dendritic Cell Proliferative Disorders (Histiocytoses)

This chapter discusses disorders of the macrophage–dendritic cell system that may prominently or predominantly involve the skin. Such massive proliferations of these cells involving the skin typically occur in three settings: neoplastic or clonal disorders, inflammatory/infectious disorders, and storage diseases secondary to a small group of metabolic diseases. The term histiocyte applies to cells with a range of cellular morphology recognized by light microscopy. Most of the syndromes previously considered 'malignant histiocytoses' are now known to be secondary to a certain infection or to T-cell proliferation, either of which may drive macrophage proliferation and prominent hemophagocytosis.

The phagocytic–dendritic system can be divided into four categories: marrow precursors, monocytes, tissue macrophage/phagocytic cells, and primarily immune accessory cells. The morphology and physiology of individual cells may depend a great deal on their microenvironment and degree of stimulation. Phagocytic cells ingest and kill parasites and senescent cells; secrete products that affect coagulation, macrophage, and lymphoid function; stimulate immune activities; present antigens; remodel tissue; or modulate tumor cell growth. Included in this category are free tissue macrophages, Kupffer cells, pulmonary alveolar macrophages, osteoclasts, and central nervous system microglia. Immune accessory cells process antigen and present it to B or T cells, induce mixed lymphocyte reactions, induce contact hypersensitivity, or stimulate cytolytic T-cell development, and they may exhibit variable phagocytic activity. When appropriately stained, such cells are typically dendritic. The immune accessory dendritic cells particularly prominent in the skin include Langerhans' cells, their indeterminate cell precursors, and dermal dendrocytes (collagen-associated dendritic cells). Langerhans' cells are a unique subset of immune accessory dendritic cells that reside in the epidermis and which possess a distinctive combination of immunologic and ultrastructural features, especially S-100, CD1a and neuron-specific enolase staining, and Birbeck granules. A recently described feature of Langerhans' cells is their specific expression of langerin, a C-type lectin that can bind and mediate the uptake of sugar-containing molecules, including mannose, *N*-acetylglucosamine, and fucose. Because it is germline encoded to recognize particular biochemical motifs, and appears to facilitate antigen presentation by CD1a, langerin is a pattern-recognition receptor of the innate immune system. Transfection of langerin can induce the formation of Birbeck granules.

PATHOGENESIS

With rare exception, the histiocytoses appear to be examples of unusual reactive proliferations or idiopathic disorders of macrophage–dendritic (histiocyte) cell lines. Because the pathogenesis of these disorders is so poorly understood, classification depends on clinical and pathologic features. Traditionally, these disorders were divided into histiocytosis X (derived from the dendritic Langerhans' cell) and the non-X histiocytoses.

In 1987, the Writing Group of the Histiocyte Society proposed a system of classification that divides the histiocytic disorders into three classes. Class I includes Langerhans' cell granulomatoses, class II includes proliferation of mononuclear phagocytes other than Langerhans' cells, and class III includes true malignancies of the macrophage–monocyte system (monocyte–macrophage-derived malignant histiocytosis), acute monocytic leukemia, and, perhaps, a subset of acute disseminated Langerhans' cell granulomatosis. The annual incidence of Langerhans' cell disease is estimated at 0.5 per 100 000 children in the United States, and at 1 per 200 000–2 million children worldwide, with a male:female ratio of 1.8:1. The male:female ratio is 3:1 for limited/nonprogressive disease, but 1:1 for chronic progressive or fatal disease. Seventy-five percent of patients are diagnosed before age 10, 90% before age 30. Except for juvenile xanthogranuloma, the class II and class III histiocytoses are rare to very rare disorders.

CLASS I: LANGERHANS' CELL GRANULOMATOSES

Clinical Manifestations

Letterer–Siwe disease, Hand–Schüller–Christian disease, and eosinophilic granuloma compose the classic clinical subsets of the Langerhans' cell granulomatoses (histiocytosis X), corresponding to acute disseminated, chronic progressive, and benign localized forms of disease, respectively. Although individual patients may have findings that do not fit neatly into a single classic type, these subsets remain a reasonable starting point for the diagnosis and treatment of Langerhans' cell proliferative disease.

Letterer–Siwe disease may be congenital, often begins within the first 6 months of life, usually develops before age 2 years, and rarely occurs in adults. This is an acute disseminated disease, associated with fever, weight loss, and generalized lymphadenopathy. Cutaneous manifestations are common, occurring in roughly half of patients at onset. The earliest lesions are translucent reddish-brown or reddish-yellow small papules, occurring primarily on the scalp (Fig. 17–1), upper trunk, and intertriginous areas (Fig. 17–2). These lesions occur in crops and may become confluent, especially on the scalp. Erythematous, crusted vesiculopustules are particularly common in infants presenting in the first 4 weeks of life, and are often mistaken as signs of infection. Individual lesions may

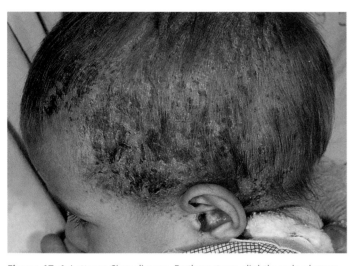

Figure 17–1 Letterer–Siwe disease. Erythematous, slightly scaly plaques are present on the scalp of this child.

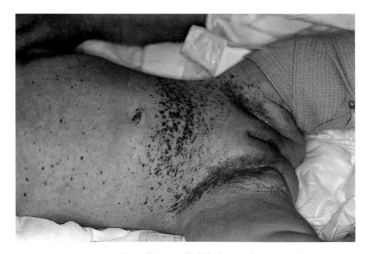

Figure 17–2 Letterer–Siwe disease. Slightly hemorrhagic erythematous papules and plaques are present in this child.

develop features of scaling, crust, pustule formation, and even hemorrhage, often in a progressive pattern. It is unfortunately not uncommon for infants with these skin manifestations to have seen several physicians and to have been treated for seborrheic dermatitis or persistent diaper dermatitis. Frequently, such lesions will undergo spontaneous regression, leaving residual scarring. Occasionally, more chronic lesions will become xanthomatous. Gingival involvement is common; mucosal ulceration or infiltration may occur. Early in the disease course, petechial skin lesions are the result of vessel inflammation, but in advanced disease purpura and hemorrhage may result from thrombocytopenia. Nail changes include paronychia, nailfold inflammation, subungual hyperkeratosis or onycholysis, and splinter hemorrhages of the nail bed. The disease commonly affects the lungs, liver, spleen, bone, and bone marrow. Bone lesions are osteolytic and occur primarily in the cranium, vertebrae, and flat bones. Before methods were available to identify Langerhans' cells reliably, Letterer–Siwe syndrome probably included a number of macrophage-monocyte disorders, such as acute monocytic leukemia, some lymphomas, and atypical vasculitic syndromes. Even though the outlook may be somewhat better with a proper diagnosis and improved treatment, Letterer–Siwe disease is still frequently life-threatening, especially if there is splenomegaly or severe liver dysfunction, and usually fatal with disease-related marrow failure (thrombocytopenia or severe anemia). In at least some infants the cytopenias may be associated with myelodysplastic changes in the bone marrow.

Hand–Schüller–Christian disease usually develops in children 2–6 years of age and almost always presents before age 30. The triad of exophthalmos, diabetes insipidus, and bone lesions defines this disease subset, but few patients have all three findings. Mucocutaneous lesions are found in about one-third of patients and may resemble those seen with Letterer–Siwe disease. Later in the disease course, lesions may occur in small numbers concentrated on the lateral scalp and on the central regions of the chest and back. Involvement of scalp or intertriginous areas may also be prominent. Mucosal lesions are often noduloulcerative, and especially involve the gingiva or vulva. The most common finding is the presence of osteolytic lesions in up to 80% of patients, primarily affecting the skull. Diabetes insipidus is present in more than half the patients, but can usually be well controlled by vasopressin. Both pulmonary involvement and exophthalmos occur in roughly 20% of cases. Unlike in Letterer–Siwe disease, hepatomegaly is rare. The progression of Hand–Schüller–Christian disease is slower than that of Letterer–Siwe disease. About half of untreated patients die of unrelated causes.

Eosinophilic granuloma is primarily an adult disease, typically presenting in patients 30–50 years of age, and in men more often than in women. Lymphadenopathy is common, but the bones and lung are the most frequently affected sites. The skull is the most involved bony location and the long bones are the least involved, but lesions can occur in any bone. Pulmonary nodule formation with fibrosis is the most common pulmonary complication, and this is seen primarily in young white men. Cutaneous disease is uncommon. Mucocutaneous lesions are usually nodules or ulcerated nodules, on or around mucosal surfaces. The periorificial, perigenital, and perianal areas are the most commonly involved, and such involvement can suggest the diagnosis, particularly when chronic weeping eruptions persist in and around the ear canal. Individual lesions may respond well to treatment. A chronic course with a good prognosis is typical for this disease subset.

Of course, many patients do not present with findings confined to or typical of these classic subsets. Some of the most difficult patients to diagnose clinically are those with skin-limited disease. Pure cutaneous disease occurs occasionally in children, and more commonly in adults (up to 50% of cases). It may be confined to one anatomic region (e.g., the genitalia). Pure cutaneous disease in adults usually progresses slowly or not at all to extracutaneous locations, and can generally be controlled with topical or local therapies.

Variants of Langerhans' Cell Disease

Congenital self-healing reticulohistiocytosis (Hashimoto–Pritzker disease) is an uncommon but perhaps underdiagnosed pediatric syndrome. Although the male:female ratio in case series has ranged from 1:2 to 4:1, when series are combined the ratio is 15:17. It presents in the newborn as solitary or multiple 2-mm to 3-cm red-brown papules or nodules, which may later crust or ulcerate. The distribution is often generalized, but mucous membranes are spared. Systemic findings may occur, including liver, bone, colon, bone marrow, and spleen, but the majority of cases are skin limited. The histologic findings include the presence of large mononucleated cells and occasional giant cells, associated with a lymphocyte- and plasma cell-rich infiltrate which extends to and may involve the epidermis. When examined by electron microscopy, 10–30% of the large cells contain Birbeck granules. The natural history is one of spontaneous regression over a 2–3-month period, occasionally leaving white atrophic scars. This syndrome is now considered a benign and self-limited variant of Langerhans' cell granulomatosis and usually requires no treatment.

Differential Diagnosis

The clinical presentation of Langerhans' cell granulomatoses can be misleading, particularly in the older child or adult. In such patients, Langerhans' cell disease is uncommon. Even when this disease occurs in adults, cutaneous findings are often not prominent or may mimic those of more common diseases. The disseminated forms in childhood are likely to be misdiagnosed as seborrheic dermatitis, eczema, Darier's disease, systemic infections (especially fungal or atypical mycobacterial), other histiocytoses, or lymphoma. The classic presentation of Hand–Schüller–Christian disease is less likely to be misdiagnosed, but xanthoma disseminatum can sometimes present with similar cutaneous findings and with diabetes insipidus. The disease in the adult patient with the classic bone or pulmonary presentation of eosinophilic granuloma also presents little problem for diagnosis, but considerable confusion may arise in those patients, especially adults, who have predominantly or exclusively cutaneous findings. Ear involvement is very easily mistaken for chronic otitis media or externa.

Histopathologic Findings

Early lesions appear as localized granulomas or areas of proliferative macrophage-like response. Some of the cells in the infiltrate are Langerhans' cells. Lymphocytes, granulocytes, and multinucleate giant cells may be present. In older lesions, eosinophilic or granulocytic infiltration may become prominent, as may areas of necrosis. Plasma cells may also become more evident, but they are a minor component of the inflammatory response. Infiltration of the dermis adjacent to the epidermis, and often the epidermis itself, is a feature commonly seen in Langerhans' cell granulomatosis, but almost never in any of the other histiocytic syndromes. Although some lesions may undergo xanthomatous change, most will become fibrotic and regress, with residual scarring.

Evaluation

The evaluation of patients with Langerhans' cell granulomatoses must be tailored to the patient's age and the type of presentation. In infants with acute disseminated disease, cutaneous biopsy specimens may be sufficient to make the diagnosis if the presence of significant numbers of Langerhans' cells can be confirmed. This will require a processing technique that identifies specific cell markers. Efforts must also be directed at excluding an associated infection. For all patients a complete history, physical examination, and laboratory studies, including a complete blood count, routine serum chemical analysis, chest X-ray studies, and usually bone films, are required to evaluate a biopsy-confirmed diagnosis properly, even in patients with apparently localized disease. Cutaneous lesions, when present, are usually the best source of diagnostic biopsy material. Particularly in the younger patient, an evaluation for subclinical diabetes insipidus may be indicated; presumed diabetes insipidus in a child should be confirmed by the appropriate use of serum and urine osmolality testing. The worst prognostic factors for Langerhans' cell disease include presentation at younger than 2 years of age; involvement of more than four organ systems; and the presence of hepatic, pulmonary, or hematopoietic dysfunction.

Treatment

The therapy for Langerhans' cell (class I) disease must be tailored to the severity of the disease and to the patient's symptoms. Patients with acute or chronic progressive multisystem disease usually require systemic chemotherapy, typically etoposide, vinblastine, or vincristine in combination with prednisone. For less acute or less extensive disease, treatment of symptoms is indicated. Examples of these therapies include the use of vasopressin analogs or radiation therapy for diabetes insipidus, and curettage, intralesional corticosteroid therapy, or radiation therapy to selected bone lesions. Symptomatic cutaneous disease may respond to treatment with topical nitrogen mustard, phototherapy (psoralen–ultraviolet A or ultraviolet B therapy), low-dose methotrexate, or electron beam or superficial radiotherapy. Both the risks of treatment and the high rate of eventual spontaneous remission or regression of less acute disease must be considered before therapy is begun. There may be a role for imatinib, a chemotherapeutic tyrosine kinase inhibitor, in both Langerhans' and non-Langerhans' cell histioctyoses, based on a very few case reports.

CLASS II AND III HISTIOCYTOSES: NON-LANGERHANS' CELL DISEASES

Clinical Manifestations

Class II histiocytoses may raise concerns of malignant disease by their widespread cutaneous or systemic involvement, but the macrophage proliferation appears to be reactive or idiopathic. Class II disease can be divided into diseases defined by their cutaneous involvement and those with multisystem involvement that may affect the skin. Features of these diseases are summarized in Table 17–1. In addition, because a number of storage disease disorders may have cutaneous and multisystem findings, Table 17–2 provides a summary of those storage disorders that on occasion might suggest class I or class II syndromes.

Indeterminate cell histiocytosis is a rare disorder in which cells share some features with Langerhans' cells. The usual presentation is in an adult (range 1 day to 67 years) with 5-mm to 1-cm red to red-brown or flesh-colored papules, plaques, or nodules on the face, upper extremities, trunk, or thighs. Mucous membranes are typically spared, but involvement has been reported. Both typical and atypical macrophage infiltrates have been described, along with the mixed infiltrate typical of Langerhans' cell disease. The macrophages are both S-100 and CD1a (OKT 6) positive; electron microscopy demonstrates comma-shaped bodies but no true Birbeck granules. The course is often indolent, sometimes with spontaneous regression, but may require chemotherapy and can be fatal. Heavy infiltration of indeterminate cells in post-scabetic nodules has been reported, suggesting that reactive proliferations of indeterminate cells may occur in previously unsuspected settings. Misdiagnosis of post-scabetic nodules as Langerhans' cell histiocytosis has also been reported.

Hemophagocytic syndrome is increasingly recognized as encompassing an expanding array of disorders, many of which were previously considered malignant histiocytoses. Familial hemophagocytic histiocytosis has been recognized since 1952 as a disease that primarily affects infants, with 90% affected by age 2. Presenting findings are irritability, anorexia, vomiting, and fever, usually with enlargement of liver or spleen, anemia, thrombocytopenia, and less often neutropenia. Central nervous system involvement, with seizures, meningitis, hemiplegia, or coma, is common later. This familial syndrome is now known to be due to inherited defects of perforin, an effector molecule of lymphocyte cytotoxicity. Interestingly, the Chediak–Higashi and Griscelli syndromes may have similar features in their 'accelerated phases,' and both of these disorders are now known to involve in part an inability to release perforin-containing cell granules. Nonfamilial settings for hemophagocytic syndromes include infection, often in immunocompromised patients (including some with autoimmune disease), malignancies (usually T-cell lymphoma), and certain drugs, especially phenytoin or lipid-rich hyperalimentation. Infections are most often viral, most typically Epstein–Barr virus, but also herpes simplex, cytomegalovirus, varicella zoster, adenovirus, human immunodeficiency virus, dengue, and parvovirus. Much less often, nonviral infections trigger hemophagocytic syndrome, including *Streptococcus, Staphylococcus, Rickettsia*, mycobacteria, *Candida*, histoplasmosis, cryptococcus, *Leishmania*, and babesiosis.

Class III histiocytoses should be limited to acute monocytic leukemia and malignant histiocytosis, both disorders in which the proliferating cell is macrophage in origin and malignant. In fact, true malignant histiocytosis (macrophage malignancy) is quite rare. In these few cases the presentation may be localized (at least initially) in the intestine, or less often the lymph nodes or skin. More often, malignant histiocytosis is generalized, and presents with findings of fever, weakness, weight loss, dyspnea, liver or spleen enlargement, and lymphadenopathy. Anemia and thrombocytopenia are expected; neutropenia and cytophagocytosis (emperipolesis) are common. Obviously, this presentation is very similar to that of familial hemophagocytic syndrome and to lymphoma- or infection-related hemophagocytic syndrome, emphasizing the importance of careful clinical and histologic/immunophenotypic assessments. Malignant histiocytosis is usually rapidly progressive despite chemotherapy, but clinical remissions of some duration may occur in up to 50% of cases.

Differential Diagnosis

The major areas of diagnostic confusion both clinically and histologically for disorders of the macrophage–dendritic cell system are caused by the inaccuracy of light microscopy alone in determining cellular lineage, and the difficulty of determining the presence or absence of malignancy from clinical or morphologic characteristics alone. Langerhans' cell markers are important in separating class I from class II or III disorders. As discussed previously, the hemophagocytic syndrome must be ruled out in most syndromes characterized by prominent macrophage proliferation. Finally, many metabolic storage disorders may have cutaneous manifestations, with macrophage accumulation or proliferation (see Table 17–2).

Evaluation

The proper evaluation of patients with cutaneous histiocytic disorders depends on a careful analysis of the features of individual cutaneous lesions, with special attention paid to variations in lesional morphology, color, or size; cutaneous distribution of lesions; and the presence of ulceration, necrosis, or evidence of involution. In addition, the examination of skin biopsy specimens requires special attention to the presence or absence of epidermal involvement, the composition of the cellular infiltrate, localization of the infiltrate to perivascular or periappendigeal locations, and special studies to evaluate the presence or absence of Langerhans' cell lineage. After a proper evaluation of the cutaneous lesions, a careful history and physical examination and knowledge of the systemic findings associated with a particular syndrome can indicate the need for further diagnostic studies. Baseline studies recom-

Table 17–1 Class II histiocytoses: mostly cutaneous non-Langerhans' cell histiocytoses

Disease & frequency	Age/Sex	Cutaneous lesions	Mucous membranes	Systemic findings	Cutaneous pathologic findings	Prognosis & treatment
Indeterminate cell histiocytosis: very rare	Adults > children	*Solitary nodular form* Soft red 1-cm nodule *Multiple papulonodular form* Widespread firm few mm to 1-cm dark red to brownish asymptomatic lesions (Can also be seen as part of nodular scabies, or at sites of healed pityriasis rosea lesions)	Spared in nearly all patients	Rare	Dermal, occasionally epidermal infiltrate; cells with large irreg folded or twisted nuclei & abundant pale eosinophilic cytoplasm. Few mitotic figures. Admixed lymphocyte clusters and occasional multinucleate giant cells seen. CD68+, S-100–, CD1a+, Factor XIIIa–; no Birbeck granules	Solitary form benign, but fatal progression described in some with widespread form. Progressive disease may respond to various chemotherapy agents, but relapse common. Some patients have developed leukemia or lymphoma
Benign cephalic histiocytosis: rare	6–12 mo (rarely onset not until age 3 yr)	Multiple 2–8-mm red to yellow-brown papules, often becoming confluent. Upper face, head initially, then upper trunk and limbs	No	No	Macrophages, rare giant cell, occasional lymphocytes or eosinophils. May infiltrate to subepidermal region; S-100 and CD1 (ODT-6) negative. EM studies show comma-shaped bodies in ~20% of macrophages	Spontaneous regression over 1–5-yr period, with temporary hyperpigmentation
Progressive nodular histiocytosis: very rare	Children > adults	Progressive development of hundreds of lesions. Most common: yellow-brown or pink 2–10-mm papules, widespread with flexural sparing. Less common: 1–5-cm red-brown dermal nodules with overlying telangiectasia. Face may be involved; ectropion and leonine facies may result	Conjunctival, oral, and laryngeal mucosa	Seldom	Dermal histiocytes with abundant, clear, vacuolated cytoplasm; variable multinucleate Touton giant cells. Intermixed lymphocytes, plasma cells. Storiform pattern possible. Older lesions may show fibrosis, lack giant cells. CD68+, Factor XIIIa+, CD1a–, S-100–. Comma-shaped granules may be seen on EM	Normolipemic, usually otherwise healthy. Spontaneous regression rare; very treatment resistant
Hereditary progressive mucinous histiocytosis: very rare	Begins in childhood or adolescence; mostly women	Few to numerous skin-colored to red-brown 1–5-mm papules or dome-shaped nodules. Symmetric, primarily face, hands, forearms, legs. Autosomal dominant inheritance	Spared	None	Nodular aggregates in papillary and mid dermis of epithelioid or spindle-shaped macrophages, large nuclei and abundant cytoplasm. May have increased mast cells. Prominent dermal mucin deposition. S-100–, CD1a–; variable staining for CD68, Factor XIIIa	Slowly progressive cutaneous course; no specific therapy

Table 17–1 Class II histiocytoses: mostly cutaneous non-Langerhans' cell histiocytoses—cont'd

Disease & frequency	Age/Sex	Cutaneous lesions	Mucous membranes	Systemic findings	Cutaneous pathologic findings	Prognosis & treatment
Generalized eruptive histiocytoma: very rare	Usually adult (infancy to adult)	Multiple 3–10-mm red, flesh-colored, or bluish papules, develop in crops on face, trunk, proximal limbs (Fig. 17–3)	Rare	Usually spared, occasional asymptomatic extracutaneous lesions noted	Dense macrophage infiltrate, occasional lymphocytes, eosinophils, and neutrophils	Spontaneous involution of individual lesions, but new lesions may arise. Ultimately, usually resolves
Papular xanthoma: very rare	Usually in children <1 yr	Multiple 2–15-mm yellow, yellow-pink papules or nodules. No confluence, no red-brown color. Face, trunk, proximal extremities, with sparing of flexural folds. In children, may resolve with anetoderma-like scars	Yes	No	Foam cells with few typical macrophages or Touton giant cells	Spontaneous involution over 1–5 years in most cases, but can be progressive
Juvenile xanthogranuloma: most common histiocytic disease	20–30% at birth; 80% by 1 yr; rare in adults	In series of 174 cases, solitary lesion in 67%, solitary subcutaneous nodule or deep soft tissue mass in 16%, multiple cutaneous lesions in 7%, solitary non-cutaneous, non-soft tissue lesion in 5%, multiple cutaneous and visceral lesions in 5%. Large nodular form: 1–2-cm translucent red nodules with surface telangiectasias. Papular/small nodular form: 2–8-mm red-brown papules, quickly changing to yellow-brown or yellow, esp involve scalp, face, trunk, proximal extremities. Pt or relative may have café-au-lait macules	Oropharynx rare	Eye most common; liver, spleen, lung, bone, colon, ovaries, testes, kidney, pericardium & muscle reported. Can be associated with neurofibromatosis, myeloid leukemia, or both. In children with both JXG and NF, the risk of myeloid leukemia is 20–32 times higher than normal, usually chronic myelocytic leukemia	Early lesions: monomorphous nonfoamy macrophages Late lesions: foam cells, Touton and other giant cells, lymphocytes, eosinophils, and neutrophils	Usual course is spontaneous resolution of lesions within 3–6 yrs. Systemic disease may prove fatal

Table 17–2 Systemic histiocytoses that may have cutaneous findings

Disease & frequency	Age/Sex	Cutaneous lesions	Mucous membranes	Systemic findings	Cutaneous pathologic findings	Prognosis & treatment
Hemophagocytic syndrome is associated with infections (viral, bacterial, parasitic), malignancies, particularly T cell, immune-deficiency states. Hemophagocytic lymphohistiocytosis (erythrophagocytic lymphohistiocytosis) may be familial (autosomal recessive) related to perforin defects or sporadic and presents in similar fashion but at <1 yr of age. Cytophagic histiocytic panniculitis emphasizes some cutaneous manifestations of HPS	Any age, but more frequent in children and young adults	20% in one series (100% in cases of cytophagic histiocytic panniculitis). Nodules or purpura most frequent, may ulcerate. Generalized or localized edema may be seen. Skin lesions in hemophagocytic lymphohistiocytosis are uncommon and nonspecific	No	Fever, constitutional symptoms, cytopenias and coagulopathy, hepatomegaly, splenomegaly, lymphadenopathy, less commonly renal failure and pulmonary infiltrates	Reaction of benign macrophages (histiocytes) is secondary to cytokines released by proliferating lymphocytes that may be benign or malignant. Infiltrate predominantly involves fat, often with fat necrosis, and affects vessels with hemorrhage, edema, vascular necrosis, or microthrombi. Cytophagocytosis by macrophages is prominent. In familial hemophagocytic lymphohistiocytosis, perforin defect leads to inability of lymphocytes to kill virus-infected cells	If caused by infection, may reverse if immunosuppressive agents withdrawn or infection treated; if caused by malignancy, course and treatment depend on tumor response to therapy. Lipid-rich hyperalimentation, Chédiak–Higashi or Griscelli syndrome may mimic in their 'accelerated phases' (see text)
Sinus histiocytosis with massive lymphadenopathy (Rosai–Dorfman disease): rare	From birth to age 74. Mean age at onset 21 yrs	Skin is most common extranodal site; rarely may occur without nodal changes. Usually consists of multiple red or yellow-brown macules, papules or nodules <4 cm, but large plaques and ulceration of nodules occur	Rare	Massive, usually painless cervical adenopathy; other nodes may be involved. Skin, eye, upper respiratory tract, and bone most common extranodal sites. Fever, anemia, leukocytosis, elevated ESR, and hypergammaglobulinemia most common findings	Characteristic macrophages have polygonal configuration, vesicular nuclei, and foamy cytoplasm and show lymphophagocytosis. Giant cells and lymphocytes also prominent; diagnostic changes seen in nodes	Usually undergoes spontaneous resolution but 7% mortality rate in one series, usually from associated immune defects

Table 17-2 Systemic histiocytoses that may have cutaneous findings—cont'd

Disease & frequency	Age/Sex	Cutaneous lesions	Mucous membranes	Systemic findings	Cutaneous pathologic findings	Prognosis & treatment
Multicentric reticulohistiocytosis (reticulohistiocytic granuloma and diffuse cutaneous reticulohistiocytosis are skin-limited variants): rare	May occur in children, but usually in adults >40 yr; M : F 1 : 3	100% cutaneous involvement. Multiple 2-mm to 2-cm translucent yellow-rose or yellow-brown papules and nodules located mainly on fingers (Fig. 17-4), hands, juxta-articular limb regions, and face. Leonine facies from nodules and cartilage destruction possible. Neurofibroma-like papules rare	Yes	Chronic destructive arthritis, especially in hands, wrists, and knees; often precedes skin involvement. Fever, pleural and pulmonary lesions reported. May rarely involve eye, thyroid, kidney, liver, muscle, or cardiovascular system. 30–58% have hyperlipidemia. Associated with malignancy in 25% (gastric, ovarian, breast, uterine); autoimmune disease in 6–17% (Sjögren, diabetes, thyroid)	Large, benign macrophages, with characteristic ground-glass appearance of cytoplasm and cytophagocytosis. Multinucleate giant cells, lymphocytes, eosinophils, neutrophils present early, later fibrosis	Disease usually becomes inactive after 5–10 yrs, but may leave significant disability. Treatment often ineffective, but cyclophosphamide, methotrexate, chlorambucil, anti-TNFα agents, and alendronate have occasionally been helpful. If associated with underlying malignancy, some patients improve in parallel with tumor response
Necrobiotic xanthogranuloma with paraproteinemia: rare	Adult (40–74 yr)	100% cutaneous involvement; <10-cm yellow or yellow-brown plaques and red nodules; overlying atrophy, telangiectasia, scarring, or ulceration; periorbital, trunk, proximal limbs, and flexural areas	No	Usually monoclonal gammopathy and leukopenia. 40% may have cryoglobulinemia. Hepatosplenomegaly in 20%	Benign macrophages and foam cells organized into inflammatory granuloma with Touton and foreign body giant cells. Necrobiosis present	Lesions poorly responsive to most therapies. Melphalan/prednisone, chlorambucil, methotrexate/prednisone occasionally helpful, but disease-related leukopenia may limit dose. Marrow dyscrasia, if present, determines prognosis
Xanthoma disseminatum	Adults more than children	100% cutaneous involvement. Multiple 2–10-mm red-brown papules, evolving to yellow-brown. Quickly become confluent. Trunk, face, proximal limbs, flexural and body fold areas. May form dark brown 'mahogany' plaques in flexural areas in adults	Yes	Upper respiratory tract infiltration can cause hoarseness or dyspnea. Eyelids, conjunctivae, or cornea may be involved. Diabetes insipidus in 50%. Growth retardation and seizures reported. May have monoclonal gammopathy, marrow dyscrasia	Benign large macrophages and foam cells. Giant cells, lymphocytes, plasma cells, eosinophils, and neutrophils often present	Diabetes insipidus may resolve spontaneously. Cutaneous lesions may involute with scarring. General health usually good; adults may have associated gammopathy or marrow dyscrasia. Treatments only occasionally helpful

Disease	Age	Skin	Mucous membranes	Other findings	Histopathology	Course
Erdheim–Chester disease: very rare	Adult (26–78 yrs)	25% involve skin. May have erythema over long bones. Xanthoma disseminatum-like presentation: lesions either red-brown papules becoming more yellow, isolated but gradually coalescing into plaques, later softening or becoming atrophic. Symmetric involvement, decreasing frequency eyelids, axillae, groin, neck, trunk, face Papular xanthoma-like presentation: less common. 2–15-mm yellow to pink-yellow papules, nodules, on back & head	Spared	Focal bone pain, esp. lower extremity, is presenting symptom in 50%. X-ray: mixed sclerotic (common) & lytic (30%). Diabetes insipidus up to 1/3 of pts. Bilat. painless exophthalmos common, renal & retroperitoneal 1/3; pulmonary 20%	Dermal infiltrate of foamy macrophages with few lymphocytes, plasma cells, neutrophils. Touton giant cells variable in number	Usually progressive with high mortality. Mean survival in one study <3 yrs. Cases of this disease with Langerhans' cell histiocytosis reported
Sea-blue histiocytosis syndrome: rare	Begins in adolescents or young adults; may be familial	Skin involved rarely. Facial macular brown hyperpigmentation; nodular lesions on face, trunk, hands, or feet. Eyelid infiltrative swelling and facial waxy plaques	Spared	Primary form: hepatosplenomegaly & bone marrow infiltration with bleeding diathesis; lung, lymph nodes > retinal or nervous system. Secondary form with marrow disorders, inherited metabolic defects such as Niemann–Pick, partial sphingomyelinase deficiency, apoE mutations, or abnormal lipid metabolism (including total parenteral nutrition): findings depend on underlying disease	Nodular lesions show dermal edema; sparse micronodular infiltrate of large, pale, macrophages containing vacuoles and granules. Granules stain with Giemsa or toluidine blue. CD 68+, S-100–; CD1a & Factor XIIIa not tested	Primary form relatively benign clinical course, but with progressive skin lesions. No known effective treatment. Secondary forms: course depends on underlying disease

Table 17-2 Systemic histiocytoses that may have cutaneous findings—cont'd

Disease & frequency	Age/Sex	Cutaneous lesions	Mucous membranes	Systemic findings	Cutaneous pathologic findings	Prognosis & treatment
Niemann–Pick disease (autosomal recessive, 4 types; infantile form involves skin)	Infant	Rare cutaneous involvement. Diffuse yellow-brown pigmentation. Xanthomas or red nodules rarely seen in juvenile form	No	Sphingomyelinase deficiency. Hepatosplenomegaly, rapidly progressive CNS disease in infantile form	Increased melanin in basal cell layer of epidermis. Large vacuolated (mulberry) foam cell characteristic but seldom seen in skin	Infantile form fatal by age 1–3 yrs
Tangier disease (autosomal recessive)	Child to adult	Rare cutaneous involvement. One patient developed truncal papules following splenectomy	Yes	α-Lipoprotein deficiency. Orange-yellow striations on enlarged tonsils, splenomegaly, peripheral neuropathy. Greatly decreased plasma HDL and cholesterol levels	Lipid stains of 'normal' skin show lipid deposits in dermis and dermal macrophages. Tonsillar lesions have foam cells	No evidence for predisposition to premature atherosclerotic disease
Lipogranulomatosis (Farber's disease, autosomal recessive)	Child	100% cutaneous involvement. Small papules to large plaques. Subcutaneous masses over wrists and ankles characteristic	Yes	Ceramidase deficiency. Involves tendon sheaths, synovium, liver, spleen, kidney, lymph nodes, and especially, CNS	Macrophages and fibroblasts in skin. Foam cells in other tissues	Progressive fatal course
Gaucher's disease (autosomal recessive, 3 types, adult form involves skin)	Adult (type I)	Common cutaneous involvement. Yellow-brown, brown, or gray-brown pigmentation on face, hands, and pretibial area	Yes	Glucocerebrosidase deficiency. Hepatosplenomegaly, bone lesions, pulmonary involvement in adults, with pathologic fractures as a result of bone lesions, and thrombocytopenic hemorrhage and neutropenic infection from hypersplenism. Yellow-brown pinguecula on bulbar conjunctivae	Increased melanin in basal cell layer of epidermis. May see increased dermal iron on special stains	Adult form slowly progressive. No known treatment

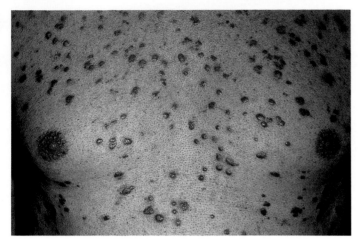

Figure 17–3 Generalized eruptive histiocytosis.

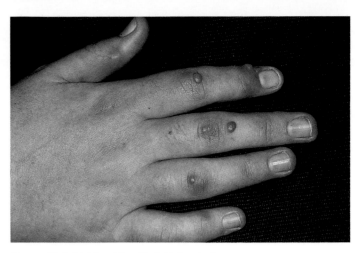

Figure 17–4 Multicentric reticulohistiocytosis.

mended by the Histiocyte Society include complete blood cell counts, liver function tests, coagulation studies, chest radiography, skeletal surveys, and urine osmolality testing.

Treatment

Treatment of class II and III histiocytoses is syndrome dependent and often not indicated or, unfortunately, not effective.

Therapeutic decisions are most critical in the setting of the hemophagocytic syndrome, in xanthoma disseminatum (where vasopressin therapy may be required), and in true malignancies (class III disease). The natural history of each class II syndrome, and the available therapy, is summarized in Table 17–1. Treatment of some class II and all class III diseases will obviously require intensive hematologic subspecialty care, as discussed under clinical manifestations.

SUGGESTED READINGS

Caldemeyer KS, Parks ET, Mirowski GW. Langerhans' cell histiocytosis. J Am Acad Dermatol 2001; 44: 509–511.

Caputo R, Marzano AV, Passoni E, Berti E. Unusual variants of non-Langerhans' cell histiocytoses. J Am Acad Dermatol 2007; 57: 1031–1045.

Chetritt J, Paradis V, Dargere D, et al. Chester–Erdheim disease: a neoplastic disorder. Hum Pathol 1999; 30: 1093–1096.

Contreras F, Fonseca E, Gamallo C, Burgos E. Multiple self-healing indeterminate cell lesions of the skin in an adult. Am J Dermatopathol 1990; 12: 396–401.

Dehner L. Juvenile xanthogranulomas in the first two decades of life: a clinicopathologic study of 174 cases with cutaneous and extracutaneous manifestations. Am J Surg Pathol 2003: 27: 579–593.

Gorman JD, Danning C, Schumacher HR, et al. Multicentric reticulohistiocytosis: case report with immunohistochemical analysis and literature review. Arthritis Rheum 2000; 43: 930–938.

Hashimoto K, Fujiwara K, Punwaney J, et al. Post-scabetic nodules: a lymphohistiocytic reaction rich in indeterminate cells. J Dermatol 2000; 27: 181–194.

Howarth DM, Gilchrist GS, Mullan BP, et al. Langerhans' cell histiocytosis: diagnosis, natural history, management, and outcome. Cancer 1999; 85: 2278–2290.

Hsu S, Ward SB, Le EH, Lee JB. Multicentric reticulohistiocytosis with neurofibroma-like nodules. J Am Acad Dermatol 2001; 44: 373–375.

Hunder RE, Sieling PA, Ochoa MT, et al. Langerhans' cells utilize CD1a and langerin to efficiently present nonpeptide antigens to T cells. J Clin Invest 2004; 113: 701–708.

Jang KA, Ahn SJ, Choi JH, et al. Histiocytic disorders with spontaneous regression in infancy. Pediatr Dermatol 2000; 17: 364–368.

Kapur P, Erickson C, Rakheja D, et al. Congenital self-healing reticulohistiocytosis (Hashimoto–Pritzker disease): ten-year experience at Dallas Children's Medical Center. J Am Acad Dermatol 2007; 56: 290–294.

Lahey ME. Prognostic factors in histiocytosis X. Am J Pediatr Hematol Oncol 1981; 3: 57–60.

Newman B, Hu W, Nigro K, Gilliam AC. Aggressive histiocytic disorders that can involve the skin. J Am Acad Dermatol 2007; 56: 302–316.

McLelland J, Chu AC. Multi-system Langerhans'-cell histiocytosis in adults. Clin Exp Dermatol 1990; 15: 79–82.

Mehregan DA, Winkelmann RK. Necrobiotic xanthogranuloma. Arch Dermatol 1992; 128: 94–100.

Mejia R, Dano JA, Roberts R, et al. Langerhans' cell histiocytosis in adults. J Am Acad Dermatol 1997; 37: 314–317.

Moretta L, Moretta A, Hengartner H, Zinkernagel RM. On the pathogenesis of perforin defects and related immunodeficiencies. Immunol Today 2000; 21: 593–594 [with reply].

Novice FM, Collison DW, Kleinsmith DM, et al. Letterer–Siwe disease in adults. Cancer 1989; 63: 166–174.

Rosenberg AS, Morgan MB. Cutaneous indeterminate cell histiocytosis: a new spindle cell variant resembling dendritic cell sarcoma. J Cutan Pathol 2001; 28: 531–537.

Stefanato CM, Andersen WK, Calonje E, et al. Langerhans' cell histiocytosis in the elderly: a report of three cases. J Am Acad Dermatol 1998; 39: 375–378.

Stein SL, Paller AS, Haut PR, Mancini AJ. Langerhans' cell histiocytosis presenting in the neonatal period: a retrospective case series. Arch Pediatr Adolesc Med 2001; 155: 788–793.

Stepp SE, Dufourcq-Lagelouse R, Le DeistF, et al. Perforin gene defects in familial hemophagocytic lymphohistiocytosis. Science 1999; 286: 1957–1959.

Surico G, Muggeo P, Rigillo N, Gadner H. Concurrent Langerhans' cell histiocytosis and myelodysplasia in children. Med Pediatr Oncol 2000; 35: 421–425.

Tani M, Ishii N, Kumagai M, et al. Malignant Langerhans' cell tumor. Br J Dermatol 1992; 126: 398–403.

Utikal J, Ugurel S, Kurzen H, et al. Imatinib as a treatment option for systemic non-Langerhans' cell histiocytoses. Arch Dermatol 2007; 143: 736–740.

Writing Group of the Histiocyte Society. Histiocytosis syndromes in children. Lancet 1987; 1: 208–209.

Langerhans' Cell Disease Confined to Skin

Hoeger PH, Nanduri VR, Harper JI, et al. Long term follow up of topical mustine treatment for cutaneous Langerhans' cell histiocytosis. Arch Dis Child 2000; 82: 483–487.

Lichtenwald DJ, Jakubovic HR, Rosenthal D. Primary cutaneous Langerhans' cell histiocytosis in an adult. Arch Dermatol 1991; 127: 1545–1548.

Meehan SA, Smoller BR. Cutaneous Langerhans' cell histiocytosis of the genitalia in the elderly: a report of three cases. J Cutan Pathol 1998; 25: 370–374.

Modi D, Schulz EJ. Skin ulceration as sole manifestation of Langerhans'-cell histiocytosis. Clin Exp Dermatol 1991; 16: 212–215.

Solano T, Espana A, Sola J, Lopez G. Langerhans' cell histiocytosis on the vulva. Gynecol Oncol 2000; 78: 251–254.

Steen AE, Steen KH, Bauer R, Bieber T. Successful treatment of cutaneous Langerhans' cell histiocytosis with low-dose methrotrexate. Br J Dermatol 2001; 145: 137–140.

Stefanato CM, Andersen WK, Calonje E, et al. Langerhans' cell histiocytosis in the elderly: a report of three cases. J Am Acad Dermatol 1998; 39: 375–378.

Vascular Neoplasms

There are a number of vascular lesions that serve as cutaneous signs of systemic disease, from the mat telangiectasias of scleroderma to the papular telangiectasias of hereditary hemorrhagic telangiectasia (Rendu–Osler–Weber syndrome) to the angiokeratomas of Fabry disease. In addition, both vascular tumors and vascular malformations are associated with syndromes ranging from Kasabach–Merritt to Sturge–Weber. Over the past two decades, an appreciation of the differences between hemangiomas and vascular malformations has grown, thanks in large part to the writings of two surgeons, John Mulliken and Anthony Young. This chapter concludes with a discussion of two malignant vascular tumors with internal manifestations, Kaposi's sarcoma and angiosarcoma.

TELANGIECTASIAS

Telangiectasias are such a common cutaneous finding that they are often overlooked or disregarded. In the head and neck region, the linear variety is most commonly due to solar damage and/or acne rosacea, whereas on the lower extremities telangiectasias are usually a sign of venous hypertension (Fig. 18–1; Table 18–1). The recurrent flushing of the face and upper trunk that occurs in patients with the carcinoid syndrome may be accompanied by linear telangiectasias; this constellation of clinical findings may result in the misdiagnosis of the erythematous form of acne rosacea.

In ataxia–telangiectasia, linear telangiectasias first appear on the bulbar conjunctivae during childhood, followed over time by similar lesions in the periocular region, ears and flexural areas, i.e., the antecubital and popliteal fossae. The telangiectasias are accompanied by cerebellar ataxia and a predilection for pulmonary infections and lymphomas. This autosomal recessive disorder is due to mutations in the *ATM* gene, but how this relates to the formation of telangiectasias is not well understood (see Chapter 34).

A rare variant of mastocytosis (see Chapter 36), referred to as telangiectasia macularis eruptiva perstans (TMEP), is characterized by multiple clusters of telangiectasias. Although somatic activating mutations in the *KIT* gene have been described in adults with urticaria pigmentosa, to date they have not been reported in patients with TMEP. Telangiectasias are classically described in association with basal cell carcinomas, but also occur within cutaneous B-cell lymphomas (Fig. 18–2).

One or two isolated papular telangiectasias are commonly seen on the face or hands of both children and adults. However, when multiple papular telangiectasias are present on the oral mucosa as well as the lips (Fig. 18–3A), face, fingers (Fig. 18–3B) and nailfolds (Fig. 18–3C), the possibility of hereditary hemorrhagic telangiectasia (HHT; Rendu–Osler–Weber syndrome) needs to be considered, especially if there is a personal or family history of epistaxis, gastrointestinal bleeding, or cerebrovascular accidents. The vascular lesions actually represent arteriovenous malformations (AVMs), which explains their propensity to bleed. By stretching the skin, an eccentric punctum with radiating branches can be visualized.

When the clinical diagnosis of HHT is made, it is important to screen individuals with a transthoracic echocardiogram bubble study (which assesses shunting) and a brain MRI with gadolinium enhancement to exclude pulmonary and cerebral AVMs, both of which are amenable to interventional vascular procedures, e.g., embolotherapy using balloons and coils, or surgical excision. It is still rather common for the diagnosis of HHT to be made clinically because it is not always possible to detect mutations in either of the responsible genes (which encode endoglin and activin receptor-like kinase-1 (ALK-1)). Patients with juvenile gastrointestinal polyposis in addition to HHT may have mutations in the *SMAD4* gene, which encodes a protein that, like endoglin and ALK-1, is involved in transforming growth factor-β signaling.

Spider nevi (also known as nevus araneus, spider angioma, and spider telangiectasia) represent dilations in ascending dermal arterioles and are characterized by both a punctum and radiating legs; occasionally, pulsations can be seen. Spider nevi can be a sign of hyperestrogenemia, and multiple lesions often appear during pregnancy and in patients with hepatic cirrhosis.

Poikiloderma is defined by the presence of (1) telangiectasias; (2) wrinkling due to epidermal atrophy; and (3) reticulated areas of hypo- and hyperpigmentation. Until recently, the easiest way to conceptualize poikiloderma was to

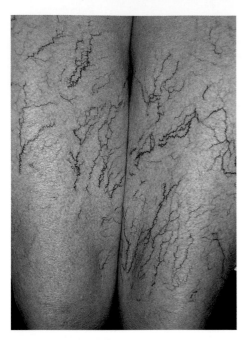

Figure 18–1 Linear telangiectasias of the lower extremities in a patient with venous hypertension.

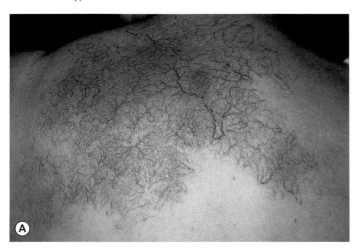

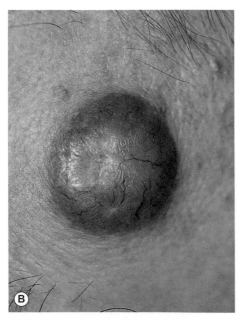

Figure 18–2 (A,B) Linear telangiectasias within lesions of cutaneous B-cell lymphoma. (A, courtesy of Yale Residents' Slide Collection.)

Table 18–1 Types and causes of telangiectasia

I. Primary cutaneous disorders
  A. Linear
    1. Acne rosacea
    2. Actinically damaged skin
    3. Venous hypertension, especially lower extremities
    4. Generalized essential telangiectasia
    5. Within basal cell carcinomas
  B. Papular
    1. Idiopathic
  C. Spider nevus
    1. Idiopathic
    2. Pregnancy
  D. Poikiloderma
    1. Ionizing radiation
    2. Poikiloderma vasculare atrophicans
  E. Stellate
    1. Unilateral nevoid telangiectasia

II. Systemic diseases
  A. Linear
    1. Carcinoid
    2. Ataxia-telangiectasia
    3. Mastocytosis (in particular telangiectasia macularis eruptiva perstans [TMEP])
    4. Within B-cell lymphomas of the skin
  B. Papular
    1. Hereditary hemorrhagic telangiectasia
  C. Spider nevus
    1. Hepatic cirrhosis
  D. Poikiloderma
    1. Dermatomyositis
    2. Xeroderma pigmentosum
    3. Other genodermatoses (e.g., Kindler syndrome, Rothmund-Thomson syndrome)
    4. Cutaneous T-cell lymphoma
  E. Mat
    1. Scleroderma
  F. Periungual
    1. Systemic lupus erythematosus
    2. Scleroderma
    3. Dermatomyositis
    4. Hereditary hemorrhagic telangiectasia

Adapted from Bolognia JL and Braverman IM. Skin manifestations of internal disease. In: Fauci AS, Braunwald E, Kasper DL, et al., eds. Harrison's principles of internal medicine, 17th edn. New York: McGraw-Hill Medical, 2008; 324.

think of the appearance of the skin years after orthovoltage irradiation. Poikiloderma can be a cutaneous sign of dermatomyositis (Fig. 18–4A), and may also be a clinical manifestation of cutaneous T-cell lymphoma. In the latter, the lesions favor the axillae and groin (Fig. 18–4B).

Telangiectasias are an important cutaneous clue to the diagnosis of autoimmune connective tissue diseases (AI-CTD), in particular mat telangiectasias and periungual telangiectasias. Mat telangiectasias are flat and often polygonal in shape, and tend to favor the face, oral mucosa, and hands (Fig. 18–5). They are a sign of scleroderma or an overlap syndrome that includes scleroderma. Of note, in the mnemonic for the more indolent, anticentromere antibody-positive CREST variant of scleroderma, the T stands for telangiectasias. Periungual telangiectasias are seen in systemic lupus erythematosus (SLE), dermatomyositis (DM), and scleroderma. In the latter two AI-CTD, individual telangiectasias appearing as swollen loops are

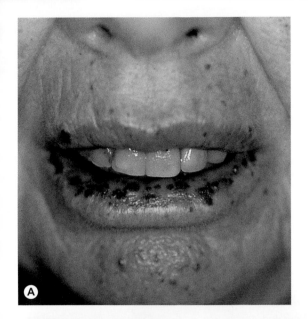

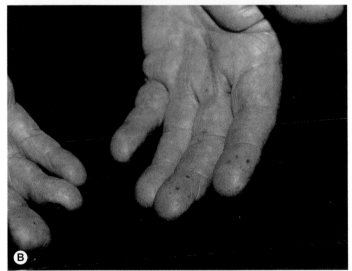

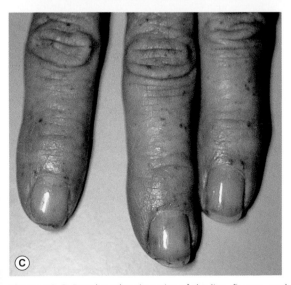

Figure 18–3 Papular telangiectasias of the lips, fingers, and nailfolds in two patients with hereditary hemorrhagic telangiectasia (HHT). (Courtesy of Yale Residents' Slide Collection.)

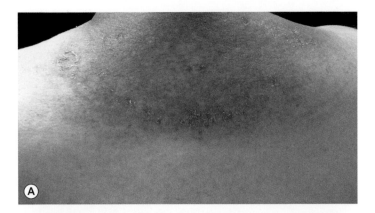

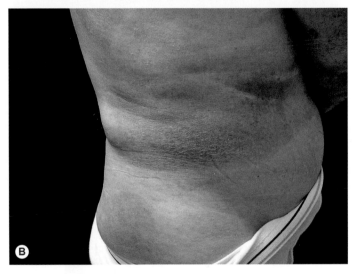

Figure 18–4 (A) Poikiloderma of the upper back (shawl sign) in a patient with dermatomyositis. (B) Poikiloderma in a patient with early cutaneous T-cell lymphoma. The latter photograph was taken over 20 years ago, and this patient has been controlled with the application of moderately potent corticosteroids.

admixed with avascular areas (Fig. 18–6), whereas in lupus the telangiectasias have an appearance that has been likened to that of renal glomeruli. Nailfold telangiectasias are accompanied by erythema in SLE, and both erythema and ragged cuticles in DM.

HEMANGIOMAS AND VASCULAR MALFORMATIONS

On the basis of biologic characteristics, vascular anomalies are divided into two major categories (Table 18–2): vascular tumors (including infantile hemangiomas), which arise by cellular hyperplasia; and vascular malformations, which result from errors in vasculogenesis (differentiation of angioblasts into a primitive vascular network) and angiogenesis (sprouting of new vessels from existing vasculature) during embryonic development and have normal cellular turnover. When vascular tumors are compared to vascular malformations, there are

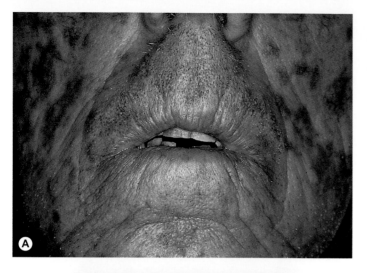

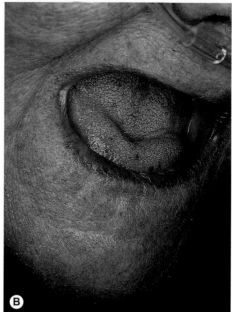

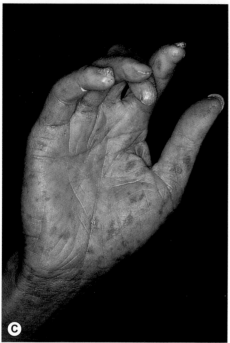

Figure 18–5 Mat telangiectasias of the face, tongue and hand in two patients with scleroderma. Note the perioral furrowing in (A) and the sclerodactyly and loss of distal digits in (C). (A and C, courtesy of Yale Residents' Slide Collection.)

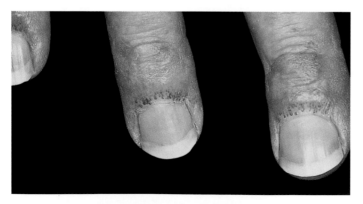

Figure 18–6 Periungual telangiectasias in a patient with dermatomyositis; note the swollen loops alternating with avascular areas.

important differences in natural history, histologic features, associated anomalies/syndromes (Table 18–3), prognosis, and treatment options. However, despite the distinct processes that govern their development, occasionally vascular tumors and malformations are associated with one another, e.g., in kindreds with autosomal dominant co-segregation of infantile hemangiomas and vascular malformations. This suggests overlap in the regulation of prenatal vascular development and postnatal angiogenesis.

Vascular Tumors

Hemangiomas are the most common tumors of infancy, with an incidence of approximately 5–10% by 1 year of age and a female-to-male ratio of 3–4 : 1. Unlike other vascular tumors

Table 18–2 Classification of benign vascular tumors and malformations

Vascular tumors
   Infantile hemangioma (hemangioma of infancy)
      Proliferative phase (superficial and/or deep components)
      Involutional phase
   Congenital hemangioma
      Rapidly involuting (RICH)*
      Noninvoluting (NICH)
   Cherry angioma (senile angioma)
   Pyogenic granuloma
   Tufted angioma*
   Kaposiform hemangioendothelioma*
   Multifocal lymphangioendotheliomatosis with thrombocytopenia
   Glomeruloid hemangioma
   Targetoid hemosiderotic hemangioma
   Spindle cell hemangio(endothelio)ma
   Angiolymphoid hyperplasia with eosinophilia**
   Reactive angioendotheliomatosis†
   Bacillary angiomatosis
   Hemangiopericytoma

Vascular malformations
   Low flow
      Capillary malformation (CM; port-wine stain; nevus flammeus)
      Venous malformation (VM)
      Lymphatic malformation (LM)
         Superficial/microcystic (lymphangioma circumscriptum)
         Deep/macrocystic (cystic hygroma)
      Combined (capillary–venous–lymphatic malformation; CVLM)
      Angiokeratoma circumscriptum
      Verrucous 'hemangioma'
      Glomuvenous malformation
   High flow
      Arterial–venous fistula (AVF)
      Arterial–venous malformation (AVM)
      Arterial malformation (AM)

*Can be associated with Kasabach–Merritt syndrome or, for RICH, a milder thrombocytopenic coagulopathy.
**Associated with peripheral blood eosinophilia, enlargement of regional lymph nodes and salivary glands.
†Can be associated with paraproteinemia, cryoglobinemia, bacterial endocarditis, and atherosclerosis (diffuse dermal angiomatosis)

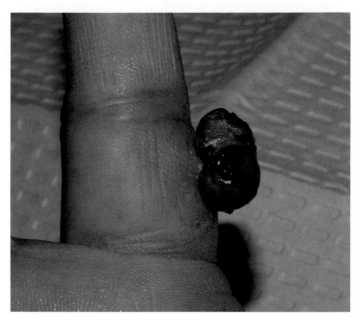

Figure 18–7 Pedunculated pyogenic granuloma of the finger at a site of trauma. The beefy red appearance is reminiscent of granulation tissue.

and malformations, infantile hemangiomas express the placental marker glucose transporter protein-1 (GLUT-1). Infantile hemangiomas typically become apparent during the first few weeks of life, and subsequently undergo a predictable course of rapid growth (proliferative phase) until 3–12 months of age, followed by slow spontaneous regression (involutional phase) that is usually complete by 5–10 years. The lesions can be described as having superficial (initially bright red in color, then dull red to gray during involution) and/or deep (often bluish in color; initially rubbery to palpation, then softer during involution) components. The term 'cavernous hemangioma,' which has been used to describe hemangiomas with both a deep component and venous malformations, has led to confusion and should be avoided. Hemangiomas can be complicated by ulceration, interference with the function of vital structures such as the eyes or airway, high-output cardiac failure, and problems related to associated structural anoma-

lies (Table 18–3). Hypothyroidism may also be observed in infants with large proliferative-phase hemangiomas, perhaps owing to the presence of increased levels of iodothyronine deiodinase within the tumors.

There are a variety of benign vascular tumors and hyperplasias other than infantile hemangiomas (Table 18–2). Congenital hemangiomas represent uncommon, GLUT-1-negative vascular tumors that are fully formed at birth (often pink to blue-violet in color, with central coarse telangiectasias and peripheral pallor) and have a natural history of either rapid involution during the first year of life or proportionate growth and failure to involute.

Cherry angiomas are small, bright-red papules representing a benign proliferation of capillaries; commonly seen on the trunk of adults, they increase in number with age. Pyogenic granulomas are rapidly developing vascular lesions that typically appear as friable papules on the face, fingers (Fig. 18–7), or mucous membranes; histologically resembling granulation tissue, lesions often occur at sites of minor trauma (fingers) or during pregnancy (gingiva).

Bacillary angiomatosis, predominantly affecting patients with AIDS but also occurring in immunocompetent individuals, is characterized by multiple red, hemangioma-like vascular proliferations in the skin as well as internal organ involvement, e.g., liver and bone. The causative organisms, *Bartonella quintana* or *henselae*, can be seen with Warthin–Starry staining of tissue specimens. Kaposiform hemangioendotheliomas and tufted angiomas are two vascular tumors that can be complicated by Kasabach–Merritt syndrome, an acute, life-threatening consumptive coagulopathy with profound thrombocytopenia and anemia (Table 18–3). Spindle cell hemangio(endothelio)mas are unusual tumors that typically develop within existing venous malformations and may

Table 18–3 Benign vascular tumors and malformations: syndromes and associations

	Syndrome/Association	Features of vascular lesion(s)	Associated clinical features
Vascular tumors	Kasabach–Merritt syndrome	Kaposiform hemangioendothelioma or tufted angioma; large, rapidly growing ecchymotic mass (cutaneous or retroperitoneal)	Thrombocytopenia, microangiopathic hemolytic anemia, consumption coagulopathy (disseminated intravascular coagulation, DIC); occurs primarily in infants; 10–30% mortality
	Diffuse neonatal hemangiomatosis	Multiple small cutaneous hemangiomas + visceral hemangiomas (liver > gastrointestinal tract, lungs, CNS)	Hepatomegaly, anemia, high-output cardiac failure
	Airway hemangiomas	Hemangiomas in 'beard' distribution	Hoarseness, stridor, respiratory failure
	PHACES syndrome	Large cervicofacial 'segmental' hemangiomas	*Posterior fossa malformations; Hemangiomas; Arterial, Cardiac, and/or Eye anomalies; Sternal/abdominal clefting*
	Spinal dysraphism, ano- or uro-genital anomalies (SACRAL/PELVIS syndrome)	Infantile hemangiomas in lumbosacral location*	Pseudotail/skin tag, abnormal gluteal cleft
	Hypothyroidism	Large infantile hemangiomas in proliferative phase and/or hepatic hemangioma	
	POEMS syndrome	Cherry angiomas, glomeruloid hemangiomas	*Polyneuropathy, Organomegaly, Endocrinopathy, M-protein (monoclonal gammopathy), Skin changes;* diffuse hyperpigmentation, edema, sclerodermoid changes
Vascular malformations[†]	Sturge–Weber syndrome (encephalotrigeminal angiomatosis)	Facial CM in V1 (+/– V2, V3) dermatomal distribution (uni- > bilateral) + ipsilateral leptomeningeal CVM and/or choroidal vascular malformation	Seizures, mental retardation, contralateral hemiplegia/hemiatrophy of the body, ipsilateral glaucoma, ipsilateral facial soft tissue/bony hypertrophy, pathognomonic radiographic feature of 'tram-track' cerebral gyral calcifications
	Bonnet–Dechaume–Blanc syndrome (Wyburn–Mason syndrome)	(Centro)facial AVM (may mimic a CM) + ipsilateral AVM of retina/intracranial optic pathway	Ipsilateral visual impairment, various contralateral neurologic manifestations
	von Hippel–Lindau syndrome	CM of head and neck	AD inheritance; skin findings in ~5%; retinal and CNS (posterior fossa, spine) hemangioblastoma, renal cell carcinoma, pheochromocytoma, renal and pancreatic cysts, polycythemia
	Klippel–Trenaunay syndrome	CVM/CVLM of lower extremity > upper extremity, trunk; 85% unilateral	Soft tissue/bony hypertrophy (or occasionally hypotrophy**) of affected limb(s), venous thrombosis and ulcers, lymphedema; occasionally gastrointestinal bleeding, hematuria and pulmonary embolism
	Parkes Weber syndrome (PKWS)	AVF +/– CM/CLM of an extremity	Soft tissue/bony hypertrophy with progressive deformity over time, high-output cardiac failure
	Capillary malformation–arteriovenous malformation	Multifocal, small, round-to-oval CM +/– AVM/AVF of face, extremities or brain	PKWS (see above); AD inheritance of *RASA1* mutations

Table 18–3 Benign vascular tumors and malformations: syndromes and associations—cont'd

	Syndrome/Association	Features of vascular lesion(s)	Associated clinical features
	Cutis marmorata telangiectatica congenita (CMTC)	Localized, segmental or generalized reticulated vascular network on extremities > trunk > face, +/– CM, +/– cutaneous atrophy	Hypotrophy (rarely hypertrophy) of affected limb/limb-length discrepancy, glaucoma, developmental delay; aplasia cutis + transverse limb defects +/– cardiac malformation (Adams–Oliver syndrome)
	Macrocephaly–CM (macrocephaly–CMTC)	Reticulated CM (not true CMTC), persistent midfacial capillary stain	Macrocephaly, asymmetry/hemihypertrophy, CNS and facial abnormalities, developmental delay, syndactyly (especially of 2nd–3rd toes), joint laxity
	Phacomatosis pigmentovascularis	CM > CMTC; +/– nevus anemicus	Dermal melanocytosis and/or speckled lentiginous nevus (nevus spilus); may have extracutaneous features of Sturge-Weber syndrome, Klippel–Trenaunay syndrome or nevus of Ota
	Blue rubber bleb nevus syndrome (Bean syndrome)	Multiple VM of skin, gastrointestinal tract > other organ systems	Gastrointestinal bleeding, anemia
	Multiple cutaneous and mucosal venous malformations	Multiple VM of skin, oral mucosa and muscles	AD inheritance of *TEK* mutations
	Cutaneous + cerebral capillary malformations	Hyperkeratotic cutaneous CVM + cerebral capillary malformations	Dominant inheritance of *KRIT1* mutations
	Maffucci syndrome	Multiple VM/VLM, most often of distal extremities; spindle cell hemangio(endothelio)ma	Multiple enchondromas of long bones (most often the metacarpals and phalanges of the hands), chondrosarcoma (15–30%), skeletal deformities, short stature
	Proteus syndrome	CM/LM/CVM/CLM, most often of extremities	Progressive, disproportionate, asymmetric soft tissue/bony overgrowth, cerebriform connective tissue nevi of soles > palms, dermal hypoplasia, lipomas, regional absence of fat, epidermal nevi, CNS abnormalities, venous thrombosis, pulmonary embolism, lung cysts
	Gorham syndrome	Multiple CVLM/LM of the skin, mediastinum, and bones	Massive osteolysis ('disappearing bones'), skeletal deformities, pathologic fractures, pulmonary and neurologic complications
	PTEN hamartoma-tumor syndrome (Bannayan–Riley–Ruvalcaba syndrome > Cowden syndrome)	Multifocal intramuscular AVF associated with ectopic fat; intracranial developmental venous anomalies	AD inheritance of *PTEN* mutations; macrocephaly, developmental delay, multiple lipomas, pigmented macules of genitalia, trichilemmomas, acral keratoses, oral papillomas, neuromas, sclerotic fibromas, intestinal hamartomatous polyps, thyroid adenoma/carcinoma
	Cobb syndrome	AVM (may mimic CM/angiokeratomas) in a dermatomal distribution + AVM in the corresponding spinal cord segment	Neurologic manifestations of spinal cord compression (e.g., paraparesis/paraplegia)

Table 18–3 Benign vascular tumors and malformations: syndromes and associations—cont'd

	Syndrome/Association	Features of vascular lesion(s)	Associated clinical features
Angiokeratomas[‡]	Fabry disease	Angiokeratoma corporis diffusum – small dark red papules symmetrically in a 'bathing trunk' distribution, +/– mucosal involvement	X-linked recessive lysosomal storage disease due to α-galactosidase A deficiency; acral paresthesias, painful crises, hypohidrosis, whorl-like corneal and lenticular opacities, progressive renal and coronary artery disease, cerebrovascular accidents
	Fucosidosis	Angiokeratoma corporis diffusum (as described above)	AR lysosomal storage disease due to α-L-fucosidase deficiency; mental retardation, spastic paresis, seizures, recurrent sinus and pulmonary infections

CM = capillary malformation; VM = venous malformation; LM = lymphatic malformation; CVLM = capillary–venous–lymphatic malformation; AVF = arterio-venous fistula; AVM = arterio-venous malformation; AD = autosomal dominant; AR = autosomal recessive; CNS = central nervous system; SACRAL = *S*pinal dysraphism, *A*nogenital anomalies, *C*utaneous anomalies, *R*enal and urologic anomalies, *A*ngioma of *L*umbosacral localization; PELVIS = *P*erineal hemangioma, *E*xternal genitalia malformations, *L*ipomyelomeningocele, *V*esicorenal abnormalities, *I*mperforate anus, *S*kin tag.
*Capillary malformations in a lumbosacral location may also be associated with spinal dysraphism.
**Referred to as Servelle-Martorell syndrome.
[†]Midfacial capillary stains have also been described in association with a variety of dysmorphic conditions, including Beckwith–Wiedemann, Roberts, and Rubinstein–Taybi syndromes.
[‡]Angiokeratoma corporis diffusum has also been reported in other lysosomal storage diseases such as galactosialidosis, GM1 gangliosidosis, and β-mannosidosis.

be associated with Maffucci syndrome (Fig. 18–8; Table 18–3).

Vascular Malformations

Classically, vascular malformations are present at birth and enlarge in proportion to the child's growth; however, some of these structural anomalies do not become clinically apparent for many years, and rapid expansion in size may occur as a result of hormonal fluctuations (e.g., puberty or pregnancy), trauma, thrombosis or infection. Histologically, vascular malformations are characterized by dilated vascular channels with abnormal walls lined by quiescent endothelium. Further categorization of vascular malformations depends upon the rate of blood flow and the predominant type of vessel involved (Table 18–2). In addition, these malformations are associated with a wide variety of syndromes with localized and systemic features (Fig. 18–9; Table 18–3).

Low-flow vascular malformations may be composed of capillaries, veins and/or lymphatic channels. Capillary malformations (port-wine stains) appear as pink to dark red patches and can serve as a cutaneous marker for internal vascular malformations, e.g., ocular and leptomeningeal (Table 18–3; see Chapter 34). Unlike the fading macular stain of infancy (stork bite, salmon patch) that is present in 30–50% of neonates and commonly located on the nape of the neck, eyelids, glabella, philtrum, and nasal tip, the port-wine stain is typically unilateral in distribution and persists throughout life, often deepening in color and becoming raised and nodular over time.

Venous malformations appear as soft, compressible swellings that are blue to violaceous in color. In the autosomal dominant blue rubber bleb nevus syndrome, multiple venous malformations are found in the skin and the gastrointestinal tract (Fig. 18–10); the latter can lead to gastrointestinal bleeding. In contrast, multiple glomuvenous malformations (caused

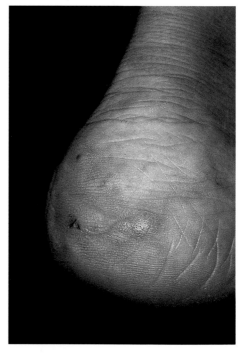

Figure 18–8 Spindle cell hemangioendotheliomas in a patient with Maffucci syndrome. (Courtesy of Yale Residents' Slide Collection.)

by autosomal dominant or paradominant inheritance of *GLMN* mutations) typically present as blue-purple nodules and plaques that are limited to the skin and subcutis, resist full compression, and are painful upon palpation. Venous and lymphatic malformations may be associated with skeletal alterations, functional impairment of involved limbs, and a low-grade, chronic, localized consumptive coagulopathy that results in thrombosis (leading to phlebolith formation) as well as bleeding. Lastly, the presence of a high-flow vascular mal-

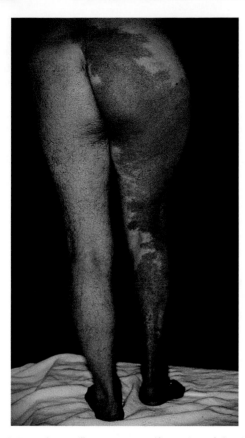

Figure 18–9 Extensive capillary–venous malformation of the right lower extremity associated with limb-length discrepancy in a patient with Klippel–Trenaunay syndrome. (Courtesy of Yale Residents' Slide Collection.)

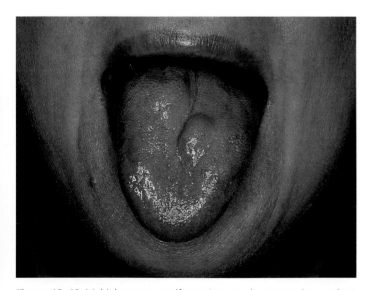

Figure 18–10 Multiple venous malformations on the tongue in a patient with blue rubber bleb nevus syndrome and gastrointestinal bleeding.

formation such as an arteriovenous malformation (AVM) is suggested by clinical signs such as warmth, a bruit, a thrill, or pulsations. In the later stages, AVMs are characterized by ulceration, intractable pain, and when located within an extremity, violet plaques of acroangiodermatitis ('pseudo-Kaposi's sarcoma'; Fig. 18–11).

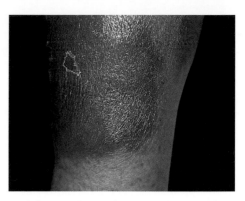

Figure 18–11 Violaceous plaque of acroangiodermatitis ('pseudo-Kaposi's sarcoma') on the distal shin of a patient with venous hypertension and chronic lower extremity edema.

Angiokeratomas

Angiokeratomas are small (1–5 mm) red to red-blue papules with distinct histologic features. When numerous, they can be a sign of inborn errors of metabolism such as Fabry disease (Table 18–3). More commonly, however, angiokeratomas are a manifestation of aging, e.g., multiple dark blue to purple papules on the scrotum and vulva, or single lesions on the lower extremity that can be mistaken for cutaneous melanoma because of their dark color.

KAPOSI'S SARCOMA

Kaposi's sarcoma was first described in 1872 by Moritz Kaposi as 'idiopathic multiple pigmented sarcoma of the skin.' Over a century later, human herpesvirus 8 (HHV-8; Kaposi's sarcoma-associated herpesvirus) was determined to be the primary and necessary agent in the pathogenesis of this vascular tumor. HHV-8 is the infectious cause of all the clinical variants of Kaposi's sarcoma, which have similar histologic features but develop in distinct patient populations and clinical settings, with different sites of involvement, rates of progression, and prognoses. These variants include: (1) classic Kaposi's sarcoma, an indolent disease that primarily affects elderly men of Mediterranean, Eastern European, or Jewish heritage; (2) African-endemic Kaposi's sarcoma, a locally aggressive cutaneous disease in adults and a fulminant lymphadenopathic disease in children; (3) human immunodeficiency virus (HIV)-associated epidemic Kaposi's sarcoma, an aggressive disease most frequently affecting men who have sex with men; and (4) iatrogenic Kaposi's sarcoma occurring in the setting of immunosuppression, in particular after solid organ transplantation.

HHV-8 DNA can be detected in virtually all Kaposi's sarcoma lesions, regardless of clinical subtype. HHV-8 encodes several genes that have been shown to independently transform cells to a malignant phenotype in vitro; this herpesvirus is also clearly associated with body cavity-related B-cell lymphoma (primary effusion lymphoma) and multicentric Castleman's disease. Both the detection of HHV-8 DNA in peripheral blood and antibody seroconversion studies have shown that HHV-8 infection precedes and is predicative of the development of Kaposi's sarcoma. Antibodies to HHV-8 can be found in 80–95% of all patients with Kaposi's sarcoma, and almost 100% of immunocompetent patients with the disease, compared to approximately 1–5% of the general population. The seroprevalence of HHV-8 infection parallels the incidence of Kaposi's sarcoma, and both the seroprevalence and the incidence are higher in geographic areas such as the Mediterranean regions and central Africa, as well as in subpopulations such as HIV-negative and HIV-positive men who have sex with men (approximately 20% and 40% HHV-8 seroprevalence, respectively). Approximately 40% of men who are seropositive for both HIV and HHV-8 develop Kaposi's sarcoma within 10 years. HHV-8 DNA has been detected in both the saliva and the semen of infected individuals, and epidemiologic evidence suggests a sexual mode of transmission.

Immunosuppression appears to be an important cofactor in the pathogenesis of Kaposi's sarcoma in HHV-8-infected individuals. HIV infection in particular may promote the development of Kaposi's sarcoma via mechanisms such as depletion of CD4+ T lymphocytes, stimulation of cytokine release, and production of mitogens such as the HIV tat protein. However, paradoxically, in the setting of the immune reconstitution inflammatory syndrome due to the institution of highly active antiretroviral therapy (HAART), new lesions can appear as well as progression of previously stable lesions.

Clinical Manifestations

Most cases of classic Kaposi's sarcoma develop after the sixth decade of life, and although the older literature reported a male:female ratio of 10–15:1, recent population-based studies have found lower ratios of 3–4:1. Classic Kaposi's sarcoma usually begins as one or more pink to deep red-purple macules on the distal lower extremities. Lesions progress slowly, expanding and coalescing to form large plaques or developing into nodular tumors (Fig. 18–12). Older lesions may become purple-brown in color and develop keratotic surface changes. The disease spreads centrally towards the trunk and often involves both lower extremities, which may become edematous as a result of lymphatic involvement and/or cytokine release; eventually, lesions can erode, ulcerate, and cause severe pain.

Kaposi's sarcoma may involve the oral mucosa and conjunctiva, and the gastrointestinal tract is the most frequent site of visceral disease; however, these lesions are usually asymptomatic. Other potential sites of internal involvement include the lymph nodes, liver, spleen, lungs, adrenal glands, and bones. Classic Kaposi's sarcoma typically has an indolent course, with patients surviving 10–15 years and eventually dying of unrelated causes; however, several studies have noted an increased incidence of lymphomas in patients with classic Kaposi's sarcoma.

African-endemic Kaposi's sarcoma most commonly affects young adults in equatorial Africa (male:female ratio 13–18:1), often with an indolent course resembling that of classic Kaposi's sarcoma, but sometimes with locally aggressive disease characterized by invasion of muscle and bone. A fulminant lymphadenopathic variant occurs in African children (male:female ratio 3:1) and is generally fatal within 2 years.

Kaposi's sarcoma develops in 0.5–5% of solid organ transplant recipients (male:female ratio 2–4:1), most often within 2–3 years of transplantation, and has also been reported in patients undergoing chronic immunosuppressive therapy for autoimmune diseases and malignancies; the incidence is highest in ethnic groups at increased risk for classic Kaposi's sarcoma. Although Kaposi's sarcoma in the setting of iatrogenic immunosuppression tends to be aggressive, lesions often undergo spontaneous regression upon reduction or discontinuation of immunosuppressive therapy. Recently, substitution of sirolimus (rapamycin) for cyclosporine was reported to lead to resolution of cutaneous lesions of Kaposi's sarcoma in kidney transplant recipients, without leading to rejection or worsening of renal function.

Kaposi's sarcoma had been reported to develop in approximately 20% of HIV-positive men who had sex with men and <1–5% of other HIV-positive patients (male:female ratio 10–20:1); however, the incidence has been decreasing over the past decade. The clinical course of HIV-associated Kaposi's sarcoma is highly variable, ranging from stable localized lesions to rapid widespread growth, but in general (with the exception of flares in the setting of the immune reconstitution inflammatory syndrome) its natural history is related to the degree of immune impairment and the overall health of the patient. As a result, most patients have CD4+ T-lymphocyte counts <500/mm³ and usually develop multicentric, progressive disease (Fig. 18–13).

In contrast to other variants of Kaposi's sarcoma, initial cutaneous lesions often develop on the face and trunk; in the latter location, lesions may be aligned with their long axes in the direction of skin folds (Fig. 18–13C). Lesions of the oral mucosa, most often involving the palate, are common and may be the first manifestation of disease. The lymph nodes are affected in approximately half of patients with HIV-associated Kaposi's sarcoma. Symptomatic gastrointestinal involvement is also common, with complications including ulceration, bleeding, perforation and ileus. Pulmonary Kaposi's sarcoma has a poor prognosis; its clinical presentation may be similar to that of opportunistic respiratory infections, with symptoms such as dyspnea, intractable cough, and hemoptysis. Radiographic findings range from discrete parenchymal nodules to bilateral perihilar infiltrates to pleural effusions.

Histopathologic Findings

A skin biopsy can confirm the diagnosis of Kaposi's sarcoma, revealing an angioproliferative neoplasm characterized by spindle-shaped tumor cells and irregular, slit-like endothelium-lined spaces containing erythrocytes. A normal vessel or adnexal structure protruding into an ectatic vascular space (promontory sign) is a hallmark for early disease; spindle cells become more prominent as the lesions progress. An inflammatory infiltrate containing lymphocytes, plasma cells, and histiocytes is typically present. Immunohistochemical staining for the latency-associated nuclear antigen (LNA-1) of HHV-8 can help to distinguish Kaposi's sarcoma from other vascular neoplasms.

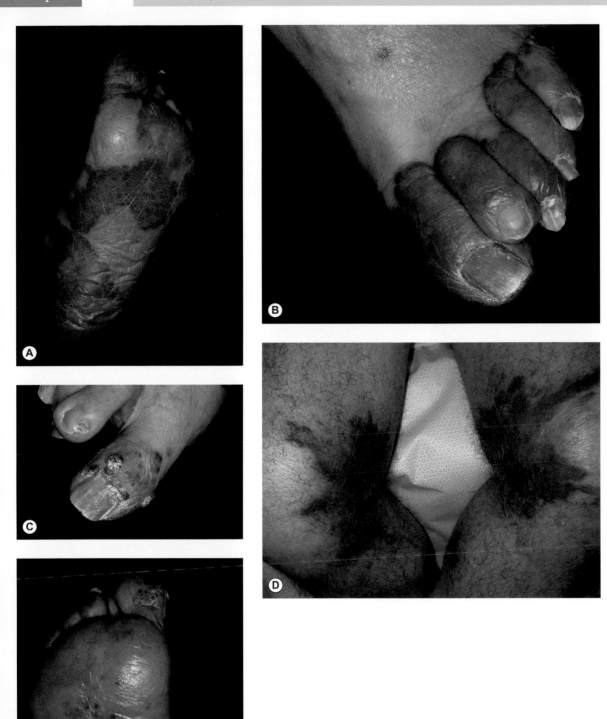

Figure 18–12 Classic Kaposi's sarcoma with involvement of the lower extremities. Violaceous patches become plaques (A, B, C) and may develop a verrucous appearance (D, E) or nodular component (C, E).

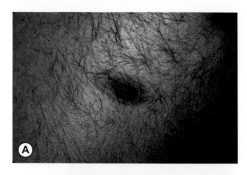

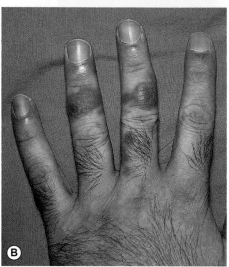

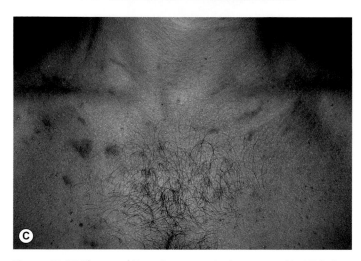

Figure 18–13 Plaques of Kaposi's sarcoma in three men with AIDS; the lesions range in color from deep purple with a rim of hemorrhage (A) to violet (B) to pink-red (C). On the chest, several of the lesions are aligned with their long axes in the direction of skin folds. (B and C, courtesy of Yale Residents' Slide Collection.)

Although the precise cell of origin of Kaposi's sarcoma is still debated, the predominant expression of endothelial markers in Kaposi's sarcoma tissues suggests development from endothelial cells of vascular or lymphatic origin. In vitro, HHV-8 can infect blood as well as lymphatic vascular endothelial cells, with induction of lymphangiogenic molecules in both cell types.

Evaluation and Treatment

The initial evaluation of a patient with Kaposi's sarcoma involves a thorough physical examination with careful attention to areas frequently affected by the disease (including the oral mucosa), testing of the stool for occult blood, and a chest X-ray. When gastrointestinal or pulmonary involvement is suspected, the work-up should include endoscopy or bronchoscopy. Additional studies include HIV testing, particularly in men who have sex with men, and other high-risk patients, and determination of HIV-1 viral load and CD4+ T-lymphocyte count in HIV-positive patients.

Treatment options in Kaposi's sarcoma depend on the extent and rate of growth of the tumor as well as the overall medical condition of the patient. Limited cutaneous disease can be treated with local excision, topical alitretinoin gel, intralesional vinblastine, radiation therapy, laser therapy, photodynamic therapy or cryotherapy. In patients with widespread disease in whom systemic therapy is warranted, liposomal anthracyclines (daunorubicin or doxorubicin) and taxanes (e.g., paclitaxel) are the treatments of choice, with high benefit-to-risk ratios and response rates of 50–80%. Vinblastine, vincristine and bleomycin, either alone or in combination, have also been shown to produce response rates of >50%. Interferon-α therapy has been widely used for HIV-associated Kaposi's sarcoma, but requires high doses that result in significant systemic toxicity. Iatrogenic Kaposi's sarcoma often regresses with reduction or modification (e.g., switch to sirolimus) of immunosuppressive therapy; however, the risk of allograft rejection may limit the first option in organ transplant recipients. Lastly, the use of HAART has been associated with a dramatic reduction in the incidence of HIV-associated Kaposi's sarcoma, as well as regression of existing lesions in most patients (see above).

Therapies currently under investigation include angiogenesis inhibitors (e.g., thalidomide, bevacizumab), tyrosine kinase inhibitors, and matrix metalloproteinase inhibitors.

ANGIOSARCOMA

Angiosarcoma represents a malignancy of endothelial cells, either vascular or lymphatic in origin, which has four clinical variants. The idiopathic form develops on the scalp and upper face, usually in older adults. The lesions range from subtle erythema of the face and scalp to obvious purple plaques and tumors the color of an eggplant (Fig. 18–14). Clinically, the more subtle forms are sometimes misdiagnosed as acne rosacea or soft tissue infections, and areas of induration can mimic cutaneous lymphoma.

In the second subtype (Fig. 18–15) tumors arise within areas of chronic lymphedema, e.g., the lower extremities of patients with congenital lymphedema (Milroy's disease), or the upper extremities of breast cancer patients who have undergone lymph node dissections. The latter form is sometimes referred to as lymphangiosarcoma of Stewart–Treves, but more recently use of the more general term angiosarcoma has been advocated, given the difficulty of determining whether the endothelial cells are vascular or lymphatic in origin.

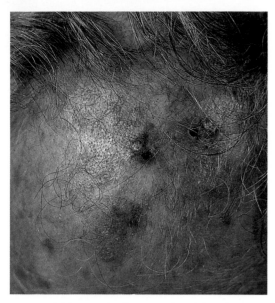

Figure 18–14 Dark blue-purple plaques and nodules of angiosarcoma on the forehead and scalp of a 70-year-old man. The circular area is the biopsy site.

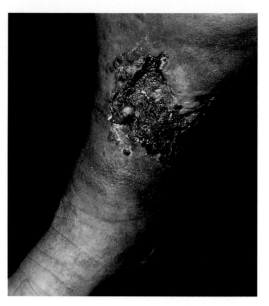

Figure 18–15 Ulcerated plaque of angiosarcoma in a woman with chronic severe lower extremity lymphedema. (Courtesy of Yale Residents' Slide Collection.)

The third type of cutaneous angiosarcoma arises within radiation ports in patients who have been treated for internal malignancies; the most common location for radiation-associated angiosarcoma is the anterior trunk, in particular the breast. With the increasing use of breast-conserving therapy (i.e., lumpectomy followed by radiation therapy) for the treatment of breast cancer, the incidence of the latter has increased, but it is still uncommon. The fourth type is an aggressive variant referred to as epithelioid angiosarcoma.

The diagnosis of an angiosarcoma may require the examination of several biopsy specimens. Histologically, anastomosing vascular channels lined by atypical endothelial cells are observed in the well-differentiated portions of the tumor. In the less well-differentiated areas, pleomorphic cells are seen, some of which are epithelioid in appearance. Positive staining of the tumor cells for CD31 serves as a diagnostic aid. Angiosarcoma must be differentiated from Kaposi's sarcoma as well as benign endothelial proliferations, including those within organizing thrombi (intravascular papillary endothelial hyperplasia).

Treatment of angiosarcoma is difficult because the tumor often extends beyond the clinically apparent margins. As a result, local recurrences are common following surgical excision. Although patients can develop metastases to regional lymph nodes and visceral organs, they often die of complications due to local disease. In addition to surgical excision, extended field radiation and chemotherapy, in particular taxanes (paclitaxel, docetaxel) and daunorubicin, can be used.

SUGGESTED READINGS

Antman K, Chang Y. Kaposi's sarcoma. N Engl J Med 2000; 342: 1027–1038.

Blockmans D, Beyens G, Verhaeghe R. Predictive value of nailfold capillaroscopy in the diagnosis of connective tissue diseases. Clin Rheumatol 1996; 15: 148–153.

Chang Y, Cesarman E, Pessin MS, et al. Identification of herpesvirus-like DNA sequences in AIDS-associated Kaposi's sarcoma. Science 1994; 266: 1865–1869.

DiLorenzo G, Konstantinopoulos PA, Pantanowitz L, et al. Management of AIDS-related Kaposi's sarcoma. Lancet Oncol 2007; 8: 167–176.

Enjolras O, Mulliken JB. Vascular tumors and vascular malformations (new issues). Adv Dermatol 1997; 13: 375–422.

Garzon MC, Huang JT, Enjolras O, et al. Vascular malformations. Part I. J Am Acad Dermatol 2007; 56: 353–370.

Garzon MC, Huang JT, Enjolras O, et al. Vascular malformations. Part II: associated syndromes. J Am Acad Dermatol 2007; 56: 541–564.

Haggstrom AN, Drolet BA, Baselga E, et al. Prospective study of infantile hemangiomas: clinical characteristics predicting complications and treatment. Pediatrics 2006; 118: 882–887.

Hunt SJ, Santa Cruz DJ. Vascular tumors of the skin: a selective review. Semin Diagn Pathol 2004; 21: 166–218.

Isovich J, Boffetta P, Franceschi S, et al. Classic Kaposi sarcoma. Cancer 2000; 88: 500–517.

Leidner RS, Aboulafia DM. Recrudescent Kaposi's sarcoma after initiation of HAART: a manifestation of immune reconstitution syndrome. AIDS Patient Care STDS 2005; 19: 635–644.

Mulliken JB, Young AE. Vascular birthmarks. Hemangiomas and malformations. Philadelphia: WB Saunders, 1988.

Naka N, Ohsawa M, Tomita Y, et al. Prognostic factors in angiosarcoma: a multivariate analysis of 55 cases. J Surg Oncol 1996; 61: 170–176.

Stallone G, Schena A, Infante B, et al. Sirolimus for Kaposi's sarcoma in renal-transplant recipients. N Engl J Med 2005; 352: 1317–1323.

Chapter | 19 |

Gary S. Wood
and Warren W. Piette

Primary Cutaneous T-cell and B-cell Lymphomas

Primary cutaneous lymphoma is a term that includes syndromes of both T- and B-cell neoplasms for which the skin is the primary organ affected during much or all of the course, despite the ability of the neoplastic cells to circulate within the body. Although most of these syndromes presumably have the potential for severe systemic involvement, a relatively indolent course is expected in many cases. These lymphomas have an estimated annual incidence of 1–1.5/100 000, and are second only to gastrointestinal lymphomas as the most common group of extranodal lymphomas. However, extranodal lymphomas as a group comprise only a small proportion of all lymphomas, which has often led to distinctive organ-specific presentations being overlooked in general classifications of lymphoma. Some systemic lymphomas or leukemias may involve the skin early in their course, but characteristically have important nodal, marrow, or other extracutaneous involvement either preceding or concomitant with cutaneous lesions. Still other hematopoietic malignancies rarely involve the skin, and then usually only late in the course of disease after extensive infiltration of other sites. Cutaneous involvement by leukemias and systemic lymphomas is discussed in Chapter 15.

The term cutaneous T-cell lymphoma (CTCL) was coined in the 1970s by Edelson to combine a variety of T-cell lymphoma syndromes characterized by early cutaneous involvement, particularly classic and variant mycosis fungoides (MF) and the closely related leukemic variant, Sézary syndrome. Since that time there have been a number of other T-cell lymphomas recognized which have early and primarily cutaneous involvement. The term CTCL can be confusing in that it is now used by some to describe mostly MF/Sézary variants, and by others (as in this chapter) to include all T-cell lymphoma syndromes that fit the definition of primary cutaneous lymphoma. The realization that B-cell lymphomas might also predominantly or exclusively involve the skin is more recent. Many lesions formerly classified as cutaneous pseudolymphoma or lymphocytoma cutis would now be considered indolent primary cutaneous B-cell lymphomas.

Most primary cutaneous lymphomas are T cell (75%); B-cell lymphomas comprise the remainder (25%). When subsets of primary cutaneous lymphomas are considered, approximately 50% are MF/Sézary variants of CTCL, 25% are other cutaneous T-cell lymphomas, and 25% are cutaneous B-cell lymphomas.

CLASSIFICATIONS OF CUTANEOUS LYMPHOMAS

The classification of lymphomas is confusing and often controversial, especially when applied to primary cutaneous lymphomas. With respect to lymphomas in general, most early classifications were based solely on morphology (e.g., Gall and Mallory, or Rappaport). Others, like the Working Formulation, relied on primarily the treatment response and survival. Still others (e.g., Kiel, Lukes, and Collins) focused particularly on cell lineage and differentiation, attempting to correlate neoplasms with recognizable morphologic differentiation stages of normal lymphocyte biology. Each scheme has advanced the recognition and treatment of lymphomas, but all have proved insufficient, and none seemed particularly useful in the diagnosis and treatment of primary cutaneous lymphomas.

The classification of extranodal lymphomas has received more attention in recent years. The Revised European–American Lymphoma (REAL) classification was devised to use morphology, immunophenotype, genetic features, and clinical features to classify all lymphomas, with an emphasis on reproducibility of diagnosis (>85% interobserver reproducibility for pathologists, >95% of cases able to be classified). For some lymphomas, a specific genetic abnormality/translocation is an important defining criterion: t(11;14) in mantle-cell lymphoma, t(14;18) in follicular lymphoma, and t(8;14) in Burkitt's lymphoma. For other lymphomas, clinical features are important, such as whether the presentation is nodal or extranodal in marginal zone lymphoma, in peripheral T-cell lymphomas, and in mediastinal large B-cell lymphoma. The REAL classification was updated in the WHO classification for all lymphomas. Unfortunately, both classifications still lump most primary cutaneous lymphomas into large histologically defined subgroups, especially the diffuse large B-cell lymphomas and the peripheral (mature) T-cell lymphomas. In response to these and other difficulties with existing classifications, the Cutaneous Lymphoma Group of the European Organization for Research and Treatment of Cancer proposed in 1997 the EORTC Classification for primary cutaneous lymphomas that was later updated as the combined WHO/EORTC Classification (see Willemze et al., 2005). This classification incorpo-

Table 19–1 WHO/EORTC classification of cutaneous T-cell lymphomas

Indolent (5-yr survival >75%)

MF and variants
LyP-CD30+ ALCL spectrum
Subcutaneous panniculitic, αβ TCR, usually CD8+
Small/medium pleomorphic, CD4+

Aggressive (5-yr survival <25%)

SS
NK/T, nasal type, CD56+ EBV+, often ulcerative
Aggressive epidermotropic, CD8+, often ulcerative
γδ, CD56+, often ulcerative
Peripheral TCL, unspecified (large CD4+ pleomorphic)
Adult T-cell leukemia/lymphoma (classic type)
(CD4+CD56+ plasmacytoid DC 'blastic NK' lymphoma)

Table 19–2 WHO/EORTC classification of cutaneous B-cell lymphomas

Indolent (5-yr survival >95%)

Follicle-center cell lymphoma
Marginal zone lymphoma (including immunocytoma)

Intermediate (5-yr survival 50–65%)

Large cell lymphoma, leg
Large cell lymphoma, intravascular
Large cell lymphoma, other

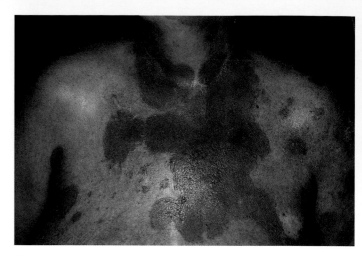

Figure 19–1 Multiple erythematous plaques with some irregular margins in a patient with mycosis fungoides.

rated cutaneous T- and B-cell lymphomas into a limited number of well-defined types comprising at least 95% of primary cutaneous lymphomas (Tables 19–1 and 19–2). It also contains a number of provisional categories for which distinctive clinical presentations or clinical outcomes have not yet been completely defined. This system places even more emphasis on clinical, immunophenotypical, and molecular criteria for final diagnosis than do earlier classifications. In some instances the histopathologic diagnosis by itself is not definitive, but instead defines a limited differential diagnosis, which is completed by evaluating the nonhistopathologic elements.

PRIMARY CUTANEOUS T-CELL LYMPHOMAS

Mycosis Fungoides and Sézary Syndrome (Classic Cutaneous T-Cell Lymphoma)

The most traditional and most common subset of cutaneous T-cell lymphoma (CTCL) is mycosis fungoides (MF). The incidence of MF in the United States is estimated at 0.36/100 000 person-years, with an incidence ratio of black to white patients of 1.7, and of Asian to white patients of 0.6. Tumor-stage MF is much less common, as is the Sézary syndrome. Despite the serious progression of disease in some patients, MF is more typically an indolent malignancy, especially in patients with patch or plaque disease only. The chance of long-term survival after the diagnosis of early disease is excellent. Thus, treatment

for early MF is usually conservative. Patients with tumoral MF, nodal or visceral disease, or Sézary syndrome require more aggressive treatment, including chemotherapeutic agents, radiation treatment, or extracorporeal photopheresis.

Clinical Manifestations

The MF subset of CTCL is typically a disease of late middle age and beyond, affecting men more commonly than women. However, patients of all ages, including children, may be affected. It often begins as a nonspecific chronic dermatitis, frequently diagnosed as atopic, contact, nummular, or photo-induced dermatitis, and it can be mimicked by these same disorders. In view of the similarity of clinical findings in early disease to those of many common inflammatory dermatoses, it should not be surprising that the median duration of symptoms before diagnosis is 48 months (range 1–648 months). MF classically begins as pruritic, macular, erythematous patches with fine scale. Lesions may show epidermal atrophy, telangiectasia, or mottled hyper- and hypopigmentation; all three features combined are termed poikiloderma. Poikiloderma is very suggestive of MF-type CTCL, but this term is also used to describe skin changes in some patients with dermatomyositis or scleroderma. Poikiloderma in these latter two diseases is somewhat different from that in MF, with dyspigmentation usually more prominent and epidermal atrophy less evident. MF tends to asymmetrically involve the trunk, buttocks, thighs, and abdomen initially. These patches may thicken, becoming more indurated with hyperkeratotic surfaces, resulting in sharply demarcated, psoriasiform plaques. They may become circinate, annular, or arciform (Figs 19–1 to 19–3). Plaques may evolve from previous patches or arise de novo.

Most patients with MF do not progress beyond patch- or plaque-type disease, but a small percentage will develop soft to moderately firm, erythematous to violaceous nodules or tumors (Figs 19–4, 19–5). Tumors gradually enlarge, often leading to necrosis and ulcer formation. They may arise de novo without evidence of pre-existing MF (tumeur d'emblée), though this is rare (Fig. 19–6). Most reports of tumeur d'emblée are now thought to represent other forms of CTCL, such as

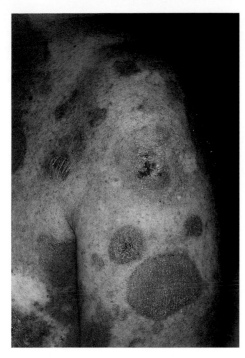

Figure 19–2 Multiple erythematous annular lesions in a patient with mycosis fungoides.

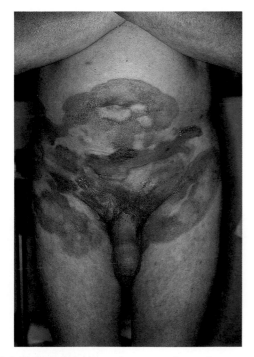

Figure 19–3 Multiple irregular erythematous plaques in a man with mycosis fungoides.

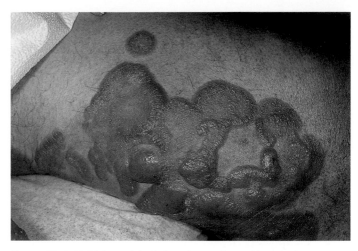

Figure 19–4 Multiple nodular lesions in a patient with mycosis fungoides.

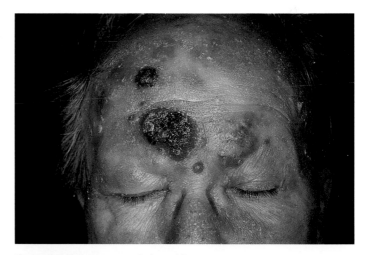

Figure 19–5 Tumor mycosis fungoides.

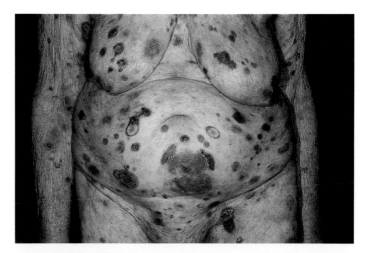

Figure 19–6 Rapid onset of multiple tumors in a patient with mycosis fungoides, representing tumeur d'emblée.

anaplastic large cell lymphoma or pleomorphic T-cell lymphomas. Both tumors and indurated plaques on the face may eventuate in a prominent brow and leonine facies (Fig. 19–7). Leonine facies is not specific to MF: similar changes may occur in patients with leprosy, chronic actinic dermatitis, and even in severe atopic dermatitis.

Progression to symptomatic systemic disease may develop at any stage of MF-type CTCL, usually beginning with peripheral lymph node involvement. Other organs, particularly the liver, lung, and spleen, may be affected. Terminal illness may result in fever, fatigue, anorexia, or cytopenias. Patients with patch/plaque MF may also progress to an exfoliative erythroderma (erythrodermic MF), but erythroderma as a manifestation of MF usually occurs de novo as Sézary syndrome, a leukemic variant of CTCL closely related to MF (Fig. 19–8). Sézary syndrome is characterized by erythroderma, circulating Sézary cells (atypical lymphocytes with hyperconvoluted or cerebriform nuclei) with or without an absolute lymphocytosis, adenopathy, and sometimes hepatosplenomegaly. In fact, at presentation it might more properly be considered a systemic lymphoma/leukemia with prominent early skin involve-

ment. Patients with Sézary syndrome have diffuse erythema with broad areas of lichenification and scale. The face and scalp are often involved, occasionally resulting in ectropion of the lower eyelids. Alopecia may develop. The palms and soles are frequently affected with erythema, thick hyperkeratosis, and painful fissures. The nails are thickened, dystrophic, and brittle. At this stage, pruritus is almost always present and is often severe and unremitting.

The patient with exfoliative erythroderma is at great risk for widespread internal involvement and serious complications. The loss of the integrity of the corneal barrier and the marked vasodilatation may result in dehydration, temperature dysregulation, high-output congestive heart failure, and increased susceptibility to infection. Patients with Sézary syndrome are also susceptible to disseminated herpes simplex infection, called Kaposi's varicelliform eruption, which can cause significant morbidity, and, in a small percentage of patients, can be associated with internal dissemination of herpes simplex. Most deaths that are caused by Sézary syndrome result from bacterial sepsis and pneumonia, but the pruritus may be so unrelenting as to provoke suicide.

In addition to the difficulties of distinguishing early MF from many inflammatory dermatoses, and vice versa, the diagnosis can be exceedingly challenging because of the great variety of unusual clinical presentations MF can assume (Table 19–3).

Follicular MF is characterized by tumor cell infiltration of hair follicles. This is usually accompanied by deposition of mucin between follicular epithelial cells. Follicular MF with mucin deposition must be distinguished from alopecia mucinosa. The syndrome of alopecia mucinosa is characterized clinically by flesh-colored or erythematous follicular papules or boggy indurated plaques with localized alopecia, and histologically by follicular deposition of mucin in the outer root sheath. Lesions are usually located on the head and neck (Fig. 19–9); however, they may become more widespread, involving the trunk and extremities. This syndrome is typically a troublesome but nonmalignant disease, but can also be a manifestation of MF/CTCL. In general, patients with only a few lesions and those who are under 40 years of age are likely to

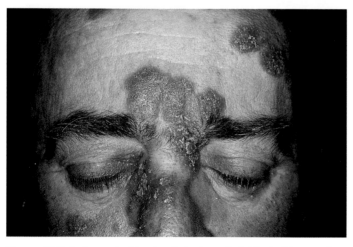

Figure 19–7 Early onset of leonine facies in an individual with mycosis fungoides.

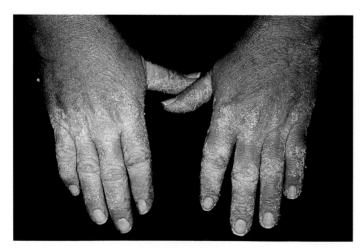

Figure 19–8 Erythrodermic mycosis fungoides.

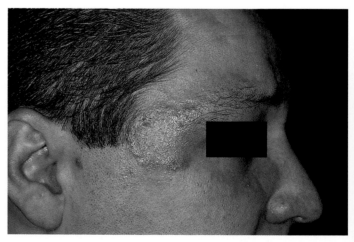

Figure 19–9 Patch of alopecia mucinosa on the lateral face.

Table 19–3 Clinical variants of mycosis fungoides-type CTCL

Presentation	Comments	Reference
Invisible MF	Pruritus with normal-appearing skin	Pujol RM et al. J Am Acad Dermatol 2000; 42: 324–328
Poikiloderma atrophicans vasculare/parapsoriasis variegata	Triad of atrophy, telangiectasia, and mottled dyspigmentation	
Hyperpigmented MF	Macular	Yamamoto T et al. Blood 1997; 90: 1338–1340
Hypopigmented MF	Macular	Akaraphanth R et al. J Am Acad Dermatol 2000; 432: 33–39
Pigmented purpuric MF (can be mimicked clinically and histologically by drug reactions)	Pigmented purpura morphology	Ameen M et al. Br J Dermatol 2000; 142: 564–567; Crowson AN et al. Hum Pathol 1999; 30: 1004–1012; Puddu P et al. J Am Acad Dermatol 1999; 40: 298–299
Folliculocentric, cystic, or comedomal MF		Hodak E et al. Br J Dermatol 1999; 141: 315–322; Fraser-Andrews E et al. Br J Dermatol 1999; 140: 141–144
Syringotropic MF		Tannous Z et al. J Am Acad Dermatol 1999; 41: 303–308
Palmar/plantar keratotic MF		Hannah M, Jacyk WK. Arch Dermatol 1998; 134: 1021–1024
Keratotic lichenoides chronica-like MF		Bahadoran P et al. Br J Dermatol 1998; 138: 1067–1069
Necrobiosis lipoidica-like MF		Woollons A et al. J Am Acad Dermatol 1999; 41: 815–819
Granuloma annulare and MF		Wong WR et al. Dermatology 2000; 200: 54–56
Nonhealing wounds, esp. feet, mimicking ischemic or diabetic foot		Goldstein LJ et al. Ann Vasc Surg 1999; 13: 305–307
Bullous MF		Pfohler C et al. Dermatology 2000; 200: 51–53; Cordoba S et al. Br J Dermatol 1999; 141: 164–166
Pyoderma gangrenosa-like MF		Ho KK et al. Br J Dermatol 2000; 142: 124–127
Granulomatous MF		Topar G et al. Acta Dermatol Venereol 2001; 81: 42–44
Woringer–Kolopp/pagetoid reticulosis		Heald PW, Glusac EJ. J Am Acad Dermatol 2000; 42: 283–285

have a shorter benign course, often with remission within 1 year. In contrast, 15% of patients with multiple lesions who are older than 40 can be expected to have or develop MF. Most patients with alopecia mucinosa-like lesions will actually be found to have follicular MF on careful histologic perusal, and only rarely will patients with histologically benign alopecia mucinosa progress to MF. Interestingly, both the benign and the MF-associated forms of follicular mucinosis usually exhibit dominant T-cell clonality, so this is not a useful differential diagnostic criterion.

Another and more rare clinical and histologic variant of MF is pagetoid reticulosis. The clinical presentation is typically a well-demarcated erythematous scaling plaque, often with evidence of central clearing and an elevated, occasionally verrucous, border. Histopathologically, there is massive epidermal infiltration of atypical lymphocytes. This extensive epidermotropism differs from plaque-stage CTCL, in which smaller intraepidermal collections of atypical cells (Pautrier's microabscesses) are expected. Also, unlike typical MF, which is CD4+, the cells may be CD4+, CD8+, or neither, and can express the CD30 antigen. Presentation as a solitary lesion has also been

termed Woringer–Kolopp syndrome. Patients with the solitary form have an excellent long-term prognosis with only lesional treatment (Fig. 19–10). A multilesional presentation, Ketron–Goodman syndrome, should be considered a more epidermotropic variant of otherwise typical MF.

Granulomatous slack skin is a rare but distinctive condition considered to be related to MF. Skin laxity and folds develop in intertriginous areas, especially axillae and groin (Fig. 19–11). Lesional histology demonstrates a dense dermal infiltrate of somewhat MF-like atypical lymphoid cells, and may show epidermotropism. Multinucleated giant cells or granulomatous tubercles are also present; elastic fibers are absent. CD4+ monoclonal T-cell proliferation has been demonstrated. Patients with this syndrome have an increased risk of Hodgkin's and non-Hodgkin's lymphoma.

Typical MF can occasionally transform into a large cell lymphoma, with a corresponding transition to a much worse prognosis (median survival as low as 1–2 years). Transformation of MF is usually to large cell pleomorphic anaplastic cell histologies (50% CD30+, 50% CD30–), with little difference in survival between the CD30-positive and CD30-negative groups.

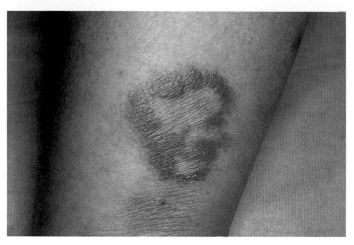

Figure 19–10 Localized intraepidermal mycosis fungoides, also known as Woringer–Kolopp disease.

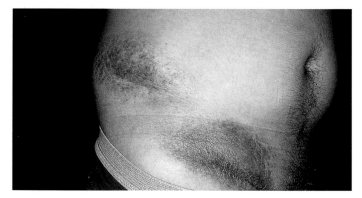

Figure 19–11 Granulomatous slack skin syndrome.

Precursor or Associated Eruptions

MF is often preceded by more distinctive dermatoses, including parapsoriasis and poikiloderma atrophicans vasculare. These disease entities may either herald the onset of or coexist with MF. Accurately identifying these eruptions may lead to earlier recognition and treatment.

The word 'plaque' in small and large plaque parapsoriasis is misleading in that both conditions usually produce lesions which are not plaques but rather patches – i.e., lesions that are neither infiltrated nor elevated. Small-plaque parapsoriasis typically presents with scaly red patches <5 cm in diameter, and mild spongiotic dermatitis on histology. Although most cases demonstrate a clonal T-cell proliferation using PCR methods, progression to clinically typical MF is extremely rare, and treatment appropriate for MF is not indicated. Digitate dermatosis is probably a variant of small-plaque psoriasis, and is characterized by elongated oval (digitate) patches or thin plaques, typically aligned in parallel along the chest, flanks, or abdomen.

Large-plaque parapsoriasis is more appropriately considered a MF-precursor dermatosis. It is characterized by large, pruritic, red-yellow, finely scaling patches, sometimes reticulated (retiform parapsoriasis), and usually truncal. The plaques are by definition large: >5 cm in diameter on the trunk, and often larger on the buttocks. Approximately 10–30% of patients with large-plaque parapsoriasis develop MF over a decade or more of follow-up. Some authors consider every case of large-plaque parapsoriasis to be early-stage MF. Histologic examination reveals mild superficial dermatitis, sometimes with mild spongiotic or interface dermatitis. As with small-plaque parapsoriasis, many cases show clonal T-cell receptor (TCR) gene rearrangements by PCR. From a biological standpoint, large-plaque parapsoriasis and MF probably exist on a continuum of progressive clonal evolution eventuating in recognizable MF. Still, many patients with this disease will never develop overt MF, and therapy for MF is usually reserved for patients whose clinicopathological findings are diagnostic.

Poikiloderma atrophicans vasculare presents clinically with patches of epidermal atrophy, telangiectasia, and mottled hypo- and hyperpigmentation. Histologically, such lesions may show the nonspecific features of large-plaque parapsoriasis, or may be diagnostic of MF. In patients with nonspecific histologic features, this clinical presentation is usually considered more likely to progress to MF than other forms of large-plaque parapsoriasis (up to 50% likelihood).

Other Cutaneous T-cell Lymphomas

Clinicopathological correlation has shown that some features of cutaneous lymphomas are more important than others in predicting their innate behavior and response to therapy. This has affected classification in the WHO/EORTC system. For example, earlier schemes that defined lymphomas as 'panniculitic' or 'angiocentric' have been supplanted by more clinically relevant groupings that divide these lymphomas into alternative categories, as discussed below.

Relatively Indolent (5-Year Survival >75%)

Lymphomatoid papulosis is a chronic eruption that most often consists of crops of recurrent erythematous papules that undergo central necrosis and crust formation. Skin lesions frequently resemble those of pityriasis lichenoides et varioliformis acuta (PLEVA). However, lesions may appear as relatively nondescript red patches or thin plaques, which resemble small-plaque parapsoriasis or pityriasis lichenoides chronica (Fig. 19–12). Uncommonly, patients may develop nodular eruptions, sometimes with ulceration, and this clinical appearance coupled with histologic changes can result in a diagnosis of lymphoma. This is explained by the fact that lymphomatoid papulosis and primary cutaneous CD30+ anaplastic large cell lymphoma represent the two ends of a spectrum of CD30+ cutaneous lymphoproliferative disorders that contains many intermediate clinical presentations. The most important aspect of correct clinical management is to recognize that a patient is within this spectrum, rather than precisely where they lie along it. Histologically, patients with lymphomatoid papulosis can exhibit variable features, including those with large Ki-1/

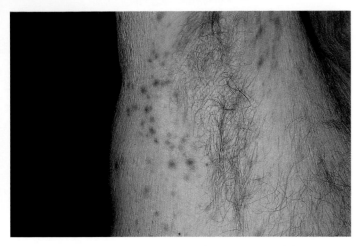

Figure 19–12 Multiple papules and nodules in a patient with lymphomatoid papulosis.

CD30+ atypical cells (type A), and those with much smaller Sézary cell-like atypical cells with hyperconvoluted nuclei (type B). A type C has been described with sheets or clusters of the large type A cells, which requires clinical correlation to distinguish from anaplastic large T-cell lymphoma. Because of these differing histologies, lymphomatoid papulosis bridges the MF and the non-MF types of CTCL, especially anaplastic large T-cell lymphoma. In patients presenting with lymphomatoid papulosis lesions, the incidence of subsequent development of clinically malignant lymphoma has ranged from 5% to 50%. The largest population study suggests that 5% is closer to the usual expected rate. In the WHO/EORTC classification (Table 19–1) lymphomatoid papulosis is considered an indolent lymphoma, but it is usually not treated as such clinically. Topical corticosteroids, tetracycline, erythromycin, phototherapy, and low-dose oral methotrexate are the principal therapies. In patients with the uncommon development of lymphoma, the size of the atypical cell is somewhat predictive of the type of lymphoma that may develop. The small cell variant is more likely to evolve to MF, the large cell to Hodgkin's disease or anaplastic large T-cell lymphoma.

Anaplastic large T-cell lymphoma CD30+, the most common form of non-MF CTCL, includes the entity previously termed 'regressing atypical histiocytosis.' Histologically, it contains predominantly CD30+ large atypical cells similar to those seen in type A and type C lymphomatoid papulosis. Clinical lesions may be red or flesh-colored plaques or nodules, and may ulcerate. Histologically, lesions consist of a dense dermal infiltrate of large atypical lymphoid cells with pleomorphic nuclei and abundant cytoplasm. It is critical to distinguish this primary cutaneous lymphoma from systemic CD30+ anaplastic large cell lymphoma. The systemic form is aggressive, is positive for anaplastic large cell kinase-1 (ALK-1) and t(2;5) translocation, may have prominent skin involvement, and requires systemic chemotherapy. The cutaneous version is more indolent, with frequent slow spontaneous resolution of cutaneous lesions, and slow or no progression to symptomatic systemic disease. It is histologically identical to the systemic form, but usually negative for ALK-1 and t(2;5) (except for some pediatric cases),

and typically is treated by local therapies or low-dose oral methotrexate.

The term subcutaneous panniculitic T-cell lymphoma is now used to refer to CD8+ T-cell lymphomas with an αβ-TCR that are centered in the subcutis and typically spare the overlying skin. They generally exhibit an indolent clinical course. Treatments include systemic corticosteroids, radiation therapy, and chemotherapy.

CD4+ small/medium pleomorphic T-cell lymphomas are often localized nodules or plaques. Lesional infiltrates consist of small to medium-sized atypical lymphoid cells with scant cytoplasm, and may contain a small number of large pleomorphic cells (less than one-third of atypical cells). Infiltrates often invade the subcutis, and may be epidermotropic. This lymphoma group has a worse prognosis than MF and the CD30+ CTCL groups, but a better prognosis than the CD30– large T-cell lymphomas.

Relatively Aggressive (5-Year Survival <25%)

CD30– large T-cell lymphoma is defined by the presence of large atypical cells with low percentage or negative CD30 staining, and plaques or nodules clinically. This is more aggressive than the CD30+ cutaneous lymphoma, with 5-year survival ranging from 10% to 20%.

Epidermotropic CD8+ cytolytic T-cell lymphomas present with localized or generalized ulcerated papulonodules containing epidermotropic infiltrates of small, medium, or large atypical T cells with a cytolytic phenotype. Median survival is less than 3 years.

Extranodal NK/T-cell lymphoma, nasal type, is associated with Epstein–Barr virus in many parts of the world, especially Asia, but not in North America. Formerly known as 'lethal midline granuloma,' this is an angiocentric lymphoma with a predilection for the skin and upper respiratory tract. Tumor cells express CD56 and multiple cytolytic proteins such as TIA-1. Therapy for NK/T-cell lymphomas is usually aggressive, to match their aggressive behavior.

Cutaneous γδ T-cell lymphomas are defined by expression of TCR-γδ rather than TCR-αβ. Patients usually present with generalized skin lesions and often mucosal involvement. Lesional infiltrates can vary in their cytologic features and may be epidermotropic or centered in the dermis or subcutis. The latter panniculitic form presents as deep subcutaneous nodules (Fig. 19–13). Fever, weight loss, and cytopenias (from hemophagocytosis) commonly accompany these lesions. Many cases were previously described as 'cytophagocytic histiocytic panniculitis,' but it is now clear that the prominent hemophagocytosis characteristic of this syndrome is often driven by a T-cell lymphoma. There is a TCR-β–δ+, cytolytic T-cell phenotype lacking both CD4 and CD8. Clonal TCR-γ gene rearrangement is present. Median survival is less than 1.5 years, and death is typically secondary to systemic complications or sepsis.

Adult T-cell leukemia/lymphoma is an aggressive lymphoma caused by HTLV-1 retrovirus. It is endemic in southern Japan and rarely seen in the United States. Tumor cells are typically CD4+ and show monoclonal integration of the HTLV-1 provirus. Several clinical variants exist, but the prognosis is generally poor.

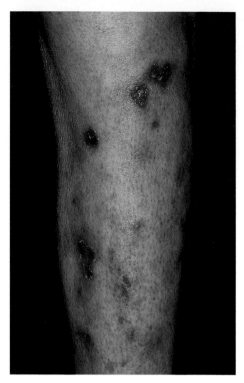

Figure 19–13 Subcutaneous panniculitis-like T-cell lymphoma.

Table 19–4 ISCL algorithm for the diagnosis of early MF: 4 points needed to establish diagnosis

Criteria	2 points	1 point
Clinical	Any 2	Any 1
Persistent and/or progressive patches and plaques plus 1) Non-sun-exposed location 2) Size/shape variation 3) Poikiloderma		
Histopathologic	Both	Either
Superficial lymphoid infiltrate plus 1) Epidermotropism 2) Atypia		
Molecular biological		Present
Clonal TCR gene rearrangement		
Immunopathological		Any 1
T-cell antigen deficiency 1) CD2,3,5 <50% 2) CD7 <10% 3) Epidermal/dermal discordance for CD2,3,5 or 7		

ISCL, International Society for Cutaneous Lymphomas.

Another tumor previously classified as 'blastic NK-cell lymphoma' is now believed to be a plasmacytoid dendritic cell neoplasm termed 'CD4+/CD56+ hematodermic neoplasm.' Half of cases present with disseminated extracutaneous disease in addition to bruise-like skin nodules. Lack of CD3 and expression of CD123 support a plasmacytoid dendritic cell relationship. Median survival is only about 1 year.

Diagnosis and Evaluation

MF is a neoplasm of T cells belonging to the skin-associated lymphoid tissue (SALT). These cells traffic between the skin and peripheral lymph nodes via the blood and lymphatics. They express the CD4 helper T-cell marker and produce Th2 cytokines such as IL-4, -5 and -10. Patients with clinical lesions suspicious for MF should have one or more skin biopsies performed. Multiple biopsies are especially indicated either when there are multiple strictly macular lesions, or when lesions of very different morphologies coexist. Clinically identical lesions may have different histologic patterns; often none or only one will be confirmatory in what ultimately proves to be early MF. Ideally, patients are preferably biopsied at a time when topical corticosteroids have not been used on the lesion for several weeks, as their application seems to alter the histopathological findings. Specimens from patch-stage MF have typical findings that include a banal dermal inflammatory infiltrate that resembles that of other benign dermatoses. Lymphocytes begin to invade the epidermis (called epidermotropism). Intraepidermal edema (spongiosis) may also be present. Atypical lymphocytes with hyperconvoluted nuclei (mycosis or Sézary cells) are usually not prominent at this stage. To facilitate the diagnosis

of early MF, the International Society for Cutaneous Lymphomas (ISCL) has published an algorithm based on a combination of clinical, histologic, immunophenotypic, and clonal features (Table 19–4). Because pseudolymphomatous drug eruptions and certain collagen vascular diseases can closely mimic early MF, they must be excluded from the differential diagnosis.

Biopsy specimens of MF plaques will usually reveal the classic pathologic findings. The epidermis is acanthotic and contains epidermotropic atypical lymphocytes, often in small collections called Pautrier's microabscesses. Spongiosis is often minimal. There is an underlying band of inflammatory cells that often contain both plasma cells and eosinophils; this band typically abuts the epidermis, unlike the narrow subepidermal infiltrate-free space (Grenz zone) typically seen in most other forms of T-cell and almost all B-cell lymphomas. Tumor lesions in MF are histopathologically characterized by large dermal and subcutaneous collections of atypical lymphocytes. The overlying epidermis is no longer thickened. The epidermis is often atrophied, and occasionally completely ulcerated. There is a concomitant decrease in epidermotropism.

Sézary syndrome may show histopathologic features similar to those of plaque-stage MF, including a dense, mixed, band-like dermal infiltrate with an epidermis that contains Pautrier's microabscesses. However, many skin biopsy specimens from Sézary syndrome patients do not show epidermotropism, and frequently show only nonspecific dermatitis.

Assessment for peripheral lymphadenopathy is important in all patients. Palpability of lymph nodes is not confirmatory of histologic involvement, however, as evidenced by the staging criteria (Table 19–5). Palpable lymph nodes are often resected.

Table 19–5 ISCL/EORTC revised TNM classification of mycosis fungoides and Sézary syndrome

Classification	Definition	
T (tumor), skin		
T1	Patches/plaques <10% body surface area (a vs b: patch only vs other)	
T2	Patches/plaques >10% body surface area (a vs b: patch only vs other)	
T3	1 or more cutaneous tumor nodules	
T4	Erythroderma	
N, lymph nodes	**Palpable nodes**	**Node patholgy**
N0	No	Negative
N1	Yes	Negative (a vs b: clone negative vs positive)
N2	Yes	Early positive (no effacement of architecture) (a vs b: clone negative vs positive)
N3	Yes	Positive (partial or complete effacement of architecture)
NX	Yes	Not done
M, visceral organs		
M0	No visceral organ involvement	
M1	Visceral involvement, pathology confirmed	
B, blood		
B0	≤5% of lymphocytes are Sézary cells (a vs b: clone negative vs positive)	
B1	>5% of lymphocytes are Sézary cells but not B2 (a vs b: clone negative vs positive)	
B2	≥1000 Sézary cells per microliter; positive clone	

However, it remains difficult to diagnose lymph node involvement with MF accurately. Reactive lymphadenopathy can be present in benign skin conditions such as eczema and psoriasis, and can even show atypical Sézary cells, which simply represent activated T cells. Unless there are sheets of Sézary cells replacing normal nodal architecture, diagnosing MF/SS by lymph node biopsy may be difficult.

The complete blood count may reveal leukocytosis in patients with Sézary syndrome, though in the early stages both the total white count and the absolute lymphocyte count may be normal. Complicating matters further is the fact that erythroderma resulting from a number of benign dermatoses may also be associated with the presence of apparent Sézary cells on peripheral blood smear. Although best visualized by electron microscopy, Sézary cells can be seen on light microscopic examination of peripheral blood smears. Sézary cell counts >1000/mm^3 in conjunction with dominant clonality satisfy the criteria for blood involvement (B2 status) and stage IVA in the new ISCL/EORTC revised staging system for MF/SS (Tables 19–5 and 19–6).

Special techniques have been devised for confirming MF in patients in whom the clinical history and the routine histopathologic findings suggest MF but are not diagnostic. Monoclonal antibodies directed against lymphocyte surface antigens can be used to identify the immunophenotypic characteristics of the infiltrating cells. A predominance of CD4+ lymphocytes is consistent with MF, but this finding alone is consistent with many inflammatory dermatoses. Deficiencies of antigens expressed by normal T cells may aid the diagnosis. CD7 and CD26 are commonly absent on MF cells in skin and blood.

Looking for expansion of a single clone of T-helper cells is another method of confirming the diagnosis of MF, and is now readily available and increasingly accurate. The mature T-cell receptor is a heterodimer of two glycoprotein chains, usually α and β, but this receptor expression usually follows gene rearrangement receptor expression for the γδ T-cell receptor. This is analogous to B-cell maturation from IgM surface expression to either IgG, IgA, or IgE. If a clonal expansion of a malignant cell occurs, over-representation of one particular T-cell receptor would be expected. This can be identified by Southern blot analysis of DNA that codes for the receptor, or by PCR which is now the standard technique. Monoclonal antibodies to different V regions have been used to stain fresh skin biopsy specimens to identify a clonal expansion of T-helper cells. When a particular anti-V region antibody stains a majority of epidermotropic cells, CTCL can be suspected. Clonal expansion of T cells is an expected finding in MF and other cutaneous T-cell lymphomas, but is not foolproof. False-negative results may result from primers which may not detect all possible gene rearrangements, from failure to target the altered gene in a clone, from deletion of the altered gene by the clone, or from clonal cell concentrations below the limits of detec-

Table 19–6 ISCL/EORTC revised staging of mycosis fungoides and Sézary syndrome

MF Cooperative Group 1979				ISCL/EORTC 2007				
	T	N	M		T	N	M	B
IA	1	0	0	IA_1	1_a	0	0	0,1
				IA_2	1_b	0	0	0,1
IB	2	0	0	IB_1	2_a	0	0	0,1
				IB_2	2_b	0	0	0,1
IIA	1–2	1	0	IIA_1	1_a or 2_a	1–2	0	0,1
				IIA_2	1_b or 2_b	1–2	0	0,1
IIB	3	0,1	0	IIB	3	0–2	0	0,1
III	4	0,1	0	IIIA	4	0–2	0	0
				IIIB	4	0–2	0	1
IVA	1–4	2–3	0	IVA_1	1–4	0–2	0	2
IVB	1–4	0–3	1	IVA_2	1–4	3	0	0–2
				IVB	1–4	0–3	1	0–2

tion. False-positive results are known in several diseases not considered lymphoma; may occur secondary to amplification of benign lymphoid subsets (pseudoclonal); or may be secondary to cross-contamination with clonal DNA for other positive controls. Benign dominant T-cell clones have been detected in the blood of some healthy elderly controls. Just as the presence of a serum monoclonal gammopathy alone does not reliably distinguish between malignant and nonmalignant B-cell proliferations, so it is that T-cell clonality is insufficient by itself to distinguish between benign and malignant T-cell disease. To confirm blood involvement, the clones detected in lesional skin and blood should match.

After the diagnosis of MF is confirmed, appropriate staging is necessary (Tables 19–5 and 19–6). Staging procedures may include a complete physical examination, with attention to the extent and type of clinical lesions and the presence of adenopathy and hepatosplenomegaly; a complete blood count with differential; and a chest X-ray. Patients with extensive patch/plaque disease or erythroderma will frequently have mild lymphadenopathy, which does not necessarily indicate malignant involvement of the node. Treating secondary infection before considering lymph biopsy node seems prudent, particularly when there is prominent crusting. The presence of asymmetric lymphadenopathy, especially if nontender, should prompt early lymph node biopsy. The bone marrow is usually spared in MF, even with Sézary syndrome, and hence a bone marrow biopsy is not routinely performed.

Diagnosis of other forms of CTCL is usually more straightforward. As these present with papules, nodules, or tumors, there is seldom a need for more than one lesional biopsy. However, sufficient material should be obtained to allow for simple histologic examination, as well as immunophenotyping and molecular diagnostics. Histologic findings are seldom subtle in these other syndromes. Special care must be used, however, in distinguishing between large cell variant lymphomatoid papulosis, and anaplastic large cell lymphoma CD30+. Staging of these forms of CTCL is less standardized, although it seems unlikely that many of these syndromes will have visceral or central node involvement in the absence of extracutaneous symptoms, peripheral adenopathy, or basic hematologic and serum chemistry screening abnormalities.

Prognosis and Treatment

Mycosis fungoides is usually a slowly progressive disease; many patients die of causes unrelated to the T-cell lymphoma. Enlargement of the peripheral nodes is usually the first sign of clinically evident extracutaneous disease, and symptomatic visceral involvement is a late manifestation, if it develops at all. In the study by van Dorn et al., patients with T1 skin stage (patch/plaque, <10% body surface area) had a 5-year survival of 99% in the absence of nodal disease. Similarly, node-negative T2 patients (>10% surface involved) had a 5-year survival of 86%. Survival at 5 years for T3 (skin tumor stage) patients was 65%. Patients with nodal involvement of any kind, regardless of skin stage, had 40–49% 5-year survival. In a similar study in the United States, Zackheim et al. found that T1 patients had the same 10-year survival as control patients. In T2 skin stage patients, 10-year survival was 67%, and most of the reduced survival appeared to be in those patients with plaque rather than patch lesions. Ten-year survivals for patients with tumor stage or erythroderma were much lower, at 39% and 41%, respectively.

Of patients dying from their disease, roughly half do so because of septicemia or serious infection, the skin being the site of initial infection. Disseminated disease resulting in ination or serious organ dysfunction accounts for most of the remaining deaths due to CTCL.

The trafficking of malignant T cells from very early in the course of patch/plaque CTCL makes the likelihood of cure of early disease improbable with skin-limited therapy alone. The usual onset of disease later in life and the high frequency of complete clinical remission following treatment with topical chemotherapy, phototherapy, or occasionally electron beam therapies, make it likely that a patient might remain apparently disease free until death from another cause. This makes claims of cures difficult to assess. In addition, aggressive systemic therapy has not been shown to be curative in this disease. Therefore, therapy in early stage I and II disease should usually be gentle and directed towards control of cutaneous disease. Although curative therapy cannot be promised, patients should be reassured by the excellent survival statistics in recent studies, and by the high incidence of clinical remission available through current therapies. Later-stage disease will require more aggressive therapy, but is also much more likely to have lower rates of complete remission, and shorter duration of remission with such aggressive therapy.

Considering the diversity of clinical patterns of MF/SS and the wide range of the severity of this disease, the diversity of the treatment approaches is not surprising. Treatment modalities have included topical nitrogen mustard, phototherapy, radiation, systemic interferon and other immunomodulators, chemotherapy, and most recently, extracorporeal photopheresis (ECP).

In addition, there remains controversy surrounding how aggressive treatment of early-stage MF should be. Kaye and associates compared the results of treatment using combined radiation and chemotherapy with more conservative topical regimens. Although the aggressive approach resulted in a slightly better initial response, these patients were plagued by serious complications and had no increase in long-term survival, regardless of the stage of disease. Thus, current management of patients with MF types of CTCL usually involves a stepwise approach, beginning with conservative treatments directed at the skin.

The treatment of early MF may begin with topically applied potent corticosteroids, nitrogen mustard (mechlorethamine hydrochloride), or phototherapy. Nitrogen mustard is applied directly to the skin daily, as either an ointment or a solution. Total body application (sometimes sparing intertriginous areas) is usually recommended, though some advocate only lesional treatment if the skin disease comprises less than 25% of the body surface area. Even if total body applications are anticipated, in patients with relatively limited cutaneous disease it is often helpful to treat only the lesions for the first few months, so as to judge the therapeutic response. It is easier to obtain patient compliance for unpleasant total body therapy if the treatment is clearly effective, and conversely it spares the patient months of overnight total body applications only to find that the therapy is ineffective or poorly tolerated. Nitrogen mustard has been shown to induce remission in 75% of patients with stage I disease, but is less useful in patients with more advanced disease. Remission occurs within 6–36 months. Side effects include a reversible hyperpigmentation and contact hypersensitivity.

Phototherapy options include UVB, narrowband UVB, and psoralen–UVA light (PUVA). Phototherapy may be given initially to patients with resistant disease or who are intolerant of nitrogen mustard. Phototherapy is given three times weekly, and remissions occur in most patients in 6–36 weeks. The therapy may then be slowly tapered to a maintenance regimen. Narrowband UVB has become the preferred phototherapy option for most MF patients, although PUVA may be useful for recalcitrant disease. In some patients, retinoids (vitamin A derivatives) or interferon may be co-administered, which may reduce the amount of UV light exposure needed. Patients who receive PUVA must wear protective glasses after treatment to avoid the development of cataracts. In addition, an increased incidence of cutaneous and genital cancers is a risk of long-term PUVA treatment.

Total skin electron beam radiation is the treatment for early-stage CTCL with the highest initial response rate. Remissions occur in 90% of treated patients. Even tumors may respond; however, erythrodermic CTCL usually does not. Patients are given 400 cGy weekly to a total of 3000–3600 cGy. The side effects, including anhidrosis (absence of sweating), alopecia, and radiodermatitis, are significant. Cutaneous cancers, often aggressive in nature, may arise years later. Electron beam therapy is not recommended for younger patients. Total body electron beam is best performed at a center which has considerable experience, and in many regions such centers may be difficult to find. Finally, the intensity of therapy is usually such that electron beam becomes a once-in-a-lifetime option. Taking these considerations together, it is prudent to reserve this form of therapy for patients who have failed less aggressive therapies and whose disease is progressing. Localized radiation therapy (electron beam or conventional radiation) can be used to supplement topical nitrogen mustard or phototherapy. Following total skin electron beam therapy, relatively rapid relapse is common unless other maintenance therapy is started soon after the radiation therapy ends.

Many regimens have been proposed for the treatment of more advanced disease. These include oral methotrexate with leucovorin rescue, prednisone plus chlorambucil, gemcitabine, fludarabine, 2-CDA, and various multidrug chemotherapies. In general, these have not been shown to lengthen survival and have significant side effects, and so they are not widely used. α-Interferon (IFN-α) has been used in high doses for advanced disease that is refractory to all treatments. In these patients, some clinical response has been noted. Side effects are significant and include fever, malaise, lethargy, weight loss, and depression. Interferons are also beneficial used in combination with other treatment modalities, especially PUVA or narrowband UVB. Interleukin (IL)-2 may be occasionally effective, but has significant toxicity. IL-12 is much less toxic, and early studies have shown some benefit. Denileukin diftitox is a fusion toxin protein combining IL-2 coding sequences with those for diphtheria toxin A chain. Vorinostat is an orally administered histone deacetylase inhibitor. These latter two agents have efficacy in 30–40% of advanced MF/SS patients.

ECP (extracorporeal photopheresis) is a procedure designed to elicit a host immune response to the circulating malignant T-helper cell. The patient receiving ECP ingests 8-methoxypsoralen, and peripheral blood is removed. Buffy coat cells are separated, irradiated with UVA light, and reinfused. ECP is performed for 2 consecutive days every 4 weeks. ECP is most effective for treating Sézary syndrome, especially within the first 2 years of the onset of the erythroderma. Marked clinical improvement can be expected in 25% of ECP-treated patients, with an additional 50% having a partial response. Efficacy is usually not noted until after 4–6 months of treatment. The erythema and scale resolve sooner than the pruritus and palmar hyperkeratosis. Survival may be lengthened, although no controlled studies to assess this have been performed. The real value of ECP is the lack of toxic side effects. The side effects are limited to a rare transient febrile reaction on reinfusion of the cells and minor fluid and electrolyte shifts during the treatment. No long-term side effects have yet been identified, and no deaths caused by the procedure have been reported.

Oral retinoids in use for acne and psoriasis have occasionally been beneficial in patients with MF CTCL. This, coupled with the beneficial effect of ALL-trans-retinoic acid in promyelocytic leukemia, led to the development of other retinoid derivatives. Bexarotene is one such retinoid used in oral and topical form for treatment of MF forms of CTCL. It is the first retinoid X receptor-selective rexinoid. Side effects of the oral agent include occasional disturbance of thyroid function, frequent hyperlipidemia, and leukopenia. When used at recommended doses of 300 mg/m²/day, many patients have developed skin erythema, fissuring, and severe xerosis. Despite this, it has been very effective in some patients resistant to other therapies. The topical form of bexarotene avoids the systemic complications but can cause local irritation, and its use has almost certainly been limited by economic constraints. A different class of topical retinoid, tazarotene, is used in the treatment of psoriasis, but early trials suggest a possible benefit in limited CTCL. Imiquimod has also been reported to be beneficial when used topically on MF lesions.

The discussion of therapy thus far has focused on MF/SS forms of CTCL. Therapies for non-MF forms of CTCL are determined primarily by their clinical behavior. For those with indolent behavior, local therapy with intralesional injection, excision, or radiation seems most appropriate. The more aggressive diseases may require systemic chemotherapies similar to those used for systemic lymphomas. The primary cutaneous CD30+ lymphoproliferative disorders often respond to low-dose oral methotrexate. Multiagent chemotherapy should be reserved only for those CD30+ cases exhibiting aggressive clinical behavior.

PRIMARY CUTANEOUS B-CELL LYMPHOMAS

Primary Cutaneous Follicle-Center Cell Lymphoma

This is the largest group of primary cutaneous B-cell lymphomas (CBCL), and includes conditions previously known as Crosti's lymphoma (Table 19–2). Lesions are typically solitary or clustered plaques or nodules on the head or trunk. Histologically, this lymphoma typically manifests as a bottom-heavy infiltrate of the entire dermis, sometimes the subcutis, with sparing of the epidermis and the Grenz zone of superficial papillary dermis. The atypical cells are usually a mixture of small cleaved and large noncleaved follicle-center cells (centrocytes and centroblasts). Earlier lesions have a follicular (nodular) architecture, whereas older lesions become more diffuse and large cells may eventually predominate. The WHO/EORTC classification treats this as clinically distinct from histologically similar large B-cell lymphomas of the legs. Unlike nodal presentations of follicle-center lymphomas, these lymphomas typically lack the t(14;18) translocation and CD10. They are BCL-2−6+. An indolent course and good response to local treatment are typical. Options include topical agents (potent corticosteroids, nitrogen mustard, imiquimod), intralesional agents (corticosteroids, anti-CD20 antibody), and local radiation therapy. For more generalized lesions, systemic agents are beneficial, including prednisone, α-interferon and anti-CD20 antibody. Some cases, primarily in Europe, are associated with *Borrelia burgdorferi* infection and respond to antibiotics.

Marginal Zone B-Cell Lymphoma/MALT-Type Lymphoma

Marginal zone B-cell lymphoma of mucosa-associated lymphoid tissue (MALT type) is a distinct entity known especially from gastrointestinal pathology. This lymphoma typically presents in skin as red to violaceous papules or nodules, erythematous red plaques, or a solitary larger nodule (tumor) of the upper extremities, trunk, head, or neck. Middle-aged to older adults are most commonly affected. Histologically, this lymphoma spares the epidermis and Grenz zone papillary dermis, but infiltrates the reticular dermis and subcutis. Reactive T cells and histiocytes are invariably present and may obscure the neoplastic cell component. Reactive B-cell follicles may be present, surrounded by neoplastic B cells. The neoplastic B cells range from small and medium-sized lymphocytes with pale cytoplasm (monocytoid B cells), to centrocyte-like cells, and occasionally larger cells. Plasma cells and plasmacytoid cells are usually present. Tumor cells are monotypic (Ig-light chain restricted) and BCL-2+6−. This lymphoma has been associated with *Borrelia burgdorferi* infection (in Europe), and with anetoderma. The course is indolent, with a good response to local therapy. Many European cases respond to antibiotics. Primary cutaneous plasmacytoma is rare and considered part of the marginal zone B-cell lymphoma spectrum. It must be distinguished from dissemination of multiple myeloma to the skin, a rare and usually very late-stage complication of myeloma. Clonal mature plasma cells characterize the primary form of plasmacytoma and the course is indolent, in contrast to myeloma-associated cases. Treatment is usually local.

Large B-Cell Lymphoma of the Leg

This lymphoma is listed separately in the WHO/EORTC classification, as distinct from the remainder of the diffuse large B-cell lymphomas that are usually follicle-center cell lymphomas. This usually presents in elderly women as a nodule or nodules on one or both legs (Fig. 19–14). The histologic pattern is one of dense diffuse dermal and sometimes subcutis infiltration by large lymphoid cells with centroblastic or immunoblastic features. Although they are t(14;18)-negative, they strongly express BCL-2, unlike CBCL follicle-center cell lymphoma. They are also BCL-6+, MUM-1+ and Fox-P1+. The lymphoma is more aggressive that the previous two categories of CBCL, with a 55% 5-year survival. Systemic therapy is required, with or without local radiation therapy.

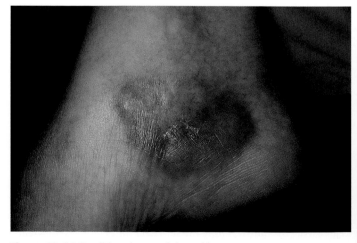

Figure 19–14 B-cell lymphoma of the ankle.

Other Cutaneous B-Cell Lymphomas

Intravascular large B-cell lymphoma is also rare. Even more rare is a T-cell counterpart previously known as 'malignant angioendotheliomatosis.' Clinical presentation is variable, with patches, plaques, or nodules, which may be painful or ulcerative. The histologic pattern of partial or complete occlusion of cutaneous vessels by large pleomorphic mononuclear cells can be overlooked on initial review of the biopsy specimen. Cerebral involvement is frequent and an important cause of death. The course is variable but often aggressive, and the optimal treatment uncertain.

Lymphomatoid Granulomatosis

Lymphomatoid granulomatosis is a disease mostly likely to affect males in their 50s, usually presenting with cough, hemoptysis, dyspnea, or chest pain. Skin lesions may precede pulmonary disease in roughly 10% of cases, and rare patients have been described who appear to have skin-limited disease. Skin manifestations include a red to violaceous papular eruption (Fig. 19–15), and nodules in dermis or fat. Other frequently involved sites include the central nervous system, kidney, and liver. Involved organs show angiocentric or angiodestructive lymphoid infiltrates of small to medium-sized lymphocytes, with interspersed larger atypical cells which are B cells. This

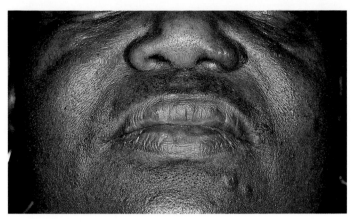

Figure 19–15 Lymphomatoid granulomatosis. This patient presented with lesions that simulated sarcoidosis.

disease has been considered a malignancy, but the cell of origin has been controversial. Consensus now seems to be that it is an angiocentric/angiodestructive T cell-rich, Epstein–Barr virus-associated B-cell lymphoma. This is unusual in that most other angiocentric lymphomas appear to derive from T or NK cells. Lymphomatoid granulomatosis usually requires aggressive therapy. However, the presence of cases with indolent cutaneous involvement suggests that there may be subsets of patients for whom less intensive therapy may be warranted.

SUGGESTED READINGS

Bekkenk MW, Geelen FAMJ, van Voorst Vader PC, et al. Primary and secondary cutaneous CD30+ lymphoproliferative disorders: a report from the Dutch cutaneous lymphoma group on the long-term follow-up data of 219 patients and guidelines for diagnosis and treatment. Blood 2000; 95: 3653–3661.

Burg G, Kempf W, Cozzio A, et al. WHO/EORTC classification of cutaneous lymphomas 2005: histological and molecular aspects. J Cutan Pathol 2005; 32: 647–674.

Cerroni L, Fink-Puches R, Back B, Kerl H. Follicular mucinosis: a critical reappraisal of clinicopathologic features and association with mycosis fungoides and Sézary syndrome. Arch Dermatol 2002; 138: 182–189.

de Coninck EC, Kim YH, Varghese A, Hoppe RT. Clinical characteristics and outcome of patients with extracutaneous mycosis fungoides. J Clin Oncol 2001; 19: 779–784.

Duvic M, Martin AG, Kim Y, et al. Phase 2 and 3 clinical trial of oral bexarotene (Targretin capsules) for the treatment of refractory or persistent early-stage cutaneous T-cell lymphomas. Arch Dermatol 2001; 137: 581–599.

Kaye FJ, Bunn PA Jr, Steinberg SM, et al. A randomized trial comparing combination electron-beam radiation and chemotherapy with topical therapy in the initial treatment of mycosis fungoides. N Engl J Med 1989; 321: 1784–1790.

Kempf W, Dummer R, Burg G. Approach to lymphoproliferative infiltrates of the skin. The difficult lesions. Am J Clin Pathol 1999; 111: S84–S93.

Kim BK, Nelson BP, Calonje E. Newly described cutaneous lymphomas. Adv Dermatol 1999; 15: 397–440.

Massone C, Kodama K, Kerl H, Cerroni L. Histopathologic features of early (patch) lesions of mycosis fungoides: a morphologic study on 745 biopsy specimens from 427 patients. Am J Surg Pathol 2005; 29: 550–560.

Massone C, El-Shabrawi-Caelen L, Kerl H, Cerroni L. The morphologic spectrum of primary cutaneous anaplastic large T-cell lymphoma: a histopathologic study on 66 biopsy specimens from 47 patients with report of rare variants. J Cutan Pathol 2008; 35: 46–53.

Olsen E, Vonderheid E, Pimpinelli N, et al. Revisions to the staging and classification of mycosis fungoides and Sézary syndrome: a proposal of the ISCL and EORTC. Blood 2007; 110: 1713–1722.

Pimpinelli N, Olsen EA, Santucci M, et al. Defining early mycosis fungoides. J Am Acad Dermatol 2005; 53: 1053–1063.

Santucci M, Biggeri A, Feller AC, et al. Accuracy, concordance, and reproducibility of histologic diagnosis in cutaneous T-cell lymphoma. An EORTC cutaneous lymphoma project group study. Arch Dermatol 2000; 136: 497–502.

van Doorn R, van Haselen CW, van Voorst Vader PC, et al. Mycosis fungoides: disease evolution and prognosis of 309 Dutch patients. Arch Dermatol 2000; 136: 504–510.

Weinstock MA, Gardstein B. Twenty-year trends in the reported incidence of mycosis fungoides and associated mortality. Am J Pub Health 1999; 89: 1240–1244.

Willemze R, Jaffe ES, Burg G, et al. WHO-EORTC classification of cutaneous lymphomas. Blood 2005; 105: 3768–3785.

Willemze R, Jansen PM, Cerroni L, et al. Subcutaneous panniculitis-like T-cell lymphoma: definition, classification, and prognostic factors: an EORTC cutaneous lymphoma group study of 83 cases. Blood 2008; 111: 838–845.

Wood GS. Benign and malignant cutaneous lymphoproliferative disorders including mycosis fungoides. In: Knowles DM, ed. Neoplastic hematopathology, 2nd edn. Baltimore: Williams & Wilkins, 2001; 1183–1233.

Wood GS. T-cell receptor and immunoglobulin gene rearrangements in diagnosing skin disease. Arch Dermatol 2001; 137: 1503–1506.

Zackheim HS, Amin S, Kashani-Sabet M, McMillan A. Prognosis in cutaneous T-cell lymphoma by skin stage: long term survival in 489 patients. J Am Acad Dermatol 1999; 40: 418–425.

Diabetes Mellitus

In recent years the incidence and prevalence of diabetes has been rising worldwide, being especially high in industrialized nations. From 30% to 71% of patients with diabetes mellitus have some type of cutaneous involvement during the course of their chronic disease. The skin microvasculature is highly affected by diabetes mellitus, as are other organs such as the kidney and the retina. This chapter outlines the major skin findings in diabetes mellitus and summarizes recent studies and reports.

DIABETIC FOOT

Description

Typically a thick callus forms under an area of repeated pressure and breaks down to form an ulcer. Infection and gangrene are potential complications (Fig. 20–1).

Pathogenesis

Diabetic foot is a consequence of diabetes-associated peripheral neuropathy (60–70%), peripheral ischemic vascular disease (15–20%), or combined clinically 1–4 significant neuropathy and vascular disease (15–20%) as the cause of the foot ulcers.

Significance

Diabetics have a 15–25% lifetime risk of developing a foot ulcer. Foot ulcers account for significant morbidity and mortality in the diabetic population and are responsible for 70% of annual lower limb amputations in the United States.

Treatment

In a setting of diminished or absent sensation, foot deformity, and adequate blood supply, neuropathic ulcers usually heal within weeks if treated with aggressive debridement and offloading with various devices, or most effectively with a total contact cast. A surgical revascularization procedure can correct the ischemic state. Adherence to principles of wound therapy effects healing. The use of topical growth factors or bioengi-

neered skin grafts cannot replace a needed revascularization procedure, debridement, and ulcer offloading. Because of the prevalence of bacterial colonization of foot ulcers, the need for antibiotic therapy rests on clinical evaluation and judgment that actual infection exists. Prevention of complications remains paramount through daily foot inspection, care guidelines, and prevention of pressure, friction, and callus formation by using appropriate footwear.

DIABETIC DERMOPATHY (SHIN SPOTS)

Description

Diabetic dermopathy lesions are circumscribed reddish to brownish lesions, typically very small, measuring 0.5–1.5 cm. Thickening of blood vessels, a perivascular lymphocytic infiltrate, and scattered hemosiderin skin deposits associated with hemorrhage are noticed on histologic examination of biopsy specimens (Fig. 20–2).

Frequency

These lesions are the most common cutaneous markers of diabetes mellitus, seen in up to 50% of diabetics. They are more prevalent in longstanding disease and are twice as common in males.

Location

Lesions occur most commonly on the shins. They occasionally affect the thighs and arms.

Pathogenesis

Microangiopathy is the reported cause of diabetic dermopathy.

Significance

Patients with diabetic dermopathy typically have other vasculopathy-associated complications of diabetes, such as retinopathy, neuropathy, or nephropathy, hence one should look for

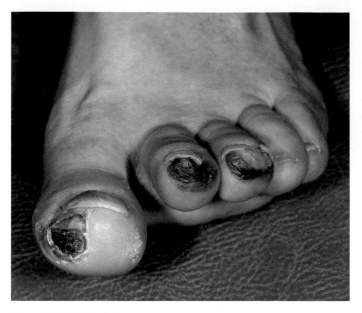

Figure 20–1 Diabetic foot.

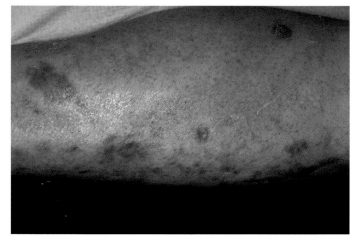

Figure 20–2 Diabetic dermopathy.

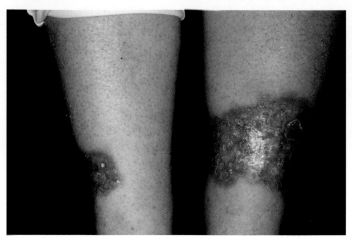

Figure 20–3 Necrobiosis lipoidica.

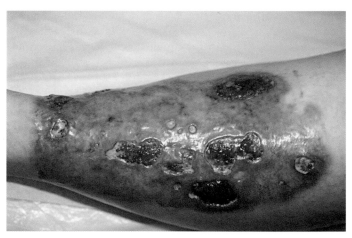

Figure 20–4 Ulcerative necrobiosis lipoidica.

NECROBIOSIS LIPOIDICA (FORMERLY NECROBIOSIS LIPOIDICA DIABETICORUM)

Description

Necrobiosis lipoidica is clinically characterized by well-circumscribed, yellow-brown, nonpainful patches with pronounced epidermal atrophy. The active border is raised and erythematous. Most lesions occur on the shin (Figs 20–3 and 20–4). In 75% of patients the condition is bilateral. Less commonly, lesions may occur on the feet, arms, trunk, or scalp. Because lesions also occur in persons without diabetes, the term diabeticorum has been eliminated from its name. Patients with insulin-dependent diabetes mellitus develop this lesion considerably earlier, at a mean age of 22 years, whereas in noninsulin-dependent diabetes mellitus and nondiabetic patients it appears at a mean age of 49 years.

Frequency

Less than 1% of diabetics develop necrobiosis lipoidica. More than 66% of patients with necrobiosis lipoidica have overt

these complications. These lesions are not specific to diabetes, but may precede frank insulin resistance, signaling early or new-onset diabetes.

Treatment

There is no effective therapy. The condition heals by itself, leaving depressed, atrophic, hyperpigmented scars. Glycemic control and the development of diabetic dermopathy are not correlated.

diabetes mellitus. This condition occurs predominantly in females.

Pathogenesis

The pathogenesis is unknown, but diabetic microangiopathy may play a role. It is a disorder histopathologically characterized by collagen degeneration surrounded by a palisaded granulomatous response, thickening of blood vessel walls, and fat deposition.

Significance

Necrobiosis lipoidica may be associated with microangiopathic changes, particularly in pretibial lesions. These changes are less common in lesions occurring elsewhere on the body, however, indicating that microangiopathy may not be necessary for the development of lesions. The lesions are typically chronic, with variable progression and scarring. Unless treated, they can enlarge to involve large areas of the skin surface. Patients with necrobiosis lipoidica should be evaluated and followed for the possibility that they will develop diabetes mellitus at a later date.

Treatment

Treatment is not very effective, and spontaneous remission is uncommon. Excellent control of the diabetes, unfortunately, is not associated with improvement. Topical and intralesional corticosteroids can lessen the inflammation of early active lesions and the active borders of enlarging lesions, but the atrophic component may take years to burn out. When the plaques ulcerate, treatment consists of the application of warm compresses and the use of systemic antibiotics. Semipermeable membrane dressings (e.g., Op Site, Vigilon, and DuoDERM) are helpful in treating painful ulcerating lesions. The ulcerative component may also benefit from compressive therapy. Attempts at local excision and grafting are usually complicated by recurrences at the borders.

ACQUIRED ICHTHYOSIFORM CHANGES OF THE SHINS

Frequency

This sign might be the commonest skin manifestation of diabetes: a study has shown a prevalence of 50% in young insulin-dependent diabetic mellitus patients.

Pathogenesis

The pathogenesis is unknown. Microangiopathy, stratum corneum adhesion defects, advanced glycosylation, and accelerated skin aging may be involved.

Significance

This finding is associated with microangiopathic complications, especially retinopathy, and scleroderma-like skin changes, and is directly related to the duration of diabetes mellitus.

ACANTHOSIS NIGRICANS

Description

Acanthosis nigricans is manifest by a velvety thickening and hyperpigmentation of the skin, usually on intertriginous surfaces (Fig. 20–5). Histopathologically, the lesions are characterized by papillomatosis, hyperkeratosis, and mild acanthosis. The dark color is related to the thickness of the keratin-containing superficial epithelium, not to any change in melanocyte number or melanin content.

Frequency

Acanthosis nigricans is very common, especially in patients with type A insulin resistance. It is commonly seen in African-Americans, Hispanics and Southeast Asian patients in association with obesity as a part of the metabolic syndrome.

Location

The most commonly affected areas are the neck, axillae, groin, umbilicus, areolae, submammary regions, and elbows. Involvement of the dorsal hands is referred to as tripe hands.

Pathogenesis

Hyperinsulinemia may activate insulin growth factor (IGF-1) receptors on keratinocytes, leading to epidermal growth.

Significance

Acanthosis nigricans is most often associated with insulin resistance. Other endocrinopathies have been reported, including hypothyroidism and adrenal insufficiency. A malignant form of acanthosis nigricans is rare: these patients are not obese and often have a glossitis (see Chapter 13).

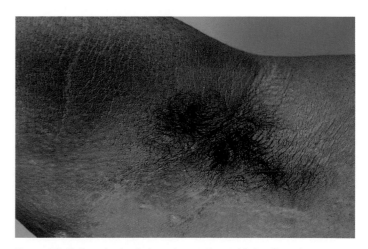

Figure 20–5 Acanthosis nigricans in a patient with insulin resistance.

Treatment

Weight reduction will often result in a reversal of the process. In addition, patients are often treated with oral metformin because of their insulin resistance, but a direct effect of this therapy for acanthosis nigricans has not been demonstrated. Topical urea-containing preparations have occasionally been useful for control of the manifestations.

SKIN TAGS

Description

Skin tags are common benign skin tumors usually occurring on the neck and major flexors of older people. In many patients they appear in conjunction with acanthosis nigricans. Some studies have shown an increased risk of diabetes mellitus in patients with multiple skin tags.

Significance

Many patients with type 2 diabetes mellitus remain undiagnosed until they develop end-organ damage, such as cardiovascular diseases, impairment of renal function, loss of visual acuity, or limb ulcers. Recognition of possible risk factors of impaired carbohydrate metabolism helps in the earlier diagnosis of at-risk patients and in prevention of these complications. The authors believe that physicians should maintain a higher level of suspicion for impaired carbohydrate metabolism in patients with multiple skin tags.

SCLERODERMA-LIKE SKIN CHANGES

Description

Distinct from scleroderma, scleroderma-like skin changes consist of thickening and induration of the skin on the dorsum of the fingers (sclerodactyly) and proximal interphalangeal joints, and may also involve the metacarpophalangeal joints (Fig. 20–6). It can extend to the forearms, arms, and back. The skin may have a waxy appearance. These changes are bilateral, symmetric, and painless. Extensive scleroderma-like skin changes of the torso and back occur in a subgroup of diabetic patients. Scleroderma-like skin changes resemble scleroderma, but do not demonstrate dermal atrophy, telangiectasia, edema, Raynaud's phenomenon, and pain, which are commonly noted in the latter entity. Scleroderma-like skin changes differ from scleredema diabeticorum because there is a greater extent of involvement, no or mild histologic evidence of mucin deposition, and the sclerodermoid change commonly appears in younger patients.

This skin manifestation occurs in many patients in conjunction with diabetic hand syndrome, which consists of joint limitations (mainly an inability to fully extend the fingers), thickened skin of the hand, and the 'prayer sign' – an inability to press the palms together completely, with a gap remaining between opposed palms and fingers (Fig. 20–7). Commonly, contractures begin in the fifth digit and progress radially to the other fingers. Palmar fascial thickening (Dupuytren's contracture) further complicates the diabetic hand syndrome.

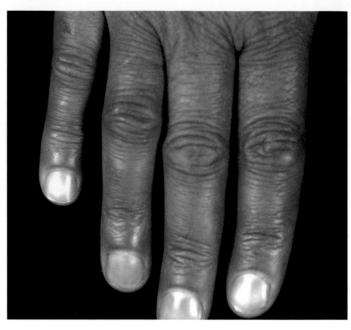

Figure 20–6 Scleroderma-like skin changes.

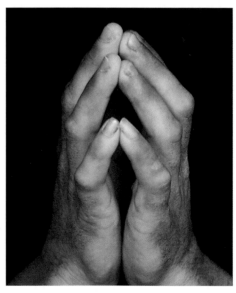

Figure 20–7 Limited joint mobility.

Frequency

Between 10% and 50% of diabetics manifest a degree of these findings. It is more common in patients with type 1 diabetes mellitus. Males and females appear to be equally affected.

Pathogenesis

Advanced glycosylation end-products are believed to cause stiffening of collagen.

Significance

The clinical course is progressive and leads to more extensive involvement and more stiffness. Patients with type 1 diabetes mellitus and severe scleroderma-like skin changes showed a twofold increased tendency of retinopathy and nephropathy compared to patients with no or mild scleroderma-like skin changes. Most studies have shown that scleroderma-like skin changes are related to disease duration but not to parameters of diabetic control. A strong association has been found with dry palms. The skin changes may occur early in the disease.

Treatment

Anecdotal reports have demonstrated that tight glycemic control with an insulin pump results in reduced skin thickness. Another treatment option used in several patients with limited joint mobility is aldose reductase inhibitors, which inhibit the accumulation of sugar alcohols. Physical therapy may be important in patients with severe disease to improve the range of motion of the joints.

Finger Pebbles

Finger pebbles, or Huntley's papules, represent a variation of diabetic thick skin and often occur in patients with type 2 diabetes. Grouped, minute papules occur on the dorsum of the hand, the knuckles, and periungual areas. Over time, the papules may coalesce into confluent plaques that feature some hypopigmentation.

SCLEREDEMA (SCLEREDEMA ADULTORUM, SCLEREDEMA DIABETICORUM OF BUSCHKE)

Description

Diffuse, symmetric, nonpitting induration of the skin with occasional erythema, mainly on the back, characterizes this disorder (Fig. 20–8).

Frequency

This is a rare disorder that tends to occur in male diabetics over the age of 40 years. These patients tend to be on insulin and have multiple complications. Scleredema not associated with diabetes mellitus is more common in females.

Location

The neck, shoulders, and upper back are typical. Rarely, the buttocks, abdomen, and thighs may be affected.

Pathogenesis

The pathogenesis is unknown. Perhaps scleredema is caused by glycosaminoglycan deposition in the dermal connective tissue. Thickening of the reticular dermis with deposition of mucin between thickened collagen bundles is noted. This phenomenon may be similar to the more prevalent waxy indura-

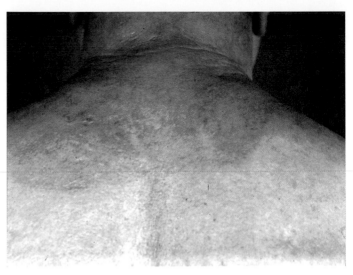

Figure 20–8 Scleredema. Erythematous, indurated area on the upper back of this diabetic patient. (Courtesy of Dr Neil A. Fenske, Tampa, FL; reprinted with permission from Callen JP, Greer KE, Paller A, Swinyer L, eds. Color atlas of dermatology: A morphological approach, 2nd edn. Philadelphia: WB Saunders, 2000.)

tion of the skin of the extremities seen in insulin-dependent diabetics.

Significance

The course is unpredictable. Typically the disease is slowly progressive and unremitting over years. Morbidity depends on the body region affected, e.g., limited range of motion, dysarthria, and difficulty closing the eyes. The process correlates with the duration of diabetes mellitus and with the presence of microvascular disease.

Treatment

There is no effective therapy and the lesions are usually asymptomatic. The condition often goes unnoticed by others and does not require treatment. In severely affected patients, typically those with poorly controlled type 2 diabetes, significant neck and back stiffness and pain occur. Glycemic control does not affect the condition.

DIABETIC BLISTERS (BULLOSIS DIABETICORUM)

Description

Diabetic blisters are tense, 0.5–3.0-cm bullae without surrounding inflammation. The lesions develop acutely and are usually painless.

Frequency

This is a rare phenomenon.

Location

Blisters occur on the fingers, hands, toes, feet, legs, or forearms. Rarely, the trunk may be involved.

Pathogenesis

The pathogenesis is unknown. Histologic analysis of lesions shows intraepidermal, nonacantholytic or, less often, subepidermal cleavage formation, the latter leading to clinical scarring. Immunopathologic studies are negative in patients with all forms of diabetic bullae.

Significance

Bullae often occur in patients with severe diabetes mellitus, diabetic neuropathy, or retinopathy. Spontaneous acral bullae may be the first sign of diabetes mellitus.

Treatment

Diabetic bullae are a self-limiting condition and lesions usually resolve within 2–4 weeks. Drainage and topical antibiotics may be required for large lesions. There is no preventive treatment.

ACQUIRED PERFORATING DERMATOSES

Description

The cutaneous perforating disorders, characterized by the transepidermal elimination of some component of the dermis, have been reported in patients with chronic renal failure, diabetes, or both. The extruded material contains degenerated collagen bundles. The lesions typically are perifollicular, dome-shaped papules or nodules featuring a central keratotic plug. They tend to be pruritic. The common denominator is usually devitalization of dermal elements (e.g., collagen, elastic fibers) due to trauma, such as from excoriation, with subsequent transepidermal elimination of the material.

Frequency

Although these conditions are usually rare, their incidence in diabetic patients undergoing renal dialysis may be in the region of 5–10%. The disorder typically occurs late in the course of the disease – 10–30 years after the diagnosis, and usually several months after initiation of renal dialysis. Some lesions have occurred before initiation of dialysis.

Location

Perforating lesions can occur almost anywhere, but are most common on the legs and back.

Pathogenesis

It has been proposed that chronic scratching and rubbing may induce more papules, as described above.

Treatment

These lesions are chronic, but may heal after months if scratching and trauma are avoided. Treatment is directed at the underlying pruritus. Topical retinoids, topical and intradermal corticosteroids, cryotherapy, and exposure to UVB light may be helpful. Renal transplantation has resulted in clearance of the dermatosis.

RUBEOSIS

Description

Rubeosis is a characteristic chronic flushed appearance of the face and neck, and even of the extremities, that occurs in diabetics.

Frequency

From 3% to 59% of diabetics experience rubeosis.

Pathogenesis

The cause may be reduced vasoconstrictor tone.

Significance

None.

Treatment

Reduced intake of vasodilators, including alcohol and caffeine, may help alleviate symptoms.

YELLOW SKIN OF DIABETICS (CAROTENODERMA)

Location

Areas of prominent sebaceous activity (e.g., the face) and areas with thick stratum corneum, such as the palms and soles, are affected. Often, the nails also have a similar yellow pigmentation.

Pathogenesis

One theory of pathogenesis of yellow skin of diabetics is that there is disproportionate accumulation of carotene in the skin owing to impairment of its hepatic conversion. Another theory attributes the yellow skin to dermal collagen glycosylation with the yellow end-stage glycosylation products.

Significance

No correlations exist.

Treatment

Better glycemic control will improve the yellow skin of diabetes mellitus.

KERATOSIS PILARIS

Description

Keratosis pilaris is a disorder of perifollicular hyperkeratosis. It is a very common benign condition that manifests as folliculocentric keratotic papules in characteristic areas of the body. Keratosis pilaris, like acquired ichthyosis, develops early in the course of diabetes (Fig. 20–9).

Treatment

General measures to prevent excessive skin dryness (e.g., the use of mild soaps) are recommended. Some available therapeutic options include emollients, lactic acid, tretinoin cream, α-hydroxy acid lotions, urea cream, salicylic acid, and topical corticosteroids.

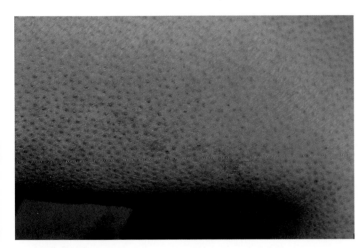

Figure 20–9 Keratosis pilaris.

ERUPTIVE XANTHOMAS

Description

Eruptive xanthomas present as multiple yellow to red-brown papules that erupt abruptly (Fig. 20–10). Histologically, the lesions show infiltration of the dermis with macrophages filled with lipid which, unlike in other forms of xanthoma, represents triglyceride rather than cholesterol esters; these macrophages are called foam cells.

Pathogenesis

Marked hypertriglyceridemia is the cause.

Treatment

Improved control of diabetes and triglyceride levels results in the resolution of the papules.

INFECTIONS

Cutaneous infections occur in 20–50% of patients with diabetes and are more prevalent in those with poorly controlled diabetes and those with type 2 diabetes than in those with type 1 disease. Poor glycemic control increases the risk of infection by causing abnormal microcirculation, reduced phagocytosis, impaired leukocyte adherence, and delayed chemotaxis.

Fungal Infections

Fungal infections are the most prevalent type of cutaneous infection in diabetic patients. Candidal infections are common and are often the first manifestation of diabetes mellitus. Candidal infections often cause angular stomatitis, paronychia, balanitis, and vulvovaginitis. Treatment of all candidal infec-

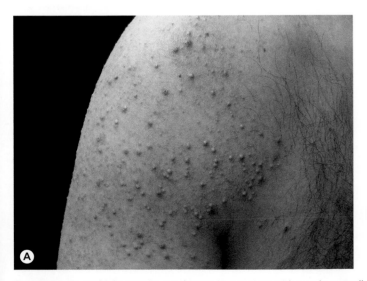

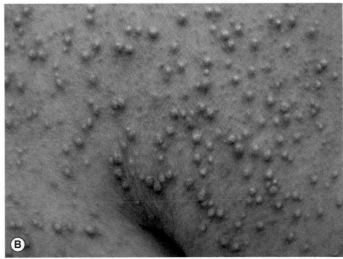

Figure 20–10 Multiple eruptive xanthomas in a patient with poorly controlled diabetes. This patient did not know that he had diabetes mellitus when he presented for evaluation. His blood glucose was 598 mg/dL (normal = 65–99) and his triglyceride level was 11270 mg/dL (normal = 0–149).

tions in diabetic patients requires the use of topical or oral antifungal agents, keeping the affected site dry, and, most important, normalization of blood glucose levels.

Dermatophyte infections can present a significant threat in persons with diabetes mellitus. Diabetic neuropathy in the distal lower extremities creates an ideal environment for dermatophyte infections, allowing benign cases of tinea pedis to become devastating. Breaks in the normal skin barrier due to tinea may lead to superficial bacterial infections, erysipelas and cellulitis, and, ultimately, to sepsis or even fungemia. Tinea pedis should be promptly and aggressively treated in patients with diabetes mellitus.

Diabetes mellitus with ketosis that is debilitating puts the patient at risk for life-threatening mucormycosis (Fig. 20–11). This occurs when various fungi of the Phycomycetes group produce an angiocentric necrotizing infection, especially in the nasopharyngeal area, that may lead to cerebral involvement and death. Prompt intensive supportive care and surgical debridement and intravenous therapy with amphotericin B are required.

Bacterial Infections

A polymicrobial etiology has been implicated in infected diabetic feet. Gram-negative infections are three times more frequent in diabetic than in nondiabetic individuals. Gram-negative bacteria such as *Pseudomonas aeruginosa* may cause severe tissue damage in diabetics, and should never be disregarded as insignificant in diabetic foot ulcers. The consequence of considering the bacteria as contaminants or commensals may result in sepsis and amputation. Antibiotic resistance in *P. aeruginosa* from diabetic foot ulcers is very common, and all the isolates

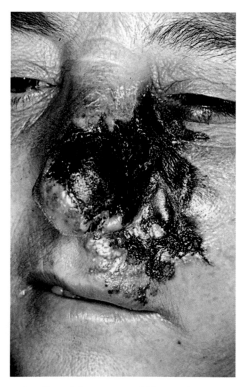

Figure 20–11 Swelling of the upper eyelid in a patient with mucormycosis.

were resistant to at least one or more antibiotics tested. β-Lactamase inhibitor antibiotics should be used as first-line agents. Other antibiotics which can be used are clindamycin plus a Gram-negative antimicrobial agent, or broad-spectrum quinolones and linezolid.

Diabetic patients are more likely to have methicillin-resistant *Staphylococcus aureus* (MRSA) colonization and MRSA-induced bullous erysipelas. Erysipelas and cellulitis are more common in diabetic patients.

Uncontrolled diabetes mellitus is an important risk factor for necrotizing fasciitis, which is the most serious skin and soft tissue infectious necrotizing process affecting adults, who are often in their 60s or 70s. Necrotizing fasciitis causes rapidly spreading necrosis of these tissues, often leading to systemic sepsis, multiorgan failure, and delayed cutaneous necrosis. In most patients with necrotizing fasciitis the causative organism cannot be isolated, and if it is isolated is commonly multimicrobial. Necrotizing fasciitis has a high mortality rate despite combined treatment with antibiotics, surgical debridement, and hyperbaric oxygen.

Malignant otitis externa is an uncommon pseudomonal infection of the external ear canal. This condition occurs more frequently in elderly patients with diabetes mellitus, causing purulent discharge and severe external ear canal pain. The cellulitic infection may spread to deeper tissues, causing osteomyelitis and meningitis. Despite aggressive treatment with debridement and antipseudomonal antibiotics, the infection is fatal in over 50% of patients.

A common uncomplicated diabetic skin infection is bacterial folliculitis, which can respond well to topical antibacterials. Recent studies have shown a significant increase in community-acquired MRSA folliculitis.

Erythrasma is characterized by nonpruritic, well-demarcated, red-tan scaly plaques in intertriginous areas. Caused by *Corynebacterium minutissimum*, erythrasma is often confused with tinea cruris or candidiasis. Wood's light examination aids in diagnosis, showing the characteristic coral-red fluorescence of erythrasma. Treatment consists of the use of topical erythromycin, clindamycin, or clotrimazole and oral erythromycin.

CUTANEOUS COMPLICATIONS OF ANTIDIABETIC THERAPY

Cutaneous reactions that occur with oral antidiabetic drugs include macular erythemas, urticaria, and erythema multiforme. In addition, tolbutamide and chlorpropamide can produce photosensitivity. Of all oral hypoglycemic medications, the sulfonylureas most often cause allergic skin reactions. Lichenoid and rosacea-like eruptions are common with oral hypoglycemic agents, which cause a reaction in 1–5% of diabetic patients. Resolution often occurs while the patient is on a maintenance drug regimen. The second-generation sulfonylureas (i.e., glimepiride, glipizide, and glyburide) cause fewer cutaneous side effects than the first-generation agents.

Lipoatrophy is characterized by circumscribed, depressed areas of skin at insulin injection sites, and occasionally at distant sites, 6–24 months after starting insulin. It seems to occur more often in children and women, and in areas of substantial fat deposits, such as the thighs. Several pathogenetic theories are proposed, including the lipolytic components of the insulin preparation. Spontaneous improvement after rotating injection sites is rare, but has been reported. Use of purified and recombinant human insulin has resulted in reduced lipoatrophy. Substituting rapidly acting insulin may be effective.

Lipohypertrophy is described as soft dermal nodules that clinically resemble lipomas. Its prevalence is 20–30% in type 1 and 4% in type 2 diabetics. It is more common with human insulin, frequent number of injections per day, higher total daily dose of insulin, reuse of needles, and missing rotation of injection sites. It may be a response to the lipogenic action of insulin. Immunologic factors may also play a role. Injection into a lipohypertrophied site can lead to a significant delay in insulin absorption, resulting in erratic glucose control and unpredictable hypoglycemia. Education of patients about correct injection techniques and the necessity for routine change of injection sites can be preventive.

Insulin allergy is relatively rare and more commonly seen with beef insulin than with pork insulin. Recombinant DNA-produced human insulins produce less allergy and lipodystrophy. Documented examples of insulin allergy include immediate hypersensitivity reactions that manifest cutaneously, such as urticaria; serum sickness-like reactions, which are often characterized by vasculitic or purpuric urticarial lesions; and delayed hypersensitivity reactions, which may present as localized nodules.

DERMATOLOGIC DISEASES ASSOCIATED WITH DIABETES MELLITUS

Disseminated Granuloma Annulare

Description

This presents with a few to hundreds of 1–2-mm papules or nodules. Lesions may coalesce into annular plaques, with peripheral extension and central clearing.

Frequency

Granuloma annulare is relatively common, but the disseminated variety is uncommon.

Pathogenesis

The pathogenesis is unknown.

Significance

The association between disseminated granuloma annulare and diabetes mellitus remains very controversial.

Treatment

Disseminated granuloma annulare is difficult to treat and lesions do not tend to resolve spontaneously. Treatment is unnecessary, but some patients seem to be greatly disturbed by the appearance of these lesions. Photochemotherapy with psoralen plus UVA light (PUVA), isotretinoin, dapsone, antimalarial agents, corticosteroids (caution because of the long-term risk and potential for rebound) and other agents have all been used with varying success.

Lichen Planus

In one series, approximately half of patients with lichen planus had glucose metabolism disturbance, and one-quarter had diabetes mellitus.

Vitiligo

Vitiligo occurs up to 10 times more frequently in diabetic patients than in the normal population. It is particularly common among women with type 2 diabetes mellitus. In insulin-dependent diabetic patients, vitiligo may be associated with anti-insulin and other autoendocrine autoantibodies.

MISCELLANEOUS CONDITIONS

Dry Scaly Palms

This disorder is reported in young patients with insulin-dependent diabetes mellitus. This does not reflect the presence of atopic dermatitis, and is associated with scleroderma-like skin changes.

Erythromelalgia

This is a syndrome characterized by erythema, burning pain, and increased skin temperature of the affected extremities. It can be either primary (idiopathic) or secondary. Diabetes mellitus is infrequently associated with the secondary form. Erythromelalgia is associated with small nerve fiber neuropathy.

Anhidrosis and Hyperhydrosis

Autonomic neuropathy may be associated with localized anhidrosis and hyperhydrosis associated with food intake.

Purpura Diabeticorum

The increasing fragility of capillary vessels associated with microangiopathy, as well as subsequent extravasation of erythrocytes and deposition of hemosiderin in macrophages (siderophages), can lead to purpura diabeticorum in later stages of disease.

Renal Calciphylaxis

The presence of diabetic nephropathy with renal insufficiency as well as secondary hyperparathyroidism can lead to localized depositions of calcium salts in the skin. This disorder is usually accompanied by livedo reticularis, severe pain symptoms, and the formation of deep central areas of necrosis. The prognosis is guarded.

SUGGESTED READINGS

Ahmed I, Goldstein B. Diabetes mellitus. Clin Dermatol 2006; 24: 237–246.

Bee YM, Ng ACM, Goh SY, et al. The skin and joint manifestations of diabetes mellitus: superficial clues to deeper issues. Singapore Med J 2006; 47: 111.

Huntley AC. Cutaneous manifestations of diabetes mellitus. Diabetes Metab Rev 1993; 9: 161–176.

Ngo BT, Hayes KD, DiMiao DJ, et al. Manifestations of cutaneous diabetic microangiopathy. Am J Clin Dermatol 2005; 6: 225–237.

Tabor CA, Parlette EC. Cutaneous manifestations of diabetes. Signs of poor glycemic control or new-onset disease. Postgrad Med 2006; 119: 38–44.

Yosipovitch G, Hodak E, Vardi P, et al. The prevalence of cutaneous manifestations in IDDM patients and their association with diabetes risk factors and microvascular complications. Diabetes Care 1998; 21: 506–509.

Chapter | **21** |
Warren R. Heymann, Ted Rosen, and Joseph L. Jorizzo

Thyroid and the Skin

Thyroid hormones influence the differentiation, maturation, and growth of many different body tissues; the total energy expenditure of the organism; and the turnover of nearly all substrates, vitamins, and other hormones. Thus, it is not surprising that the thyroid gland plays an important role in both skin development and the maintenance of normal cutaneous function. In general, the biologic effects of thyroid hormones require binding to specific nuclear receptors with subsequent alteration of gene transcription and stimulation of messenger RNA synthesis. It is postulated that, in addition to nuclear receptors, subcellular receptors exist in mitochondria and plasma membranes. It has been clearly demonstrated that thyroid activity directly affects oxygen consumption, protein synthesis, mitosis, and the thickness of the epidermis. Thyroid activity is also considered essential for the formation and growth of hair, and for sebum secretion. Dermal effects are less well defined.

The impact of thyroid hormone activity on the integument, however, is more notable during deficiency or excess states than during normal physiologic processes. With several important exceptions (discussed later), the majority of cutaneous changes accompanying thyroid disease are neither unique nor pathognomonic. However, in patients with thyroid dysfunction, even such nonspecific cutaneous findings and associations often provide important clues that aid in the diagnosis of previously unsuspected thyroid disease. Examination of the skin and its appendages, the thyroid gland, and the body habitus may also suggest thyroid disorders without evidence of hormone excess or deficiency. Finally, some syndromes with cutaneous or mucosal lesions are associated with an increased risk for thyroid tumors (e.g., Cowden's disease and multiple mucosal neuroma syndromes).

The thyroid gland, which weighs an average of 20–25 g in adults, actively secretes thyroxine (T_4) and triiodothyronine (T_3) from the intraluminal thyroglobulin of its follicular cells. The latter are derived primarily from median midpharyngeal tissue during embryologic development. It is worth noting that about 80% of the T_3 produced daily actually results from hepatic and renal deiodination of T_4, rather than from direct thyroid secretion. Thyroxine has a lower metabolic clearance rate and longer serum half-life than T_3 because it binds more

tightly to serum-binding proteins than does T_3. The half-life of T_3 is less than a day, whereas the half-life of T_4 is about 7 days. Furthermore, although only 0.02% of the total plasma T_4 and 0.30% of the total plasma T_3 are free (i.e., not protein bound), the free forms both determine the thyroid 'status' and maintain the negative feedback regulatory system involving the hypothalamopituitary–thyroid axis.

Calcitonin is secreted from thyroid parafollicular cells (C cells). This hormone is involved in the metabolism of calcium and phosphorus, leading to decreasing serum calcium by inhibiting osteoclast bone resorption, compared to parathyroid hormone, which increases bone resorption. The parafollicular cells are derived embryologically from the neural crest, becoming incorporated within the ultimobranchial pharyngeal pouch.

There are numerous methods to assess thyroid function. Any evaluation should commence with a careful physical examination of the gland. Laboratory tests of direct thyroid function include total and free T_4 and T_3, free T_4 index, T_3 or T_4 resin uptake (now termed the thyroid hormone-binding ratio), and radioactive iodine uptake. An evaluation of thyroid gland function is characteristically based on thyrotropin levels (thyroid-stimulating hormone – TSH), being elevated in patients with primary causes of hypothyroidism (e.g., Hashimoto's thyroiditis) or reduced in patients with primary forms of hyperthyroidism (e.g., Graves' disease). Other less commonly used tests assessing thyroid gland regulatory mechanisms include the thyrotropin-releasing hormone infusion test, and the T_3 suppression test. The thyroid may undergo anatomic evaluation by a thyroid scan, ultrasonography, or fine-needle aspiration or surgical biopsy. Finally, tests for autoimmune thyroid disease include serum thyroid peroxidase (antimicrosomal), thyroid-stimulating, or antithyroglobulin antibody determination. Following thyroidectomy for carcinoma, increases in serum thyroglobulin are considered suspicious for recurrent disease.

The cutaneous manifestations of thyroid disease are often considered in such categories as follows: (1) specific lesions that contain thyroid tissue; (2) signs and symptoms of hyperthyroid and hypothyroid states; and (3) other skin or systemic disorders associated with thyroid disease.

199

SPECIFIC LESIONS

Thyroglossal Duct Cysts

During embryonic life, the developing thyroid gland descends in the neck while possibly maintaining its connection to the tongue by a narrow tube of undifferentiated epithelium, the thyroglossal duct. This structure may activate later in life, and the cells then differentiate into columnar, ciliated, or squamous epithelium, or even into overt glandular tissue. Thyroglossal duct cysts account for 70% of the congenital cystic abnormalities of the neck. They usually present in the first decade of life as a cystic midline mass containing mucoid material. Occasionally, part of the duct will form a sinus tract extending to the skin surface at, or just lateral to, the midline. These anomalies are classified according to their location with respect to the hyoid bone: 65% infrahyoid; 20% suprahyoid; and 15% juxtahyoid. Thyroglossal duct cysts are usually mobile and nontender, unless complicated by infection. Malignancies develop within these structures in less than 1% of cases; 80% of such neoplasms are papillary adenocarcinomas. It is essential that clinicians be certain that these cysts are distinguished from ectopic thyroid tissue, which on occasion may be the only functioning thyroid tissue present.

Cutaneous Metastases

Papillary thyroid carcinoma accounts for the majority of thyroid malignancies in early life. It metastasizes to regional lymph nodes, but only rarely distantly (including to the skin). By contrast, follicular carcinoma usually appears in middle-aged or elderly individuals, and distant metastases are more frequent. Anaplastic tumors – the giant or spindle cell subtypes – occur almost without exception in those over 60 years of age, grow rapidly, and possess a propensity for both nodal and distant metastases. Albeit rare, all histologic types of thyroid cancer have been reported to metastasize to the skin. Such metastatic lesions tend to favor the head and neck region, may be either solitary or multiple, and are generally painless. In this respect, metastases from thyroid neoplasms do not differ significantly from those originating in other sites. Thyroid cancer metastases have been reported from 2 to 10 years after the discovery of the primary tumor. Although such lesions usually occur in patients with a known history of malignancy, they may be the initial presentation of a cancer. In those cases where a biopsy was performed and the routine histology is equivocal, immunohistochemical stains may allow for a precise diagnosis to be made.

Medullary carcinoma of the thyroid originates from parafollicular cells (C cells); these are of neural crest origin. Medullary thyroid carcinoma is familial in 20% of cases, occurring as an autosomal dominant trait as part of multiple endocrine neoplasia (MEN) syndrome type 2a or 2b, caused by mutations in the RET proto-oncogene. In this setting, thyroid cancer is associated with mucosal neuromas, pheochromocytomas, neurofibromas, diffuse lentigines, and café-au-lait macules. Cutaneous macular (or lichen) amyloidosis can occur in association with MEN 2a. Another autosomal dominant disorder that predisposes to thyroid carcinoma is Cowden's disease, also known as multiple hamartoma syndrome. The syndrome shows a dominant inheritance pattern, with a variable penetrance. Various germline mutations in the PTEN gene have been found in more than 80% of patients. Features of this disease include facial trichilemmomas, oral papillomatosis, acral and palmar keratoses, and an increased risk of developing breast carcinoma. Thyroid involvement is common in Cowden's syndrome, with as many as 60% developing benign thyroid lesions, such as multinodular goiter, and follicular adenomas. The risk for thyroid cancer (typically follicular, but occasionally papillary) is approximately 10%.

Hyperthyroidism may be seen in patients who develop widespread metastatic lesions from a primary thyroid malignancy, regardless of the histologic type. The occurrence of this phenomenon, albeit rare, correlates with a large tumor load. Successful therapy for the tumor and possible metastatic lesions results in a resolution of the symptoms of hyperthyroidism.

HYPERTHYROIDISM

General

Excessive quantities of circulating thyroid hormones produce a hypermetabolic state known as hyperthyroidism or thyrotoxicosis. The prevalence of this condition is about 2.5% in women and less than 0.2% in men. Graves' disease accounts for 85% of all cases of hyperthyroidism. However, there are many other causes of this disorder, including toxic multinodular goiter, toxic follicular adenoma, subacute thyroiditis, ingestion of excess thyroid hormone (factitious thyrotoxicosis), tumors secreting hormones that stimulate the thyroid (e.g., TSH-secreting pituitary tumor, choriocarcinoma, and embryonal testicular carcinoma), and tumors that directly secrete thyroid hormone. Etiologies of hyperthyroidism are listed in Table 21–1. The most common symptoms accompanying hyperthyroidism, regardless of the exact cause, are systemic rather than cutaneous. These include nervousness, emotional lability, weight loss despite an increased appetite, heat intolerance, hyperhidrosis, 'weakness,' palpitations, and/or tremor. Patients often speak rapidly and complain bitterly about heat intolerance. Common clinical signs in thyrotoxic patients include sinus tachycardia; atrial fibrillation; increased systolic and lowered diastolic blood pressures; fine to coarse resting or intention tremors; proximal muscle weakness; and changes in the skin, hair, and nails (Table 21–2).

The skin is described as being moist and warm, the result of vasodilation and increased cutaneous perfusion. It is further characterized as soft and velvety in texture, comparable to that of an infant. The skin is usually less oily, and hyperthyroidism in adolescence is associated with a reduced incidence of acne. Palmar erythema, episodic flushing over the face and thorax, increased capillary fragility, and persistent erythema of the elbows may also occur. Hyperhidrosis may be either generalized or localized to the palms and soles.

Diffuse hair loss is present in 20–40% of hyperthyroid patients, although the severity of alopecia does not correlate

Table 21–1 Causes of hyperthyroidism

Autoimmune
Graves'
Inflammatory/destructive
Postpartum thyroiditis
Painless thyroiditis
Subacute thyroiditis
Thyroid infarction
Radiation thyroiditis
Ectopic production
Struma ovarii
Hypothalamopituitary axis dysregulation
TSH-secreting adenoma
Thyrotropic resistance to thyroid hormone
Trophoblastic tumor
Hyperemesis gravidarum
Gestational thyrotoxicosis
Autosomal dominant hyperthyroidism
Extrinsic consumption
Exogenous thyroid consumption
Dietary iodine excess
Drug-induced thyroiditis
Intrinsic overproduction
Thyroid carcinoma
Toxic adenoma
Toxic multinodular goiter

Reproduced with permission from Cokonis CD, Cobb CW, Heymann WR, Hivnor CM. Cutaneous manifestations of hyperthyroidism. In: Heymann WR, ed. Thyroid disorders with cutaneous manifestations. London: Springer Verlag, 2008.

Table 21–2 Dermatological manifestations of hyperthyroidism

Skin	Fine, velvety, or smooth Warm and moist (increased sweating), rarely dry Hyperpigmentation (localized or generalized) Vitiligo Urticaria or dermatographism Pretibial myxedema and thyroid acropachy
Hair	Fine, thin Alopecia (diffuse and mild; rarely severe) Alopecia areata
Nails	Onycholysis Koilonychia Clubbing with thyroid acropachy

with the severity of thyrotoxicosis. The hair itself is typically fine, soft, straight, and unable to retain a permanent wave.

Nail changes, present in about 5% of cases of hyperthyroidism, are often reversible following successful therapy. The nails are described as rapidly growing, soft, and friable. Although not truly pathognomonic for thyrotoxicosis, the nails often assume a 'scoop shovel' configuration and/or demonstrate striking onycholysis. Such nails are referred to as Plummer nails. Any or all the fingernails and toenails may be involved.

Pigmentary changes associated with hyperthyroidism include localized hyperpigmentation (facial, in scars, or in palmar creases), generalized hyperpigmentation, which may be in an Addisonian pattern, or vitiligo. Hyperpigmentary states are believed to be caused by an increased release of adrenocorticotropic hormone in compensation for an accelerated rate of peripheral cortisol degradation. Vitiligo is associated with a variety of autoimmune disorders, the most frequent being autoimmune thyroid disease (including both Graves' disease and Hashimoto's thyroiditis).

Graves' Disease

Graves' disease is an autoimmune disorder that develops as a result of susceptibility genes and presumed exposure to environmental factors. To date, no unique susceptibility genes specific to pretibial myxedema or Graves' ophthalmopathy have been identified. The hyperthyroidism of Graves' disease appears to be caused by the binding of thyroid-stimulating autoantibodies to the TSH receptor. Activation of the TSH receptor by the autoantibody results in excessive production of thyroid hormones.

In addition to demonstrating the nonspecific signs and symptoms discussed previously, patients with Graves' disease often demonstrate several distinctive features, e.g., pretibial myxedema (0.5–10%) and thyroid acropachy (1%). Pretibial myxedema is often, albeit not invariably, associated with ophthalmopathy. It may also be seen with Hashimoto's thyroiditis and Graves' disease. The status of thyroid function bears no direct relation to the development of pretibial myxedema, and the condition may develop after treatment. Although the pretibial location is most typical, lesions may occur on the arm, shoulder, and thigh. For this reason, the term 'thyroid dermopathy' is preferred.

Early lesions of pretibial myxedema appear as bilateral, raised, asymmetrical, firm plaques and nodules (Fig. 21–1). A peau d'orange appearance, caused by dermal infiltration by the glycosaminoglycans hyaluronic acid and chondroitin sulfate, may be noted (Fig. 21–2). The lesions may be pink, violaceous, or flesh-colored and have a waxy translucent quality. They may enlarge and coalesce to form grotesque arrays. Topical and intralesional corticosteroids are the mainstay of therapy. Compression therapy is valuable. Plasmapheresis was reported to be of transient benefit in some patients; surgery yields equivocal results, and is not routinely recommended. Although

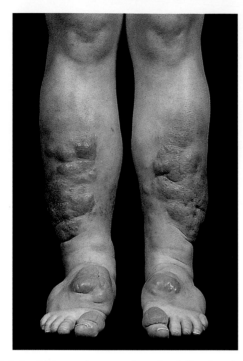

Figure 21–1 Pretibial myxedema manifested as infiltrative plaques in a woman 10 years after thyroidectomy for Graves' disease.

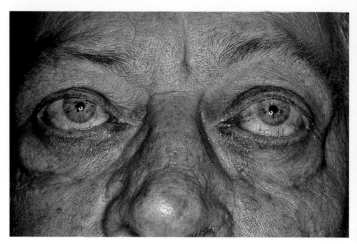

Figure 21–2 An example of the ophthalmopathy associated with Graves' disease. (Reproduced with permission from Cokonis CD, Cobb CW, Heymann WR, Hivnor CM. Cutaneous manifestations of hyperthyroidism. In: Heymann WR, ed. Thyroid disorders with cutaneous manifestations. London: Springer Verlag, 2008).

HYPOTHYROIDISM

General

Hypothyroidism results from a deficiency of thyroid hormones and, like hyperthyroidism, is much more likely to be seen in women, with a female-to-male ratio of 7:1. The disorder is particularly likely to affect women between the ages of 40 and 60 years. Almost 95% of all cases can be classified as either primary acquired or idiopathic. About 5% are the result of pituitary or hypothalamic dysfunction; the remainder are caused by the congenital absence of thyroid tissue, inherited deficiency in thyroid hormone-synthesizing enzymes, or severe iodine deficit. Rarely, hypothyroidism results from drugs (e.g., lithium and sulfonamides) or from irradiation of the neck region. The cause for the disease in the majority of patients affected by primary acquired hypothyroidism is Hashimoto's thyroiditis or iatrogenic thyroid ablation (^{131}I therapy or surgical thyroidectomy). Table 21–3 lists the causes of hypothyroidism.

The term thyroiditis actually covers a number of histologically distinct entities, including acute suppurative thyroiditis, subacute granulomatous thyroiditis, and chronic sclerosing thyroiditis of Riedel. Nonetheless, the majority of patients are classified as having Hashimoto's or chronic lymphocytic thyroiditis. This disorder is believed to have an autoimmune-mediated pathogenesis, as illustrated by the many patients who have circulating antithyroglobulin or antiperoxidase (microsomal) antibodies. There is also a strong genetic predisposition to develop this disease among those with the HLA-B8 and -DR3 haplotypes.

The clinical manifestations of hypothyroidism, regardless of the exact cause, can be attributed to both a deceleration of cellular metabolic processes and/or myxedema, the accumulation of acid mucopolysaccharides in various organs, such as the skin, vocal cords, and oropharynx. The exact pathogenesis of myxedema remains obscure, but most authorities have

lesions persist, most patients will improve slowly with time, typically over many years.

Thyroid acropachy is rare, with fewer than 100 cases being reported. Ninety-five percent of patients develop acropachy after therapy for Graves' disease. This disorder consists of a triad of clubbing of the fingers and toes; periosteal proliferation of the phalanges and long bones; and swelling of the soft tissue overlying bony structures. The most common manifestation of acropachy is clubbing of the fingernails and toenails, which occurs in 19% of patients who have thyroid dermopathy. The first, second, and fifth metacarpals, the proximal phalanges of the hand, and the first metatarsal and proximal phalanges of the feet are most often affected. Bone scanning is the most sensitive objective test to detect thyroid acropachy. No therapy is indicated because the condition is usually asymptomatic. Patients who smoke should be encouraged to quit, as smoking has been associated with all extrathyroidal manifestations of Graves' disease, including thyroid acropachy.

In patients with suspected Graves' disease, examination of the neck may reveal obvious thyromegaly. Examination of the eyes will reveal mild changes (exophthalmos) to severe changes (proptosis), along with congestion of the sclerae. Exophthalmos occurs in nearly all patients with Graves' disease and may be the first sign of hyperthyroidism (Fig. 21–2). The complaints accompanying this problem include 'protruding' eyes, easy tear production, photophobia, and the sensation of a foreign body in the eye. This disorder is caused by infiltration of retrobulbar tissues and extraocular muscles by mononuclear cells and mucopolysaccharides, but the precise factor(s) responsible remain unidentified.

Table 21–3 Causes of hypothyroidism

Primary	Defects in thyroid hormone biosynthesis
	  Congenital defects in hormone synthesis
	  Inheritable enzyme defects
	  Iodine deficiency
	  Iodine excess
	  Anti-thyroid medications (lithium,
	    amiodarone, goitrogens, bexarotene)

	Reduced functional thyroid tissue
	  Hashimoto's (chronic autoimmune thyroiditis)
	  Thyroid surgery
	  Radioiodine (^{131}I) therapy
	  Radiation to head and neck
	  Infiltrative diseases: sarcoidosis,
	    hemochromatosis, systemic sclerosis,
	    amyloidosis, Riedel's thyroiditis, cystinosis
	  Viral infections: subacute thyroiditis
	  Postpartum thyroiditis
	  Thyroid dysgenesis/agenesis

Central (pituitary/
hypothalamic)
	Reduced pituitary/hypothalamic tissue
	  Tumors: pituitary adenoma,
	    craniopharyngioma, meningioma, glioma,
	    metastases
	  Vascular: ischemic necrosis, hemorrhage
	    (Sheehan's syndrome), internal carotid
	    artery aneurysm, compression of pituitary
	    stalk
	  Trauma: head injury, radiation, surgery
	  Infectious: brain abscess, tuberculosis,
	    syphilis, toxoplasmosis
	  Infiltrative: sarcoidosis, hemochromatosis,
	    histiocytosis
	  Chronic lymphocytic hypophysitis
	  Congenital abnormalities: pituitary
	    hypoplasia, basal encephalocele
	  Genetic mutations in TRH receptor, TSH
	    receptor, and Pit-1

Reproduced with permission from Kopp SA et al. Cutaneous manifestations of hypothyroidism. In: Heymann WR, ed. Thyroid disorders with cutaneous manifestations. London: Springer Verlag, 2008.

Table 21–4 Dermatological manifestations of hypothyroidism

Skin	Dry, rough, or coarse; cold and pale; puffy, boggy, or edematous (myxedema) Yellow discoloration as a result of carotenemia Ichthyosis and palmoplantar hyperkeratosis Easy bruising (capillary fragility) Eruptive bruising (capillary fragility) Eruptive and tuberous xanthomas (rare)
Hair	Dull, coarse, and brittle Slow growth (increase in telogen or resting hairs) Alopecia (lateral third of eyebrows, rarely diffuse)
Nails	Thin, brittle, striated Slow growth Onycholysis (rare)

uronic acid and chondroitin sulfate). The entire skin appears swollen, dry, waxy, and pale. The cutaneous pallor is due both to vasoconstriction and to the increased water and mucopolysaccharide content in the dermis, which alters the refraction of incident light. The skin is also 'boggy' but nonpitting, especially around the eyes, lips, and acral portions. The skin is cool to the touch and may be so xerotic as to develop an acquired ichthyosis. The palms and soles are hypohidrotic and may demonstrate a keratoderma. Carotenemia may also be encountered on the volar and palmar surfaces as a result of reduced hepatic conversion of β-carotene to vitamin A.

The hair in patients with hypothyroidism is dull, coarse, and brittle. The growth rate is slowed, with an increase in telogen (resting) hairs. Although diffuse alopecia may be seen in patients with hypothyroidism, the classic pattern of hair loss is the loss of the lateral third of the eyebrows (madarosis).

The nails are affected to some degree in 90% of all patients. They are typically thin, brittle, slow growing, and striated (either in longitudinal or transverse fashion). Onycholysis, more commonly seen in hyperthyroid states, has also been reported to accompany myxedema.

Congenital Hypothyroidism

When the thyroid gland fails to secrete sufficient hormone in utero or during the early perinatal period, congenital hypothyroidism (cretinism) occurs. This phenomenon appears in one of every 3000–4000 live births. The overwhelming majority of cases are sporadic, although some 15% are genetic, secondary to dyshormonogenesis. This disease becomes clinically apparent by 6 weeks of age, although no single clinical feature can be said to be pathognomonic.

The earliest symptoms of cretinism are nonspecific and include lethargy, poor feeding, constipation, persistent neonatal jaundice, and respiratory difficulty as a result of myxedema of the oropharynx and larynx. The characteristic puffy facies, macroglossia, umbilical hernia, and hypotonia are not evident until 3–4 months of age. The presence of a clavicular fat pad at birth may suggest cretinism. As in adult hypothyroidism, the skin tends to be cold, dry, and pale; the hair is coarse, dry, and brittle. A reduced metabolic rate causes reflex peripheral vasoconstriction, which may result in cutis marmorata. Growth

abandoned the hypothesis that it is the result of increased levels of TSH, which occurs in response to low thyroid hormone levels. The extracutaneous features of hypothyroidism include pleural and pericardial effusions, bradycardia and reduced cardiac output, weight gain secondary to fluid retention, hoarseness, swollen lips and tongue, rheumatoid-like polyarthritis, and a wide variety of neurologic problems (such as slowed mentation). When hypothyroidism develops in adolescence, delayed sexual maturation occurs; in adults, impotence, oligospermia, and amenorrhea are common. The symptoms often include weakness and fatigue, anorexia, cold intolerance, voice changes, muscle cramps, and the swelling of extremities. Such symptoms may easily be overlooked or mistakenly ascribed to aging.

Alterations in the skin, hair, and nails occurring in hypothyroidism are summarized in Table 21–4. The most characteristic sign is generalized myxedema, which is caused by the dermal deposition of acid mucopolysaccharides (notably hyal-

retardation and mental retardation occur if therapy is not instituted at an early stage.

MISCELLANEOUS CUTANEOUS DISORDERS AND THE THYROID

Thyroid diseases need to be considered as contributing to the clinical picture in patients with a host of systemic and dermatologic disorders, many of which are classified as autoimmune. Alopecia areata occurs in up to 8% of patients with thyroid disease. Bullous pemphigoid and various forms of pemphigus have been linked statistically to autoimmune thyroid disease. About one-third of all patients with dermatitis herpetiformis have either clinical thyroid disease or abnormal thyroid function test results. Most connective tissue–vascular diseases have an increased frequency of autoimmune thyroid disorders.

Atopic dermatitis may be linked to Graves' disease, as may acanthosis nigricans. Sweet's syndrome (acute febrile neutrophilic dermatosis) has been reported in conjunction with several different thyroid disorders. Generalized granuloma annulare has occurred in patients with autoimmune thyroiditis. In one study of patients who developed typical melasma, the frequency of thyroid dysfunction was four times that of a control group. Both myxedema and thyrotoxicosis have been reported with pseudoxanthoma elasticum. Hyperthyroidism and psoriasis may also be statistically associated.

Finally, it should be noted that pruritus may be severe in up to 5% of patients with Graves' disease, especially those with attendant chronic idiopathic urticaria associated with thyroid autoantibodies Pruritus may also be associated with the xerotic skin that occurs in hypothyroidism, and there are a number of reports in which the urticaria resolved only when the underlying thyroid problem was treated.

SUGGESTED READINGS

Ai J, Leonhardt JM, Heymann WR. Autoimmune thyroid diseases: etiology, pathogenesis, and dermatologic manifestations. J Am Acad Dermatol 2003; 48: 641–659.

Alsanea O, Clark OH. Treatment of Graves' disease: the advantages of surgery. Endocrinol Metab Clin North Am 2000; 29: 321–337.

Bijlmer-Iest JC, van Vloten WA. Thyroid and the skin. Curr Probl Dermatol 1991; 20: 34–44.

Heymann WR. Cutaneous manifestations of thyroid disease. J Am Acad Dermatol 1992; 26: 885–902.

Heymann WR, ed. Thyroid disorders with cutaneous manifestations. London: Springer Verlag, 2008.

Leonhardt JM, Heymann WR. Thyroid disease and the skin. Dermatol Clin 2002; 21: 473–481.

Chapter | 22 |

Sarah L. Taylor,
Kenneth E. Greer, and
Joseph L. Jorizzo

Lipids

Lipids are a heterogeneous group of fats or fat-like substances that are insoluble in water but soluble in fat solvents. They include compounds such as fatty acids, neutral fats, waxes, and steroids. When compounded, lipids also include lipoproteins, glycolipids, and phospholipids. Owing to their insolubility, lipids travel in the circulation as complexes of lipoproteins and specific apoproteins. These protein complexes also serve as ligands to specific receptors, facilitate transmembrane transport, and regulate enzymatic activity. Lipoproteins are classified according to their density, as follows: chylomicrons, very-low-density lipoproteins (VLDL), intermediate-density lipoproteins (IDL), low-density lipoproteins (LDL), and high-density lipoproteins (HDL). Defects in the metabolism of lipoproteins can produce clinical disease that can be the result of overproduction or insufficient removal of lipoproteins from the circulation.

DISORDERS OF LIPID METABOLISM

The disorders of lipid metabolism with cutaneous manifestations are primarily the hyperlipoproteinemias (hyperlipidemias), and they have been defined as primary (single-gene disorders that are transmitted by autosomal dominant or recessive mechanisms) or secondary (multifactorial disorders with both genetic and environmental factors) (Tables 22–1 and 22–2). At times it is difficult to differentiate primary from secondary hyperlipoproteinemias because of the similar clinical and laboratory findings.

Distinguishing between these two categories is important for therapeutic reasons. Xanthomas represent the major cutaneous change of lipid disease, and are especially important because their recognition can lead to the investigation, diagnosis, and treatment of the various hyperlipidemias. This is significant because abnormalities of plasma lipoprotein levels can result in a predisposition to premature coronary artery disease, pancreatitis, and neurologic disease. Various classification schemas have been proposed, based primarily on the genetics of the syndromes and the lipoprotein patterns (see Table 22–1). However, numerous synonyms have been used to describe the different disorders, making a precise classification difficult.

The diagnosis is based on the history (including the family history); the presence, type, and distribution of xanthomas; fasting levels of serum triglycerides, cholesterol, and HDL-cholesterol (LDL and VLDL can then be calculated from these values); and the 'refrigerator test.' In this test, plasma or whole blood is stored in the refrigerator overnight. If a creamy layer forms over the clear plasma beneath, chylomicrons are present. When there is a high concentration of VLDL or remnant lipoprotein (IDL), the entire plasma is turbid. A finding of clear plasma rules out disorders of chylomicrons, VLDLs, and IDLs. Pathophysiologically, the disorders are caused by increased production or deficient removal of the various lipoproteins (chylomicrons, VLDL, LDL, and IDL). The estimated frequency of occurrence of the primary hyperlipidemias ranges from relatively common (1 : 100 for type III familial dysbetalipoproteinemia) to extremely rare (1 : 1 000 000 for autosomal recessive apoprotein C-II deficiency).

Hyperchylomicronemia

Two genetically determined defects of triglyceride removal lead to hypertriglyceridemia and hyperchylomicronemia: these are autosomal recessive lipoprotein lipase deficiency (also known as type I or Bürger–Grütz disease) and familial apoprotein C-II deficiency. However, the majority of patients with high levels of chylomicrons and triglycerides have acquired or secondary forms of hyperlipidemia. Pancreatitis and bouts of abdominal pain are common in severe type I disease, often beginning in early childhood. In addition, these children develop hepatosplenomegaly, eruptive xanthomas, and lipemia retinalis, especially when the triglyceride levels exceed 4000 mg/dL. Premature atherosclerotic vascular disease does not occur in type I disease. Patients with an absence of lipoprotein lipase activator (apoprotein C-II) first develop symptoms after adolescence. Patients with type V disease have elevations of both chylomicrons and VLDLs – so-called familial combined hyperlipidemia. The symptoms usually begin in adult life, and as is true for many patients with primary hyperlipidemia, secondary

Table 22–1 Primary hyperlipoproteinemias

Elevated lipoprotein class	Synonyms and primary disorders
Chylomicrons	Type I, familial lipoprotein lipase deficiency, familial apoprotein C-II deficiencies
Chylomicrons and VLDLs	Type V, familial combined hyperlipidemia
VLDLs	Type IV, endogenous familial hypertriglyceridemia
LDLs	Type IIa, familial hypercholesterolemia, familial combined hyperlipidemia
LDLs and VLDLs	Type IIb, familial multiple lipoprotein-type hyperlipidemia, combined hyperlipidemia
IDLs	Type III, remnant hyperlipidemia, familial dysbetalipoproteinemia

VLDL = very-low-density lipoprotein, LDL = low-density lipoprotein, IDL = intermediate-density lipoprotein.

Table 22–2 Secondary hyperlipoproteinemias

Secondary hypercholesterolemia

Acute intermittent porphyria
Cholestasis
Hypothyroidism
Pregnancy

Secondary hypertriglyceridemia

Alcoholism
Diabetes mellitus
Drugs: estrogens, isotretinoin, targretin, acitretin, corticosteroids
Oral contraceptive use

Pancreatitis

Paraproteinemia, e.g., myeloma, Waldenström's macroglobulinemia, cryoglobulinemia, lymphoma
Primary biliary cirrhosis
Renal disease, e.g., nephrotic syndrome, uremia

factors, such as alcohol intake, obesity, associated renal disease, or diabetes mellitus, are frequently involved in the exacerbation of the disease.

Increased VLDLs

Endogenous familial hypertriglyceridemia (type IV disease) results primarily from accelerated production of VLDL in the liver. This autosomal dominant disorder is common. The symptoms first appear in adulthood, frequently being precipitated by the ingestion of large amounts of carbohydrate or alcohol. Not uncommonly, patients with this disorder are obese, diabetic, and hyperuricemic. In addition, they appear

to have an increased risk of coronary artery disease. Eruptive xanthomas are common, and xanthoma striatum palmares can also occur. As mentioned previously, VLDLs may be elevated along with chylomicrons in type V disease. Patients with elevations of both VLDL and LDL have type IIb disease. Some patients with type IIb disease have an elevated triglyceride concentration in addition to higher cholesterol levels, but the VLDL level is insufficient to produce milky or turbid plasma as determined by the refrigerator test.

Increased LDLs

LDLs (β-lipoproteins) alone are elevated in the plasma in type IIa disease (familial hypercholesterolemia), and are elevated together with VLDLs in type IIb disease. There are several different phenotypic genetic conditions of familial hypercholesterolemia, and the severity of the clinical manifestations varies considerably. Xanthomas, especially the tendinous and tuberous types, are prominent, and there is a significant increase in the incidence of coronary artery disease, often beginning in early adulthood.

Elevated IDLs

Patients with high levels of cholesterol and triglycerides, carried in remnant lipoproteins (IDLs), have type III or broad-β disease (familial dysbetalipoproteinemia). Type III hyperlipoproteinemia is inherited as an autosomal dominant disease, although similar remnant lipoprotein accumulation in the plasma has been seen as a secondary phenomenon in hypothyroidism. The disorder appears to be related to a defect in the removal of these remnants from the circulation. Clinically, patients with broad-β disease are usually obese; are glucose intolerant; have xanthomas (tuberous xanthoma in 80%, xanthoma striatum palmare in 64%, and tendinous xanthoma in 25%); and have peripheral atherosclerotic vascular and coronary artery disease.

Secondary Hyperlipoproteinemias

The diagnosis of a specific type of hyperlipoproteinemia cannot be made on the basis of the clinical type of xanthoma found in a patient because these same xanthomas occur in various lipid disorders, primary or secondary. Secondary or acquired hyperlipidemias result from disease in various organs (e.g., liver, kidney, thyroid, or pancreas) and are caused by a disturbance in the metabolism of triglycerides and cholesterol. In fact, the majority of cases of xanthomatosis are secondary, rather than the primary familial disorders listed in Table 22–1. Eruptive xanthomas may appear when hypertriglyceridemia develops in patients with uncontrolled diabetes mellitus, and in patients with the nephrotic syndrome. Tuberous and eruptive xanthomas can be seen in patients with hypothyroidism, but only rarely. Infants with biliary atresia and adults with biliary cirrhosis may develop any of the four types of xanthoma (Figs 22–1 and 22–2). Diffuse plane xanthomas are associated primarily with malignancies of the reticuloendothelial system, including

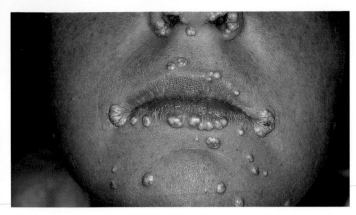

Figure 22–1 Primary biliary cirrhosis. Multiple xanthomas are present, but in addition there is a brown color to the skin.

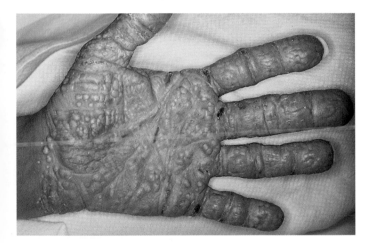

Figure 22–2 Primary biliary cirrhosis with palmar xanthomas.

multiple myeloma and lymphoma, and with various other paraproteinemias.

Normolipemic Xanthomatosis

Xanthomas may occur in disorders with histiocytic proliferation and secondary uptake of fat, rather than with an error of lipid metabolism. Blood lipid levels are normal in these disorders, which include nevoxanthoendothelioma, xanthoma disseminatum, and cerebrotendinous xanthomatosis. This group of diseases is collectively known as the normolipemic xanthomatoses. Nevoxanthoendothelioma, also known as juvenile xanthogranuloma, is a benign proliferation of lipid-laden histiocytes that occurs primarily in infancy and is usually characterized by one or a few nodules that are yellow-brown and vary from a few millimeters to several centimeters in diameter. They are especially common on the scalp, face, or extensor extremities, and although they usually disappear spontaneously over several months, they may persist for many years. Involvement of visceral organs is rare, but the lesions may occur in the iris and ciliary body of the eye, and in the lung, heart, and oropharynx. Xanthoma disseminatum is a rare and

unusual disease characterized by xanthomatous nodules in the axillae, the antecubital and popliteal fossae, the intertriginous areas, and the oropharynx and upper respiratory tract. The disorder is discussed in Chapter 17. Approximately 20 cases of familial cerebrotendinous xanthomatosis have been described. The deposition of cholestanol and cholesterol in all tissues of the body begins in childhood. Xanthomas in the Achilles tendon are characteristic, but the major damage results from sterol deposition in the brain and lungs.

Hypolipoproteinemias

Abnormally low levels of cholesterol and triglyceride may be observed in patients with malabsorption, parenchymal liver disease, or cachexia, but primary or familial cases of hypolipoproteinemia are extremely rare and include such diseases as Tangier disease (α-lipoprotein deficiency), hypo- or abetalipoproteinemia, and lecithin-cholesterol acyltransferase deficiency. Cutaneous lesions are not specific in these disorders, but patients with Tangier disease have characteristic yellow-orange tonsils.

CLINICAL MANIFESTATIONS

With respect to the skin, xanthomas represent the major cutaneous manifestation of disorders of lipid metabolism, occurring primarily as a result of hyperlipoproteinemia. Xanthomas are localized accumulations of lipid that contain foamy histiocytes and are usually found in the dermis or tendons. They have been categorized as tendinous, tuberous, planar, or eruptive. Cholesterol is the major lipid found in xanthomas, although sterols and triglycerides may accumulate in significant quantities in certain xanthomas. Xanthomas can occur in persons of any age, but usually occur in those over 50; males and females are equally affected. The morbidity and mortality of xanthomas are related primarily to associated atherosclerosis and pancreatitis.

Xanthomas

Tendinous Xanthomas

Tendinous xanthomas are produced by a diffuse infiltration of lipid within tendons, ligaments, and occasionally, fasciae. They appear as slowly enlarging subcutaneous nodules related to the tendons or the ligaments. They are deeply situated, smooth, firm nodules with normal overlying skin that is freely movable over the lesions. Classically, they affect the extensor tendons of the hands, knees, and elbows, and the Achilles tendons, where they may be confused with rheumatoid nodules or gouty tophi. Trauma is thought to be a predisposing factor in xanthoma formation, although the unique distribution of the lesions in the various forms of hyperlipoproteinemia is unexplained. Tendinous xanthomas are usually associated with hypercholesterolemia and increased levels of LDL, and they may occur in association with other cutaneous xanthomas, especially xanthelasmas and tuberous xanthomas. Rarely, however, tendinous xanthomas may occur in normolipemic xanthomatosis, especially in cerebrotendinous xanthomatosis. Patients with tendinous xanthomas have an extremely high incidence of atherosclerotic vascular disease.

Tuberous Xanthomas

Tuberous xanthomas begin as small, soft, yellow, red, or flesh-colored papules, and usually develop in pressure areas such as the extensor surfaces of the body, including the elbows, knees, and buttocks. They are painless and frequently coalesce to form large globular masses (Figs 22–3 and 22–4). Their presence usually suggests an elevation of serum cholesterol and LDL, but they may also be seen with triglyceride elevation. They can be associated with familial dysbetalipoproteinemia and familial hypercholesterolemia, and may be present in some of the secondary hyperlipidemias (e.g., nephrotic syndrome, hypothyroidism). As with tendinous xanthomas, patients with tuberous xanthomas also have an extremely high incidence of atherosclerotic vascular disease.

Planar Xanthomas

Planar xanthomas are by far the most commonly encountered xanthomas. These yellow, soft, macular to barely palpable lesions occur in three forms: xanthelasma, xanthoma striatum palmare, and diffuse plane xanthoma.

Xanthelasmas are soft, velvety, flat, yellow, polygonal papules that appear in the eyelid area, most commonly in the medial canthus (Fig. 22–5). At least 50% of patients with xanthelasmas will have normal plasma lipid levels. If the lipid levels are abnormal, serum cholesterol is usually elevated. This is especially true in younger patients. An associated finding in many of these patients is corneal arcus, which may also occur in the older population in the setting of normal lipid levels. Some secondary hyperlipoproteinemias, such as cholestasis, may also be associated with xanthelasmas.

Xanthoma striatum palmare are flat, yellow to orange lesions in the palmar creases (Fig. 22–2) that occur only in patients with abnormal serum lipid levels, including elevations of cholesterol and triglycerides. There have been a few reports in the literature of this type of xanthoma occurring in individuals with primary biliary cirrhosis.

Diffuse plane xanthomas usually cover large areas of the face, neck, thorax, and arms. Individuals may or may not have hyperlipidemia (hypertriglyceridemia in particular), but frequently have paraproteinemia, including multiple myeloma.

Eruptive Xanthomas

Eruptive xanthomas appear suddenly, usually in crops, and unlike the other forms of xanthoma may be pruritic and/or tender. Eruptive xanthomas are characterized by their yellow color, small size (1–4 mm in diameter), palpability, and the erythematous halo around their base. They occur most commonly over pressure points and extensor surfaces of the arms, legs, and buttocks (Figs 22–6 and 22–7). Rarely, they may be diffusely scattered over the trunk or on the mucous membranes. They occur exclusively in association with elevated triglyceride levels. A frequent circumstance is their occurrence with hypertriglyceridemia secondary to uncontrolled diabetes mellitus. Treatment of the diabetes mellitus can lead to subsequent resolution of the xanthomas.

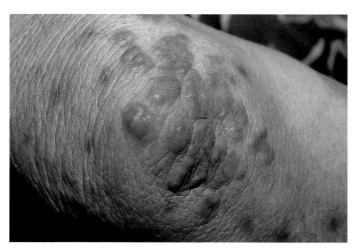

Figure 22–3 Tuberous xanthomas of the elbows.

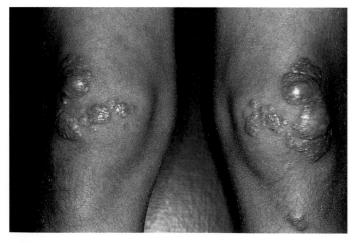

Figure 22–4 Tuberous xanthomas of the knees.

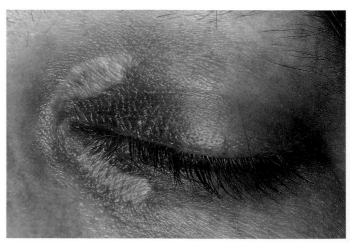

Figure 22–5 Planar xanthomas (xanthelasmas of the eyelids).

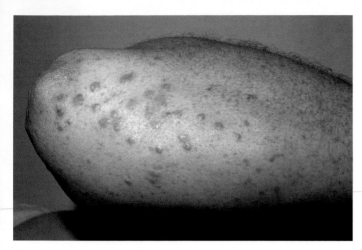

Figure 22–6 Eruptive xanthomas.

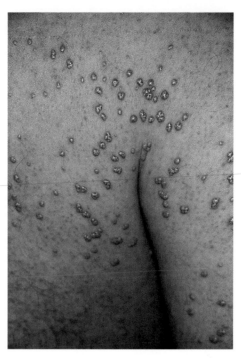

Figure 22–7 Eruptive xanthomas: multiple yellow papules appeared over several weeks in this man with insulin-dependent diabetes mellitus.

TREATMENT

The therapy of disorders of lipid metabolism depends on the underlying lipoprotein abnormality and is directed toward returning the lipids to normal levels. Attempts should also be made to find any underlying secondary disease causing the hyperlipidemia so that it can be addressed. Dietary manipulation and lipid-lowering agents such as statins, fibrates, bile acid-binding resins, probucol, and nicotinic acid are the mainstays of therapy for primary hyperlipidemias, but there is no effective therapy for the normo- or hypolipemic conditions. The lipid-lowering effects of these agents have been well studied, but few studies mention the efficacy of these drugs for resolving xanthomas. Eruptive xanthomas usually resolve within weeks of initiating systemic treatment, and tuberous xanthomas usually resolve after months, but tendinous xanthomas take years to resolve or may persist indefinitely. The main goal of therapy for hyperlipidemia is to reduce the risks of atherosclerotic cardiovascular disease, whereas in patients with severe hypertriglyceridemia the goal is to prevent pancreatitis and its complications.

Surgery or locally destructive modalities can be used for idiopathic or unresponsive xanthomas. Xanthelasmas are often treated with topical trichloroacetic acid, electrodesiccation, laser therapy, and excision, but recurrences may occur. Although these therapies can be effective in clearing the xanthomas, the goal is to attempt to reverse or slow the associated atherosclerotic process (lipid-laden plaques collecting on the intima of blood vessels), the most serious complication of lipid disorders. A full discussion of therapy is beyond the scope of this chapter.

SUGGESTED READINGS

Basar E, Oguz H, Ozdemir H, et al. Treatment of xanthelasma palpebrarum with argon laser photocoagulation. Argon laser and xanthelasma palpebrarum. Int Ophthalmol 2004; 25: 9–11.

Bergman R. Xanthelasma palpebrarum and risk of arteriosclerosis: a review. Int J Dermatol 1998; 37: 343–345.

Borelli C, Kaudewitz P. Xanthelasma palpebrarum: treatment with the erbium:YAG laser. Lasers Surg Med 2001; 29: 260–264.

Burnside NJ, Alberta L, Robinson-Bostom L, Bostom A. Type III hyperlipoproteinemia with xanthomas and multiple myeloma. J Am Acad Dermatol 2005; 53: S281–S284.

Fujita M, Shirai K. A comparative study of the therapeutic effect of probucol and pravastatin on xanthelasma. J Dermatol 1996; 23: 598–602.

Hayes BB, Boyd AS. Eruptive xanthomas. Papules may indicate underlying lipid disorder. Postgrad Med 2005; 118: 11–12.

Haygood LJ, Bennett JD, Brodell RT. Treatment of xanthelasma palpebrarum with bichloracetic acid. Dermatol Surg 1998; 24: 1027–1031.

Hollman G, Olsson AG, Ek AC. Disease knowledge and adherence to treatment in patients with familial hypercholesterolemia. J Cardiovasc Nurs 2006; 21: 103–108.

Hsu JC, Su TC, Chen MF, et al. Xanthoma striatum palmare in a patient with primary biliary cirrhosis and hypercholesterolemia. J Gastroenterol Hepatol 2005; 20: 1799–1800.

Kashyap AS, Kashyap S. A young man with dry skin and nodules on elbows and buttocks. Postgrad Med J 2000; 76: 109–111.

Marcoval J, Moreno A, Bordas X, et al. Diffuse plane xanthoma: a clinicopathologic study of 8 cases. J Am Acad Dermatol 1998; 39: 439–442.

Raulin C, Schoenermach MP, Werner S, Greve B. Xanthelasma palpebrarum: treatment with ultrapulsed CO_2 laser. Lasers Surg Med 1999; 24: 122–127.

Sato-Matsumura KC, Matsumura T, Yokoshiki H, et al. Xanthoma striatum palmare as an early sign of familial type III hyperlipoproteinemia with an apoprotein E genotype e2/e2. Clin Exp Dermatol 2003; 28: 321–322.

Sibley C, Stone NJ. Familial hypercholesterolemia: a challenge of diagnosis and therapy. Cleveland Clin J Med 2006; 73: 57–64.

Zech LA Jr, Hoeg JM. Correlating corneal arcus with atherosclerosis in familial hypercholesterolemia. Lipids Health Dis 2008; 7: 7.

Adrenal, Androgen-related, and Pituitary Disorders

Hormones of the steroid family (glucocorticoids, androgens and other sex steroids, and mineralocorticoids) are critical in the control of homeostasis and cell differentiation. These hormones are produced by the adrenal gland and gonads, and are regulated by pituitary secretions. They control cell growth, differentiation, and metabolism by binding to intracellular receptors that act directly at the DNA level to produce changes in gene expression.

ADRENAL DISORDERS

Excessive Glucocorticoid Activity (Cushing's Syndrome)

Hypercortisolism is most commonly the result of the administration of glucocorticosteroids, but similar cutaneous findings are also present in patients with endogenous hypercortisolism, e.g., pituitary adrenocorticotropic hormone (ACTH) production (Cushing's disease), adrenal tumors, or ectopic ACTH secretion. The findings may be dramatic or subtle. The systemic alterations may include hypertension, myopathy, obesity, osteopenia, and psychiatric disturbances. The association of these features with cutaneous atrophy has led to the aphorism: 'the presence of thin skin, thin muscle, and thin bones in a fat person should raise the possibility of Cushing's syndrome.'

The constellation of cutaneous findings seen in hypercortisolism includes cutaneous atrophy, striae, purpura, telangiectasia, and acne. Cutaneous atrophy is caused by a reduction in both epidermal and dermal components. There is thinning of the epidermis, and collagen synthesis is reduced. There is also loss of elastic fibers and dermal mucopolysaccharides. The weakened dermis and the obesity result in the development of prominent striae (Fig. 23–1). The skin is injured easily by minor trauma. This may result in purpura or ulcerations that heal slowly (as a result of the inhibition of wound healing by hypercortisolism).

The deposition of subcutaneous fat over the face and trunk contributes to the characteristic facies and body habitus. Erythrocytosis, telangiectasia, and cutaneous atrophy also contribute to the characteristic facial appearance, resulting in a plethoric moon facies. Steroid acne may also occur (Fig. 23–2).

This is characterized by red papules and pustules, which are uniform in their stage of development, without a comedonal component. The usual distribution is on the trunk, shoulders, and arms, with sparing of the face. Patients with hypercortisolism are also predisposed to the development of chronic fungal infections of the skin (tinea versicolor and dermatophytes). When the hypercortisolism is caused by increased ACTH production, hyperpigmentation may occur, as in adrenal insufficiency.

Cortisol levels can be increased in several disorders other than Cushing's syndrome. This condition is known as pseudo-Cushing's syndrome. Possible causes include physiologic stress, obesity, major depressive disorder, and, in rare cases, chronic alcoholism. Patients with pseudo-Cushing's syndrome seldom display the cutaneous findings associated with Cushing's syndrome.

Laboratory abnormalities observed in hypercortisolism include hypokalemia and hyperglycemia, but these are not specific. Screening for hypercortisolism begins with a 24-hour urine collection for cortisol excretion. If urinary cortisol excretion is not unequivocally increased, the measurement of serum or salivary cortisol late in the evening is a reliable means of clarifying the diagnosis. In the past, the overnight dexamethasone suppression test was widely used for screening; however, this test is limited by a reduced sensitivity in patients with mild disease.

After hypercortisolism is discovered, the cause must be determined. Most cases of endogenous hypercortisolism are the result of excessive secretion of ACTH by a pituitary tumor. Other causes include adrenal tumors and ACTH production from nonpituitary tumors, the most common of which are oat cell carcinoma of the lung, carcinoid, gastrinoma, malignant thymomas, pheochromocytomas, and medullary carcinoma of the thyroid. The treatment of hypercortisolism depends on the detection and correction of the underlying cause.

Insufficient Glucocorticoid Activity (Addison's Disease)

Adrenal insufficiency may result from a number of processes that cause atrophy or extensive destruction of these glands.

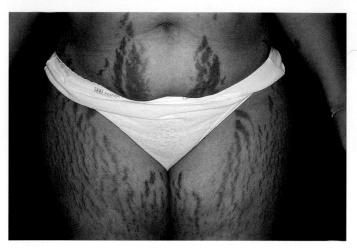

Figure 23–1 Striae in a patient with Cushing's syndrome.

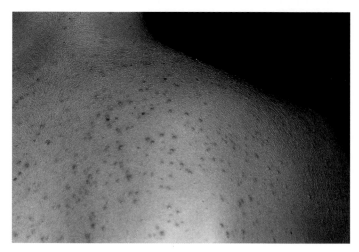

Figure 23–2 Steroid-induced acne in an adolescent male with iatrogenic Cushing's syndrome.

Prolonged administration of synthetic glucocorticoids with subsequent discontinuation is by far the most common cause of adrenal insufficiency. Other major causes include autoimmune adrenalitis (more common in women and whites), infections (primarily tuberculosis and deep fungal infections), and metastatic disease. Less common causes include drugs and hemorrhage. The systemic antifungal medication ketoconazole inhibits steroidogenesis, but only rarely causes clinical hypocortisolism. Other medications that inhibit cortisol biosynthesis include the antiepileptic drug aminoglutethimide, the anesthetic–sedative drug etomidate, and the antiparasitic drug suramin.

The clinical manifestations of this condition are exceedingly diverse. Constitutional symptoms include malaise, reduced energy, weight loss, and a feeling of ill health. Other systemic manifestations are hypotension, weakness and fatigue, gastrointestinal symptoms (anorexia, nausea, and abdominal pain), and psychiatric symptoms.

The primary dermatological manifestation is hyperpigmentation of the skin and mucous membranes (Fig. 23–3). The hyperpigmentation of adrenal insufficiency is induced by high levels of ACTH (and melanocyte-stimulating hormone), which

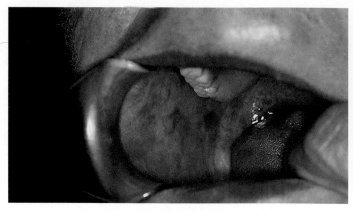

Figure 23–3 Pigmented macules on the buccal mucosa and lips in Addison's disease.

result from primary adrenal failure. Hyperpigmentation is therefore not present in hypocortisolism secondary to pituitary failure. Because adrenal insufficiency often has an insidious onset, the increased pigmentation may go unnoticed by the patient. The areas commonly involved include sun-exposed areas, the skin over the joints, old scars, the axillae, the perineum, and the nipples. Darkening of the palmar creases is considered a nearly specific sign for adrenal insufficiency in whites. Pigmentation of the tongue is another useful sign. The hair may become darker, and pigmented longitudinal bands may develop on the nails. New nevi can appear and old nevi darken.

Adrenal insufficiency is associated with other skin manifestations as a part of polyglandular autoimmune syndrome type I (chronic mucocutaneous candidiasis) and type II (vitiligo). A rare manifestation of adrenal insufficiency is fibrosis and calcification of the ear cartilage.

The laboratory abnormalities seen in adrenal insufficiency include hyponatremia and hyperkalemia. Screening for adrenal insufficiency includes two tests: basal plasma ACTH level, and cortisol level 30 minutes after an ACTH stimulation test. Primary adrenal insufficiency manifests as a high basal ACTH combined with a blunted cortisol response to the ACTH stimulation test. Low cortisol and low basal ACTH levels suggest either secondary (i.e., pituitary) or tertiary (i.e., hypothalamic) adrenal insufficiency; in this instance, a corticotropin-releasing hormone (CRH) stimulation test is necessary to distinguish between the two etiologies. After the diagnosis of hypocortisolemia is determined, the cause of adrenal failure must be found.

The treatment of adrenal insufficiency is long-term replacement of glucocorticoids. Prednisone and dexamethasone have replaced shorter-acting agents such as cortisone or hydrocortisone because the longer duration of action provides a smoother physiologic effect. Mineralocorticoid replacement can be achieved with fludrocortisone. In times of physiologic stress induced by illness or surgery, glucocorticoid replacement must be increased.

Pheochromocytoma

Pheochromocytoma is a catecholamine-producing tumor arising from chromaffin cells of the sympathetic nervous system. The majority of pheochromocytomas develop in the medulla of one or both adrenal glands. Other sites of origin include para-aortic sympathetic ganglia, the walls of the urinary bladder, the chest, and, extremely rarely, sympathetic tissue in association with intracranial branches of the vagus nerve. There are inherited disorders with associated pheochromocytomas, including neurofibromatosis and Sipple's syndrome. More than 90% of the tumors are benign, and they occur most frequently during the fourth and fifth decades of life.

The most distinctive clinical feature of pheochromocytoma is hypertension, although the tumors account for less than 0.1% of patients with diastolic hypertension. The hypertension is usually paroxysmal and occurs in association with palpitations, tachycardia, a feeling of apprehension, and sweating. These symptoms can be reproduced experimentally by the injection of norepinephrine (noradrenaline) and epinephrine (adrenaline). These episodes may occur at weekly intervals or as frequently as 20 times a day, and may be precipitated by emotional upset, eating, and exercise, and especially by activities that compress the tumor (such as bending). The only significant cutaneous manifestation of pheochromocytoma is flushing, which appears to occur primarily when the tumor secretes larger amounts of epinephrine than norepinephrine. The flushing occurs paroxysmally and is most prominent on the face, chest, and upper extremities. In addition, pheochromocytomas may complicate the course of patients with neurofibromatosis. In some patients with hypertension, recognition of the café-au-lait spots led to the appropriate diagnosis.

The diagnosis of pheochromocytoma can be established by assaying catecholamine levels and their metabolites in the plasma or urine, especially during paroxysmal attacks. In patients in whom the episodes are very brief, establishing the diagnosis becomes much more challenging, and, occasionally, diagnostic inducement of attacks with intravenous glucagon or histamine is performed. Treatment involves the use of adrenergic antagonists, such as phentolamine and phenoxybenzamine, and surgical removal of the tumors.

ANDROGEN-RELATED DISORDERS

Excess Androgen Activity

Excess androgen activity is reflected in precocious puberty in children and degrees of virilization in women; men are asymptomatic. In women, the cutaneous signs of virilization include hirsutism, acne, and androgenic alopecia; these may have devastating psychosocial consequences. Some increase in androgen levels in women at adolescence is normal, however, and is responsible for the development of axillary and pubic hair.

Hirsutism is defined relative to cultural and environmental norms as more facial and body hair than is considered acceptable. It is a common complaint, with a prevalence estimated to be as high as one-third of menstruating and 75% of postmenopausal women. Objective measurement of hirsutism is possible using the Ferriman–Gallwey scale (Fig. 23–4), which quantifies the extent of hair growth in androgen-dependent areas. Using this scale, mild hirsutism is defined by a score of 8–15; >15 is considered moderate or severe. Hirsutism occurring in the absence of increased androgens is termed idiopathic

hirsutism. This must be distinguished from hypertrichosis, which is generalized excess hair growth not limited to androgen-sensitive sites. Hirsutism may or may not be associated with other signs of virilization, including worsening acne, male-pattern alopecia, and menstrual irregularity.

Acne vulgaris is a common disorder. Nevertheless, some authors recommend an evaluation of androgen levels in all women with acne; others disagree. Most women exhibit a degree of scalp hair loss over time, generally in the form of hairline recession. More extensive alopecia, with marked thinning of hair on the central scalp, may be associated with androgen excess.

Androgen excess may be caused by a wide variety of conditions of both adrenal and ovarian origin. These include adrenal tumors, Cushing's syndrome, congenital (or late-onset) adrenal hyperplasia (discussed later), polycystic ovaries, ovarian tumors, ovarian hyperplasias, and other nonadrenal, nonovarian neoplasms. Adrenal androgens include androstenedione, testosterone, dehydroepiandrosterone (DHEA), and DHEA sulfate (DHEAS). Androstenedione and testosterone are also produced by the ovaries.

In patients with mild hirsutism and regular menses who lack any further signs to suggest androgen excess, laboratory testing may not be necessary given the high likelihood that the hirsutism is idiopathic. If hirsutism is moderate or severe or there are features of a secondary cause, then testing for androgen levels is essential. Testing for plasma free testosterone, the bioactive portion of plasma testosterone, is more sensitive than testing for total testosterone. Testosterone is bound to albumin by sex hormone-binding globulin, low levels of which may result in an elevated plasma free testosterone level despite a normal total testosterone. Routine testing for other androgens is of little use. If a neoplasm is suspected, ultrasonographic evaluation of the adrenal glands, ovaries, or both may be useful.

An abrupt onset of signs of virilization, DHEAS levels > 700 ng/dL, and free testosterone levels > 200 ng/dL suggest an androgen-producing tumor. Patients with polycystic ovary syndrome have elevated androgen levels associated with elevated luteinizing hormone (LH) levels and lower than expected follicle-stimulating hormone (FSH) concentrations; the LH:FSH ratio is high. The laboratory investigation of congenital adrenal hyperplasia is discussed later.

The treatment of these signs of elevated androgens is multifaceted. The most common approach includes cosmetic and physical measures. Hirsutism may be treated by bleaching; by temporary hair removal mechanisms, such as shaving, plucking or waxing, or depilatory creams (these do not cause thickening or increase the growth of hair); by the hair growth inhibitor eflornithine hydrochloride cream; by laser therapy (most effective in women with lightly pigmented skin and dark terminal hairs); or by the permanent hair removal method of electrolysis.

Systemic treatment may include estrogen–progestin oral contraceptives, antiandrogens, glucocorticoids, and other hormonal therapies. Oral contraceptives can arrest the progression of hirsutism from various causes and reduce by half the need for shaving; contraceptives with nonandrogenic progestins are preferred. Substantial reduction of hirsutism requires the use of antiandrogens. Spironolactone is the first choice; it is started

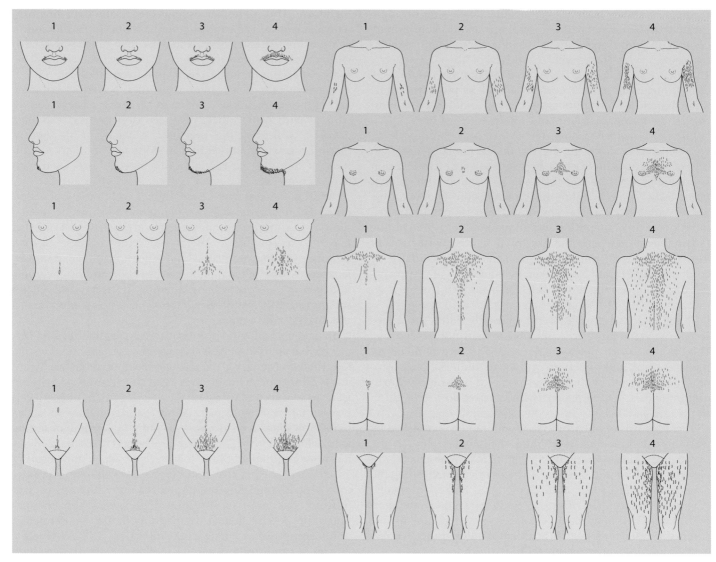

Figure 23–4 The Ferriman–Gallwey scoring system for hirsutism. (Reproduced with permission from Hatch R, Rosenfield RL, Kim MH, Tredway D. Hirsutism: implications, etiology, and management. Am J Obstet Gynecol 1981; 140: 815–830.)

at 75–100 mg/day in two divided doses. Hydration must be maintained, and patients with risk factors for hyperkalemia must be closely monitored. There may be troublesome increases in menstrual bleeding. Other androgen antagonists include cyproterone acetate and flutamide. Flutamide is rarely used for hirsutism because of its risk for hepatotoxicity. Prednisone therapy at bedtime doses of 5–7.5 mg may improve hirsutism but is associated with serious side effects. The 5α-reductase inhibitor finasteride may be beneficial. In addition to the above therapeutic options, psychosocial support is an important aspect of treatment.

Deficient Androgen Activity

The cutaneous manifestations of androgen deficiency depend on the age at onset of the deficiency, because maintenance of sexual hair is less dependent on androgen than is the development of sexual hair. If androgen deficiency occurs prior to puberty, the development of sexual hair and sebaceous and

apocrine glands will be limited. Acne and androgenic alopecia do not occur. The skin shows pallor, the penis is small, the scrotum is smooth, and fine wrinkling occurs around the eyes and lips. There is poor muscular development, and delayed closure of the epiphyses results in increased height.

With the development of androgen deficiency after puberty, sexual hair remains present but grows slowly. The sebaceous glands atrophy, and acne will improve or clear. Vasomotor phenomena (hot flashes) may occur. All the cutaneous manifestations of androgen deficiency are reversible with replacement therapy.

Adrenogenital Syndromes

Adrenogenital syndromes result from genetically determined defects in the synthesis of cortisol. An increase in ACTH production occurs because of the deficiency in cortisol production; the increased adrenal stimulation from increased ACTH levels combined with the blockade in the cortisol production pathway results in massive accumulation of adrenal androgens. This causes virilization in women and sexual precocity in males. Some of the genetic defects are associated with salt wasting and early death. 'Partial' 21-hydroxylase deficiency can present with hirsutism, even in older women.

These conditions can be diagnosed by the finding of increased levels of steroid precursors and androgens and reduced levels of cortisol. The plasma 17-hydroxyprogesterone level is measured before and after ACTH administration to detect patients with partial 21-hydroxylase deficiency. The treatment is glucocorticoid administration to suppress completely the ACTH secretion initially, followed by maintenance doses that control the level of cortisol precursors. Surgery may be required to match the phenotypic sexual characteristics to the genotypic sex; psychosocial support is another important facet of treatment of this condition.

DISORDERS OF STEROID HORMONE RECEPTORS

Receptors for glucocorticoids, androgens, and other steroid hormones form a family of related proteins. These receptors contain a domain responsible for steroid hormone binding and a domain responsible for DNA binding and effector function. Genetic defects in both the glucocorticoid and androgen receptors have been described.

In male patients with familial glucocorticoid resistance, cutaneous findings have not been described; female patients may develop hirsutism, androgenic alopecia, and menstrual abnormalities. Both sexes have hypercortisolism and elevated ACTH levels without other features associated with Cushing's syndrome. Laboratory abnormalities may also include hypertension and hypokalemic acidosis. The virilization is the result of elevated adrenal androgen levels secondary to chronic ACTH overstimulation. The treatment is dexamethasone, which normalizes the ACTH, cortisol, and androgen levels without excessive mineralocorticoid stimulation.

Androgen insensitivity syndrome is asymptomatic in female carriers. Genotypic male patients may have involvement from subtle (infertility and azoospermia) to profound (a female phenotype); the latter has been termed the testicular feminization syndrome. The cutaneous manifestations in these patients include an absence of acne or androgenic alopecia, and sparse development of sexual hair. Mild cases of androgen insensitivity can be treated with surgical repair of hypospadias if present, and supplementation of androgens; in severe cases, patients may be best treated by considering them as infertile females and removing the abdominal gonads to prevent the development of gonadal malignancy.

PITUITARY DISORDERS WITH CUTANEOUS MANIFESTATIONS

Hyperpituitarism (Acromegaly)

Acromegaly results from hypersecretion of growth hormone by a pituitary tumor or by hyperplasia of the eosinophil cells of the anterior pituitary. The term gigantism refers to the same process, but this occurs in prepubertal children before fusion of the epiphyses, resulting in excessively tall stature. Hyperpituitarism occurs more commonly in adults and leads to exaggerated growth of acral parts, especially the head, hands, and feet, although the excess growth hormone affects all organs and tissues. The onset of acromegaly is usually insidious, and even before the changes in appearance are noticed, patients may complain of arthralgias, hyperhidrosis, pain, paresthesias of the slowly expanding fingers and toes, headache, and loss of libido.

The clinical picture of well-developed acromegaly is easily recognized by physical examination. The skin is thickened and doughy, owing to an increase in connective tissue and to interstitial fluid. The skin pores are usually prominent. The skin of the face is oily as a result of increased sebum production, and there is an increase in both apocrine and eccrine sweating. Early in the course of the disease there may be an increase in body and scalp hair, and the hair is coarse. Additional cutaneous findings in some patients include acanthosis nigricans, hyperpigmentation, and a variety of nail changes. The face is often elongated, and there may be furrowing of the brow with accentuation of the skin folds. Macroglossia is present, and the enlarged nose is often triangular. One of the key diagnostic features is enlargement of the hands, and patients often note a significant increase in ring and glove sizes.

Systemic findings in acromegaly include organomegaly (e.g., liver, spleen, heart, thyroid, and kidneys); nerve entrapment, which may lead to the carpal tunnel syndrome; visual impairment; hypertension; insulin resistance and diabetes mellitus; and galactorrhea. The course is extremely variable and may be fulminant, leading to death in a matter of a few years, or benign, lasting 50 years or longer. The diagnosis involves an evaluation of both growth hormone levels and growth hormone-dependent circulating molecules IGF-1 and IGFBP-3. Once growth hormone hypersecretion has been confirmed, magnetic resonance imaging of the pituitary is recommended. The treatment may include surgery, pituitary radiation, or medical management. Long-acting somatostatin analogs comprise the first line of medical therapy. Dopamine agonists and growth hormone receptor antagonists may also be beneficial.

Hypopituitarism

Hypopituitarism may manifest as an isolated deficiency of one or many anterior pituitary hormones, resulting in secondary atrophy of the gonads, thyroid, and adrenal cortex. Panhypopituitarism (Simmonds' disease) implies total absence of all known pituitary hormones, including growth hormone, thyrotropin, prolactin, corticotropin, and two gonadotropins (FSH and LH). The most common cause of hypopituitarism in adult life is chromophobe adenoma. Other tumors, infections (syphilis or tuberculosis), sarcoidosis, basal skull fracture, infarcts (postpartum necrosis of Sheehan), and a variety of other disorders may disrupt the normal function of the gland and lead to hypopituitarism.

The endocrine manifestations of hypopituitarism vary with the type, age of development, and degree of hormonal deficiency. At least 75% of the gland must be destroyed before the wide variety of signs and symptoms become clinically manifest. Cutaneous changes may be the first clue to the diagnosis. The skin and subcutaneous tissues are thin, body hair is scant, and the skin is usually pale or yellowish in color. Signs of hypothyroidism may be evident, and there may be symptoms of gonadotropin deficiency, especially a reduction in libido.

After the diagnosis has been established by appropriate laboratory studies, the treatment includes the replacement of a variety of hormones.

SUGGESTED READINGS

Feingold KR, Elias PM. Endocrine-skin interactions. J Am Acad Dermatol 1988; 19: 1–20.

Jabbour SA, Miller JL. Review article: endocrinopathies and the skin. Int J Dermatol 2000; 39: 88–99.

Melmed MB. Acromegaly. N Engl J Med 2006; 355: 2558–2573.

Moghetti P, Tocsano V. Treatment of hirsutism and acne in hyperandrogenism. Best Pract Res Clin Endocrinol Metab 2006; 20: 221–234.

Niemann LK, Chanco Turner ML. Addison's disease. Clin Dermatol 2006; 24: 276–280.

Rosenfield RL. Hirsutism. N Engl J Med 2005; 353: 2578–2588.

Shibli-Rahhal A, Van Beek M, Schlechte JA. Cushing's syndrome. Clin Dermatol 2006; 24: 260–265.

Chapter 24

Julia R. Nunley,
Marc E. Grossman,
and Warren W. Piette

Porphyrias

The porphyrias (Table 24–1) are a heterogeneous group of inherited or acquired disorders, each characterized by a partial deficiency of a specific enzyme in the heme biosynthetic pathway (Fig. 24–1). Porphyria cutanea tarda (PCT), the most common disorder of porphyrin metabolism in Europe and North America, will be the major focus of this chapter. Erythropoietic protoporphyria (EPP), as well as the other less common cutaneous porphyrias, will be briefly discussed. The clinical expression of the porphyrias is variable for most of the syndromes, suggesting a strong interplay between genetic inheritance and environmental exposures. Except for the very rare syndrome of X-linked sideroblastic anemia, phenotypic expression of the porphyrias occurs either as episodic neurovisceral disease, chronic photosensitivity, or both (Fig. 24–1).

Normal heme biosynthesis, which takes place in the bone marrow and liver, begins with the formation of δ-aminolevulinic acid (ALA) catalyzed by the rate-limiting enzyme of hepatic heme synthesis, ALA synthetase. Two molecules of ALA combine to form porphobilinogen (PBG); four molecules of PBG are converted to uroporphyrinogen III. Four decarboxylations of uroporphyrinogen I or III, catalyzed by uroporphyrinogen decarboxylase (UPG-D, which is reduced in patients with PCT and with hepatoerythropoietic porphyria), result in coproporphyrinogen. Subsequently, protoporphyrinogen and protoporphyrin are synthesized. Ferrochelatase (reduced in EPP, variegate porphyria, and lead poisoning) is the final enzyme required for the conversion of protoporphyrin to heme, and may be the rate-limiting enzyme for bone marrow heme synthesis.

In cases of porphyria, each enzyme deficiency results in accumulation of the substrate of that specific enzyme and other precursors. These excess porphyrins can be found in the urine, feces, or erythrocytes (Table 24–2). Irreversible nonenzymatic oxidation of these colorless, nonphotoactive heme precursor porphyrinogens to the corresponding photoactive porphyrin byproducts then occurs. The porphyrins are capable of absorbing light energy maximally in the 400–410-nm wavelength (Soret band). These wavelengths penetrate human epidermis; therefore, porphyrins present in the skin become unstable excited-state molecules that mediate oxidative damage. Cutaneous photosensitivity and its symptoms result when the absorbed energy is released by lipid peroxidation and/or complement activation, with the destruction of cell membrane integrity and leakage of cellular contents. Although the pathogenesis of the inherited porphyrias has been defined at the molecular level, there remains a great heterogeneity of clinical expression with each porphyria.

PORPHYRIA CUTANEA TARDA

PCT, first described by Waldenström in 1937, is the most common disorder of porphyrin metabolism. The disease is a photocutaneous syndrome classified as a hepatic porphyria because the overproduction of porphyrins occurs in the liver. The primary defect in PCT is reduced activity of the enzyme UPG-D.

Pathogenesis

In normal heme biosynthesis, UPG-D affects the sequential decarboxylation from uroporphyrinogen (8-carboxylic side groups) to coproporphyrinogen (4-carboxylic side groups). Reduced levels of UPG-D result in large increases in uroporphyrin and smaller increases in coproporphyrin in urine and plasma and produce isocoproporphyrin, an unusual 4-carboxylic porphyrin, in feces.

PCT is the only porphyrin disorder with both a familial and an acquired (sporadic) form. The less common familial form, inherited as an autosomal dominant trait, is characterized by heterozygous gene expression for UPG-D, resulting in a partial enzyme deficiency (usually 50% reduced activity). Homozygous inheritance of the genetic defect results in UPG-D enzyme activity that is less than 10% of normal and produces the more severe condition hepatoerythropoietic porphyria (HEP). Many different gene mutations have been described, and many clinical cases, phenotypically identical to HEP, are actually heteroallelic, with a different mutated allele inherited from each parent. The gene locus for UPG-D has been assigned to the short arm of human chromosome 1.

In familial PCT, UPG-D deficiency is present in both erythrocytes and hepatocytes, whereas in the more common acquired form only the hepatocytes have diminished

217

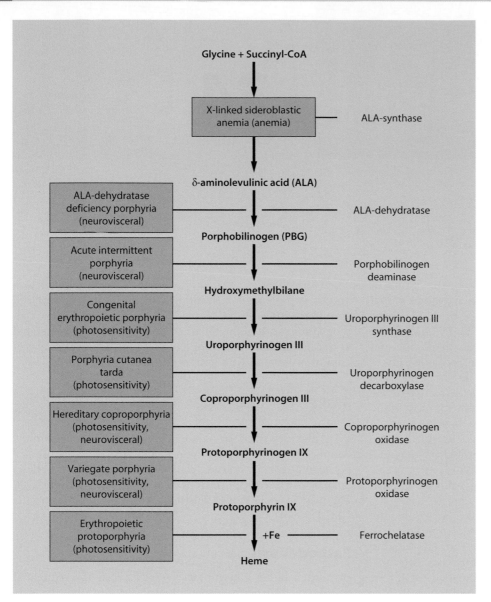

Figure 24–1 Heme biosynthetic pathway.

Table 24–1 The porphyrias

	Cutaneous disease	Neurovisceral disease	Cutaneous and neurovisceral disease
Hepatic	Porphyria cutanea tarda Hepatoerythropoietic porphyria	Acute intermittent porphyria δ-Aminolevulinic acid dehydrogenase deficiency	Hereditary coproporphyria Variegate porphyria
Erythropoietic	Hepatoerythropoietic porphyria		Congenital erythropoietic porphyria Erythropoietic protoporphyria

enzymatic activity. In the past, true cases of acquired PCT were probably missed because erythrocyte UPG-D activity was used as the diagnostic test.

Clinical Manifestations

PCT usually presents with characteristic cutaneous features that suggest the diagnosis. Lesions occur predominantly in sun-exposed areas, most frequently on the dorsal hands (Fig. 24–2), although in women the legs, feet, and chest (Fig. 24–3) may be affected. Vesicles and bullae are the most common primary lesions and vary in size from 2 mm to 3 cm (Fig. 24–4). They can be flaccid or tense and contain straw-colored, pink, or hemorrhagic fluid. Blisters may not be noticed by the patient, who instead complains of increased skin fragility. Again, this is most often noted on the dorsa of the hands

Table 24-2 Characteristic biochemical findings in the porphyrias

Type of porphyria	Urine				Feces			Erythrocytes			Plasma
	ALA	PBG	URO	COPRO	URO	COPRO	PROTO	URO	COPRO	PROTO	
Acute porphyrias											
Acute intermittent porphyria	++ to ++++	++ to ++++	+++	++	N to +	N to –	N to +	N	N	N	N
Variegate porphyria	++ to +++	++ to +++	+++	+++	N	+++	++++	N	N	N	N
Hereditary coproporphyria	N to ++	N to ++	++	++++	++	++++	N to +	N	N	N	N
ALA-D deficiency porphyria	+++	N	+	++	N	+	+	N	N	++	ALA, COPRO & PROTO ↑
Non-acute porphyrias											
Porphyria cutanea tarda	N	N	++++	++	++	ISOCOPRO	+	N	N	N	URO ↑
Erythropoietic protoporphyria	N	N	N	N	N	++	++ to ++++	N	N to +	++++	PROTO ↑
Congenital erythropoietic porphyria	N	N	++++	++	+	+++	+	++++	+++	+++	URO & COPRO ↑
Hepatoerythropoietic porphyria	N	N	+++	ISOCOPRO	N	ISOCOPRO	N	N	+	++++	URO ↑

ALA-D = aminolevulinic acid dehydratase; N = normal; + = above normal range; ++ = slightly elevated; +++ = highly elevated; ++++ = very highly elevated; ↑ = increased. ALA = δ-aminolevulinic acid; PBG = porphobilinogen; URO = uroporphyrin; COPRO = coproporphyrin; PROTO = protoporphyrin; ISOCOPRO = isocoproporphyrin.
Courtesy of Frank J, Poblete-Gutiérrez P. Porphyria. In: Bolognia JL, Jorizzo JL, Rapini RP, eds. Dermatology, 2nd edn. London: Mosby, 2008.

219

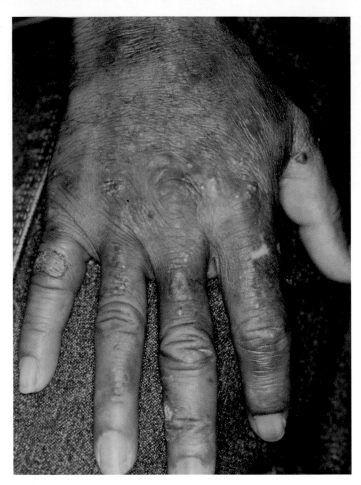

Figure 24–2 Vesicles, bullae, crusts, and milia on the dorsal hand.

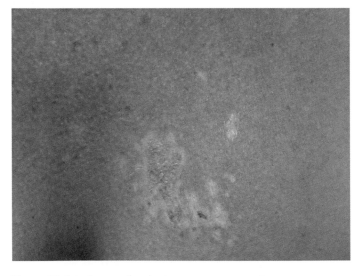

Figure 24–3 Lesions on the chest are more common in women.

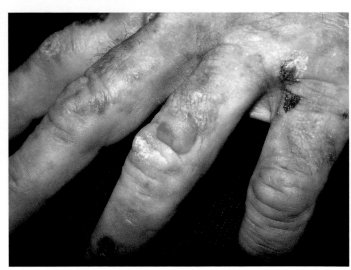

Figure 24–4 At times large bullae may be seen in porphyria cutanea tarda.

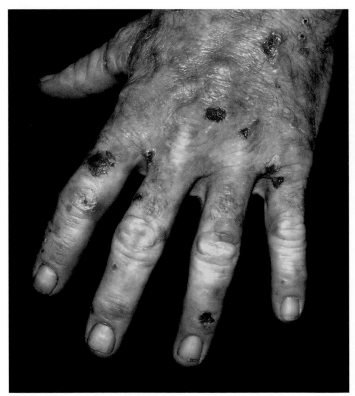

Figure 24–5 Significant erosions may develop as a result of increased skin fragility.

and forearms, areas subject to repeated trauma (Fig. 24–5). After minor trauma the skin shears away, leaving sharply marginated eroded areas. Most patients do not associate sun exposure with the development of skin lesions, despite their localization to sun-exposed areas.

Facial hypertrichosis, more noticeable in women, is a striking sign, and at times may be the presenting complaint (Fig. 24–6). Hyperpigmentation, developing as a mottled brown-black pigmentation in the periorbital and malar regions of the face, mimics melasma. Rarely, melanosis is so widespread that it simulates Addison's disease or hemochromatosis.

Repeated episodes of blistering often heal with scarring and milia formation (Fig. 24–7). Patients with active PCT often

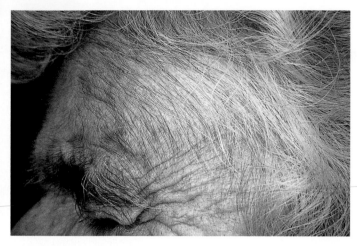

Figure 24–6 Facial hypertrichosis in a man with porphyria cutanea tarda.

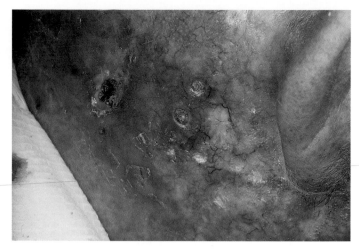

Figure 24–8 Sclerodermoid changes in a patient with porphyria cutanea tarda.

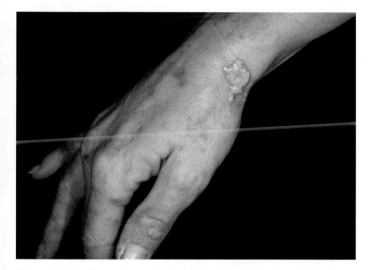

Figure 24–7 Milia en plaque in a patient with porphyria cutanea tarda.

exhibit lesions in all stages of development and involution simultaneously (Fig. 24–2). A distinctive scarring alopecia with saucer-shaped scars or crater-like depressions (Fig. 24–8) can occur in areas of repeated blistering. Dystrophic calcification and nonhealing preauricular ulcers are characteristic of PCT. Calcification also occurs on the scalp, neck, and dorsal aspect of the hands.

Scleroderma-like changes can develop in patients with PCT and may be the sole cutaneous finding. These hypopigmented pale-yellow plaques are histopathologically indistinguishable from scleroderma. Curiously, they are not limited to the sun-exposed areas and may occur on covered areas such as the back and chest.

Whereas PCT occurs predominantly in adults, HEP presents in childhood. With its severe mutilating photodestructive lesions, HEP is clinically indistinguishable from congenital erythropoietic porphyria (CEP).

Etiologic Associations

Exposure to a number of factors can trigger the onset of PCT, including alcohol ingestion, estrogen therapy, iron overload, and environmental or occupational exposure to hepatotoxic polychlorinated aromatic hydrocarbons. PCT is also seen in association with other diseases such as hemochromatosis, lupus erythematosus, infiltrating hepatic tumors, and granulomatous hepatitis due to sarcoidosis. Conditions and triggers associated with PCT are listed in Table 24–3.

The link between PCT and hepatitis C viral infection (HCV) is now firm. However, the incidence of PCT associated with HCV varies significantly with the prevalence of HCV in a geographic region, and possibly with the prevalence of the hemochromatosis gene. Thus, the percentage of PCT patients with HCV is 70–90% in southern Europe, 56% in the United States, but only 20% in northern Europe, Australia, and New Zealand, where HCV is less prevalent and the hemochromatosis gene mutation is more prevalent. The High Fe (HFE) gene for hemochromatosis has two distinct mutations (C282Y and H63D), both associated with iron overload. Almost 40% of PCT patients of northern European origin carry one or more alleles for hemochromatosis. However, iron overload, even in the absence of hemochromatosis, is common in PCT and further enhances the expression of PCT. Hepatic iron alone may worsen liver injury and hasten fibrosis or cirrhosis.

PCT has been associated with other infections and systemic diseases (Table 24–3), including human immunodeficiency virus (HIV) infection. Diabetes mellitus or glucose intolerance occurs in 18–33% of patients with PCT, an incidence three to six times higher than that in the normal population. Chronic cutaneous, subacute cutaneous, and systemic lupus erythematosus have each been described with PCT. Often the association is recognized only after the initiation of antimalarial therapy, as a treatment for lupus, precipitates the porphyria. Various theories exist regarding the coexistence of these conditions, ranging from a possible genetic linkage to porphyrin-induced photosensitivity triggering lupus.

Hepatocellular carcinoma occurs with increased frequency in patients with PCT, even in the absence of other risk factors. A hepatic malignancy should be screened for in all individuals with PCT if they present over the age of 60, or if they have HCV, cirrhosis, atypical urinary porphyrins, an unexplained

Table 24–3 Conditions and trigger factors associated with PCT
Alcohol ingestion

Medications
   Estrogen therapy
   Antimalarials
   Phenytoin

Polychlorinated aromatic hydrocarbons
Iron overload
Hemochromatosis (homozygous or heterozygous)
Hepatitis C
Human immunodeficiency virus
Cytomegalovirus
Diabetes mellitus
Hepatic sarcoidosis
Chronic kidney disease

Hepatic tumors
   Primary
   Metastatic

Lupus erythematosus
   Chronic cutaneous
   Subacute cutaneous
   Systemic

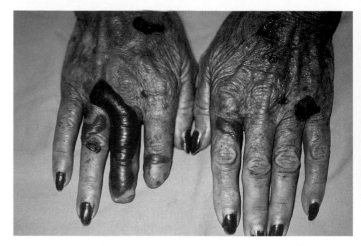

Figure 24–9 Pseudoporphyria in a patient with chronic renal failure. This condition is also known as bullous dermatosis of renal failure.

exacerbation of previously quiescent disease, or if the usual precipitating factors are absent.

Evaluation

Laboratory confirmation of PCT begins with examination of the urine. When present in large quantities, porphyrins give the urine a red or brown color. Using a Wood's light, excess urinary porphyrins can be visualized owing to their fluorescence, which can be intensified with acidification. The diagnosis is confirmed by quantitative porphyrin analysis from a 24-hour urinary collection, which will reveal elevated levels of uro- and coproporphyrin, the former elevated several times more than the latter. The same porphyrins in a similar ratio will be elevated in the plasma. In the stool there is a greater excretion of copro- than uroporphyrin, and increased levels of isocoproporphyrin are detected. Laboratory evaluation should also include a hemogram; iron studies, including serum ferritin; liver function tests; as well as hepatitis and HIV serologies, if risk factors exist. Under special circumstances patients may need an antinuclear antibody test, a 5-hour glucose tolerance test, a liver–spleen scan, and a liver biopsy. Measurement of serum α-fetoprotein may be useful to screen for hepatocellular carcinoma. Because of the association between the hemochromatosis gene, iron overload, and PCT, it is prudent to look for the HFE gene mutations, especially in populations where these mutations are more prevalent.

Although skin biopsy findings can be consistent with PCT, they are not diagnostic. Similar findings are seen in other cutaneous porphyrias, pseudoporphyria, and some primary blistering disorders.

Differential Diagnosis

The various photocutaneous changes of PCT may also occur in patients with HEP, hereditary coproporphyria (HCP), variegate porphyria (VP), and also chronic kidney disease, or in those on hemodialysis (Fig. 24–9). The vesiculobullous component of PCT may be mimicked by epidermolysis bullosa acquisita, bullous amyloidosis, bullous lupus, and reactions to various medications. The occurrence of cutaneous lesions that closely mimic PCT with no biochemical abnormality in porphyrin metabolism has been called pseudoporphyria. Although most cases can be attributed to nonsteroidal anti-inflammatory drugs (NSAIDs), tetracyclines, and furosemide, many other medications have also been implicated (Table 24–4). Lastly, the use of photodynamic therapy can at times result in a temporary PCT-like disease.

Treatment

The treatment of PCT begins with the elimination of alcohol, estrogen, or iron and with avoidance of environmental toxins that might have triggered the disease. Sun avoidance and protection are crucial; patients should be advised that sunscreens alone may not be adequate.

Phlebotomy is the most effective and most commonly used therapy. It can be performed as an outpatient procedure in otherwise healthy patients by removing 1 unit of blood weekly or biweekly, until either the total urinary porphyrin content begins to diminish or the hemoglobin level decreases to 10 g/dL. Clinical improvement occurs in a delayed fashion, beginning 3–6 months after the initiation of phlebotomy. Blistering disappears first, followed by an improvement in cutaneous fragility. Facial hypertrichosis and hyperpigmentation clear more slowly. Sclerodermoid changes do not seem to be improved by phlebotomy.

Phlebotomy may be contraindicated in patients with coronary artery disease, pulmonary disease, or pre-existing anemia, or in those with poor venous access. Treatment with low-dose oral antimalarials may be an alternative. Hydroxychloroquine sulfate (200 mg) or chloroquine phosphate (125–250 mg)

Table 24–4 Medications associated with pseudoporphyria

Anti-infectives
   β-Lactams
   Nalidixic acid
   Tetracyclines
   Voriconazole

Diuretics
   Chlorthalidone
   Bumetanide
   Furosemide
   Hydrochlorothiazide/triamterene

Nonsteroidal anti-inflammatory agents
   Diflunisal
   Ketoprofen
   Nabumetone
   Naproxen
   Oxaprozin

Retinoids
   Etretinate
   Isotretinoin

Miscellaneous
   Amiodarone
   Cyclosporine
   5-Fluorouracil
   Flutamide
   Dapsone
   Pyridoxine

may be given in low doses once or twice per week to avoid acute toxicity (manifested as fever, malaise, abdominal pain, nausea, vomiting, and marked elevation of hepatocellular enzymes) caused by rapid flushing of porphyrins from the liver. The dose may be escalated cautiously.

Plasmapheresis, cholestyramine, vitamin E, metabolic alkalinization, and iron chelators have been used with varying success in PCT. Erythropoietin in conjunction with phlebotomy may be effective for patients with significant anemia, including those on hemodialysis. Cases of hemodialysis-associated pseudoporphyria have also been successfully treated with oral *N*-acetylcysteine. For those with HCV, iron overload should first be addressed by phlebotomy; patients should subsequently be considered for treatment with interferon–ribavirin regimens. PCT may remit with treatment for HCV; however, there are reports of interferon exacerbating PCT.

ERYTHROPOIETIC PROTOPORPHYRIA

EPP, the most common childhood porphyria, was not characterized until 1961. Reduced activity of the enzyme ferrochelatase results in an accumulation of protoporphyrin, particularly in circulating red blood cells. Inheritance is autosomal dominant, but evidence suggests that coinheritance of an additional partial mutation of the ferrochelatase gene may partly explain the marked variability of disease expression between patients. Over 125 genetic mutations have been identified. Family studies show that fewer than 10% of gene carriers have clinically overt disease.

Clinical Manifestations

The cutaneous manifestations of EPP begin in childhood with acute photosensitivity. Patients complain of burning and pruritus within minutes to hours of sun exposure; subjective symptoms precede the development of photodistributed erythema and edema. Chronic sun exposure causes a thickened, weather-beaten, or cobblestone appearance, especially over the knuckles. A waxy thickening of the skin is also described. Perioral rhagades and shallow elliptic scars on the face are characteristic. Histopathologic examination of skin biopsy specimens reveals the deposition of an amorphous hyaline-like material around the capillaries and scattered throughout the dermis. Albeit less common, prolonged or intense sun exposure may result in vesicles and crusting over the bridge of the nose, cheeks, lips, and dorsal aspects of the hands.

The systemic manifestations of EPP include anemia, gallstones, and liver disease, ranging from benign cholestasis to fatal hepatic failure.

Diagnosis

The diagnosis is based on the demonstration of abnormal levels of protoporphyrin in red blood cells, plasma, and stool. Because protoporphyrin is not water soluble, urinary porphyrins in patients with EPP are not increased. All material collected for laboratory analysis must be completely protected from light to avoid photo-inactivation of protoporphyrin and erroneous results.

Treatment

Avoidance of sunlight and sun-protective clothing are helpful in managing these patients. Sunscreens are of limited benefit, but should be used.

The most effective treatment for the cutaneous symptoms of EPP is oral β-carotene given in doses of 60–300 mg/day. Increased solar tolerance develops slowly over 1–2 months. The photoprotective effect of β-carotene can be attributed to the quenching of excited molecules, such as singlet oxygen. The only side effect, other than mild gastrointestinal distress, is a visible yellowing of the skin from carotenoderma. β-Carotene does not affect the level of protoporphyrin. However, cholestyramine can diminish enterohepatic recirculation of porphyrins, thereby reducing photosensitivity and hepatic protoporphyrin content. Rare severe hepatic complications have required liver transplantation.

CONGENITAL ERYTHROPOIETIC PORPHYRIA

Congenital erythropoietic porphyria inheritance is as a recessive trait. Although milder variants have been described with adult-onset disease, this very rare condition usually presents in childhood with severe burning and blistering and, ultimately, with scarring and mutilation of light-exposed skin and mucous membranes. Pink or red-brown staining of diapers due to high urinary porphyrins may be the first clue to the diagnosis. Hypertrichosis of the face and extremities is often prominent, along with skin thickening and dyspigmentation. Erythrodontia is the reddish-brown discoloration of teeth caused by porphyrin deposition; the teeth also fluoresce bright red on exposure to ultraviolet light. Severely affected individuals must avoid all solar radiation (360–500 nm). Hemolysis is common, and anemia can be severe if the bone marrow is unable to compensate. Adults may develop significant bone loss, resulting in skeletal abnormalities. If measured, uroporphyrinogen I and coproporphyrinogen I are elevated in red cells and in urine; however, uroporphyrinogen III synthetase activity can now be measured directly.

Sun avoidance is paramount. Oral β-carotene has limited benefit. Oral α-tocopherol and ascorbic acid may reduce oxygen free radicals, limiting photodamage. Oral superactivated charcoal and cholestyramine may reduce plasma porphyrins by hindering their reabsorption; hypertransfusion may slow heme production, but relief is only temporary. Bone marrow transplantation has been met with variable results.

VARIEGATE PORPHYRIA AND HEREDITARY COPROPORPHYRIA

The cutaneous features of these two porphyrias are similar to those of PCT, but may be less intense. Patients with either disease may also present with acute attacks identical to those of acute intermittent porphyria (AIP), with abdominal pain, vomiting and constipation, acute neurologic or psychiatric symptoms, tachycardia, and hypertension. Attacks are less frequent in these conditions than in AIP. Skin lesions accompany the acute attack in about half of patients with VP and perhaps one-third of those with HCP; occasionally, the skin lesions may be the sole presentation for either of these syndromes.

Several different mutations in the protoporphyrinogen oxidase gene are found in VP, which is inherited in a autosomal dominant fashion; 60% of carriers are asymptomatic. VP is more likely than HCP to show photosensitivity. Most cases of VP present after puberty; however, a homozygous variant presents in childhood with short stature, clinodactyly, and moderately severe photosensitivity. Although porphyrin levels may be normal when the disease is quiescent, characteristic porphyrins are elevated during attacks. A plasma fluorescence test with a diagnostic peak at 625–627 nm can be used to confirm the diagnosis and to screen adult family members; this test is less reliable in children. If plasma fluorescence is not available, urine and fecal analysis should show porphobilinogen higher than aminolevulinic acid and increased coproporphyrinogen III in the urine, and protoporphyrin IX levels greater than the elevation in coproporphyrinogen III and porphyrin X. For both of these syndromes, increased urinary porphobilinogen and aminolevulinic acid may occur only during neurovisceral attacks, returning to normal between episodes.

HCP is more likely than VP to present with acute attacks; cutaneous findings occur in only a minority of patients. Like VP, HCP is autosomal dominantly inherited and typically presents in adulthood. A homozygous condition has been associated with childhood syndromes with severe photosensitivity rivaling that of congenital erythropoietic porphyria. Urine may show elevations of porphobilinogen and ALA (as in VP), and additionally increased coproporphyrinogen III in both urine and stool.

Unlike PCT, the skin lesions of VP and HCP do not respond to antimalarials or phlebotomy. Acute neurovisceral episodes due to AIP, VP, and HCP are managed by reducing heme biosynthesis and porphyrin production using heme arginate infusions along with oral and intravenous glucose. Tin protoporphyrin infusion is an experimental therapy thought to repress heme synthesis, and may prolong remission induced by heme arginate. However, its use is complicated by cutaneous photosensitivity and potential toxicity.

SUGGESTED READINGS

Badiu C, Cristofor D, Voicu D, Coculescu M. Diagnostic traps in porphyria: case report and literature review. Rev Med Chir Soc Med Nat Iasi 2004; 108: 584–591.

Cooke NS, McKenna K. A case of haemodialysis-associated pseudoporphyria successfully treated with oral N-acetylcysteine. Clin Exp Dermatol 2007; 32: 64–66.

Galossi A, Guarisco R, Bellis L, Puoti C. Extrahepatic manifestations of chronic HCV infection. J Gastrointest Liver Dis 2007; 16: 65–73.

Kohgo Y, Ikuta K, Ohtake T, et al. Iron overload and cofactors with special reference to alcohol, hepatitis C virus infection and steatosis/insulin resistance. World J Gastroenterol 2007; 13: 4699–4706.

Kostler E, Wollina U. Therapy of porphyria cutanea tarda. Expert Opin Pharmacother 2005; 6: 377–383.

Lambrecht RW, Thapar M, Bonkovsky HL. Genetic aspects of porphyria cutanea tarda. Semin Liver Dis 2007; 27: 99–108.

Lim HW. Pathogenesis of photosensitivity in the cutaneous porphyrias. J Invest Dermatol 2005; 124: xvi–xvii.

Peitsch WK, Lorentz K, Goebeler M, Goerdt S. Subacute cutaneous lupus erythematosus with bullae associated with porphyria cutanea tarda. J Dtsch Dermatol Ges 2007; 5: 220–222.

Poblete-Gutiérrez P, Wiederholt T, Merk HF, Frank J. The porphyrias: clinical presentation, diagnosis and treatment. Eur J Dermatol 2006; 16: 230–240.

Sassa S. Modern diagnosis and management of the porphyrias. Br J Haematol 2006; 135: 281–292.

Schanbacher CF, Vanness ER, Daoud MS, et al. Pseudoporphyria: a clinical and biochemical study of 20 patients. Mayo Clin Proc 2001; 76: 488–492.

Sebastiani G, Walker AP. HFE gene in primary and secondary hepatic iron overload. World J Gastroenterol 2007; 13: 4673–4689.

Seth AK, Badminton MN, Mirza D, et al. Liver transplantation for porphyria: who, when, and how? Liver Transpl 2007; 13: 1219–1227.

Cutaneous Diseases Associated with Gastrointestinal Abnormalities

There are a number of diseases of the gastrointestinal tract that feature recognizable cutaneous diseases as part of their spectrum. This discussion includes cutaneous associations of the following disorders: gastrointestinal hemorrhage, polyposis, malabsorption, and inflammatory bowel disease. The genetic basis of many of these diseases has now been elucidated (Table 25-1).

GASTROINTESTINAL HEMORRHAGE

Extensive gastrointestinal hemorrhage may occasionally be related to systemic disorders that are easily recognized by their cutaneous findings. Pseudoxanthoma elasticum and Rendu–Osler–Weber syndrome will be discussed.

Pseudoxanthoma Elasticum (OMIM #264800 and #177850)

Pseudoxanthoma elasticum (PXE) is a rare inherited disorder of elastic tissue that occurs in 1 : 70 000–100 000 births. Recent studies show an autosomal recessive mode of inheritance. Many cases appear to be new mutations. It is characterized by progressive calcification of tissue rich in elastin fibers, including the skin, retina, and blood vessels. There is significant heterogeneity in the age of onset as well as the severity of organ system involvement.

Pathogenesis

Pseudoxanthoma elasticum is an inherited disorder in which both autosomal dominant and recessive inheritance have been described in the past. Current research supports an autosomal recessive inheritance for PXE. The affected individuals are homozygous or compound heterozygous for a number of mutations, confirming the recessive nature of the disease. PXE is caused by mutation in ATP-binding cassette transporter C6 (ABCC6), also known as multidrug resistance-associated protein 6 (MRP6) gene. The gene has been mapped to chromosome 16p13.1. At least one ABCC6 mutation can be found in 80% of affected individuals. ABCC6 protein is largely expressed in the liver and kidney. The ABCC6 gene encodes for a cellular transport protein, giving rise to the concept that PXE may be a systemic metabolic disorder rather than purely a structural disorder of connective tissue.

The elastic fibers are abnormal in the affected tissues. Changes include fragmentation (elastorrhexis) and calcification of degenerated elastic tissue fibers in the middle and deep reticular dermis. Progressive accumulation of calcium within the core of elastic fibers leads to fracture and destruction. The earliest detectable change on electron microscopy is calcification of normal-appearing elastic fibers. Calcification of elastic fibers results in laxity and yellowish discoloration of the skin. Submucosal vessels of the gastrointestinal tract develop fragmentation of the elastic media, with subsequent rupture. Gastrointestinal bleeding may occur in areas affected by other diseases, such as peptic ulcer disease. Gastric bleeding may occur early before ocular and cutaneous changes are fully developed. Diffuse superficial erosions rather than focal bleeding are often found in the gastrointestinal tract. As PXE progresses, yellow papular lesions have been noted in the gastrointestinal tract. Peripheral arteries in the extremities may become so calcified that there is an actual reduction of pulses. Reports suggest an increased risk of gastrointestinal hemorrhage during pregnancy due to a progression of vascular degeneration.

Presentation

Cutaneous findings usually begin in the second to third decades. Affected skin reveals progressive yellowish coalescent papules on the neck, axilla, and groin, which may give a peau d'orange appearance. These yellow papules have been described as having a 'plucked chicken skin' appearance. In severe cases, the skin appears loose and wrinkled (Figs 25–1, 25–2).

The earliest eye changes are angioid streaks. These present as linear and branching networks of grayish discoloration radiating from the optic disc. Angioid streaks are larger in caliber than blood vessels and represent choroidal neovascularization in the elastic lamina of Bruch's membrane of the retina. Retinal

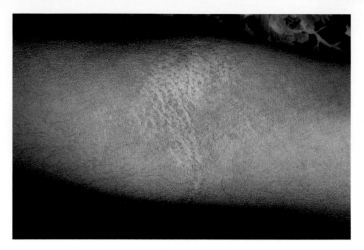

Figure 25–1 Pseudoxanthoma elasticum.

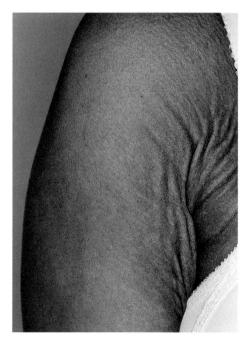

Figure 25–2 Pseudoxanthoma elasticum with lax skin evident in the axilla.

Table 25–1 Genetic links to gastrointestinal diseases
Pseudoxanthoma elasticum: ATP-binding cassette transporter C6 (ABCC6)
Hereditary hemorrhagic telangiectasia 1: endoglin (ENG)
Hereditary hemorrhagic telangiectasia 2: activin A receptor, type II-like kinase 1 (ACVRL1)
Gardner's syndrome: adenomatous polyposis coli (APC)
Peutz–Jeghers syndrome: serine/threonine kinase (STK11)
Cowden's disease: phosphatase and tensin homolog (PTEN)
Acrodermatitis enteropathica: solute carrier family 39 (zinc transporter) member 4 (SLC39A4)

pigmentation is frequently present, and chorioretinal scarring may result. Both scarring and hemorrhage lead to a loss of visual acuity, which is a common presenting symptom.

Fragmentation of the elastic media of medium-sized blood vessels produces either bleeding or vascular occlusion. Calcification of the elastic media of blood vessels results in hypertension, peripheral vascular disease, coronary artery disease, aneurysms, and cerebral hemorrhage. PXE affects the elastic tissue of the cardiac valves, the myocardium, and the pericardium. Gastrointestinal hemorrhage occurs in approximately 10% of patients with PXE, and may occur in areas affected by other diseases such as peptic ulcer disease. Gastric bleeding may occur early before ocular and cutaneous changes are fully developed. Pregnancy accentuates the degenerative disruption of elastic tissue and may predispose the patient to upper gastrointestinal bleeding.

Evaluation

The diagnosis is confirmed by the clinical picture and by the demonstration of fragmented, calcified elastic fibers on biopsy. Histologic evidence of calcified elastic fibers is essential for diagnosis. The gold standard of diagnosis is a histological examination of a skin biopsy with a von Kossa stain. Skin biopsy of flexural skin or scars is warranted in both suspected cases and potentially involved family members. Examination of the skin lesions by light microscopy demonstrates fragmentation and irregular clumping of elastic tissue in the middle to deep dermis. Involved skin shows characteristic black staining of clumped elastic fibers with Verhoeff's stain. Staining for calcium frequently shows significant elastic tissue calcification. Although such findings are classically present in involved skin, clinically normal-appearing skin of the flexural areas may show similar findings. Biopsy may confirm a diagnosis of PXE in patients with angioid streaks and minimal cutaneous findings.

The diagnosis is suggested by retinal findings in the second decade of life, by premature vascular disease, or by a positive family history. The earliest ophthalmologic findings are angioid streaks, but these are not sufficient for the diagnosis. However, they are highly suggestive of the disease in patients with a positive family history. In 85% of patients with skin findings, angioid streaks are present in the eye grounds. If PXE is suspected, detailed examination by an ophthalmologist is essential. Because eye changes are seen early in life, funduscopic examination is also recommended for screening of relatives of known patients.

Patients with PXE need to be monitored closely for evidence of vascular complications. Melena should be evaluated by endoscopy in view of the potentially catastrophic nature of gastrointestinal bleeding. If endoscopy fails to locate a source of bleeding, selective angiography may be necessary to identify the site of hemorrhage. Hypertension occurs in young patients, the evaluation of whom should include PXE in the working differential. Accelerated coronary artery disease occurs in the presence of hypertension. Angina pectoris is common, and the potential for myocardial infarction needs to be considered at an early age if symptoms of coronary insufficiency develop. Claudication is a common symptom of peripheral arterial insufficiency in young patients with PXE. In summary, close attention needs to be paid to the vascular complications of the disease, as they are potentially fatal.

Recently, genetic testing for the ABCC6 gene has become available, but not widely so. Genetic testing has limitations, and therefore should be accompanied by genetic counseling.

Differential Diagnosis

The characteristic yellowish papules of PXE may be confused with solar elastosis. The neck is a common site for both, but PXE also occurs in the axilla, groin, and popliteal and antecubital fossae. Solar elastosis produces abnormal elastic tissue that is described histologically as dense masses in the upper dermis. The abnormal elastic tissue of solar elastosis does not stain for calcium. PXE shows fragmented clumps of elastic tissue in the mid to lower reticular dermis. Patients with pseudoxanthoma-like cutaneous changes have been recognized in some acquired conditions. D-Penicillamine may produce elastic fiber damage, but this damage lacks the characteristic calcification of PXE. Eruptive xanthomas present as yellowish papules, but they usually affect the buttocks and thighs. Xanthelasma characteristically involves the eyelids. Histologically, xanthomas demonstrate foam cells filled with lipid droplets that stain positively for fat.

Angioid streaks are valuable markers for the diagnosis of PXE, but are not pathognomonic findings. Angioid streaks are seen in numerous disorders (Table 25–2), but are most commonly related to sickle cell anemia or Paget's disease of the bone. No fundamental pathogenetic relationship between the disorders causing angioid streaks has been established.

Table 25–2 Differential diagnosis of angioid streaks
Paget's disease of the bone
Sickle cell anemia
Thalassemia
Ehlers–Danlos syndrome
Tuberous sclerosis syndrome
Sturge–Weber syndrome
Neurofibromatosis
Hemolytic anemia
Diabetes
Hemochromatosis
Hyperphosphatasemia
Hypercalcinosis
Lead poisoning
Pituitary disorders
Myopia
Traumatic choroidal rupture

Treatment

There is no effective therapy for the basic defect in PXE. Limiting dietary calcium and phosphorus to minimum daily requirements has been recommended by some authors. Any intervention in calcium metabolism or deposition would necessarily involve long-term prospective study. A lack of understanding of the underlying metabolic defect makes attempted intervention empirical at best. Hemorrhage and vascular occlusive disease with PXE is managed medically.

Successful surgical removal of redundant skin for cosmetic reasons has been reported. Plastic surgery is helpful for loose folds. Complications included slow healing, extrusion of calcium particles through scars, and widening of surgical scars. The majority of patients were highly satisfied with the results.

Hereditary Hemorrhagic Telangiectasia (Rendu–Osler–Weber Syndrome) (OMIM #187300)

Hereditary hemorrhagic telangiectasia (HHT) is an autosomal dominant trait characterized clinically by multisystem vascular dysplasia. Telangiectasias are permanent dilatations of capillaries that usually blanch when pressure is applied. However, if the vascular network is extreme, strangulation of vessels may trap blood and give a nonblanching appearance. In HHT, telangiectasias begin on the mucous membranes of the nose and mouth during early childhood. Recurrent epistaxis is a common complaint in the first two decades and the severity increases with age. Involvement with telangiectasia then extends to the face, upper extremities, palms, soles, and viscera. There may not be substantial numbers of lesions until the third decade. Telangiectasias of HHT are best demonstrated by stretching the mucosal surface of the lower lip between the thumb and the forefinger, revealing 2–3-mm punctate red macules that may become papular with age (Fig. 25–3). These lesions are prone to hemorrhage with little or no trauma. Potentially fatal problems with gastrointestinal bleeding warrant close attention. In

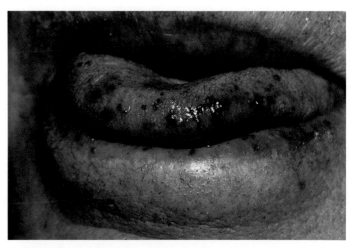

Figure 25–3 Hereditary hemorrhagic telangiectasia. Multiple, small telangiectatic mats on the lips and tongue.

young adults with HHT, an excess mortality has been attributed to HHT.

Pathogenesis

The prevalence of HHT is 1 per 10 000 population, which is much more common than previously thought. The mode of inheritance is autosomal dominant with a penetrance of approximately 97%. Two molecular subtypes of HHT are now recognized. Both HHT-1 and HHT-2 are multisystem vascular dysplasias caused by specific gene mutations found through linkage studies. The two subtypes reported have distinctions in the severity of disease and genetics markers.

HHT-1 is associated with a higher prevalence and increased severity of arteriovenous malformations. These patients have a higher risk of developing complex vascular abnormalities in the lungs and central nervous system at an early age. A mutation in the endoglin (ENG) gene has been described in HHT-1. Endoglin, which is a transforming growth factor-β (TGF-β)-binding protein, is expressed on capillaries, veins and arteries. The ENG gene maps to chromosome 9q34.1.

HHT-2 is associated with a milder phenotype, reduced penetrance, and a later age of onset. Pulmonary arteriovenous malformations are less common in HHT-2 than in HHT-1. Activin A receptor, type II-like kinase 1 (ACVRL1) is the mutated gene described in HHT-2. The ACVRL1 gene maps to chromosome 12q11-q14. ACVRL1 is detected in highly vascularized tissues and expressed primarily on endothelial cells.

Histopathologically, irregularly dilated capillaries and venules develop in the papillary dermis. There is a lack of perivascular support, including reduced pericytes, smooth muscle, and elastic fibers. A breakdown appears at the junction between endothelial cells, forming gaps that subsequently fill with thrombus. Abnormally large collagen bundles with irregular banding have also been described. Vessels with defective perivascular support are especially sensitive to insult in the gastrointestinal tract, where the epithelium is not cornified.

Presentation

Telangiectasias develop on the undersurface of the tongue and floor of the mouth at puberty. Spontaneous and recurrent epistaxis is the most common presentation in childhood, with 90% of patients affected. Vascular abnormalities of the gastrointestinal, pulmonary, and nervous systems do not manifest themselves until after the fourth decade of life. Telangiectatic lesions in the gastrointestinal tract manifest as bleeding in 20–30% of patients. Onset of gastrointestinal bleeding is usually in the fourth to sixth decades. Gastrointestinal hemorrhage may be asymptomatic in 15% of cases. Peptic ulcer disease is common in HHT patients, but bleeding is more frequently from telangiectatic mucosa that has spontaneously eroded. Gastrointestinal hemorrhage tends to be progressive. Spontaneous remission is unlikely. With advancing age, gastrointestinal bleeding leads to severe anemia requiring blood transfusions.

Elevated transaminases, γ-glutamyl transferase, and alkaline phosphatase have been reported in up to 30% of patients with HHT. Arteriovenous malformations of the liver are likely if there is hepatomegaly or a bruit over the liver. Characteristic random focal fibrovascular lesions are seen. Cirrhosis of HHT is described as abnormal dilated vessels and changing stroma throughout the liver. Bleeding from hepatic arteriovenous fistulae is rare.

Pulmonary arteriovenous fistulae have been found in 15–33% of patients. Some investigators have estimated that up to 50% of all pulmonary arteriovenous fistulae are associated with HHT. Reduced exercise tolerance may be noted in the history. Cyanosis, clubbing, and dyspnea are late signs of arteriovenous fistulae. Most lesions are detected with a combination of chest radiography and measurement of PaO_2.

High cardiac output states secondary to severe anemia and systemic arteriovenous shunting may produce biventricular failure. Multiple arteriovenous fistulae may present with CNS findings, including transient ischemic attacks, brain abscess, and cerebrovascular accidents. Cerebrovascular anomalies include arteriovenous malformation, capillary angiomas, and telangiectasias. It is estimated that cerebral arteriovenous malformations occur in 5–10% of patients with HHT. Focal neurologic defects may result from these vascular malformations of the brain, spinal cord, and meninges. Patients with pulmonary and/or cerebral arteriovenous malformations risk early death from rupture of the diseased vessels.

Evaluation

The clinical diagnosis of HHT is based on the presence of telangiectasias and on a family history of HHT. Four criteria for the diagnosis of HHT include epistaxis, telangiectasia (lips, oral cavity, fingers, nose), visceral lesions, and a family history. The diagnosis is definitive with three or four criteria, but cannot be established with fewer than two. HHT lesions occur as multiple 2–4-mm, usually symmetric, punctate, blanching macules, and as minimally elevated papules on the lips, face, nasal and oral mucosa, hands, feet, and upper extremities. The mode of inheritance is autosomal dominant, so a family history of bleeding is common.

If the characteristic telangiectasias are present on the skin or mucous membranes, a detailed family history and history of bleeding episodes are essential. Clinical telangiectasias may be few, especially in children and adolescents; therefore, close physical examination is necessary. Recurrent epistaxis at a young age may precede obvious telangiectasias by many years, and this makes family history especially important. Examination of family members should focus on the wide spectrum of HHT.

The source of mucosal bleeding should be evaluated. Hematemesis or nasogastric intubation positive for blood is an indication for endoscopy, and signs of hematochezia warrant colonoscopy. In half of the patients with HHT the source of bleeding is localized in the stomach or the duodenum. Telangiectasia will appear as small, well-defined lesions surrounded by an anemic halo. Colonic telangiectasias have been found only in 10% of patients with HHT. Selective angiography may locate a source of brisk bleeding from enteric telangiectasias. Scanning with an infusion of labeled red blood cells may be necessary when gastrointestinal bleeding is very slow. Barium examinations of the upper and lower gastrointestinal tract are not helpful in identifying the lesions of HHT. Demonstration of the lesions of HHT at surgery without prior localization is difficult, even during episodes of massive bleeding. When searching for an anatomic site of bleeding, it is necessary to remember that ingested blood from recurrent epistaxis may produce melena.

The method of screening for pulmonary arteriovenous fistulae is a combination of chest radiography and measurement of PaO_2. If hypoxemia is present, shunt measurement with 100% oxygen helps demonstrate right-to-left shunting through a pulmonary arteriovenous malformation. Arterial oxygen desaturation with 100% oxygen signifies right-to-left shunting. Evidence of vascular malformations of the central nervous system should be pursued vigorously if focal neurologic symptoms develop.

Differential Diagnosis

There are a large number of diseases that can produce cutaneous vascular abnormalities. Telangiectatic mats with similar distributions appear in CREST syndrome (calcinosis, Raynaud's phenomenon, esophageal disease, sclerodactyly, and telangiectasia) and scleroderma. However, bleeding, vascular malformation, and a positive family history are absent in scleroderma. Sclerodactyly is a common finding in CREST. Patients with CREST syndrome frequently have antinuclear and anticentromere antibodies. These findings help to distinguish HHT from scleroderma.

Generalized essential telangiectasia consists of extensive, sometimes symmetric, sheets of linear telangiectasias, predominantly on the limbs or trunk. Mucosal lesions and hemorrhage are unusual. Hereditary benign telangiectasia is clinically similar to generalized essential telangiectasia, but occurs in an autosomal dominant inheritance pattern.

Sunlight and ionizing radiation may produce localized linear telangiectasias in sun-exposed areas. Traumatic lesions are usually linear, or occasionally spider-like and localized. The telangiectasias of acne rosacea are linear, limited to the face and nose, and spare mucous membranes. Cherry angiomata occur as papules on the chest, but are rare on the lips and mucous membranes. Nevoid telangiectatic syndromes are characterized by segmental involvement of body areas with reticular vascular proliferation. One feature of chronic liver disease is spider angiomata with a characteristic central arteriole and branching.

Angiokeratomas are keratotic papules that blanch poorly on diascopy. Idiopathic solitary lesions occur on the penis and scrotum. Angiokeratomas associated with Fabry's disease are usually truncal and not mucosal. Venous lakes are deep blue, soft papules and nodules occurring on the lips and ears that blanch only partially on diascopy, are usually few in number, and are not associated with mucosal lesions.

Treatment

Treatment should be directed at controlling complications of arteriovenous malformations before they become symptomatic. Epistaxis can be controlled with nasal packing or with electrocautery. Coagulation may only offer temporary relief.

Laser therapy with argon or neodymium : YAG (Nd : YAG) laser is known to control bleeding. The placement of a split-thickness skin graft to protect fragile telangiectatic vessels has been successful in 25–64% of patients. However, telangiectatic vessels recur at the mucosal border of the graft. Prophylactic lubrication of the nasal mucosa may provide relief. There is a tendency to reduce epistaxis with estrogen therapy.

If the site can be identified, then the gastrointestinal bleeding responds to electrocautery or laser via endoscopy. If these treatments are unsuccessful, surgical resection of involved bowel segments may be necessary. Low-dose combinations of estrogen and progesterone have successfully treated severe blood loss from enteric telangiectasias.

Significant arteriovenous fistulae in any location are usually controlled by resection. Embolization with both detachable balloons and coils may significantly reduce the morbidity in pulmonary arteriovenous malformations. Cerebral arteriovenous malformations have been treated with balloon and coil embolization, stereotactic surgery, or conventional neurosurgery to prevent disabling hemorrhage.

POLYPOSIS SYNDROMES

There are two recognized groups of hereditary polyposis. Adenomatous polyposis syndromes have proven malignant potential. Hamartomatous polyposis syndromes represent malformation of the connective tissue of the intestinal mucosa. Even though they are classified as hamartomas, they still possess some risk of cancer.

Familial adenomatous polyposis refers to multiple adenomatous polyps numbering more than 100, and this condition predisposes to colorectal cancer with almost 100% certainty. Familial adenomatous polyposis is characterized by autosomal dominant inheritance of colorectal polyposis without extracolonic manifestations. Considered to be a variant of familial adenomatous polyposis, Gardner's syndrome (OMIM #175100) is characterized by an autosomal dominant inheritance with high penetrance and variable expressivity. Gardner's syndrome entails colorectal polyposis with multiple epidermoid cysts (Fig. 25–4), subcutaneous fibromas, lipomas, desmoid tumors, and osteomas of the facial bones and skull. If not treated, patients with these syndromes develop colon cancer from the ages of 20–30.

Pathogenesis

Familial adenomatous polyposis and Gardner's syndrome show an autosomal dominant inheritance with a high penetrance. However, there may be considerable variation in phenotypic expression. Both sexes are equally affected. The prevalence of familial adenomatous polyposis has been estimated to be from 1 : 8000 to 1 : 10 000, making it one of the most common hereditary diseases.

Familial adenomatous polyposis and Gardner's syndrome are caused by a highly heterogeneous spectrum of point mutations and represent a germline mutation in the adenomatous polyposis coli (APC) gene, located on chromosome 5q21. The APC gene encodes a multidomain protein that plays a role in

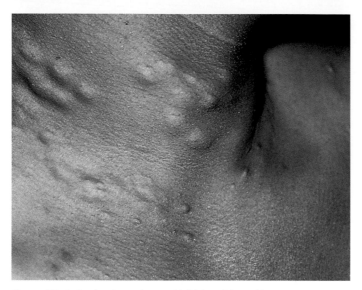

Figure 25–4 Gardner's syndrome. Multiple epidermoid cysts are present in this patient with adenomatous colonic polyps.

tumor suppression by antagonizing the WNT signaling pathway. At least 70% of patients with familial polyposis coli and Gardner's syndrome have mutations in this gene. The APC gene acts as a tumor suppressor gene, and more than 800 mutations in the gene have been identified in families with familial adenomatous polyposis. There is growing evidence that different APC gene mutations correlate with specific phenotypes.

Presentation

The inherited adenomatous polyposis syndromes are well characterized: familial polyposis coli, Gardner's syndrome, and Turcot's syndrome. Familial polyposis coli was originally separated from Gardner's syndrome solely on the basis of the absence of cutaneous findings in familial polyposis coli. Adenomatous polyps from both syndromes appear histologically, pathologically, and developmentally similar. There is great variation in the age of onset and in the number and location of polyps in both disorders. It may be impossible to diagnose intestinal polyposis before the age of 16, but the extracolonic manifestations of Gardner's syndrome can be recognized in infancy or early childhood.

The original description of Gardner's syndrome included significant extraintestinal manifestations: osteomas, epidermal inclusion (epidermoid) cysts, and subcutaneous fibromas in combination with intestinal polyposis. In general, osteomas precede the development of polyps. Osteomas, particularly of the mandible, may be palpable in puberty. Young children may have many small 3–5-mm cysts on the chest, back, and upper arms. Subcutaneous encapsulated fibromas occur on the scalp, shoulders, arms, and back.

Desmoid tumors and dental abnormalities have a significant impact on patients with Gardner's syndrome. Desmoid tumors represent benign, diffuse proliferation of soft fibrous tissue. They are abdominal wall tumors that may grow to several centimeters in size. They frequently occur at sites of trauma or surgery, but may arise de novo. Desmoid tumors are

locally aggressive and have led to death. Mesenteric fibrosis occurs in a similar fashion. The dental abnormalities include odontomas, unerupted teeth, and supernumerary teeth. Lesions of the retinal pigmented epithelium have also been described in up to 90% of patients.

Differentiation between Gardner's syndrome and sporadic epidermoid cysts is based primarily on the large numbers of lesions and on a positive family history in Gardner's syndrome patients. The presence of desmoid tumors should prompt consideration of the diagnosis of Gardner's syndrome.

Evaluation

Patients with cutaneous findings suggestive of Gardner's syndrome should have a detailed family history taken in the hope of confirming the diagnosis. Panoramic X-rays of the mandible may detect occult osteomas. Colonoscopy and biopsy may then confirm the diagnosis. Patients affected with both familial adenomatous polyposis and Gardner's syndrome have a lifetime risk of intestinal polyps transforming into adenocarcinoma at a rate approaching 100%.

Annual colonoscopic examination in high-risk individuals (family members) should be routine. In general, a preventive examination for the first generation of family members with Gardner's should begin during the 10th to 15th years of life. Colonoscopy is then continued every year until age 35. Sequencing of the gene has provided a genetic diagnosis, which is now possible in 95% of individuals with a predicted accuracy >98%. One benefit of molecular diagnosis is the elimination of the need for annual endoscopic screening in those who test negatively for a previously identified mutation in that family. The use of genetic testing linked to adenomatous polyposis coli should be accompanied by genetic counseling to avoid adverse effects on patients and families.

Differential Diagnosis

Inherited hamartomatous polyposis syndromes are characterized by the presence of multiple hamartomatous polyps of the gastrointestinal tract and have an autosomal dominant mode of inheritance. Hamartomatous polyps are malformations of the intestinal mucosa that have undergone excessive growth.

Peutz–Jeghers syndrome (OMIM #175200) consists of hamartomatous polyps in the gastrointestinal tract and mucocutaneous pigmentation of the lips, buccal mucosa, palms, and soles. Lentigines of the lips, buccal mucosa, and digits may appear in infancy or early childhood. Multiple hamartomatous polyps occur in any region of the gastrointestinal tract, but are particularly common in the small intestine. Gastrointestinal bleeding, obstruction, and intussusception are frequent complications. Uncommon cases of carcinoma affecting the entire gastrointestinal tract warrant close surveillance. Ovarian tumors and breast tumors have been reported with increasing frequency in this syndrome. Women with Peutz–Jeghers syndrome should be followed closely for associated ovarian and breast cancer. Once the diagnosis of Peutz–Jeghers syndrome is suspected, the gastrointestinal tract must be investigated with endoscopy every 2 years. Endoscopic or surgical removal of all polyps has been recommended. Screening for pancreatic cancer should be considered. Peutz–Jeghers syndrome is linked to mutations in the serine/threonine kinase STK11 gene, mapped to chromosome 19p13.3.

Cowden's disease (OMIM #158350) is characterized by multiple hamartomas of the skin, mucous membranes, breast, and thyroid. Facial trichilemmomas are flesh-colored, elongated verrucous papules in a periorificial and centrofacial distribution. Papillomatosis is found on the labial, gingival, and buccal mucosae. Less common associations are acral keratoses, palmoplantar keratoses, lipomas, hemangiomas, and neuromas. Hamartomatous polyps may be present throughout the gastrointestinal tract. The hamartomas have a potential for malignant transformation. There is a high frequency of breast cancer, and close surveillance for malignancy is warranted. Autosomal genome scanning using DNA markers on affected families have linked to chromosome 10q22-q23, encoding phosphatase and tensin homolog (PTEN).

The Cronkhite–Canada syndrome (OMIM #175500) consists of polyposis of the stomach, small intestine, and colon. Nail atrophy, alopecia, and skin pigmentation are characteristic cutaneous findings. Alopecia is rapidly progressive and leads to complete hair loss. The nail dystrophy involves all nails, with a unique pattern of an inverted triangle of normal nail bordered by dystrophy and onycholysis. The pigmentation is diffuse rather than spotted as in Peutz–Jeghers syndrome. All cases have been sporadic. Prognosis is poor.

Treatment

Once polyps are detected in a patient with familial polyposis coli, total colectomy is the treatment of choice. Malignant changes in the colon have been reported as early as age 9. The incidence of carcinoma in preadolescent polyposis patients is about 5%, and nearly 100% by the age of 30. If patients undergo a prophylactic colectomy with ileorectal anastomosis, there remains a risk of cancer in the remaining rectum. Close surveillance by a gastroenterologist is essential.

Desmoid tumors are locally aggressive. Although they do not metastasize, they have led to death. Their infiltration into surrounding muscle and fascia may require excision, which is technically difficult because of poorly defined margins. Epidermal cysts and fibromas can be removed surgically if desired. There appears to be no increased risk of malignant degeneration in such lesions.

MALABSORPTION

Malabsorption may be associated with characteristic cutaneous findings, as seen in dermatitis herpetiformis and zinc deficiency. The pathognomonic cutaneous findings usually allow for diagnosis of the bowel abnormality. Less specific cutaneous signs of malabsorption are frequently present independent of the cause of the malabsorption. These include stomatitis and glossitis related to vitamin B deficiencies; angular cheilitis; purpura as a result of vitamin C and vitamin K deficiencies; asteatotic eczema-like eruption of uncertain cause; patchy hyperpigmentation; and slowed nail and hair growth as well as alopecia secondary to protein malnutrition.

Acrodermatitis Enteropathica (OMIM #201100)

Acrodermatitis enteropathica is characterized by the intestinal malabsorption of zinc. Classic cases are genetic in origin. Acquired forms may develop in patients who are treated with total parenteral nutrition deficient in zinc, or in association with other malabsorption syndromes. The causes are summarized in Table 25–3. Oral administration with larger than normal amounts of zinc is curative.

Pathogenesis

Acrodermatitis enteropathica is transmitted in an autosomal recessive mode mapped to gene locus 8q24.3, with evidence that the phenotype is caused by mutation in the intestinal zinc-specific transporter, solute carrier family 39 (zinc transporter) member 4 (SLC39A4). Zinc deficiency results from intestinal malabsorption. Serum zinc levels, urinary excretion of zinc, and levels of zinc metalloenzymes are persistently low.

The histologic appearance of acrodermatitis enteropathica is nonspecific. The epidermis is acanthotic, with pallor and dyskeratosis of keratinocytes. Intraepidermal vesicles, subcorneal pustules, and vacuolar alteration of the dermoepidermal junction have been present in affected skin. Neutrophils may infiltrate the epidermis with extensive crusting.

Zinc is needed in various metalloenzymes for protein and DNA synthesis and for cell division. Zinc deficiency has profound effects on the immune system, including effects on T-helper cell function, T-suppressor cell function, and natural killer cell activity. Zinc also affects neutrophil chemotaxis. These abnormalities may be responsible for significant problems with intercurrent infection. Thymic hypoplasia and cortical atrophy have been reported in children. These effects are reversible with zinc supplementation.

In addition to the inherited form of zinc deficiency, there is a variety of other causes (see Table 25–3). Dietary zinc deficiency is prevalent in underdeveloped countries and may be present to a moderate degree in the United States, especially

Table 25–3 Causes of zinc deficiency
Genetic: acrodermatitis enteropathica
Dietary deficiency
Excessive alcohol ingestion
Malabsorption
Inflammatory bowel disease
Anorexia nervosa
Acquired immunodeficiency syndrome
Prolonged diarrhea
Total parenteral nutrition
Chelating agents (penicillamine)
Chronic renal disease
Pediatric 'short bowel syndrome'

in infants. Meat is the best source of dietary zinc. Consumption of unrefined cereals containing high levels of phytate renders zinc unavailable for absorption. Sources of inadequate dietary intake include refusal to eat (for example in anorexia nervosa) and limited diet selection (e.g., vegetarian diets). Alcohol intake induces hyperzincuria by poorly understood mechanisms and produces clinical zinc deficiency states.

Zinc deficiency occurs with steatorrhea from any cause. Fat malabsorption produces an alkaline environment in the bowel. Zinc forms insoluble complexes with the fat and phosphates, resulting in an increased loss of zinc in the stool. Exudation of large amounts of zinc protein complexes into the intestinal lumen from the pancreas and intestinal mucosa contributes to the reduction in plasma zinc concentration in inflammatory bowel disease and in severe chronic diarrhea. Zinc deficiency has also been reported following intestinal bypass surgery, presumably by similar mechanisms.

Failure to include zinc in fluids for total parenteral nutrition has caused severe zinc deficiency with the clinical features seen with the autosomal recessive form of acrodermatitis enteropathica. Severe zinc deficiency has also been reported following therapy with penicillamine or other chelating agents.

Presentation

Clinical findings of zinc deficiency are similar in both genetic and acquired forms. However, the cutaneous presentation of zinc deficiency is polymorphic. Findings consist of acral, perioral, and perirectal vesiculobullous, pustular, and eczematous skin lesions (Figs 25–5 and 25–6). Red scaly patches with crusting develop on the face, groin, flexures, and acral skin. Angular cheilitis and stomatitis accompany the acral lesions. Nail dystrophy with nail thinning may develop. Alopecia is generalized, but alopecia of the scalp, eyelashes, and eyebrows is prominent. Diarrhea, irritability, and failure to thrive develop simultaneously with the cutaneous eruptions in zinc deficiency, confirming clinical suspicion.

The onset of symptoms of genetic zinc deficiency usually occurs from 3 weeks to 18 months in infancy, after changing

from breast milk to cow's milk. Low-molecular-weight binding factor transports zinc into the epithelial cells of the intestine and is present in human breast milk. Low-molecular-weight zinc-binding factor in breast milk is responsible for the superior absorption of zinc from human milk. Zinc deficiency has also been reported with the absence of zinc-binding factor in deficient breast milk. Alopecia, diarrhea, growth retardation, neuropsychiatric disorders, and recurrent infections ensue if the disorder goes unrecognized.

Evaluation

Measurement of plasma zinc concentration is diagnostic, provided the sample is not hemolyzed or contaminated. Particular care needs to be taken to ensure that test tubes and other measurement equipment are free of zinc. Lowered zinc levels in plasma may occur in the absence of true zinc deficiency. Levels fall nonspecifically in the acute phases of cardiac, hepatic, renal, pulmonary, neurologic, infectious, and malignant disorders. Zinc levels in red blood cells and hair may also be assessed to determine body zinc status, but these are generally less reliable tests. Urinary excretion of zinc is reduced as a result of zinc deficiency. Determination of 24-hour urinary zinc helps to diagnose hyperzincuria and plasma zinc deficiency caused by excessive alcohol intake and chronic renal disease. Alkaline phosphatase as a zinc-dependent enzyme is frequently depressed in the zinc deficient.

Differential Diagnosis

Classic acrodermatitis enteropathica is clinically characteristic when the perioral, perirectal, and digital areas are affected. Incomplete expression of these skin findings may be confused with perioral dermatitis, hand dermatitis, candidiasis, and pustular

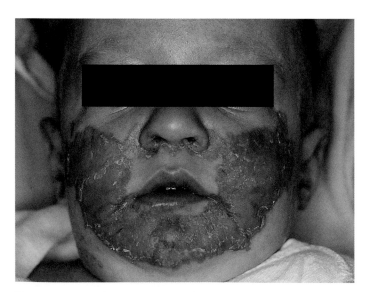

Figure 25–5 Acrodermatitis enteropathica.

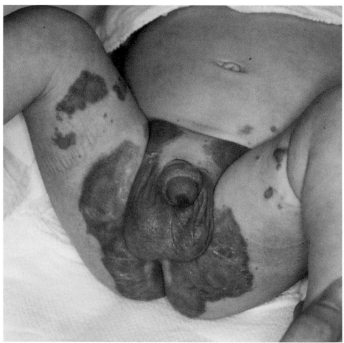

Figure 25–6 Acrodermatitis enteropathica.

psoriasis. As the dermatitis worsens, secondary colonization and infection with bacteria and *Candida albicans* can occur.

Biotin deficiency may present as periorificial dermatitis and alopecia. It occurs in those who consume an unbalanced diet containing excessive amounts of raw egg whites. Biotin binds to avidin found in egg whites, resulting in malabsorption of biotin from the intestinal tract. The perioral and intertriginous localization of early glucagonoma syndrome may also be confused with zinc deficiency.

Zinc deficiency can be corrected easily by oral supplementation. If the intake of animal protein is adequate, 15–30 mg daily of zinc sulfate is adequate. If dietary protein intake is predominantly in the form of cereals, 50–200 mg daily may be needed. Response to therapy is dramatic. Skin lesions, diarrhea, and behavioral abnormalities reverse within days to weeks. Hair growth and growth retardation improve over the course of months.

Dermatitis Herpetiformis

Dermatitis herpetiformis (DH) is a cutaneous manifestation of celiac disease. It is a lifelong disease of grouped erythematous papules and vesicles over the extensor surfaces of the forearms, elbows, knees, and buttocks. Biopsy reveals a blister at the basement membrane with the accumulation of neutrophils in dermal papillary tips. The diagnosis is confirmed with a biopsy of perilesional skin revealing deposition of granular immunoglobulin A in dermal papillary tips.

More than 85% of patients with DH demonstrate some degree of small bowel inflammation on jejunal biopsy, which is generally less severe than that in celiac disease. The attendant symptoms and signs of malabsorption are proportional to the severity of the gluten-sensitive enteropathy. DH is discussed in detail in Chapter 12. The present discussion of DH will be limited to the association with malabsorption.

Pathogenesis (OMIM 601230)

More than 90% of DH patients have a characteristic HLA genotype (DQ2A*501B*201). This carries with it an increased frequency of atrophic gastritis, achlorhydria, intrinsic factor deficiency, and resultant systemic deficiency of vitamin B_{12}. This clinical constellation of findings occurs in up to 10% of cases of DH. Ten percent of patients with DH have associated endocrine or connective tissue diseases. Endocrine diseases associated with DH include type 1 diabetes mellitus, thyroid disorders, and Addison's disease.

Over 90% of DH patients have some degree of gluten-sensitive enteropathy, which varies in severity from a mononuclear infiltrate in the lamina propria with minimal villous atrophy to complete flattening of the small intestinal mucosal cells. The enteropathy may be patchy, requiring multiple biopsy specimens for documentation. Less than 10% of DH patients have severe malabsorption. These patients represent the extreme of celiac disease, with prominent mucosal flattening. The clinical signs of malabsorption in severely affected patients are directly attributable to gluten sensitivity. Symptoms of malabsorption, including steatorrhea and foul-smelling stools, are present in a minority of patients. Clinical findings of weight loss, xerosis, alopecia, and steatorrhea are found only in the

most severe cases. Many more complain of cramping, abdominal pain, and bloating after eating. These milder symptoms may only be recognized by their cessation after the institution of a gluten-free diet.

The villous atrophy does not correlate with the severity of the skin disease. Many patients with histologically significant small bowel atrophy appear well nourished and even obese. In addition, the villous atrophy is not affected by dapsone therapy, which improves the skin disease. The small bowel atrophy is caused by gluten. Celiac disease and DH improve with a gluten-free diet. The enteropathy recurs with reinstitution of a regular diet.

Evaluation

Because virtually all patients with DH have gluten-sensitive enteropathy, it can be questioned whether small bowel biopsy is ever necessary. Although we do not perform this procedure routinely, it may be helpful to confirm the bowel abnormality. The real proof of gluten-sensitive enteropathy comes with improvement of symptoms on gluten-free diet therapy.

Between 10% and 20% of patients have abnormal D-xylose absorption, but this finding adds little when the diagnosis of gluten-sensitive enteropathy has already been made. Complete blood count is mandatory, and if anemia is seen (in the absence of dapsone-induced hemolysis), measurements of serum iron, folate, and vitamin B_{12} levels are indicated to rule out malabsorption as a cause of deficiency. Low serum vitamin B_{12} levels necessitate a Schilling's test with and without intrinsic factor administration, to differentiate between vitamin B_{12} malabsorption, secondary to enteropathy and intrinsic factor deficiency associated with atrophic gastritis.

Approximately 70% of DH patients on a regular diet have immunoglobulin A antibodies directed against endomysium. The endomysial antigen has been found to be tissue transglutaminase. These antibody tests are the most specific and sensitive serologic markers for celiac disease. The level of IgA tissue transglutaminase antibody correlates with the severity of the jejunal atrophy and returns to normal with adherence to a gluten-free diet. Antibody tests to gluten and gliadin are of little value in the diagnosis of DH because of a very high rate of false positives and false negatives.

Differential Diagnosis

The diagnosis is confirmed with the characteristic immunopathology of granular IgA deposition in perilesional skin. Previously, patients with linear IgA deposition along the basement membrane were included in the diagnosis of DH, but most investigators now consider this to be a separate disorder. The differential diagnosis of DH includes pemphigus, bullous pemphigoid, linear IgA disease, bullous lupus erythematosus, bacterial folliculitis, and eczematous processes.

Treatment

Supplementation with vitamin B_{12}, folate, or iron is indicated, depending on the results of the screening evaluation. The skin disease may be treated effectively with oral dapsone. Dapsone has been used to control DH successfully for over 50 years.

Black patients and those of southern European origin should be evaluated for glucose-6-phosphate dehydrogenase deficiency to avoid catastrophic hemolytic anemia. Monitoring with complete blood count and liver function tests is necessary owing to the hepatic and dose-related hematologic effects of dapsone. Both the skin and the bowel disease respond to gluten restriction, but a minimum 6-month trial should be undertaken before evaluating the effectiveness of gluten restriction. Maintenance on dapsone therapy is usually needed until gluten restriction has had its effect. Dapsone can then gradually be tapered and discontinued.

INFLAMMATORY BOWEL DISEASE

Inflammatory bowel disease is a general term for a group of idiopathic chronic inflammatory conditions that affect the bowel. Ulcerative colitis and Crohn's disease are distinct polygenic disorders that do not follow simple mendelian models. In genome-wide screening for susceptibility genes, linkage studies have linked inflammatory bowel disease to chromosomes 16p12-q13 and 12p13. Ulcerative colitis begins in the rectum and spreads proximally to involve the colon. Crohn's disease may involve any area of the intestinal tract and is frequently discontinuous.

Presentation

Multiple extraintestinal manifestations of inflammatory bowel disease may occur (Table 25–4). Metastatic Crohn's disease is characterized by cutaneous granulomas that occur distant from the gastrointestinal tract (Fig. 25–7). Oral aphthae occur in association with Crohn's disease and ulcerative colitis in 6–8% of cases. Aphthae seem to be related to actively inflamed bowel. Their onset coincides with relapse of the intestinal

disease. These lesions are not specific, as up to 20% of the normal population have aphthae. Malabsorption of iron, folic acid, and vitamin B_{12} occurs with inflammatory bowel disease. Correction of these deficiencies may result in improvement of the associated aphthosis.

The incidence of pyoderma gangrenosum with inflammatory bowel disease is 1–5%. Inflammatory bowel disease is the single most common cause of pyoderma gangrenosum, being responsible for between 15% and 25% of cases (Figs 25–8, 25–9). Other inflammatory diseases associated with pyoderma gangrenosum are rheumatoid arthritis, chronic hepatitis, leukemia, mycosis fungoides, polyarteritis nodosa, and cryoglobulinemia. Pyoderma gangrenosum is characterized as a sterile chronic ulceration with a violaceous undermined border. It may involve peristomal and incision sites, extremities, chest, back, abdomen, and head and neck. Rapid evolution of the

Table 25–4 Some cutaneous associations of inflammatory bowel disease

Specific lesions

Fissures and fistulae
Metastatic Crohn's disease
Mucosal lesions

Reactive lesions

Aphthous ulcers
Pustular vasculitis (bowel-associated dermatosis-arthritis syndrome)
Pyoderma gangrenosum
Erythema nodosum
Vasculitis
Erythema multiforme
Urticaria
Sweet's syndrome

Other associations

Epidermolysis bullosa acquisita
Vitiligo
Alopecia areata
Fingernail clubbing

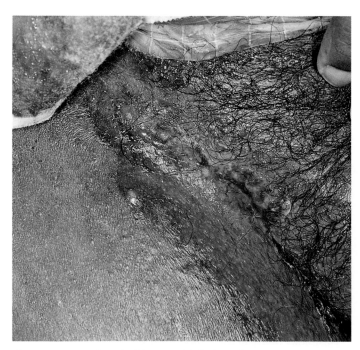

Figure 25–7 Extraintestinal (metastatic) Crohn's disease.

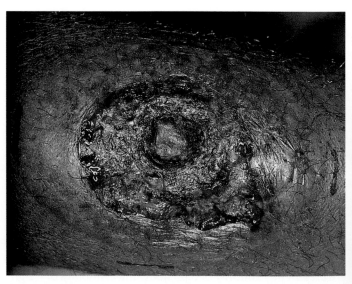

Figure 25–8 Pyoderma gangrenosum in a patient with ulcerative colitis.

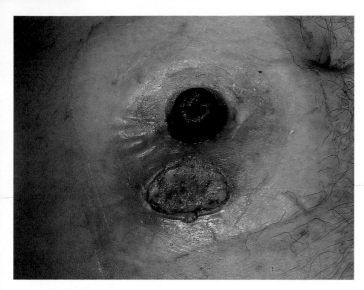

Figure 25–9 Peristomal pyoderma grenosum. This patient's colon was removed for chronic ulcerative colitis more than 10 years prior to the onset of this lesion.

ulcer is a hallmark of the disease. Exclusion of arterial/venous disease, leukocytoclastic vasculitis, and infection is crucial. Histology from the border shows endothelial injury, fibrinoid necrosis, and a prominent infiltration of neutrophils in the dermis. The activity of pyoderma gangrenosum parallels the activity of bowel disease. Response to systemic immunosuppressive treatment and lack of response to conventional wound care is characteristic. Cyclosporine has been highly effective in pyoderma gangrenosum.

Erythema nodosum may occur in 1–5% of patients with inflammatory bowel disease, and is frequently accompanied by peripheral arthritis in patients with Crohn's disease. The prevalence of erythema nodosum is higher in Crohn's disease than in ulcerative colitis. However, the majority of patients with erythema nodosum do not develop inflammatory bowel disease. They should still be questioned about signs and symptoms of bowel disease.

Additional reactive dermatoses discussed elsewhere in the book may occur in inflammatory bowel disease. These reactive dermatoses include: Sweet's syndrome, erythema multiforme, urticaria, leukocytoclastic vasculitis, polyarteritis nodosa, and epidermolysis bullosa acquisita. Thrombophlebitis, alopecia areata, vitiligo, and digital clubbing may also occur. Many of the cutaneous changes seen in patients with inflammatory bowel disease are due to nutritional deficiencies secondary to malabsorption.

Treatment

The activity of the extraintestinal manifestations of inflammatory bowel disease often parallels the course of the intestinal disease. Active inflammatory bowel disease produces inflammatory cytokines, which stimulate these reactive dermatoses. Therapy of cutaneous associations in inflammatory bowel disease is best directed at the underlying disease. Therapies often include sulfasalazine, corticosteroids, and immunosuppressants. Colectomy may produce clinical remission of extraintestinal manifestations of ulcerative colitis in many patients

Management of erythema nodosum includes bed rest, compression stockings, naproxen, indometacin, prednisone, colchicine, and potassium iodide. Cutaneous Crohn's disease may respond to metronidazole, prednisone, mesalamine, cyclosporine, and tumor necrosis factor inhibitors such as infliximab. Treatment of pyoderma gangrenosum includes topical, systemic and biologic agents. Topical therapies include occlusive hydrocolloid dressings, high-potency corticosteroids, intralesional steroids, and topical tacrolimus. Refractory pyoderma gangrenosum can be treated with cyclosporine, prednisone, azathioprine, infliximab, and adalimumab.

SUGGESTED READINGS

Bayrak-Toydemir P, Mao R, Lewin S, McDonald J. Hereditary hemorrhagic telangiectasia: an overview of diagnosis and management in the molecular era for clinicians. Genet Med 2004; 6: 175–191.

Callen JP, Jackson JM. Pyoderma gangrenosum: an update. Rheum Dis Clin North Am 2007; 33: 787–802, vi.

Chassaing N, Martin L, Calvas P, et al. Pseudoxanthoma elasticum: a clinical, pathophysiological and genetic update including 11 novel ABCC6 mutations. J Med Genet 2005; 42: 881–892.

Fry L. Dermatitis herpetiformis: problems, progress and prospects. Eur J Dermatol 2002; 12: 523–531.

Gregory B, Ho VC. Cutaneous manifestations of gastrointestinal disorders. Part I. J Am Acad Dermatol 1992; 26: 153–166.

Gregory B, Ho VC. Cutaneous manifestations of gastrointestinal disorders. Part II. J Am Acad Dermatol 1992; 26: 371–383.

Haitjema T, Westermann CJ, Overtoom TT, et al. Hereditary hemorrhagic telangiectasia (Osler–Weber–Rendu disease): new insights in pathogenesis, complications, and treatment. Arch Intern Med 1996; 156: 714–719.

Hall RP 3rd. Dermatitis herpetiformis. J Invest Dermatol 1992; 99: 873–881.

Lebwohl M, Neldner K, Pope FM, et al. Classification of pseudoxanthoma elasticum: report of a consensus conference. J Am Acad Dermatol 1994; 30: 103–107.

Maverakis E, Fung MA, Lynch PJ, et al. Acrodermatitis enteropathica and an overview of zinc metabolism. J Am Acad Dermatol 2007; 56: 116–124.

Miksch S, Lumsden A, Guenther UP, et al. Molecular genetics of pseudoxanthoma elasticum: type and frequency of mutations in ABCC6. Hum Mutat 2005; 26: 235–248.

Nakano A, Nakano H, Nomura K, et al. Novel SLC39A4 mutations in acrodermatitis enteropathica. J Invest Dermatol 2003; 120: 963–966.

Shovlin CL, Guttmacher AE, Buscarini E, et al. Diagnostic criteria for hereditary hemorrhagic telangiectasia (Rendu–Osler–Weber syndrome). Am J Med Genet 2000; 91: 66–67.

Chapter | **26** |

J. Mark Jackson,
Jeffrey P. Callen, and
Kenneth E. Greer

Cutaneous Hepatology

A number of cutaneous stigmata are associated with hepatic disease, but none is specific. Even jaundice, classically associated with liver immaturity (neonatal jaundice) or failure, may occur with hemolysis and in the setting of perfectly normal hepatic function. The cutaneous changes of hepatic disease may be related to primary diseases of the liver; to cutaneous diseases with associated hepatic abnormalities; and to a wide variety of disorders with changes in many organs, including the liver and skin. A number of drugs commonly used for the treatment of cutaneous disease may produce hepatic damage, such as methotrexate, ketoconazole, itraconazole, terbinafine, retinoids, and vitamin A. Finally, several drugs produce hypersensitivity reactions characterized by fever, lymphadenopathy, hepatitis, and cutaneous lesions. Drugs in this category include phenytoin, phenobarbital, carbamazepine, dapsone, minocycline, and allopurinol (see Chapter 41).

Classically, cutaneous manifestations have been associated with such primary hepatic diseases as alcoholic cirrhosis and hemochromatosis, but other disorders, including Wilson's disease, viral hepatitis, and primary biliary cirrhosis, produce similar changes. Porphyria cutanea tarda and erythropoietic protoporphyria, known primarily for their cutaneous manifestations, are associated with hepatic abnormalities. Patients with porphyria cutanea tarda have frequently been found to have hepatitis C virus infection. Gianotti–Crosti syndrome was originally felt to be associated with viral hepatitis, but this association may only be more prevalent in southern Europe. Lichen planus has also been associated with hepatitis C infection. Miscellaneous diseases that affect many organ systems and involve the liver and the skin include syphilis, sarcoidosis, Gaucher's disease, polyarteritis nodosa, and cytophagic histiocytic panniculitis. Finally, with the increased incidence of liver transplantation, the skin becomes an important organ for the early recognition of a graft-versus-host reaction. Many of these disorders are discussed elsewhere in this book, and others occur too infrequently to be discussed in detail here.

Cutaneous symptoms, such as pruritus and jaundice, may be important evidence for considering the diagnosis of hepatic disease, especially in conjunction with nonspecific symptoms such as fatigue, anorexia, vomiting and weight loss, diminished libido, and right upper quadrant abdominal discomfort. In addition to these symptoms, certain physical findings, espe-

cially when considered collectively, suggest the diagnosis of hepatic disease. Mucocutaneous lesions are often prominent and include scleral icterus, spider telangiectases, palmar erythema, excoriations (e.g., neurotic excoriations, and prurigo nodularis), xanthelasmas, alopecia, nail lesions, gynecomastia, and prominence of the cutaneous veins in the epigastrium. Any patient with symptoms of pruritus, and findings of neurotic excoriations and/or prurigo nodularis (Fig. 26–1), in the absence of a primary cutaneous disease should be evaluated for liver disease.

CIRRHOSIS

Cirrhosis of the liver implies an irreversible alteration of the liver's architecture, consisting of hepatic fibrosis, areas of nodular regeneration, and a loss of a considerable number of hepatocytes. Although alcohol is one of the most common causes of cirrhosis (Laënnec's cirrhosis) in the United States, cirrhosis can be caused by drugs and other toxins such as acetaminophen and alcohol; infections (especially hepatitis C virus); biliary obstruction (e.g., carcinoma of the pancreas or bile duct, gallstones, cystic fibrosis); metabolic diseases (e.g., hemochromatosis and Wilson's disease); chronic right-sided heart failure; and a group of miscellaneous diseases such as sarcoidosis, primary biliary cirrhosis, and jejunoileal bypass. There are also a number of cases of cirrhosis that are idiopathic. Individuals with cirrhosis usually present in one of two general ways, i.e., (1) with evidence of acute hepatocellular necrosis with jaundice; or (2) with evidence of the complications of cirrhosis, brought on primarily by the rise in intrahepatic vascular resistance and subsequent portal hypertension (i.e., ascites, splenomegaly, bleeding varices, and encephalopathy). Patients not infrequently present with a mixed picture of these two pathophysiologic pathways.

The dermatological stigmata of cirrhosis are well recognized and include changes in the skin, nails, and hair. Vascular lesions are common and include spider angiomas and other telangiectases; palmar erythema; and dilated abdominal wall veins, which occur in patients with portal hypertension and represent the development of portal systemic collaterals (Figs 26–2 to 26–4). Spider angiomas occur in a majority of patients

237

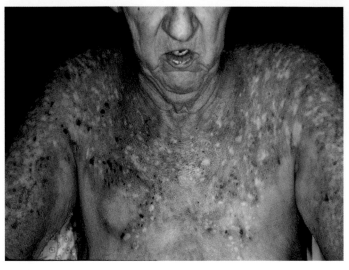

Figure 26–1 Pruritus of hepatic disease manifest as neurotic excoriations.

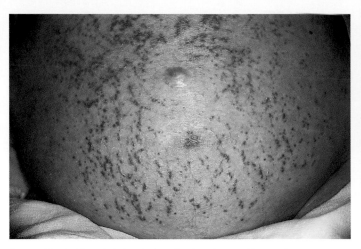

Figure 26–4 Dilated abdominal wall veins along with xerotic eczema associated with cirrhosis and portal hypertension. (Courtesy of Dr Neil Fenske, Tampa, FL.)

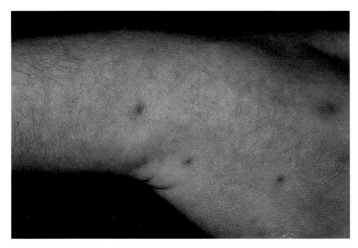

Figure 26–2 Spider angioma on the arm.

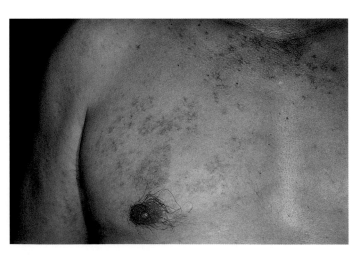

Figure 26–3 Unilateral nevoid telangiectasia in a male patient with cirrhosis of the liver due to hepatitis C.

with cirrhosis, but they are not pathognomonic of the disease because they occur commonly in young children, pregnant women, and otherwise healthy adults. They are so named because of their central pulsatile arterial punctum with radiating branching vessels. They occur almost exclusively on the upper half of the body, especially on the face, neck, and upper trunk. The spider is formed by a coiled arteriole that spirals up to a central point and then branches out into thin-walled vessels that merge with normal capillaries. The pathogenesis of these unusual vascular malformations is unknown, but they do not appear to be related to portal hypertension, which is responsible for one of the most serious complications of cirrhosis: bleeding esophageal and gastric varices. They may also be related to estrogen excess, which occurs as a result of reduced hepatic metabolism of estrogens. Palmar erythema, manifested as diffuse or splotchy erythema on the thenar and hypothenar eminences and tips of the fingers, frequently accompanies the development of the spider angiomas. Palmar erythema also occurs in healthy individuals and in association with nonhepatic diseases such as human immunodeficiency virus (HIV) infection. There may be a widespread appearance of thin, wiry telangiectases in some patients, and occasionally the lesions appear in a unilateral distribution (see Fig. 26–3).

Various forms of nail disease have been described in patients with cirrhosis, including the classic white nails of Terry. Terry's nails are characterized by a nail plate that is opaque white with the exception of the distal portion, which retains its normal pink color (Fig. 26–5). In addition, patients may develop transverse white bands (Muehrcke's nails), clubbed nails, or koilonychia (spoon-shaped nails), but none of these changes is specific for hepatic disease. Changes in body hair are common and are noted primarily in men. The axillary, pubic, and pectoral hair is usually sparse, but thinning of all body hair is common also. There is often the development of a female pubic hair pattern, coinciding with other evidence of feminization, including testicular softening and gynecomastia. This is in contrast to the hypertrichosis seen in patients with porphyria cutanea tarda and liver disease.

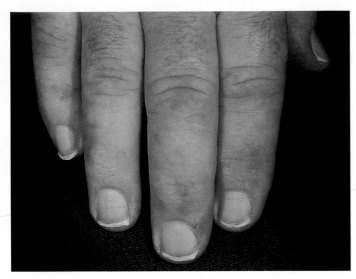

Figure 26–5 Opaque white nails of Terry in a patient with cirrhosis.

There are a number of nonspecific systemic symptoms associated with cirrhosis of the liver, especially weakness, anorexia, nausea, weight loss, and abdominal discomfort. Pruritus is less common in patients with intrahepatic cholestasis and occurs in diseases such as primary biliary cirrhosis, sclerosing cholangitis, and chronic extrahepatic biliary obstruction. The cirrhotic liver is usually small, firm, and nodular, and the spleen is often enlarged. Ascites may cause a remarkable distension of the abdominal cavity. Low albumin occurs in the setting of chronic hepatic dysfunction which results in edema, especially of the lower extremities. This can lead to stasis dermatitis and xerosis of the skin in areas of chronic edema. Owing to impaired hepatic function, a prothrombin deficiency may develop, resulting in cutaneous purpura, epistaxis, and gingival bleeding. This deficiency also causes difficulty in controlling the bleeding from varices. The use of intramuscular vitamin K to help reverse the prothrombin deficiency has led to recent – albeit rare – reports of unusual annular erythematous reactions surrounding the injection site.

A review of the diagnosis, course, treatment, and prognosis of cirrhosis is beyond the scope of this chapter. There is, however, one additional point concerning cirrhosis that is especially important for dermatologists, and this is the inducement of the disease with methotrexate in the treatment of psoriasis. Methotrexate-induced cirrhosis appears to be related primarily to the total dosage of methotrexate therapy, and is more likely to occur in patients who have been receiving the drug for more than 5 years. Cirrhosis is unusual in patients treated with methotrexate who do not have other risk factors for hepatic disease. Factors that increase the propensity for cirrhosis in patients taking methotrexate include obesity, hepatosteatosis, diabetes mellitus, hyperlipidemia, hepatitis A, B, or C, concomitant potentially hepatotoxic medications such as acetaminophen, statins, systemic antifungals, and/or excessive alcohol intake. It has recently been suggested that in the absence of other risk factors, patients on methotrexate may not need liver biopsies until a cumulative dose of 3 g is reached. There are well-established guidelines for liver biopsies, and,

more recently, noninvasive scanning techniques have been used to follow hepatic function in patients receiving long-term methotrexate therapy. Levels of the amino terminal peptide of type III procollagen have been used extensively in Europe, particularly the United Kingdom, for evaluation of the liver in order to detect early fibrosis, but this test is not available in the United States. There are two tests, known as the Fibrosure for hepatitis C and Fibrosure for steatohepatitis, which are used to follow patients with either disorder. The Fibrosure for steatohepatitis might prove useful in following patients on methotrexate, but this is not currently an approved use and studies are pending.

PRIMARY BILIARY CIRRHOSIS

Primary biliary cirrhosis, a relatively uncommon form of cirrhosis which occurs most frequently in women 40–60 years of age, deserves special recognition because the combination of pruritus, jaundice, hyperpigmentation, and xanthomas is specific for the disease. It is believed that the destruction of the small intrahepatic bile ducts – the primary defect in primary biliary cirrhosis – occurs on an immunologic basis. Abnormalities have been detected in both B- and T-cell function. Primary biliary cirrhosis may occur in patients with other autoimmune diseases, such as rheumatoid arthritis, thyroiditis, and the CREST (calcinosis, Raynaud's phenomenon, esophageal dysmotility, sclerodactyly, telangiectasia) syndrome, and it may be familial. The first and often the foremost symptom of primary biliary cirrhosis is pruritus, which is the presenting complaint in one half of patients. Patients may have multiple excoriations, and it is not unusual to see a pattern of postinflammatory hyperpigmentation in the so-called butterfly configuration on the back. This pattern results from the fact that patients have difficulty reaching the skin of the upper central back but can readily scratch the periphery. The skin in the central area appears relatively normal, whereas the border is hyperpigmented and, not infrequently, lichenified. Lichen planus may be more frequent in patients with primary biliary cirrhosis. Patients also develop jaundice, hyperpigmentation, and xanthomas, which are caused by the associated hyperlipidemia. The xanthomas may be striking and include xanthelasma, planar xanthomas in palmar creases (Fig. 26–6) and in scars, tuberous xanthomas over the extensor aspects of joints and pressure areas, and, rarely, tendinous xanthomas. Late in the course of the disease, patients may develop osteomalacia (secondary to diminished absorption of vitamin D), portal hypertension, and hepatic failure.

HEMOCHROMATOSIS

Hemochromatosis, also known as bronze diabetes, is an autosomal recessive disease characterized by cutaneous hyperpigmentation, diabetes mellitus, and cirrhosis of the liver. There is a basic defect in iron metabolism, resulting in increased absorption of iron from the intestine and deposition of iron in various tissues, especially the skin, liver, heart, pancreas, and endocrine organs. There are also secondary forms of hemo-

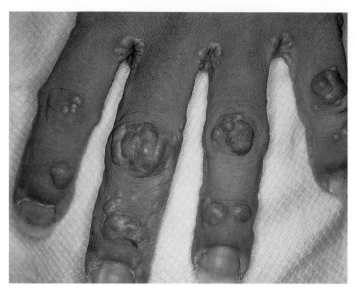

Figure 26–6 Multiple xanthomas with hyperpigmentation in primary biliary cirrhosis.

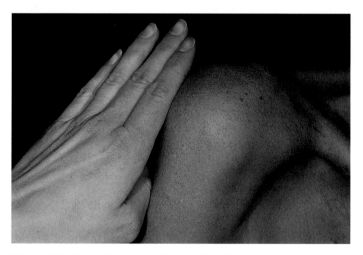

Figure 26–7 Generalized hyperpigmentation of hemochromatosis.

chromatosis that may result from excessive oral intake of iron, from repeated transfusions in patients with refractory anemia, or from a congenital transferrin deficiency. Unlike in primary biliary cirrhosis, 90% of patients with hemochromatosis are male. The disease usually becomes clinically apparent between the ages of 40 and 60 years.

The hyperpigmentation is generalized but accentuated in exposed areas (Fig. 26–7). A small percentage of patients will develop pigmentation of oral mucous membranes and on the conjunctivae, which is similar to the pattern of pigmentation seen in Addison's disease. Hyperpigmentation is the presenting manifestation in one-third of patients, and it is usually a distinctive metallic gray, although it may be brown. It results from an increase in melanin in the skin, presumably as a result of stimulation of the melanin-producing system by the excessive iron stores. The skin tends to be dry and scaly, and patients may develop other changes in the skin, hair, and nails identical to those seen with cirrhosis of the liver. Common extracutaneous features include diabetes mellitus, gonadal deficiency,

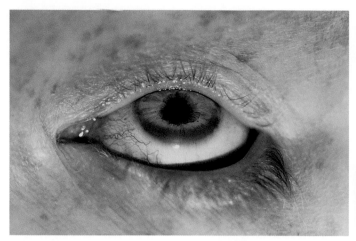

Figure 26–8 Pigmented band (Kayser–Fleischer ring) at the periphery of the cornea in Wilson's disease.

cardiac disease, and a distinctive arthropathy with chondrocalcinosis. Unlike many other forms of cirrhosis, there is an effective form of therapy for some patients with hemochromatosis, namely, removal of iron stores by repeated phlebotomy.

WILSON'S DISEASE

Wilson's disease (hepatolenticular degeneration) is also a rare autosomal recessive disease associated with cirrhosis, but its clinical and pathologic manifestations result from an excessive accumulation of copper in many tissues, especially the brain, liver, corneas, and kidneys. The triad of basal ganglia degeneration, cirrhosis of the liver, and a pathognomonic pigmentation of the corneal margins (Kayser–Fleischer ring) is characteristic of the disease. The Kayser–Fleischer ring is a golden-brown or greenish-brown circle of pigment produced by the deposition of copper in Descemet's membrane at the periphery of the cornea (Fig. 26–8). This ocular finding can be important diagnostically, but the majority of patients present with either neurologic symptoms or hepatic insufficiency. The prognosis of Wilson's disease is often grave because of a delay in early diagnosis, which allows irreparable damage to be done to the liver and nervous system. One other physical finding that might suggest the diagnosis of Wilson's disease is the presence of blue lunulae, although this azure color can be seen in normal individuals and in patients taking phenolphthalein or antimalarials. Wilson's disease is often treated with D-penicillamine, which is associated with many cutaneous problems, but in particular, elastosis perforans serpiginosa may develop from use of this drug.

CUTANEOUS DISEASE ASSOCIATED WITH VIRAL HEPATITIS

Viral hepatitis is caused by several agents, and the clinical course varies from subclinical and inapparent infections to severe and fulminant disease with hepatic failure and death. Some viruses preferentially attack the hepatocyte, especially hepatitis viruses A, B, and C; however, other viruses are commonly associated with acute hepatitis, including the Epstein–Barr virus (infectious mononucleosis), cytomegalovirus, rubella, herpes simplex, herpesvirus 6, and yellow fever viruses.

The hepatitis virus most frequently associated with dermatologic syndromes is hepatitis C virus, but hepatitis B virus has also been associated with some cutaneous findings. The incidence of new infections with hepatitis B has lessened with the widespread use of immunization and the testing of blood products. Hepatitis B has been associated with reactive erythemas such as urticaria and vasculitis. In Italy, hepatitis B infection has been linked to papular acrodermatitis of childhood (Gianotti–Crosti syndrome).

Hepatitis C (HCV) has become the most common cause of infectious hepatitis. Hepatitis C is spread primarily by parenteral routes, either by overt inoculation (e.g., transfusion or infection with a contaminated needle) or by intimate personal contact, including contact between sexual partners, and between affected patients and healthcare professionals. Patients infected with HCV usually develop a chronic infection, either in association with demonstrable hepatic disease or in otherwise seemingly healthy carriers. There are at least six serotypes of HCV and they vary in their association with progressive disease and its severity. In addition, the ingestion of alcohol is a significant cofactor that may result in more severe and more rapidly progressive liver disease. Unfortunately there is no vaccine available for this virus, as the immune response that occurs with naturally acquired infection is not protective.

Several dermatological conditions have been associated with hepatitis C infection, including a serum sickness-like prodrome, essential mixed cryoglobulinemia, porphyria cutanea tarda (Fig. 26–9), livedo reticularis, and lichen planus. Less commonly associated findings are urticaria, vitiligo pyoderma gangrenosum, polyarteritis nodosa, and alopecia areata.

There are many other extrahepatic manifestations of HCV infection, including autoimmune thyroid disease, sialadenitis resulting in xerostomia, autoimmune thrombocytopenic purpura, aplastic anemia, neuropathy, serum sickness reactions, and non-Hodgkin's B-cell lymphoma. Palpable purpura or small-vessel (leukocytoclastic) vasculitis (Fig. 26.10), erythrocyanosis, and Raynaud's phenomenon may occur in patients with essential mixed cryoglobulinemia. It seems prudent to test patients with porphyria cutanea tarda, small-vessel (leukocytoclastic) vasculitis, polyarteritis nodosa, and possibly lichen planus for the presence of HCV. Patients with oral ulcerative lichen planus (Fig. 26–11) and those with chronic and diffuse disease are more commonly seen to have HCV in association with their cutaneous findings.

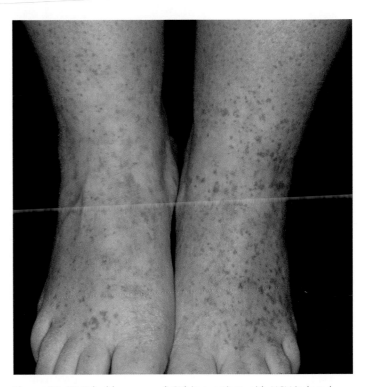

Figure 26–10 Palpable purpura (LCV) in a patient with HCV-induced cryoglobulinemia.

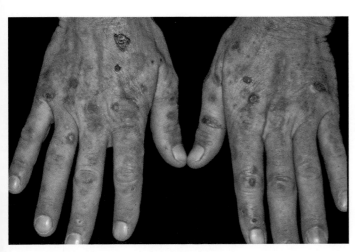

Figure 26–9 Porphyria cutanea tarda in a patient with HCV infection.

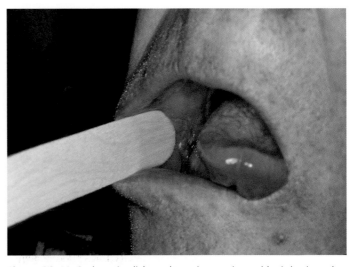

Figure 26–11 Oral erosive lichen planus in a patient with cirrhosis and HCV infection.

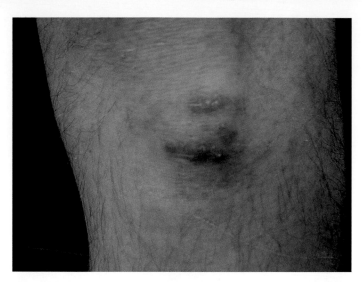

Figure 26–12 Sarcoidal granulomas developing in scars of patient with HCV on therapy with interferon.

Therapy of HCV infection involves the use of interferon and ribavirin, but a sustained response may occur only in the minority of patients. Also, it is not currently known whether intervention with these therapies will prevent cirrhosis or hepatic carcinoma.

Patients with mixed cryoglobulinemia and resulting cutaneous vasculitis often benefit from therapy with interferon and ribavirin, as the viral antigens cause the protein complexes that deposit in the vessels, resulting in inflammation and vascular destruction. Therapy for HCV results in a reduced viral load, thereby reducing the protein complexes and their resulting deposition. Most of the other cutaneous findings noted in patients with HCV infection do not improve dramatically with the therapy, other than lichen planus, which has a variable response.

Patients undergoing therapy for hepatitis C may also have cutaneous manifestations related to therapy. These include worsening or new-onset psoriasis, vitiligo, and cutaneous/systemic sarcoidosis in sites of old trauma (Fig. 26–12).

Screening for hepatitis C should be performed in all patients prior to initiating therapy with any potentially hepatotoxic medication. Patients infected with HCV may have normal liver functions, thus a routine hepatic function panel is not an adequate screening tool. Patients testing positive for HCV should have a confirmatory test via polymerase chain reaction (PCR), as false positives do occur with the routine serum screen; however, if the screen is negative, one can feel assured that there is no HCV, as few false negatives occur. Diagnosing hepatitis C at an early stage is important in order to prevent end-stage hepatic cirrhosis, which can progress to hepatocellular carcinoma.

SUGGESTED READINGS

Bonkovsky HL, Mehta S. Hepatitis C: a review and update. J Am Acad Dermatol 2001; 44: 159–179.

Cartwright GE, Edwards CQ, Kravitz K, et al. Hereditary hemochromatosis. N Engl J Med 1979; 301: 175–179.

Garden JM, Ostrow JD, Roenigk HH Jr. Pruritus in hepatic cholestasis. Arch Dermatol 1985; 121: 1415–1420.

Jackson JM. Hepatitis C and the skin. Dermatol Clin 2002; 20: 449–458.

Lauer GM, Walker BD. Hepatitis C virus infection. N Engl J Med 2001; 345: 41–52.

Sarkanv I. The skin-liver connection. Clin Exp Dermatol 1988; 13: 151–159.

Zachariae H. Liver biopsies and methotrexate: a time for reconsideration? J Am Acad Dermatol 2000; 42: 531–534.

Pancreatic Disease

The cutaneous manifestations of pancreatic disease may be secondary to either the exocrine/endocrine functions of the pancreas or to pancreatic carcinomas. Until 20 years ago, the majority of reports concerned patients who had cutaneous changes related to acute or chronic pancreatitis, and, only rarely, to metastatic nodules from carcinoma of the pancreas. Since 1966, most reports in the dermatological literature have dealt with patients who have glucagonoma syndrome, with its cutaneous manifestation necrolytic migratory erythema. However, the cutaneous lesions resulting from disorders of the pancreas are variable and include hemorrhage, panniculitis, thrombophlebitis, metastatic nodules, and necrolytic migratory erythema, which consists of lesions involving both the skin and mucous membranes (Table 27–1). Recently, there have been few additions to the existing literature on the cutaneous manifestations of pancreatic diseases.

The exocrine pancreas secretes large quantities of enzymes in response to duodenal secretin and cholecystokinin. The enzymes are grouped into those that digest starch (amylase), fat (lipase), and protein (trypsin and other proteolytic enzymes). These enzymes are thought to cause pancreatitis via autodigestion; many etiologic factors are implicated in pancreatitis. Endocrine tissue accounts for less than 1% of the weight of the gland, and it is composed of small islets that release either insulin from β cells or glucagon from α cells. Cutaneous consequences of β-cell dysfunction are many, as seen in diabetes mellitus (see Chapter 20). Patients with abnormal α-cell function as in the glucagonoma syndrome may possess cutaneous lesions that are now well recognized. Cutaneous manifestations of other pancreatic tumors include specific metastatic nodules in addition to nonspecific signs and symptoms related to pancreatic carcinoma or pancreatic endocrine tumors, excluding glucagonomas.

CUTANEOUS LESIONS ASSOCIATED WITH PANCREATITIS

Pancreatitis is classified as acute or chronic, based on whether the patient recovers after an acute episode or continues to have pain or evidence of insufficient exocrine or endocrine pancreatic secretion. Cutaneous disease is most often associated with acute pancreatitis, which has many causes, such as alcohol ingestion, diabetes, infections (including paramyxovirus and hepatitis), biliary tract disease (primarily gallstones), trauma, and drugs (including thiazide diuretics, azathioprine, sulfonamides, and estrogens). Abdominal pain and tenderness, nausea, vomiting, fever, and hypotension are common clinical findings in patients with acute pancreatitis, and the diagnosis can be established with the finding of an elevation of a single laboratory parameter, the serum amylase level. Two main types of cutaneous lesion may be seen in patients with acute pancreatitis: purpura and panniculitis.

The first account of what was considered to be a specific cutaneous manifestation of acute pancreatitis was recorded by Grey Turner in 1919. He reported a bluish patch of discoloration of the flank in a patient with pancreatitis. Initially believed to be the result of fat necrosis, Turner's sign is, in reality, an ecchymosis arising from the subcutaneous extravasation of peritoneal hemorrhagic fluid (Fig. 27–1). This may be observed in as many as 5% of cases of acute pancreatitis, and may be seen occasionally in patients with other causes of hemorrhage into the peritoneum. Anatomically, hemorrhagic fluid flows through the anterior and posterior pararenal space into the subcutaneous tissues in the flank. Hemorrhagic discoloration around the umbilicus (Fig. 27–2), described by Cullen in 1918 in association with ectopic pregnancy, may also occur in patients with acute pancreatitis and other disorders that cause retroperitoneal bleeding. This occurs as hemorrhagic fluid extends from the gastrohepatic ligament and across the falciform ligament to the periumbilical tissues. Incidentally, this pathway parallels the lymphatic drainage of the region and may explain the periumbilical metastases frequently referred to as Sister Mary Joseph's nodules. As evidenced by Cullen's original citing, neither Turner's nor Cullen's sign is specific for acute pancreatitis. Abdominal and truncal livedo reticularis (Walzel's sign) has been reported in association with pancreatitis, and, rarely, purpura or hemorrhage below the inguinal ligament has been seen (Fox's sign).

Panniculitis is associated with both pancreatitis and pancreatic carcinoma, and has been described as subcutaneous or nodular fat necrosis. The precise etiology is not clear. Most accepted theories center around the action of enzymes (predominantly lipase) that are released into the circulation from

Table 27–1 Nondiabetic cutaneous manifestations of pancreatic disease

Cutaneous changes related to pancreatitis
    Cutaneous hemorrhage (Cullen's, Turner's and Fox's signs)
    Panniculitis
    Livedo reticularis (Walzel's sign)

Cutaneous changes related to pancreatic endocrine tumors (glucagonoma syndrome)
    Necrolytic migratory erythema

Cutaneous changes related to pancreatic carcinoma
    Metastatic nodules, especially to umbilicus
    Panniculitis
    Migratory thrombophlebitis

the damaged pancreas, producing the breakdown of subcutaneous fat. However, lipase alone does not appear to be sufficient to induce the panniculitis, and there are probably other enzymes (colipase, phospholipase, and trypsin). Further confounding any relationship between lipase and pancreatic panniculitis is the occurrence of panniculitis lesions in patients with normal serum lipase values. There may be a predisposing host factor involving adipocytes and/or endothelial cells in the subcutis that play a role.

The resulting inflammatory subcutaneous nodules or plaques, 1–5 cm in diameter, occur especially on the thighs and lower legs, but also on the arms, buttocks, or trunk (Figs 27–3 and 27–4). The lesions are frequently painful; in severe cases they rupture spontaneously, discharging a viscous, sterile material containing free and esterified cholesterol, neutral fats, soaps, and free fatty acids. In mild cases the plaques involute within 2–3 weeks, leaving depressed hyperpigmented scars, but new crops tend to occur. Patients with extensive panniculitis are often febrile and have associated joint disease (synovitis, especially of small joints), abdominal pain, and vomiting.

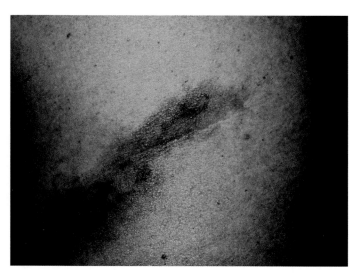

Figure 27–1 Purpura of the left flank (Turner's sign) in a patient with acute hemorrhagic pancreatitis.

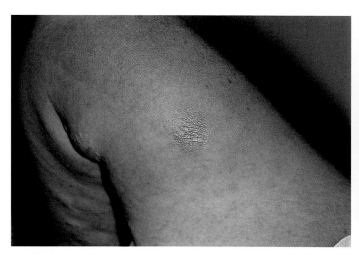

Figure 27–3 Large erythematous indurated area of the posterior arm as a result of panniculitis.

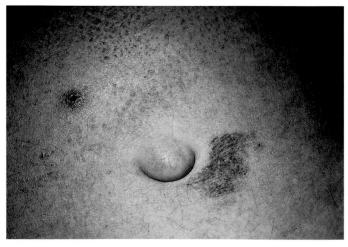

Figure 27–2 Periumbilical purpura (Cullen's sign) associated with acute hemorrhagic pancreatitis.

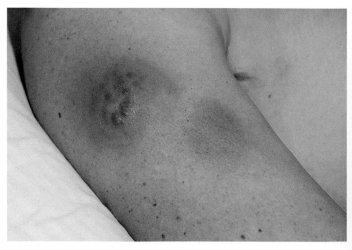

Figure 27–4 Painful nodules and plaques as a result of subcutaneous fat necrosis.

Panniculitis associated with pancreatitis usually occurs in patients in their mid 30s or 40s, whereas patients with cancer are usually significantly older and are also more likely to have blood eosinophilia and only slightly elevated (or occasionally normal) levels of serum amylase and lipase. The clinical differential diagnosis of pancreatic panniculitis includes erythema nodosum, nodular vasculitis, periarteritis nodosa, and other forms of lobular panniculitis, including cold/equestrian panniculitis, α_1-antitrypsin deficiency, and lupus profundus.

Histologically, the findings of panniculitis associated with pancreatic disease are distinctive. These pathognomonic changes include foci of fat necrosis with 'ghost-like' anucleate cells having thick 'shadowy' walls and a surrounding inflammatory infiltrate of neutrophils, eosinophils, lymphocytes, histiocytes, and foreign body giant cells. Hemorrhage and secondary calcification are not uncommon, but vasculitis is not a part of pancreatic panniculitis. The detection of these findings should prompt an exhaustive search for underlying pancreatic disease. Therapy is supportive and is primarily directed at the underlying pancreatic disease. The diagnosis of this disorder is important, because the underlying pancreatic disease may be carcinoma.

CUTANEOUS CHANGES RELATED TO PANCREATIC ENDOCRINE TUMORS

The majority of reports of cutaneous disease produced by non-diabetic pancreatic endocrine disorders discuss the glucagonoma syndrome. There are, however, pancreatic tumors that can synthesize a variety of hormones other than glucagon and insulin, and which produce or are associated with cutaneous signs or symptoms. These tumors are usually benign, and the hormones secreted by the tumors include gastrin (Zollinger–Ellison syndrome), somatostatin (somatostatinomas), adreno-corticotropic hormone (ACTH, Cushing's syndrome), and prostaglandin and serotonin (pancreatic carcinoid). Patients with the carcinoid syndrome have typical flushing episodes. Patients or family members of patients with Zollinger–Ellison syndrome have been reported to have an increased incidence of multiple lipomas. Patients with Cushing's syndrome as a result of ACTH-secreting pancreatic islet cell tumors usually have less severe clinical manifestations than do those with Cushing's syndrome that is the result of other causes, but the cutaneous changes, which are well known, may be prominent. Other hormone-secreting tumors may produce diarrhea, weight loss, and anemia, which may affect the skin indirectly and nonspecifically.

The cutaneous eruption of glucagonoma syndrome is known as necrolytic migratory erythema, and in the majority of cases is a distinctive cutaneous marker of a tumor of pancreatic α cells. The syndrome, first described by Becker and colleagues in 1942, was associated with carcinoma of the pancreas by McGovran in 1966, and was called glucagonoma syndrome by Maltinson and coworkers in 1974. In 1971 Wilkinson named the distinctive cutaneous changes 'necrolytic migratory erythema.' Glucagonomas, which are usually malignant, occur more frequently without the typical cutaneous manifestations of the full syndrome. In addition, rare reports cite necrolytic

migratory erythema occurring in patients without a pancreatic tumor or elevated levels of plasma glucagon. The majority of patients with glucagonoma syndrome have an insidious onset of symptoms, usually 1.5–2 years before the diagnosis is made. By the time of diagnosis, however, the majority of patients have glucagonomas with metastases to the liver and regional lymph nodes. The disease has a predilection for middle-aged persons and has been reported more frequently in women.

There is considerable similarity of patients with glucagonoma syndrome. In addition to the necrolytic migratory erythema, patients frequently have stomatitis or glossitis, glucose intolerance, normochromic anemia (which may be profound and require repeated transfusions), weight loss, and diarrhea. Recurrent venous thrombosis, also a feature of non-endocrine-secreting tumors of the pancreas, and depression have been associated with glucagonoma syndrome. Fasting plasma glucagon levels (normally 50–200 pg/mL) are elevated in almost all patients and may be 5–10 times the normal level. Reduced blood amino acid levels are also common.

The most distinctive feature of the syndrome is necrolytic migratory erythema, which usually occurs cyclically and has a characteristic distribution. The cutaneous eruption is frequently widespread but is most prominent in perioral and intertriginous areas, especially the perineum. The distal extremities and lower abdomen are also common sites of involvement. Superficial necrosis of the epidermis produces an erosive and occasionally a vesiculobullous dermatosis with crusting and eventual shedding of the skin. The base of the lesions is usually remarkably erythematous, and the borders are frequently annular or serpiginous. The active inflammatory process appears to cycle every 7–14 days.

As with other cutaneous markers of pancreatic disease, necrolytic migratory erythema is not specific for pancreatic glucagonoma and has been seen in jejunal or rectal adenocarcinoma, advanced cirrhosis, villous atrophy of the small intestine, and even myelodysplastic syndrome. The differential diagnosis of well-developed cutaneous lesions includes pemphigus, bullous pemphigoid, acrodermatitis enteropathica, essential fatty acid deficiency, and pellagra. However, the eruption frequently begins insidiously and may mimic numerous cutaneous disorders, including eczema, contact dermatitis, configurate erythemas, moniliasis, psoriasis, and staphylococcal pyoderma. In addition, there are a number of reports of patients with glucagonomas in whom there was no mention of a skin eruption.

Histologically, biopsy of early cutaneous lesions may be helpful in establishing the diagnosis of glucagonoma syndrome. Marked spongiosis, pallor of the upper epidermis, frank necrolysis of the upper epidermis, vacuolization of keratinocytes and accumulation of neutrophils in the epidermis are characteristic. Occasionally, clefting and intraepidermal bullae are seen, but acantholysis does not occur. The mild inflammatory infiltrate in the superficial dermis is composed primarily of mononuclear cells and is predominantly perivascular. The same changes have been described in patients with pellagra and acrodermatitis enteropathica. The pathogenesis of the cutaneous eruption is unknown, but there have been reports of improvement of the cutaneous process after the intravenous administration of amino acids.

After the possibility of the diagnosis of glucagonoma syndrome has been raised (based usually on the cutaneous lesions and elevated plasma glucagon levels), the search should be made for a pancreatic tumor. In addition, consideration should be given to other endocrine neoplasias in these patients and other family members, because familial glucagonoma has been reported in the setting of multiple endocrine neoplasias (MEN), particularly MEN-1. Resection of the tumor before metastatic spread occurs is the goal, but partial removal of large tumors or metastases may result in significant clinical improvement. A number of chemotherapeutic agents have been used with some success to treat patients with metastatic glucagonomas.

CUTANEOUS CHANGES RELATED TO NONHORMONE-SECRETING PANCREATIC CARCINOMA

Carcinoma of the pancreas is the fourth most common cancer that causes death in the United States, accounting for more than 20 000 deaths per year. The high mortality rate is largely due to the fact that more than 85% of the tumors have metastasized at the time of the diagnosis. More than 90% are adenocarcinomas, with 65% involving the head of the pancreas, 30% involving both the body and tail, and 5% involving the tail alone. The classic symptoms of pancreatic carcinoma are weight loss, abdominal pain, anorexia, and jaundice.

The three most common cutaneous manifestations of nonhormone-secreting pancreatic adenocarcinomas are metastatic cutaneous nodules; migratory thrombophlebitis; and panniculitis, specifically subcutaneous or nodular fat necrosis. Panniculitis occurs most frequently with pancreatitis, but it has also been described in patients with adenocarcinoma of the pancreas and, rarely, with pancreas divisum, a congenital pancreatic ductal abnormality. Cutaneous metastases, especially to the umbilicus, are not common from pancreatic carcinoma, but approximately 10% of umbilical metastases (Sister Mary Joseph's nodule) occur from pancreatic tumors. Migratory thrombophlebitis of both superficial and deep veins is also uncommon (Fig. 27–5). The association of this form of superficial phlebitis with carcinoma is attributed to Trousseau and was described in 1865. Interestingly, the presenting manifesta-

tion of the gastric cancer that led to Trousseau's death was venous thrombosis.

Carcinoma of the pancreas accounts for approximately 30% of the tumors associated with thrombophlebitis, and in this it is second only to carcinoma of the lung. Classically, the phlebitis occurs in short segments of superficial veins and is distributed on the trunk and neck and on the extremities. Involvement of the veins of the upper extremities is not uncommon, though it is an unusual location in thrombosis unassociated with a malignant condition. The phlebitis is often resistant to anticoagulant therapy and may lead to a life-threatening embolic phenomenon. The inflammatory changes may resolve spontaneously within a few weeks, only to recur in the same or distant veins. Recurrent and migratory thrombophlebitis may be the presenting symptom of malignancy. The pathogenesis is unknown, although cancer patients are suspected to have abnormalities in platelets, coagulation factors, and the fibrinolytic system.

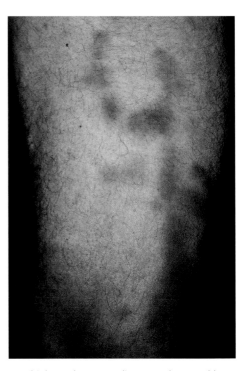

Figure 27–5 Multiple erythematous linear cords caused by superficial migratory thrombophlebitis.

SUGGESTED READINGS

Bem J, Bradley EL 3rd. Subcutaneous manifestations of severe acute pancreatitis. Pancreas 1998; 16: 551–555.

Kasper CS. Necrolytic migratory erythema: unresolved problems in diagnosis and pathogenesis. A case report and literature review. Cutis 1992; 49: 120–128.

Powell FC, Cooper AJ, Massa MC, et al. Sister Mary Joseph's nodule: a clinical and histologic study. J Am Acad Dermatol 1984; 10: 610–615.

Sibrack LA, Gouterman IH. Cutaneous manifestations of pancreatic disease. Cutis 1978; 21: 763–768.

Ward SK, Roenigk HH, Gordon KB. Dermatologic manifestations of gastrointestinal disorders. Gastroenterol Clin North Am 1998; 27: 615–636.

Christina L. Haverstock,
Mary Gail Mercurio,
Boni E. Elewski, and
Joseph L. Jorizzo

Chapter | **28**

Cutaneous Manifestations of Systemic Viral, Bacterial, and Fungal Infections and Protozoan Disease

The cutaneous manifestations of systemic infections in adults, including those caused by viruses, bacteria (spirochetes, rickettsia, mycobacteria), and fungi are the subject of this chapter. Often, cutaneous manifestations are characteristic of infectious diseases and allow for prompt diagnosis and institution of therapy. This chapter focuses on those characteristic cutaneous findings.

VIRUSES

Viruses produce a variety of cutaneous changes, including morbilliform (measles-like), papular and vesicular eruptions. It is often difficult to distinguish viral exanthems from morbilliform drug eruptions; however, subtle distinguishing features may enable differentiation.

Measles (Rubeola)

Measles (rubeola) is caused by a single-stranded RNA paramyxovirus. Humans are the only known reservoir for infection, although other primates may become infected. Transmission occurs via respiratory secretions. Routine administration of live attenuated vaccine is currently recommended by the Centers for Disease Control and Prevention (CDC) for all infants, college entrants, and medical personnel without serologic evidence of past infection. The incidence of measles infection has decreased dramatically with the introduction of widespread vaccination; however, a gradual increase has occurred in recent years in the United States. Some of those affected were previously vaccinated, although more parents are choosing not to vaccinate, resulting in small but significant local outbreaks. Two distinct forms of the disease are modified measles, which occurs when an individual is infected when they have passive immunity (during breastfeeding or with remaining transplacental antibodies), and atypical measles, which largely affects persons immunized with the killed vaccine during the 1960s. Live attenuated vaccine given at 15 months of age is preventative.

Clinical Manifestations

The viral prodrome consists of fever (may exceed 104°F), cough, coryza, conjunctivitis, photophobia, and myalgias, and lasts about 1 week. The classic exanthem consisting of erythematous confluent macules and papules is usually apparent at 2 weeks. The cutaneous eruption spreads cephalocaudally over 3 days, and resolves with fine desquamation and a brown hyperpigmentation. Koplik spots are pathognomonic and appear on the buccal, labial, and gingival mucosae just prior to the exanthem. They are 1–2-mm bluish macules on an erythematous base. Measles infection is usually benign and self-limited.

The most common complication of measles is secondary bacterial infection resulting in otitis media, pneumonia, laryngitis, encephalomyelitis, and thrombocytopenia purpura. Pneumonia is the most serious of these, is more frequent in children, and is the most common cause of death associated with the virus. Postinfectious encephalitis carries a high mortality of 15%.

Atypical measles is a characteristic clinical syndrome seen in recipients of the killed vaccine that was used in the United States from 1963 to 1967. The cutaneous eruption begins on the wrists, arms, and soles, and then spreads centrally to the extremities and trunk. The lesions are initially morbilliform and then become vesicular, purpuric, or hemorrhagic. Koplik spots are rarely present. Complications include pneumonia, hepatosplenomegaly, hyperesthesia, or paresthesia.

Diagnosis

The clinical presentation is often classic; however, confirmation may be made with viral culture, diagnostic biopsy of affected skin, or serology.

Treatment

The treatment is supportive. Immune serum globulin may be given to exposed susceptible persons who are immunocompromised. Some studies suggest the use of ribavirin in immunocompromised hosts may be beneficial.

Rubella

Rubella (German measles) is a common self-limited childhood infection caused by an RNA togavirus. Rubella generally produces a mild exanthematous illness, except when it is transmitted in utero. The incidence of rubella has decreased dramatically since the introduction of a live attenuated vaccine in 1968. Transmission occurs by inhalation of infected respiratory droplets, with increased incidence during the spring months.

Clinical Manifestations

Illness begins with a mild prodrome consisting of malaise, anorexia, fever, and headache, and coryza may occur. The cutaneous eruption appears first on the forehead and rapidly spreads inferiorly to involve the face, trunk, and extremities. The lesions consist of pink macules and papules which may become confluent, creating a scarlatiniform eruption (scarlet fever-like macular erythema). Pruritus may be present. The time course of the rubella exanthem is 3 days, which is a differentiating point from the usual 6-day course of the rubeola exanthem. The exanthem of rubella also does not desquamate. There may be tender, postauricular, suboccipital, and posterior cervical lymphadenopathy. Petechiae on the soft palate, or Forschheimer spots, may also be present. Arthritis and arthralgia are common complications of infection, especially in females. Joints may be erythematous, tender, and swollen for 1 month post infection.

Widespread vaccination against rubella was developed largely for the prevention of congenital rubella syndrome. Maternal infection during the first 16 weeks of gestation results in a 65% risk for congenital rubella. Skin manifestations include extramedullary hematopoiesis (blueberry muffin baby), thrombocytopenia, cataracts, deafness, and patent ductus arteriosus. The impact of maternal infection on the fetus drops precipitously after 20 weeks of gestation. Infection in healthy children or young adults is typically self-limited without sequelae. The most common complication is arthritis.

Diagnosis

The diagnosis of rubella is made clinically and confirmed serologically. The virus can be isolated by culture from the oropharynx or joint aspirate.

Treatment

Treatment is supportive care.

Erythema Infectiosum

Erythema infectiosum (fifth disease) is an acute childhood exanthem caused by human parvovirus B19. Most cases develop during the winter or spring, and transmission is by respiratory droplets. Although there is a parvovirus vaccination available for canines, no human vaccine is yet available.

Clinical Manifestations

Most infections due to parvovirus B19 are asymptomatic; however, in school-aged children erythema infectiosum is common. A mild prodrome of low-grade fever and headache may present initially during viremia. Soon thereafter the characteristic asymptomatic bilateral erythema of the cheeks, often referred to as a 'slapped cheek,' appears. This may be accompanied by pharyngitis, myalgia, diarrhea, nausea, or conjunctivitis. Within a few days the exanthem extends to the body and is described as an evanescent reticulated erythema of the trunk and extremities. A unique cutaneous manifestation of parvovirus B19 infection is the papular purpuric 'gloves and socks' syndrome. This affects young adults and results in symmetric swelling and pain in the distal feet and hands, followed by the purpuric eruption. Complications are much more common in adults than in children, and include arthritis, hemolytic anemia, encephalopathy, and aplastic crisis. Parvovirus infection during pregnancy has been reported to cause spontaneous abortion and hydrops fetalis.

Diagnosis

The diagnosis is usually made on clinical grounds. Serum parvovirus-specific immunoglobulin M can be measured.

Treatment

Treatment is supportive care. Chronic anemia and aplastic crises may require treatment with immunoglobulin or blood transfusion.

Hand, Foot, and Mouth Syndrome

Hand, foot, and mouth syndrome is a combination of an exanthem and enanthem that primarily affects toddlers. The etiologic agent is a Coxsackie virus, most commonly A16, but also A5, A10, B1, or B3, and enteroviruses can cause the eruption. Coxsackie viruses are small RNA viruses of the picornavirus family. Outbreaks are characteristically limited to the summer and early fall months.

Clinical Manifestations

This syndrome is characterized by the abrupt onset of sore mouth, cutaneous eruption, and fever. Malaise, diarrhea, joint pains, and lymphadenopathy may be present. The typical acral lesions are few in number and consist of oval to linear or football-shaped red papules and vesicles located over the dorsal and lateral aspects of the fingers and toes. The palmar and plantar surfaces may also be involved (Fig. 28–1). An exanthem or red papules over the proximal extremities may also be present. The oral and oropharyngeal lesions consist of papules and vesicles that become erosions scattered over the soft palate, tonsillar pillars, and posterior pharynx (Fig. 28–2). Hand, foot, and mouth syndrome is generally a self-limited disease lasting less than 1 week.

Diagnosis

The eruption is usually characteristic. In some cases, viral culture of the stool or throat washings can be used to confirm the diagnosis. Acute and convalescent sera can also be assessed for Coxsackie viral titers.

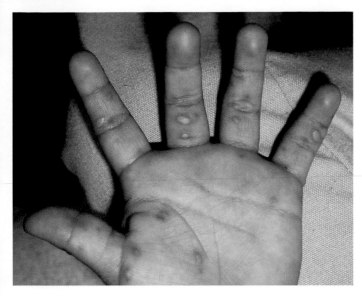

Figure 28–1 Erythematous papules and pustules in a patient with hand, foot, and mouth syndrome.

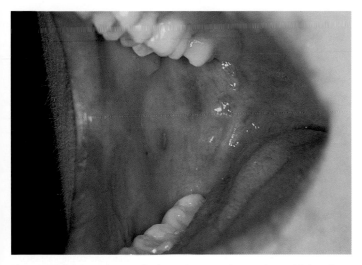

Figure 28–2 Ulceration on the buccal mucosa in a patient with hand, foot, and mouth syndrome. (Courtesy of Dr R. Schosser, Lexington, KY.)

Treatment

Treatment is supportive care.

Roseola Infantum/Exanthem Subitum (Human Herpesvirus 6)

Human herpesvirus 6 (HHV 6) is genetically and pathogenetically similar to cytomegalovirus. HHV 6 has been demonstrated to be the cause of exanthem subitum (also known as roseola infantum, or sixth disease). HHV 6 infects more than 90% of the population in early childhood, and may cause fever and/or cutaneous eruption. The presumed route of transmission is by respiratory tract secretions.

Clinical Manifestations

A prodromal syndrome with fever typically occurs 7–15 days after exposure to this virus. Constitutional symptoms, including malaise, coryza, sore throat, headache, anorexia, and nausea, appear with the exanthem in a few days. The exanthem consists of discrete pink macules and papules distributed primarily over the trunk, buttocks, and neck, which may coalesce to confluent erythema. A ring of pallor surrounds the individual lesions. Complete resolution occurs in 1–4 days. Infection is benign and self-limited with infrequent complications, the most common being febrile seizures. Other viruses that mimic roseola include Coxsackie viruses B1, B5, E11, E16, and E25.

In adults, this virus has been linked to an infectious mononucleosis-like syndrome and pneumonitis in immunocompromised hosts. There may also be a link to hepatitis, lymphoproliferative diseases, and chronic fatigue syndrome.

Diagnosis

The classic feature of an isolated high fever preceding the eruption of the exanthem is usually sufficient to make the diagnosis. Serologic studies are available for absolute confirmation.

Treatment

Treatment is supportive.

Epstein–Barr Virus

Epstein–Barr virus (EBV), a herpesvirus, is the primary etiologic agent in the clinical syndrome infectious mononucleosis. Infection with EBV usually occurs in childhood or adolescence and is generally mild and self-limited. The association of infection by this virus with the subsequent development of nasopharyngeal carcinoma and Burkitt's lymphoma is well recognized. In addition, many patients who are immunosuppressed have developed a B-cell lymphoma, which is often self-limiting.

Clinical Manifestations

The incubation period of EBV is long: 3–7 weeks. Following this, acute infection is characterized by fever, pharyngitis, and lymphadenopathy. Eyelid edema and hepatosplenomegaly are often prominent. Mucocutaneous manifestations are more common in younger children. There may be an exanthem on the trunk and upper arms consisting of macules, urticarial plaques, petechiae, or purpura. An enanthem consisting of palatal petechiae at the border of the soft and hard palate is common. A distinctive and pathognomonic copper-colored morbilliform pruritic eruption may develop in infected patients treated with ampicillin or other semisynthetic penicillins (Fig. 28–3). Gianotti–Crosti syndrome manifests as symmetric lichenoid papules on the distal extremities and face which resolve after 1 month. EBV infection is usually self-limited. Late manifestations of EBV-related disease can occur and are manifest as lymphoproliferative disease, which might affect the skin on rare occasions.

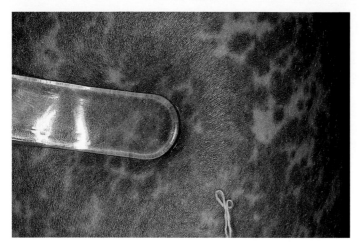

Figure 28–3 Ampicillin eruption in a patient with infectious mononucleosis.

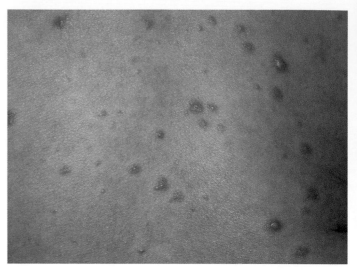

Figure 28–4 Small vesicular lesions surrounded by a slight erythematous hue, representative of acute varicella.

Diagnosis

Examination of a peripheral blood smear reveals lymphocytosis with atypical lymphocytes. Mild thrombocytopenia is common, and there may be elevated liver transaminases. The presence of heterophile antibodies (monospot) or a rise in EBV-specific antibodies can confirm the diagnosis. The virus can be cultured from the oropharynx.

Treatment

Treatment is supportive care. Ampicillin should be avoided. Occasionally, systemic corticosteroids are indicated for severe complications, such as pharyngeal edema causing airway obstruction.

Varicella

Varicella (chicken pox) is a ubiquitous childhood infection caused by the varicella-zoster virus (VZV), a member of the herpesvirus family. Transmission occurs by airborne droplets and by direct contact.

Clinical Manifestations

The exanthem typically occurs 2 weeks after exposure, begins abruptly on the head, and spreads caudally. The primary lesion is an erythematous papule that evolves into a clear fluid-filled vesicle on an erythematous base, commonly described as a 'dewdrop on a rose petal' (Figs 28–4 and 28–5). The vesicles subsequently evolve into pustules and, eventually, crusts. Additional crops occur, resulting in lesions in all stages of evolution present simultaneously, allowing easy differentiation from smallpox, where all the lesions are in the same stage of evolution. The palms and soles are typically spared. Vesicles and erosions are often present on the palate. Mild constitutional symptoms often accompany the exanthem and are more prominent with increasing age. In children, varicella is typically a self-limited disease but may be complicated by secondary infection. Primary infection in adults or in immunocompromised hosts may be complicated by pneumonia,

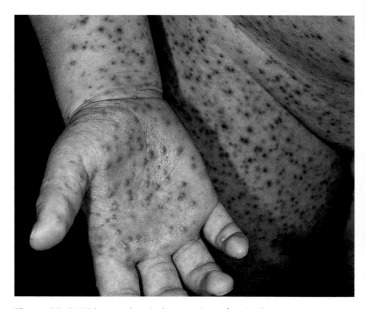

Figure 28–5 Widespread vesicular eruption of varicella.

encephalitis, or myocarditis. Mortality in adult patients is 10% when immunocompetent and 30% in immunosuppressed patients. Maternal infection with primary VZV produces congenital varicella syndrome, which includes limb defects, cortical atrophy, low birthweight, and ocular abnormalities. The risk is greatest when infection occurs in the first trimester, with about 2% of fetuses exposed before 20 weeks' gestation being affected. The differential diagnosis of varicella includes disseminated herpes simplex virus, disseminated herpes zoster, exanthem vaccinatum, bullous impetigo, vesicular pityriasis rosea, and bullous drug eruption. Vaccination with a live attenuated virus is routinely performed now, providing a 96% seroconversion rate, and is nearly 100% effective at preventing serious disease.

Diagnosis

Cytologic evaluation of the fluid or the floor of a vesicle (Tzanck preparation) reveals characteristic herpesvirus-induced changes, consisting of acantholytic balloon cells with one or several nuclei. This diagnostic procedure is highly interpreter-dependent, and positivity depends on the stage of the lesion, with vesicles having the highest positivity. Viral culture or polymerase chain reaction (PCR) techniques can confirm the diagnosis.

Treatment

In immunocompetent patients, infection with the varicella virus is self-limited, requiring supportive care only. Aciclovir produces a slightly milder disease if begun within 24 hours of the cutaneous eruption (80 mg/kg/day in four divided doses), but it does not block a normal immunologic response. It is often used for patients under 2 years of age, or those who are immunosuppressed. Acyclovir therapy in pregnancy may benefit the mother, but it may not affect fetal outcome. Varicella-zoster immunoglobulin is indicated for prophylaxis in susceptible pregnant women and in neonates whose mothers became infected shortly prior to delivery. Almost one-third to half of individuals who received varicella-zoster immunoglobulin still develop clinical disease.

Herpes Zoster

Herpes zoster infection is also caused by VZV and represents reactivation of the latent virus from prior varicella infection.

Clinical Manifestations

A severely painful prodrome often precedes the cutaneous eruption, which is typically confined to a single dermatome (Fig. 28–6). The eruption consists of grouped vesicles that may appear purpuric and which later ulcerate and crust. The sites of predilection, in descending order, are thoracic, trigeminal, lumbosacral, and cervical dermatomes. Mild constitutional symptoms may be present. Immunosuppression and advanced age are risk factors for herpes zoster. In patients with acquired immunodeficiency syndrome (AIDS) the eruption may be multidermatomal or disseminated and recurrent. Secondary infection of cutaneous lesions may be associated with scarring. Urinary retention and conjunctival scarring may complicate genital and periocular infections, respectively. There is currently a vaccine for the prevention of zoster in patients of advanced age that has been shown to reduce the incidence, duration, and post-herpetic neuralgia associated with herpes zoster.

Diagnosis

The diagnosis may be clinically obvious because of the characteristic dermatomal distribution of clustered vesicular lesions. Tzanck preparation reveals characteristic herpesvirus-induced changes. Viral culture can confirm the diagnosis. Immunoperoxidase studies using monoclonal antibodies and PCR detection of viral DNA can be useful for diagnosis in atypical cases.

Treatment

Herpes zoster infection is typically self-limited in immunocompetent patients. Local care to prevent secondary bacterial infection and analgesics for pain control are usually adequate treatment. Oral acyclovir at a dose of 800 mg five times per day for 7–10 days, valacyclovir 1 g three times daily for 7 days, or famciclovir 500 mg three times daily for 7 days have all been shown to hasten the healing time and to reduce the acute pain when initiated within 48 hours of onset of the cutaneous eruption. They may also lessen the chance of post-herpetic neuralgia and may reduce its severity and duration. Immunocompromised persons should be treated with intravenous acyclovir to prevent dissemination of the infection. In older individuals who are at higher risk of developing post-herpetic neuralgia, the use of oral antiviral agents alone or, as advocated by some, the concomitant administration of systemic corticosteroid in a tapering dose, reduces the risk of this complication. Treatment of post-herpetic neuralgia is difficult. The pain often decreases with time. Topical capsaicin may help some patients. Oral amitriptyline, gabapentin, and pregabalin may also be useful. In patients who fail these measures, the intrathecal injection of methylprednisolone has been demonstrated to be effective.

In 2006 a vaccine for herpes zoster was approved for use by the FDA. Zostavax contains live varicella-zoster virus and is indicated in patients over 60, and has been shown to reduce the incidence of zoster by 51% and the incidence of post-herpetic neuralgia by 66%.

Herpes Simplex Virus

Herpes simplex virus types 1 and 2 enter the host through mucosal surfaces or breaks in the skin. The most common entry sites are oral (HSV type 1 more than HSV type 2) and genital (HSV type 2 more than HSV type 1) via close contact

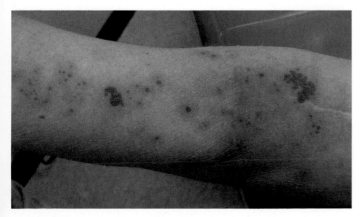

Figure 28–6 Herpes zoster. Grouped hemorrhagic blisters in a dermatomal distribution.

with an infected person. The hallmark of infection with the herpes simplex virus is its ability to establish a latent infection.

Clinical Manifestations

Herpes simplex infection commonly occurs in immunocompetent persons as a recurrent painful vesicular eruption, most commonly affecting the oral and perioral (anterior soft palate, lips, or gingival) or genital regions (Fig. 28–7). Skin-to-skin contact, such as in wrestlers, may allow for transmission of a herpes simplex viral infection known as herpes gladiatorum. Occupational exposures in medical and dental personnel can produce lesions on the hands or digits, referred to as herpetic whitlow. Recurrent eruptions are often triggered by exogenous factors, including local trauma or sunburn. The primary infection with the herpes simplex virus often produces a more severe systemic reaction, including high fever, regional lymphadenopathy, and malaise, which is different from the reactivated form of the disease. Neonatal herpes simplex infection is one of the most life-threatening of all newborn infections and is acquired by ascending infection from an infected birth canal. It can be localized to the skin, eyes/mouth, result in encephalitis without cutaneous disease, or present as disseminated infection affecting multiple organs, most commonly the liver and adrenals. Rapid and severe progression of herpes simplex virus infection may occur in patients who are immunocompromised secondary to transplant (Fig. 28–8), or who have underlying diseases such as leukemia (Fig. 28–9) or HIV infection. A generalized herpetic infection of the skin may occur in persons with a pre-existing cutaneous disorder, such as atopic dermatitis or psoriasis, and is termed eczema herpeticum or Kaposi's varicelliform eruption (Fig. 28–10). Periocular involvement requires ophthalmologic evaluation to rule out herpetic keratoconjunctivitis. Herpes keratitis it is the most common infectious cause of corneal blindness in the United States and requires prompt recognition and treatment. Herpes simplex virus is the usual infectious agent to trigger recurrent erythema multiforme.

Despite the wide variation in clinical syndromes with varying severity, herpetic lesions share the appearance of

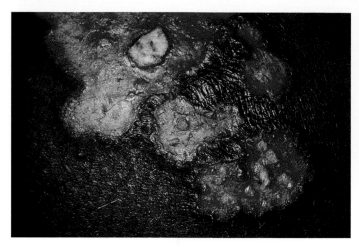

Figure 28–8 Chronic herpes simplex in a renal transplant recipient.

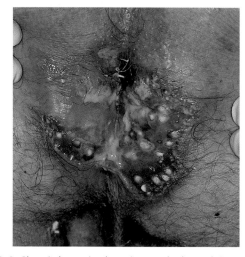

Figure 28–9 Chronic herpetic ulceration on the buttock in a patient with chronic lymphocytic leukemia.

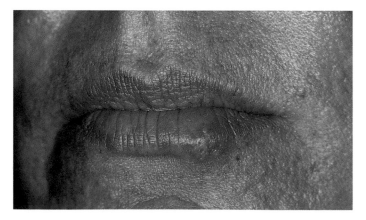

Figure 28–7 Typical appearance of herpes labialis on the lower lip in a patient with recurrent herpes simplex infection.

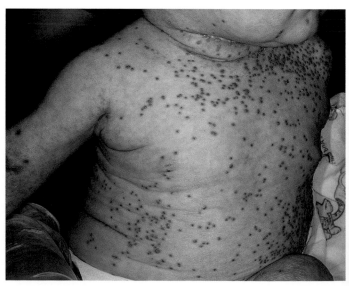

Figure 28–10 Kaposi's varicelliform eruption on a patient with eczema (also known as eczema herpeticum).

grouped vesicles on an erythematous base. Location is a critical feature in differentiating the various syndromes, with relatively well-localized recurrent infection producing a cluster of vesicles in the perioral or genital areas typifying infection with herpesvirus types 1 and 2. Lesions in immunocompromised patients may present as chronic ulcerations or vegetative lesions resembling malignancy.

Diagnosis

Culture of the virus has been the 'gold standard' of diagnosing herpes simplex virus infection. The Tzanck preparation reveals characteristic herpesvirus-induced changes. Immunoperoxidase techniques using monoclonal antibodies or DNA hybridization techniques are rapid diagnostic methods. Serologic testing plays a minor role and is useful in the diagnosis of primary infection, or is helpful if the result is negative, making infection with this virus unlikely.

Treatment

In healthy individuals, herpes simplex infection is self-limited and requires only local care to prevent bacterial superinfection and to alleviate pain. Primary oral or genital infections are often associated with significant morbidity. A course of systemic acyclovir (200 mg orally five times a day, or 400 mg three times a day), valacyclovir (2 g twice a day for 1 day), or famciclovir (1.5 g in one dose) has been shown to reduce the duration of viral shedding and pain, and speed the healing of lesions. For patients with frequent attacks, continuous suppressive therapy with acyclovir (400 mg orally twice daily), valacyclovir (1 g daily) or famciclovir (250 mg twice daily) has been shown to be highly effective without evidence of cumulative toxicity or resistance. Severe infections in immunocompromised patients or neonates require parenteral acyclovir therapy. The emergence of herpes simplex virus resistance to acyclovir in patients with AIDS and others is a problem with important ramifications. Intravenous foscarnet is currently the drug of choice in this situation.

Cytomegalovirus

Cytomegalovirus (CMV) is another member of the herpesvirus group. This organism accounts for about 10% of mononucleosis syndrome cases, and mononucleosis is the major clinical form of acquired CMV disease. Studies of antibodies to CMV indicate that infections with this virus are ubiquitous and that patients are asymptomatic. Congenital infection can occur by transplacental transmission of virus from an infected mother.

Clinical Manifestations

CMV mononucleosis is associated with an exanthem in about one-quarter of patients. It is characteristically a morbilliform erythema that primarily affects the face and trunk and lasts for 2–5 days. Occasionally, petechiae are present. There is no associated enanthem. Fever and tonsillar enlargement, malaise, and myalgia are often associated with infection, but sore throat and adenopathy are typically absent. Low-grade hepatitis with elevated liver enzyme levels is often present. The course of CMV mononucleosis is protracted, lasting weeks to months. The administration of ampicillin dramatically increases the likelihood of morbilliform eruption, as occurs with EBV mononucleosis.

Diagnosis

Culture of the urine and serologic titers for CMV are the most effective means of confirming the diagnosis. Cellular inclusions can often be detected by examining the urine. Biopsy specimens of the skin may reveal a neutrophilic vascular reaction histopathologically.

Treatment

In the nonimmunosuppressed host, treatment is supportive care. Retinitis in immunocompromised patients is treated with ganciclovir or cidofovir.

Herpangina

The etiologic agent in herpangina is a Coxsackie virus: A2, A4, A5, A6, A8, and A10 are the most frequently identified culprits.

Clinical Manifestations

Herpangina is characterized by the abrupt onset of fever, sore throat, anorexia, dysphagia, and vomiting. The exanthem is a morbilliform erythema with generalized pink papules, most prominent on the buttocks. Occasionally, petechiae are present. Oral lesions consist of 1–8-mm erosions with erythematous borders located on the soft palate, uvula, posterior pharyngeal wall, tongue, or anterior tonsillar pillars. Although oral lesions are usually few in number, they typically produce severe pain. Genital ulcerations are noted occasionally. Herpangina is a mild illness, lasting only a few days. Rarely, the course is complicated by parotitis.

Diagnosis

Viral culture of stool or throat washings can be used to confirm the diagnosis. Acute and convalescent sera can also be assessed.

Treatment

Treatment is supportive care.

BACTERIA

Systemic diseases caused by bacteria produce a variety of cutaneous changes. Dermatologic sequelae may result from bacterial toxins, from hypersensitivity reactions, or from direct cutaneous spread of organisms. Often, the changes produced are highly characteristic and allow for a prompt diagnosis and institution of therapy.

Streptococcal Infections

Scarlet Fever

The characteristic eruption of scarlet fever typically follows infection with an erythrogenic toxin produced by group A β-hemolytic streptococci. Specific antibodies synthesized in response to the toxin confer immunity.

Clinical manifestations

Scarlet fever occurs predominantly in children and typically follows streptococcal pharyngitis or tonsillitis. The characteristic cutaneous eruption consists of punctate erythematous papules, resulting in a sandpaper texture. The eruption begins on the neck and spreads caudally to involve the trunk and extremities. The palms and soles are generally spared. The face appears flushed, with a circumoral pallor. Petechiae may be present in creases of the elbows, groin, and axillae, a finding commonly referred to as Pastia's lines. The eruption begins to fade after 4–5 days with residual desquamation. A 'white strawberry' tongue, consisting of prominent, swollen red papillae (Fig. 28–11), appears in the first few days of the illness. This is followed by desquamation leading to the 'red strawberry' tongue. Cervical adenopathy and fever are usually present.

Diagnosis

The diagnosis can be confirmed by positive culture showing infection with group A streptococci. Increases in serum levels of antistreptolysin O and anti-DNase B also help confirm recent streptococcal infection.

Treatment

Penicillin is currently the treatment of choice. Erythromycin may be used in penicillin-sensitive patients.

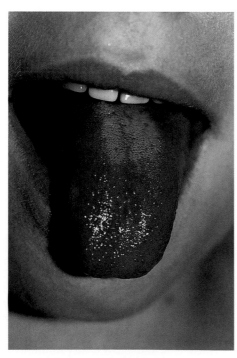

Figure 28–11 Scarlet fever – mucosal lesions.

Rheumatic Fever

Rheumatic fever is a sequela of an upper respiratory infection with group A streptococci. The disease is characterized by inflammatory lesions affecting the joints, heart, skin, and central nervous system. The peak age incidence is 5–15 years. The mechanism by which group A streptococci elicit the inflammatory response remains unknown. The recurrence rate in affected individuals is high.

Clinical manifestations

The clinical manifestations of acute rheumatic fever include erythema marginatum, subcutaneous nodules, polyarthritis, carditis, and chorea. The latency period between the antecedent streptococcal pharyngitis and the onset of symptoms of acute rheumatic fever is about 3 weeks. Erythema marginatum begins as an erythematous macule or papule that extends centrifugally as the central areas clear. Adjacent lesions may coalesce and form a serpiginous pattern. The lesions are evanescent, but the overall eruption may persist for weeks. The subcutaneous nodules are firm, painless lesions varying in size from a few millimeters to a few centimeters. The overlying skin is freely movable and is not inflamed. These lesions occur in crops over bony prominences or tendons.

Diagnosis

There is no definitive diagnostic test for rheumatic fever. Recognition of the diverse clinical manifestations of the disease is essential. The diagnostic criteria originally defined by Duckett Jones use major and minor criteria to support the diagnosis with a high degree of probability.

Treatment

Treatment with penicillin within 1 week of the onset of sore throat may prevent the subsequent onset of rheumatic fever. Antibiotics do not modify the course of an acute rheumatic attack. Acute rheumatic fever may be treated with systemic corticosteroids or supportively with nonsteroidal anti-inflammatory drugs (NSAIDs). Prophylaxis with low-dose penicillin effectively prevents recurrence.

Erysipelas

Erysipelas is a superficial dermal infection with group A streptococci.

Clinical manifestations

In adults the infection is usually found in the vicinity of a wound or ulceration. It may also affect the facial skin, presumably following some minor trauma. The characteristic cutaneous lesion is edematous, well demarcated, and dusky red, and may have prominent vesicles and bullae at the advancing edge. The patient may have toxemia and a high fever. Recurrent erysipelas has been associated with the development of lymphedema as a result of the accompanying lymphangitis. Erysipelas may also recur in lymphedematous extremities, such as after surgical intervention for breast carcinoma.

Diagnosis

Biopsy specimens of the skin reveal marked edema and a perivascular and diffuse, primarily acute, infiltrate. Intraepidermal vesicle formation may be present. Although not common, this infection has a characteristic clinical appearance. Attempts to culture organisms from tissue aspirates usually fail. Streptococcal cellulitis is a similar process; however, the skin lesions are not as well defined, and the process is not as acute. Systemic toxicity is less frequent.

Treatment

Penicillin, given intravenously, usually for 10–14 days, is the antibiotic of choice. In penicillin-sensitive individuals, erythromycin may be used.

Staphylococcal Infections

Impetigo

Impetigo is a superficial skin infection caused by *Staphyolococcus aureus* or *Streptococcus* species. Most cases today are caused by *Staphylococcus*. It is most common in children, and has the propensity to spread rapidly from one person to the next.

Clinical manifestations

Impetigo usually begins as a small cluster of blisters filled with yellow fluid. These rapidly break, leaving behind a characteristic yellow/honey-colored crust. In rare cases, lesions may remain blisters and coalesce into bullae (bullous impetigo). Lesions tend to be extremely pruritic, and scratching leads to rapid inoculation of the infection to other cutaneous sites.

Diagnosis

Bacterial culture from affected areas will yield the causative organism. Clinical suspicion warrants treatment.

Treatment

Limited cases may be adequately treated with topical antibiotic creams and ointments such as mupirocin; however, extensive lesions or those caused by methicillin-resistant *Staphylococcus aureus* require systemic antibiotics. Penicillinase-resistant penicillins or cephalosporins are a good first-line therapy until culture results are available.

Staphylococcal Scalded Skin Syndrome

Staphylococcal scalded skin syndrome (SSSS) is an acute life-threatening disease of infants caused by an exotoxin produced by *Staphylococcus aureus*, most commonly group II phage type 71. A predisposing factor for adult infection is either renal compromise or immunosuppression.

Clinical manifestations

The infection is heralded by the sudden onset of fever and diffuse tender, blanchable erythema. The eruption ordinarily begins perorally, with a rapid spread to the remainder of the body. Flaccid blistering occurs within 24–48 hours, with subsequent exfoliation in large sheets leaving extensive superficially denuded skin (Fig. 28–12). Layers of adjacent epidermis may easily peel off with rubbing (Nikolsky positive). The palms, soles, and mucous membranes are spared. Unless secondary bacterial infection occurs, the skin heals without scarring.

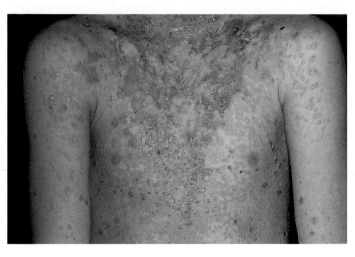

Figure 28–12 Crusted and vesiculated lesions in a patient with staphylococcal scalded skin syndrome.

Diagnosis

SSSS can be confirmed by a biopsy of the skin demonstrating an upper epidermal cleavage plane without dermal inflammation, which distinguishes this from toxic epidermal necrolysis. The organism cannot be cultured from bulla fluid because the lesions are caused by a toxin and the staphylococcal infection in general is present at a distant focus. Recovery of *Staph. aureus* from a bulla suggests a diagnosis of bullous impetigo. Recovery of *Staph. aureus* from the blood, urine, pharynx, nose, conjunctiva, umbilicus, or other sites confirms the diagnosis.

Treatment

The treatment of choice is a penicillinase-resistant penicillin. Systemic corticosteroids are contraindicated. Supportive measures include local care to skin blisters and erosions to prevent secondary bacterial infection. Close monitoring of fluid balance is required.

Toxic Shock Syndrome

Toxic shock syndrome is a multisystem illness whose diagnosis is based on the clinical case definition from the CDC: fever >38.9°C, diffuse erythematous macules or erythroderma with acral desquamation, hypotension, and involvement of three or more organ systems. It is caused by toxin-producing strains of *Staph. aureus*, and most reported cases have involved tampon use in menstruating women. Cases related to infected wounds, contraceptive devices, and nasal packing after rhinoplasty have also been reported.

Clinical manifestations

The majority of reported cases have occurred in young women during their menstrual periods. The initial symptoms include fever, abdominal pain, vomiting, diarrhea, reduced urine output, and alterations in mental status. The cutaneous eruption is generally a diffuse scarlatiniform erythema, which may progress to erythroderma. Desquamation occurs about 1 week after the onset of the cutaneous eruption, and may be acral or generalized. The conjunctivae and pharynx are typically infected. Strawberry tongue and/or oral erosions may also be features of toxic shock syndrome.

Diagnosis

In cases related to tampon use, a positive vaginal culture for *Staph. aureus* can usually be obtained. Blood cultures are less commonly positive.

Treatment

Treatment consists of systemic administration of antistaphylococcal antibiotics, such as penicillinase-resistant penicillins. Aggressive fluid and electrolyte therapy is crucial. Removal of tampons or nasal packing or drainage of an infected site is a key part of the management.

Gram-Negative Infection

Meningococcemia

Meningococcemia is one of the most important diseases for the physician to recognize because of its ability to rapidly lead to patient demise. The etiologic agent in meningococcemia is the Gram-negative diplococcus *Neisseria meningitidis*. Various clinical syndromes are associated with meningococcal sepsis, the most life-threatening being acute meningitis with septicemia. Meningococcal vaccine is now routinely recommended for children aged 11–12. It is also recommended for children entering high school who have not been previously vaccinated, military recruits entering boot camp, college freshmen planning to live in dormitories, and patients who have had a splenectomy or who have terminal complement deficiencies, as well as for tourists traveling to epidemic areas, including sub-Saharan Africa and areas in the Middle East, India, and Nepal. If the vaccine is for travel reasons, it should be administered at least 1 week prior to departure.

Clinical manifestations

The hallmark of acute meningococcemia is a petechial eruption accentuated in areas generally covered by tight clothing. The lesions may coalesce and appear as large areas of confluent purpura (Figs 28–13 and 28–14). Other cutaneous manifestations include a viral exanthem-like eruption, hemorrhagic vesicles, and pustules. Profound ischemic necrosis known as purpura fulminans may accompany meningococcal sepsis, which is often fatal.

Diagnosis

The diagnosis is confirmed by the detection of organisms on Gram stains of cutaneous lesions followed by culture of the organism (blood and cerebrospinal fluid produce the highest yield). Biopsy specimens of the skin reveal an acute neutrophilic vascular reaction, and in most instances meningococci can be demonstrated on tissue Gram stains.

Treatment

Antibiotic management with ceftriaxone is currently the treatment of choice for all forms of meningococcal disease. The correction of hemodynamic instability, often in an intensive care unit, is of paramount importance. Even with treatment, neurologic sequelae are possible.

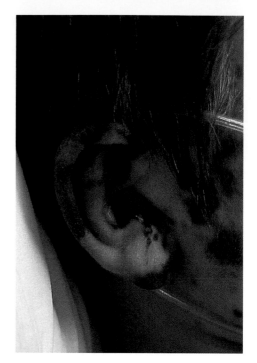

Figure 28–13 Meningococcemia.

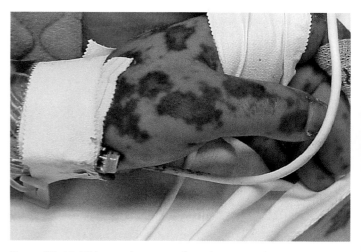

Figure 28–14 Widespread purpura of meningococcemia.

Cat Scratch Disease

Cat scratch disease is a benign self-limited infection caused by a cat scratch or bite, which consists of a primary lesion and subsequent development of regional adenopathy. The etiologic agent has recently been reported to be the pleomorphic Gram-negative rod *Bartonella henselae*.

Clinical manifestations

The initial manifestation of cat scratch disease is a papule, pustule, or vesicle at the site of trauma. Mild fever, malaise, and anorexia may be associated features, and regional lymphadenopathy develops. Lymph nodes are usually solitary, moderately tender, and freely movable. If the conjunctiva is the primary inoculation site, the patient may present with con-junctivitis and ipsilateral preauricular adenopathy; this unusual presentation is called the oculoglandular syndrome of Parinaud.

Diagnosis

Culture of a causative organism for cat scratch disease is cur-rently not possible. Indirect fluorescent antibody testing has low sensitivity but high specificity. Rising IgG titers indicate recent infection. Biopsy specimens from a primary lesion reveal frank dermal necrosis with surrounding epithelioid cells, giant cells, and eosinophils. The organism can best be identified with the Warthin–Starry stain.

Treatment

Localized cat scratch disease is benign and self-limited. Occa-sionally, surgical drainage of a suppurative node is indicated. For severe disease or disease in immunocompromised hosts, both rifampin (600–900 mg/day) and azithromycin are effec-tive for short courses of treatment.

Spirochetes

As the causative agent of syphilis, *Treponema pallidum* is dis-cussed in Chapter 29. The only spirochetal organism addressed in this chapter is *Borrelia burgdorferi*.

Lyme Disease

Lyme disease is a multisystem infection caused by the spiro-chete *B. burgdorferi*. It is the most common tick-borne illness in the United States and is most prevalent along the northeast coast, northern midwest, and west coast. The primary arthro-pod vector in the northeast and midwest is the deer tick *Ixodes scapularis*. *I. pacificus* is the vector on the west coast.

Clinical manifestations

The characteristic cutaneous eruption erythema migrans is the earliest manifestation and best clinical marker of this systemic disease. It occurs 1–2 weeks after the infectious bite and is often accompanied by flu-like symptoms. The eruption begins with erythema at the site of the bite and expands as an ery-thematous palpable ring. The lesion gradually expands circum-ferentially, and the central area may clear or become necrotic (Fig. 28–15). Erythema migrans is asymptomatic, and there-fore the eruption may be missed by the patient. Approximately 20% of patients develop multiple annular lesions at distant sites secondary to *Borrelia* dissemination. Fever, malaise, arthralgias, and myalgias typically accompany the cutaneous lesions. If untreated, further dissemination of the organism may occur, resulting in chronic arthritis and neurologic or cardiac complications. Acrodermatitis chronica atrophicans is an uncommon cutaneous disease that may occur with chronic *Borrelia* infection, primarily in Europe, and is characterized by erythematous atrophic lesions on the extremities.

Diagnosis

The presence of the classic erythema migrans lesion is diagnos-tic for Lyme disease and treatment should be started. This is

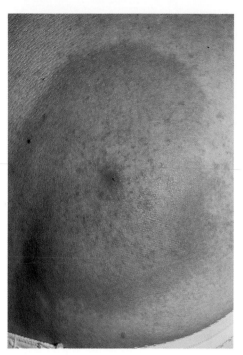

Figure 28–15 Erythematous annular lesion of erythema chronicum migrans.

because serologies do not become positive for 4–6 weeks after the initial infection. An enzyme-linked immunosorbent assay (ELISA) is the usual method of testing. There may still be a problem of reproducibility of results from one laboratory to another. False-positive serologic results may occur in patients with other infections, such as subacute bacterial endocarditis, mononucleosis, leptospirosis, or syphilis, or in patients with systemic lupus erythematosus. For these reasons, interpreta-tion of serologic results can be difficult. For example, the CDC does not recommend serologies in endemic areas when the classic eruption is present. At the same time, when the pretest probability is low, the CDC also does not recommend sero-logic testing as a positive result does not necessarily implicate Lyme disease as a cause of the patient's symptoms.

Treatment

Antibiotic management with oral doxycycline, usually for 21 days, is currently the treatment of choice in limited disease. Meningitis or cardiac involvement is treated with intravenous ceftriaxone. Amoxicillin is also effective and is preferred for children and for pregnant or lactating women.

Rickettsia

Rickettsiae are obligate intracellular organisms containing both DNA and RNA whose natural reservoirs are a variety of arthropods. The organisms specifically infect vascular endothe-lial cells. Cutaneous small-vessel vasculitis is often a promi-nent manifestation of these disabling febrile illnesses. The spectrum of clinical manifestations ranges from benign and self-limited to fatal. Serologic examination is the most useful method of diagnosis for the varied rickettsial infections. Often the organism can be found by PCR in biopsy specimens.

Rocky Mountain Spotted Fever

Rocky Mountain spotted fever (RMSF) is the most frequently reported rickettsial disease in the United States, and is the most severe. Without treatment RMSF has a 30% mortality rate; with effective treatment this drops to 3–5%. The causative agent, *Rickettsia rickettsii*, is transmitted by an infectious tick. The principal offender in the western United States is the wood tick *Dermacentor andersoni*, and in the eastern United States is the dog tick *D. variabilis*.

Clinical manifestations

After an incubation period of about 5–10 days, nonspecific symptoms, including severe headache, fever, and myalgias, develop, prompting an initial visit to the primary care physician. Early cutaneous findings include discrete rose-colored blanching macules of the wrists, ankles, palms, and soles (Fig. 28–16), which are present in 85% of affected patients. The lesions subsequently spread to the trunk and head, become petechial, and may slough, forming ulcerations. The palms and soles are involved in at least 50% of patients, but in 10% no cutaneous findings are evident. Without prompt treatment, systemic manifestations, including renal insufficiency, meningitis, disseminated intravascular coagulation, hepatic failure, and death, can occur.

Diagnosis

The diagnosis must be made clinically and treatment should never be delayed. Confirmation of the diagnosis can be achieved by serologic testing, the gold standard of which is an indirect immunofluorescence assay. Other serologic tests such as ELISA, immunoblot and latex agglutination are available. Demonstration of rickettsiae in a biopsy specimen of the skin by a direct immunofluorescence microscopic technique using a specific antibody is also possible.

Treatment

The treatment of choice in adults and children is doxycycline, with chloramphenicol being used in selected patients such as pregnant women.

Endemic Typhus

Endemic or murine typhus is caused by *R. typhi* and is transmitted by the rat flea *Xenopsylla cheopis*, the same vector that propagates plague. This disease occurs worldwide, mainly in urban areas.

Clinical manifestations

After a 12-day incubation period, a prodrome consisting of fever, chills, severe headache, and nausea develops. A few days later, a morbilliform, often petechial, cutaneous eruption appears and primarily involves the trunk. Splenomegaly and regional or widespread lymphadenopathy may be present. The course is usually mild, resulting in underdiagnosis. Systemic large-vessel vasculitis is a rare complication.

Diagnosis

The diagnosis can be made by complement fixation tests or by indirect fluorescence antibody studies using acute and convalescent sera. The Weil–Felix reaction is positive.

Treatment

Antibiotic therapy consisting of tetracycline or chloramphenicol is the current treatment of choice.

Epidemic Typhus

Epidemic typhus is caused by *R. prowazekii* and is transmitted by the human body louse, *Pediculus humanus* var. *corporis*. Transmission occurs as a result of louse defecation during feeding, with subsequent inoculation caused by scratching. The only animal reservoir that has been implicated is the flying squirrel, *Glaucomys volans*.

Clinical manifestations

After a 12-day incubation period the disease is heralded by fever, chills, headache, and weakness. A few days later a truncal macular eruption appears and spreads distally, sparing the face, palms, and soles. These macular lesions may subsequently become hemorrhagic and are more severe than those of endemic typhus. They may lead to gangrene.

Diagnosis

Complement-fixing antibodies allow for differentiation between the rickettsial species. Indirect fluorescence antibodies are demonstrable during convalescence, but do not differentiate between species.

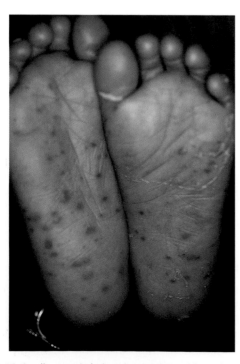

Figure 28–16 Small purpuric lesions in a patient with Rocky Mountain spotted fever.

Treatment

The current treatment of choice is doxycycline or chloramphenicol. Vaccination is suggested for high-risk groups.

Rickettsial pox

Rickettsial pox is a mild febrile disease caused by *R. akari* and is transmitted by the house mouse mite *Allodermanyssus sanguineus*.

Clinical manifestations

A primary erythematous papular lesion occurs at the site of the mite bite, followed by fever, headache, myalgias, and a generalized varicella-like vesicular cutaneous eruption. Generalized lymphadenopathy and splenomegaly may be present. Rickettsial pox is a benign illness, and recovery occurs without therapy.

Diagnosis

Complement fixation and indirect fluorescence demonstrate antibodies.

Treatment

The current treatment of choice is doxycycline or chloramphenicol.

Scrub Typhus

Scrub typhus, or tsutsugamushi fever, is caused by *Orientia tsutsugamushi*. Infection is transmitted through the bite of larvae of certain trombiculid mites (chiggers), and is most common in Southeast Asia, Japan, Korea, and Australia. The classic tsutsugamushi disease occurs during the summer, has a high mortality rate, and is transmitted by *Leptotrombidium akamushi*. The so-called new type of tsutsugamushi disease is milder than the classic form and is transmitted by *Leptotrombidium deliense*.

Clinical manifestations

After the bite a primary lesion is usually detectable at the site. This consists of an enlarging erythematous papule that undergoes central necrosis and then forms an eschar within 1–2 weeks. Regional adenopathy is associated. A few days later, a truncal morbilliform rash, resembling roseola or rubella, develops and spreads peripherally. It is often accompanied by high fevers and myalgia. Pneumonia, thrombocytopenia, and hypofibrinogenemia have been described in scrub typhus, and most deaths are the result of severe disseminated intravascular coagulation. The presence of bradycardia relative to the elevated temperature is a unique feature.

Diagnosis

Complement fixation and indirect fluorescence demonstrate antibodies.

Treatment

The current treatment of choice is doxycycline or chloramphenicol.

MYCOBACTERIA

Tuberculosis

Tuberculosis of the skin can be divided into exogenous and endogenous forms. The cell-mediated immune response modulates the form of infection in a given patient.

Exogenous Infection

Clinical Manifestations

Exogenous infection occurs when *Mycobacterium tuberculosis* is inoculated directly into the skin of a nonimmune host. The primary lesion is typically a verrucous papule that may be crusted or eroded (tuberculous chancre) and is associated with regional lymphadenopathy. The diagnosis can be confirmed by biopsy of the skin and culture. 'Sporotrichoid spread,' in which progressive lesions develop along lymphatic drainage channels, is another pattern of cutaneous disease that can occur following primary cutaneous inoculation. This may be more common with atypical mycobacterial infection.

Inoculation of *M. tuberculosis* into the skin of a person who has previously been infected by this organism results in tuberculosis verrucosa cutis. The primary lesion is a papule with a violaceous halo that evolves into a hyperkeratotic, warty plaque. Lesions occur most commonly on the dorsolateral hands and fingers, are usually discrete, and are not associated with lymphadenopathy. This form of tuberculosis must be differentiated from other hyperkeratotic verrucous processes, such as blastomycosis, chromoblastomycosis, Madura foot, Majocchi's granuloma, iododerma, bromoderma, atypical mycobacterial infection, and botryomycosis.

Endogenous Infection

Clinical Manifestations

Lupus vulgaris is another skin lesion found in patients with previous exposure to *M. tuberculosis*. Found primarily on the head and neck, it is characterized by groups of 'apple jelly'-colored nodules due to deep dermal infiltration with tuberculous granulomas. Nodules coalesce into large plaques (Fig. 28–17) and lead to scarring and distortion and destruction of underlying cartilaginous structures. A large percentage of patients with lupus vulgaris have underlying tuberculosis in other organs, with hematogenous spread to the skin.

Scrofuloderma is produced by direct extension of tuberculosis to the skin from an underlying structure (lymph nodes, bones, or joints). The clinical lesion is characterized by a firm subcutaneous nodule that suppurates, becoming a boggy plaque. The most commonly involved areas are the head and neck. Hematogenous secondary extension to the skin may result in the formation of metastatic tuberculous 'cold' abscesses that break down to form ulcers and fistulae.

Acute miliary tuberculosis represents dissemination of the organism to the skin on all parts of the body, particularly the trunk, and consists of a morbilliform-like exanthem or vesicular purpuric lesions. This is rare and usually occurs in severely

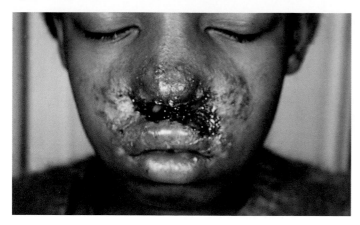

Figure 28–17 Crusted plaques in a malar distribution also involving the nose and the mustache area in a patient with cutaneous tuberculosis (lupus vulgaris).

immunocompromised patients. Unlike other cutaneous lesions of cutaneous tuberculosis, granulomas may be absent histopathologically. A high index of suspicion is required to make this diagnosis.

Diagnosis

Cutaneous tuberculosis produces variable histopathologic changes, depending on the type and age of the lesion. Tuberculous organisms can often be identified by acid-fast stains. Patients with cutaneous tuberculosis should be evaluated for disseminated disease and for predisposing risk factors. Culture often confirms the diagnosis. Skin testing, using the intradermal Mantoux test to purified protein derivative, can be performed to support the clinical diagnosis. Reactivity to the tuberculin protein is impaired in medical conditions in which cellular immunity is deficient, and a negative test finding does not exclude tuberculosis. When tuberculosis is confirmed it is essential to notify the local Department of Health.

Treatment

Various antituberculous therapeutic agents are available, including isoniazid, rifampin, and ethambutol. Recommendations for the exact combination and duration of treatment change periodically. Localized lesions may be amenable to surgical excision. Thorough evaluation for systemic involvement is warranted in patients who present with cutaneous disease.

Atypical Mycobacterial Infections

In healthy individuals, cutaneous involvement by atypical mycobacteria is caused primarily by *M. marinum*. This organism is found in aquatic environments and is usually inoculated into the skin following an abrasion. Thus, the lesion occurs primarily in persons exposed to fish tanks, boats, stagnant pools, and so forth. Lesions for the most part occur on the hands and arms.

The primary lesion of *M. marinum* infection is chancriform, hyperkeratotic, and occasionally ulcerative (Fig. 28–18). Sec-

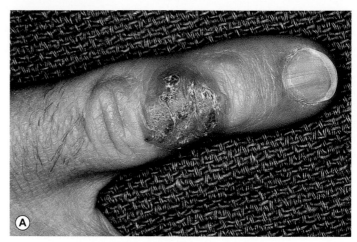

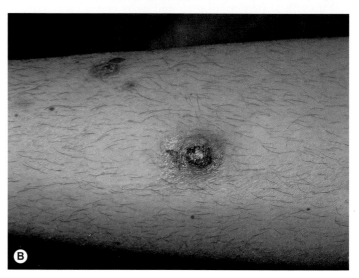

Figure 28–18 Ulcerated nodular lesion representative of atypical mycobacterial infection (swimming pool granuloma). (Courtesy of Dr W. Barkey, Flint, Michigan.)

ondary lesions may spread in a sporotrichoid fashion along the regional lymphatic vessels. The disease is self-limited and usually resolves within 1–2 years.

A rare cutaneous lesion is Buruli's ulceration, an extensive ulcerative process that results from infection with *M. ulcerans*. Most of these lesions are solitary and are on the lower extremities. This diagnosis should be considered if the patient has traveled to an endemic area (Uganda, Mexico, or Australia) and has a large ulcerative cutaneous lesion with associated paresthesiae.

M. avium intracellulare and other atypical mycobacteria can produce nonspecific cutaneous lesions following dissemination. This is a particular problem in patients who have AIDS.

Diagnosis

Biopsy of a swimming pool granulomatous lesion (*M. marinum*) reveals granulomatous dermatitis, and acid-fast stains will demonstrate organisms in some cases. Failure to demonstrate acid-fast organisms does not exclude the diagnosis of atypical mycobacteriosis. Biopsy of Buruli's ulcer reveals cutaneous ulceration with necrosis and a sparse infiltrate. Acid-fast stains will demonstrate organisms in the ulceration. Biopsy of skin lesions of *M. avium intracellulare* may reveal granulomatous inflammation with myriad acid-fast organisms within the cytoplasm of histiocytes. A high index of suspicion is required so that the laboratory can perform cultures on appropriate media.

Treatment

A variety of treatments can be used for *M. marinum* infection, including the local application of heat, local excision, and oral therapy with minocycline, trimethoprim–sulfamethoxazole, or antituberculous drugs such as rifampin. Treatment for other atypical mycobacteria depends on the organism.

Leprosy

Leprosy is a chronic granulomatous disease caused by *M. leprae*, an acid-fast-positive bacterial rod found primarily within histiocytes. Despite historic beliefs, the disease is not highly communicable. The method of transmission is not clearly defined, but probably involves direct contact or fomites. The cutaneous lesions include a panoply of findings that indicate the type of host response induced by the infection. Leprosy affects the relatively cool areas of the skin; lesions are therefore most apt to occur on exposed surfaces, such as the earlobes or distal extremities. A high proportion of individuals are immune to infection with the organism, which accounts for its relatively infrequent presentation. An important reservoir of *M. leprae* in the United States is the nine-banded armadillo, found frequently in Texas and other southwestern states. The World Health Organization has long been trying to reduce the prevalence of leprosy in all countries to <1:10 000 persons. As of 2006 all but six nations (Brazil, Congo, Madagascar, Mozambique, Nepal, and Tanzania) had achieved this goal through early recognition and treatment strategies.

Clinical Manifestations

The earliest cutaneous lesions occur as indeterminate leprosy, which is characterized by ill-defined macules. As the disease advances to one of the more clearly defined stages, these early lesions may fade.

Patients with tuberculoid leprosy have active cellular immunity to *M. leprae* and a strongly positive lepromin test (a cutaneous response to standardized extracts of infected tissue). The lesions may be single or multiple and are variable in size, clearly defined, and frequently hypopigmented (Fig. 28–19). Paresthesia is common within these lesions secondary to the neurotropism of the organism, with sensation to temperature being the first sensation lost. Neurotropism may also lead to nerve enlargement, particularly of the ulnar and greater auricular nerves. Enlargement may be to the point at which these nerves are grossly visible during a general physical examination.

In patients with a reduced cellular immune response to *M. leprae*, cutaneous disease evolves into lesions that are typical of lepromatous leprosy. Lepromatous leprosy represents an immune state in which there is anergy and a negative lepromin

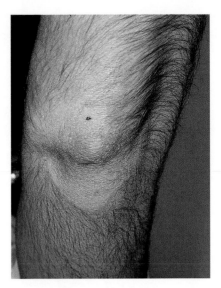

Figure 28–19 Hypopigmented anesthetic skin in an Indian physician with tuberculoid leprosy.

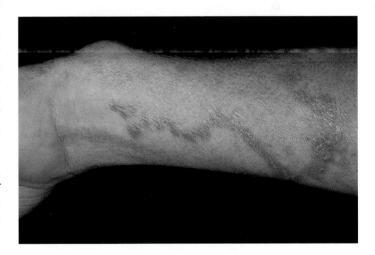

Figure 28–20 Annular lesions of lepromatous leprosy.

reaction. The cutaneous lesions are pleomorphic and range from macules to nodules, plaques, and diffuse infiltrative lesions (Figs 28–20 and 28–21). Patients may develop leonine facies, in which there is diffuse facial thickening associated with loss of eyebrows (madarosis) and eyelashes. The lesions are usually widespread and multiple. A rare form of lepromatous leprosy is the diffuse leprosy of Lucio. This is characterized by a diffuse skin infiltrate and ulcerations, with few localized stigmata of leprosy.

Borderline, or dimorphous, leprosy can present a spectrum of cutaneous lesions, including those similar to lepromatous leprosy. Infiltrative annular lesions are characteristic of borderline leprosy. The lepromin reaction is variable. The lesions in a given patient can vary from one extreme to the other as the immune response of the host alters. If there is a shift towards the tuberculoid pole, the patient may have a reversal reaction in which the cutaneous lesions may redden and become tender, with painful swelling and enlargement of the nerves. If there is a shift towards the lepromatous pole, the patient

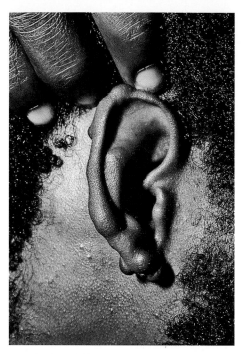

Figure 28–21 Multiple nodules present in lepromatous leprosy.

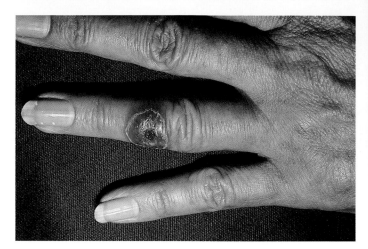

Figure 28–22 A chancriform lesion on the digit in a patient with sporotrichosis.

may experience a downgrading reaction heralded by widespread lesions of erythema nodosum leprosum (painful red nodules that clinically mimic those of erythema nodosum), which is accompanied by fever and other constitutional symptoms. Downgrading reactions are frequently chronic and may be disabling.

Diagnosis

Biopsy specimens of the skin reveal a spectrum of findings, depending on the type of disease. Specimens from indeterminate leprosy are not diagnostic and contain a minimal inflammatory infiltrate. A slit smear (a small superficial skin incision with expression of tissue fluid that is stained with acid-fast or the Fite stain) can be used to confirm the diagnosis from borderline tuberculoid to lepromatous leprosy (in cases in which ample quantities of organisms are present in tissue). Appropriate neurologic, otolaryngologic, ophthalmologic, and surgical evaluation should be performed, depending on the symptoms and signs exhibited by the patient. Results from skin biopsies dramatically reduce the list of diagnostic possibilities.

Treatment

Therapy mainly involves the use of at least two drugs, as monotherapy leads rapidly to organism resistance. The WHO uses dapsone and rifampin in cases of paucibacillary leprosy, and a triple-agent treatment with rifampin, dapsone, and clofazimine for multibacillary disease. Thalidomide is the treatment of choice in erythema nodosum leprosum. There are of course many variations in the treatment of this complex disease. Patients must be followed for prolonged periods, and coordination of care with infectious disease specialists is of paramount importance.

FUNGI

Cutaneous fungal infections with systemic involvement include a variety of subcutaneous and systemic mycoses. The subcutaneous mycoses (i.e., sporotrichosis) are often referred to as 'fungi of implantation' because they are typically acquired by inoculation from an infected object; however, with sporotrichosis, and to a lesser extent with chromoblastomycosis, subsequent dissemination to other organs can occur. The systemic fungal infections are divided into true pathogens (histoplasmosis, blastomycosis, coccidioidomycosis, and paracoccidioidomycosis) and opportunistic infections (candidiasis, aspergillosis, zygomycosis, and cryptococcosis). The largest group of fungi to infect the skin is dermatophytes, but because they seldom produce systemic involvement they will not be discussed.

Subcutaneous Mycoses with Systemic Manifestations

Sporotrichosis

Sporotrichosis is a fungal infection caused by *Sporothrix schenckii*. Sporotrichosis is worldwide in distribution but occurs most commonly in temperate and tropical zones, where high humidity and warm temperatures favor its saprophytic growth. The organism typically gains access to the skin of its host by traumatic inoculation from objects that have been contaminated by the fungus (e.g., sphagnum moss, thorny plants, baled hay). Rarely, direct inhalation into the lungs is the mode of acquisition, with subsequent dissemination to the skin.

Clinical manifestations

The classic disease begins as a small painless papule/subcutaneous nodule at the site of inoculation (Fig. 28–22). This lesion becomes violaceous and ulcerates to expose a ragged necrotic base, forming a sporotrichotic chancre. Local extension may occur via lymphatic channels. This results in the proximal spread of subcutaneous nodules, which suppurate

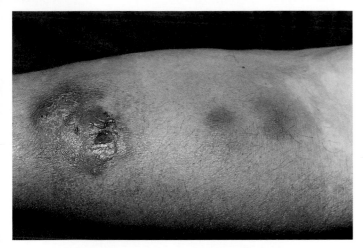

Figure 28–23 Lymphangitic spread in a patient with sporotrichosis.

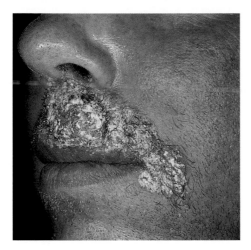

Figure 28–24 Facial lesions of sporotrichosis.

and ulcerate along the lymphatic channel (Fig. 28–23). Lesions are most common on the hands and arms, but occasionally the face may be inoculated (Fig. 28–24).

Disseminated sporotrichosis is rare and usually results from hematogenous dissemination of a primary lesion. The most common extracutaneous sites are the bones and joints, lungs, meninges, genitourinary tract, and eyes. Risk factors include hematologic and lymphoreticular malignancies, chronic alcoholism, immunosuppressive drugs, and AIDS.

Diagnosis

Because of the paucity of organisms usually found in tissue, histopathologic examination is of only modest value in evaluating sporotrichosis. At room temperature, culture is possible on Sabouraud's agar. Microscopic examination of material from cultures reveals conidiophores developing at right-angles from the hyphae. These culture plates should be examined only in facilities that specialize in mycologic diagnosis, because the spores could be inhaled.

Treatment

Itraconazole is the current CDC-recommended treatment of choice for localized disease in nonpregnant adults. Oral iodide

is the treatment of choice for disease resistant to itraconazole. Treatment for disseminated disease is liposomal amphotericin B, and itraconazole can be used as a stepdown therapy once the patient is stabilized.

Other Subcutaneous Mycoses

Less common subcutaneous mycoses, such as chromoblastomycosis and mycetoma, are typically limited to cutaneous and subcutaneous regions; however, dissemination to other organs may occur in immunocompromised patients. Further discussion of these rare mycoses is beyond the scope of this chapter.

Systemic Mycoses

Pathogenic Fungal Infections: Respiratory Dimorphic Mycoses

Respiratory dimorphic fungal infections are acquired by inhaling the causative organism from the mold state in nature, resulting in a primary pulmonary infection. The organism appears in a different state in the tissue than in nature, with the exception of coccidioidomycosis, which has endosporulating spherules in tissue. The dimorphic mycoses are mostly yeasts in tissue (except for *Coccidioides immitis*) and mold at room temperature, hence the name 'dimorphic.'

Blastomycosis

North American blastomycosis is caused by the fungus *Blastomyces dermatitidis*. Most cases occur in the states surrounding the Mississippi and Ohio Rivers, where soil is rich in decomposing organic substances; however, cases also occur in persons with high exposure to wooded areas (farmers, hunters, campers, forestry workers).

Clinical manifestations

Approximately 50% of infected patients are symptomatic at disease onset. Symptoms include fever, chills, myalgia, arthralgia, and cough. Patients who fail to recover completely from the illness may develop chronic infection of the lungs, bones, or skin. In fact, the skin is the most common extrapulmonary site of involvement. Cutaneous lesions begin as papules or pustules, most commonly affecting the head, neck, or extremities. They then evolve into ulcers with undermined or verrucous borders and central atrophic scars (Figs 28–25 and 28–26). Without treatment the lesions continue to enlarge and may be disfiguring. Most of these are presumed to be the result of disseminated pulmonary infection, though some primary inoculum cases of cutaneous blastomycosis have been reported.

Diagnosis

Acute respiratory infection is confirmed by a sputum examination. Histopathologic findings with special stains and culture confirmation can be performed on cutaneous lesions. Interestingly, wet-mount KOH preparation from pustules may reveal the organism, which has characteristic broad-based budding. At room temperature, this organism grows rapidly in Sab-

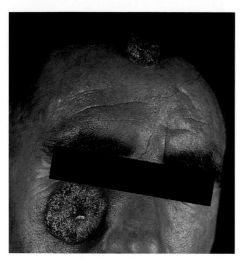

Figure 28–25 Verrucous plaque on the cheek in a patient with North American blastomycosis.

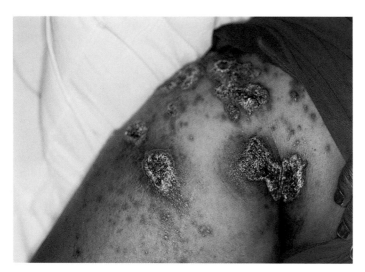

Figure 28–26 Verrucous plaques on the arm of a patient with blastomycosis.

ouraud's glucose agar. Methenamine silver or periodic acid–Schiff stains facilitate identification of these organisms.

Treatment

Pulmonary disease is most often treated with amphotericin B. For limited cutaneous disease, oral itraconazole has been shown to be highly effective. Duration of treatment is guided by the extent of dissemination, with treatment courses lasting as long as 12 months in patients with osteomyelitis.

Histoplasmosis

Histoplasmosis is caused by the dimorphic fungus *Histoplasma capsulatum*. Infection is most commonly seen in the eastern and central United States, where starling guano is thought to be an important reservoir. Pulmonary infection follows the inhalation of conidia. The majority of cases are subclinical; however, immunosuppression, malignancy, and HIV all predispose to more severe disseminated disease.

Clinical manifestations

Inhalation of spores leads to the initial infection, which is often asymptomatic (90% of patients). Cutaneous lesions of histoplasmosis result from dissemination through the bloodstream from a primary pulmonary focus. Mucous membrane lesions are more common than are lesions of glabrous skin. Cutaneous lesions are nonspecific, with a broad variety of morphologies, including macules, papules, pustules, abscesses, plaques, ulcers, purpuric lesions, dermatitic lesions, and vasculitic lesions. Erythema multiforme and erythema nodosum are commonly associated reactive dermatoses. These usually occur during the primary exposure phase or simultaneously with dissemination.

Diagnosis

The diagnosis can be confirmed by a demonstration of dimorphic fungal growth in culture. Biopsy specimens of the skin reveal perivascular inflammation containing lymphocytes, plasma cells, and the characteristic parasitized histiocytes. The cells contain intracellular *H. capsulatum* in the yeast state with narrow neck budding. In patients with disseminated disease, bone marrow biopsy and culture may lead to the correct diagnosis. Immunodiagnostic studies are helpful and include polysaccharide antigen testing, histoplasmin skin testing, and a serologic determination of antibody response.

Treatment

The treatment of choice for severe pulmonary infection or disseminated disease is intravenous amphotericin B. Pneumonitis in immunocompetent patients is treated conservatively with supportive care.

Coccidioidomycosis

Coccidioidomycosis (also known as Valley Fever) is caused by infection with *Coccidioides immitis*, the most virulent of fungal pathogens. The organism is a soil saprophyte endemic to the southwestern United States, northern Mexico, Central America, and South America. Since 1993 the incidence of infection has risen more than 300% in Arizona. Infection occurs after inhalation of arthroconidia, and occurs with greater frequency in persons routinely exposed to dry desert soil (farm workers, archaeologists, and constructions workers), pregnant women, and African-Americans. Epidemics have also occurred as a result of natural disasters that stir up desert sands (earthquakes, dust storms). Immunocompromised states, including lymphoproliferative disease and AIDS, are risk factors for dissemination.

Clinical manifestations

Primary coccidioidomycosis is a disease of the lungs that produces fever, cough, chest pains, and myalgias in 40% of patients. The remaining 60% remain asymptomatic at the time of infection. A morbilliform erythema may accompany the acute episode. Within 2 weeks painful subcutaneous nodules of erythema nodosum may appear on the legs: this is a positive prognostic indicator. Erythema multiforme may also be observed. All of these are nonspecific cutaneous reactions, so

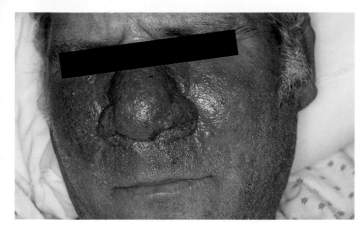

Figure 28–27 Erythematous, cellulitic-appearing eruption on the malar skin and the nose in a man with coccidioidomycosis.

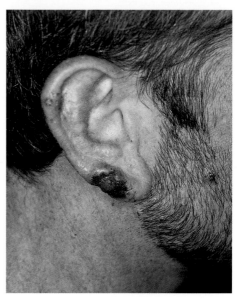

Figure 28–28 Nodular, ulcerated lesions of disseminated cryptococcosis in an HIV-infected patient.

a high clinical suspicion of coccidioidomycosis must be present to confirm the diagnosis. In normal hosts, the infection clears within a month; however, occasionally coccidioidomycosis may produce chronic and disseminated disease. The cutaneous lesions seen in patients with disseminated disease represent a highly variable clinical picture, including papules, pustules, subcutaneous abscesses, granulomatous plaques, and ulcers (Fig. 28–27). Primary coccidioidomycosis of the skin is rare. Widespread dissemination of specific coccidioidomycosis to internal organs is possible, and must be excluded in patients with disseminated cutaneous disease.

Diagnosis

Skin tests to coccidioidin antigen are positive in most patients after 2 weeks of illness, and antibody tests become positive later. Fungal culture in a standard medium containing cyclo-heximide will yield the dimorphic fungus, but must be performed in specialized laboratories because of the ability of the organism to infect laboratory personnel. Biopsy specimens show epidermal hyperplasia, a polymorphic infiltrate, and occasional fungal organisms that appear in the tissue as endo-sporulating spherules.

Treatment

Most of the time the disease resolves on its own; however, treatment of patients at risk for dissemination is often advocated. Fluconazole and itraconazole have both been shown to be efficacious. Amphotericin B is the treatment of choice for disseminated disease.

Opportunistic Fungal Infections

Opportunistic fungal infections are most commonly caused by two groups of yeasts (*Candida* and *Cryptococcus*) and two groups of molds (Zygomycota and *Aspergillus*). However, most fungi could cause systemic disease in immunocompromised patients.

Cryptococcosis

Cryptococcosis is a systemic infection caused by the fungus *Cryptococcus neoformans*. Evidence indicates that the organism is acquired by inhalation. There is an increased incidence of infection in patients who are immunosuppressed (e.g., as a manifestation of AIDS, from corticosteroid or cytotoxic therapy in association with lymphoma or connective tissue disorders, or in association with sarcoidosis)

Clinical manifestations

Cryptococcus produces a pneumonia-like illness consisting of shortness of breath and fever. Central nervous system manifestations are the most severe and the most common initial presentation. Cutaneous lesions are not uncommon, and may be solitary papules, some with central dells, pustules, nodules, cellulitic lesions, or ulcers (Fig. 28–28). The face and scalp are the most common locations, and lesions may resemble those of molluscum contagiosum, basal cell carcinoma, and a variety of other cutaneous lesions.

Diagnosis

Cryptococcal antigen tests are available for both blood and CSF. In tissue, the organism can be identified by its positivity with Mayer's mucicarmine, which stains the yeast's capsule red but does not stain other fungi that have similar morphologic characteristics. Because skin involvement is most often a result of dissemination, affected internal foci, particularly the central nervous system, must be identified. The presence of disseminated cryptococcal infection may reflect endogenous immunosuppression, such as that noted in AIDS.

Treatment

The treatment of choice for meningitic cryptococcosis is systemic amphotericin B combined with flucytosine. Fluconazole is used for prophylaxis in HIV patients with a history of cryptococcal meningoencephalitis. In milder, non-CNS disease, fluconazole may also be used.

Zygomycosis

Zygomycosis is caused by fungi belonging to the phylum Zygomycota. The most common organisms causing opportunistic zygomycosis are in the genera *Rhizopus*, *Absidia*, and *Mucor*. The common etiologic organisms are ubiquitous saprophytic molds found in soil and decaying matter. Infection typically occurs in patients with uncontrolled diabetes or immunocompromised patients as a result of organ transplantation or hematologic malignancy. It has a mortality rate of 50%, often due to the extent of infection at diagnosis. This group of fungi is angiotropic, leading to extensive necrosis and rapid dissemination.

Clinical manifestations

There are five major forms of zygomycosis: rhinocerebral, pulmonary, gastrointestinal, cutaneous, and disseminated. Rhinocerebral disease is the most commonly encountered variant and involves infection of the nasal sinuses, eyes, brain, and meninges. It has a particular affinity for patients with diabetic ketoacidosis and may cause palsy of cranial nerves II, III, IV, and VI. Rhinocerebral zygomycosis is characterized by acute development of orbital or facial swelling, a bloody nasal discharge, and black necrotic ulcers over the nasal septum. Rapid invasion into the orbit and sinuses can occur. In most cases, cutaneous lesions result from dissemination from the lung, but primary inoculation of the skin can occur. Cutaneous lesions are nonspecific but can resemble those seen in ecthyma gangrenosum. Necrosis of skin is commonly observed.

Diagnosis

The diagnosis of zygomycosis can be made by identification of broad, right-angle branched, nonseptate hyphae in KOH-prepared tissue smears or tissue biopsy specimens. Culture of the organism, which is typically fast growing and cottony or woolly, is necessary to identify the specific organism.

Treatment

Early surgical debridement is an essential aspect of disease management. Liposomal amphotericin B is the treatment of choice for serious infections; however, posaconazole is an option for patients with less severe infection or those intolerant to amphotericin.

Aspergillosis

Aspergillosis results from infection by fungi in the genus *Aspergillus*. The two most common species responsible for opportunistic infection are *A. fumigatus* and *A. niger*. Cutaneous aspergillosis may occur as a primary or secondary infection. Primary aspergillosis is caused by direct inoculation from contaminated materials. Secondary cutaneous metastasis from the lung is more common. Patients with leukemia, those receiving immunosuppressive medications, and children with chronic granulomatous disease and cystic fibrosis are at the highest risk for systemic aspergillosis.

Clinical manifestations

Aspergillosis causes four syndromes: allergic bronchopulmonary aspergillosis, chronic necrotizing pulmonary aspergillosis, aspergilloma, and disseminated aspergillosis. Cutaneous dissemination usually results from lymphohematogenous dissemination from a primary pulmonary focus. Dissemination may also produce endocarditis, endophthalmitis, or abscesses of internal organs. Primary cutaneous aspergillosis is typically associated with contaminated adhesive dressings, intravenous lines, and central venous catheters, or contaminated wounds secondary to burns or other trauma. The cutaneous lesions are nonspecific, including macules and papules, hemorrhagic bullae, and ulcerations (Fig. 28–29). A cellulitis-like reaction unresponsive to systemic antibiotics may also occur.

Diagnosis

Culture of appropriate clinical material reveals septate hyphae with unbranched conidiophores. Biopsy specimens of the skin show a neutrophilic infiltrate, often with areas of necrosis and granuloma, and septate hyphae with branching at acute angles. A galactomannan assay and *Aspergillus* precipitin antibody tests are also available for serologic confirmation.

Treatment

Voriconazole has recently become the treatment of choice as a result of increased tolerance and survival. Amphotericin B is effective and a good first-line agent if the diagnosis is unconfirmed and any chance of zygomycosis is possible (as zygomycetes do not respond to voriconazole).

Candidiasis

The genus *Candida* contains several species that have significant potential for causing a variety of opportunistic infections. The degree of immune impairment and debilitation accounts for the variability in clinical disease and determines the risk of life-threatening infection.

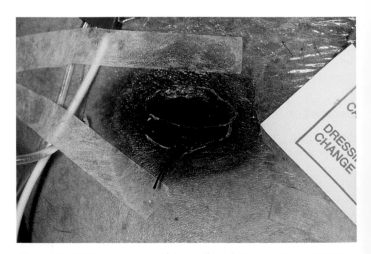

Figure 28–29 Nodular lesions of aspergillosis following a bone marrow transplant.

Clinical manifestations

Localized infections of skin and mucous membranes with *Candida* species are common and include oropharyngeal candidiasis (thrush), vaginitis, balanitis, intertrigo, paronychia, and diaper dermatitis. Predisposing factors include heat, occlusion, and moisture, impairment of epithelial barrier function, such as trauma induced by dentures, antibiotic use, and use of corticosteroids. Diabetes mellitus facilitates colonization by *Candida*. In immunocompetent persons the host defense mechanisms limit infection. In some, these localized infections, particularly persistent oral candidiasis and chronic vaginal candidiasis, may be a harbinger of malignancy or AIDS. *Candida* can affect any skin surface; however, there is a predilection for skin folds, including the axillae, the groin, under a panniculus, beneath the breasts, and in interdigital spaces. The clinical appearance is usually moist and 'beefy' red, often with satellite pustules (Fig. 28–30). The features of oral candidiasis include a white thick exudate on the oral mucosa, usually the tongue (Fig. 28–31). At presentation, patients often complain of dysphagia.

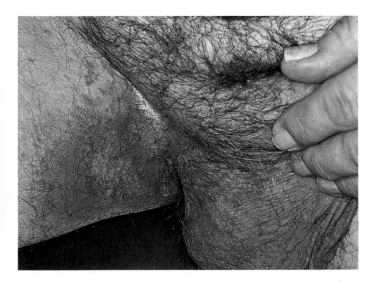

Figure 28–30 Erythematous scaly plaque in the groin characteristic of *Candida* intertrigo.

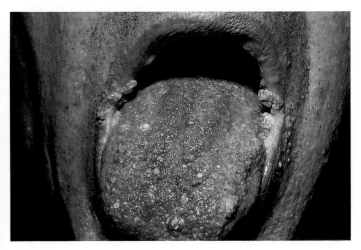

Figure 28–31 Mucosal surface involvement with chronic mucocutaneous candidiasis.

Systemic candidiasis, usually resulting from a primary gastrointestinal source, is a life-threatening infection that afflicts immunocompromised hosts. The majority of cases are caused by *Candida albicans*, followed in frequency by *C. tropicalis*. *C. tropicalis* is the most common species of *Candida* to disseminate to the skin. Severe prolonged neutropenia, antibiotic suppression of resident flora, and central venous catheters permit fungal overgrowth. The cutaneous lesions are nonspecific and include erythematous to violaceous macules, papules, pustules, or vasculitic lesions.

Chronic mucocutaneous candidiasis is found in association with a heterogeneous group of disorders often characterized by the failure of T-cell lymphocyte function in response to candida antigen. The majority of patients have disease onset in childhood. Skin, nails, and mucous membranes are the most commonly affected sites. By definition, the infection is chronic and resistant to therapy; autoantibody-mediated endocrine dysfunction may be associated with one of the recessively inherited forms.

Diagnosis

Localized disease can be diagnosed with a potassium hydroxide preparation which, when performed in appropriate clinical specimens, reveals budding yeast or pseudohyphae. Whenever fungemia is suspected, blood cultures should be performed.

Treatment

Localized infection with *Candida* species can often be managed topically. In patients who are immunodeficient with disseminated infection, systemic therapy with fluconazole or an echinocandin is indicated. Patients who have been on prolonged prophylaxis (such as after a bone marrow transplant) where resistance is an issue, or those who are infected with *C. glabrata* or *C. krusei*, are often treated with micafungin.

PROTOZOAN DISEASE

The parasitic diseases, such as the helminthic diseases, are of critical importance in many areas of the world. However, a review of these conditions is beyond the scope of this text. Scabies and pediculosis are important dermatological diseases, but are not dermatologic signs of systemic disease. The next section focuses briefly on an overview of leishmaniasis and amebiasis.

Leishmaniasis

Leishmania is a genus of dimorphic protozoa found within the cells of the reticuloendothelial system as amastigotes in the mammalian host. The disease leishmaniasis is transmitted by the sandfly.

Clinical Manifestations

The most common forms of leishmaniasis (cutaneous leishmaniasis of the Old World, cutaneous leishmaniasis of the New World, and diffuse cutaneous leishmaniasis) are localized cutaneous lesions produced by *Leishmania tropica*, *L. brazilien-*

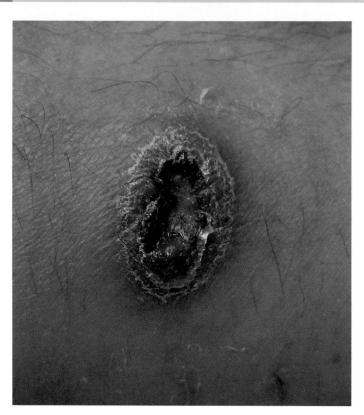

Figure 28–32 Necrotic ulcerative plaque on the arm in a patient with leishmaniasis.

sis, and *L. mexicana*, respectively (Fig. 28–32). Lesions may occur along draining lymphatic channels (i.e., sporotrichoid spread). Infection by *L. donovani* produces visceral leishmaniasis, which in turn can be associated with characteristic cutaneous changes. The primary inoculation site in visceral leishmaniasis is usually not apparent. The clinical manifestations vary, but usually include the insidious onset of abdominal discomfort, fever, weakness, and pallor. Organomegaly develops, and the spleen may become dramatically enlarged. Many cutaneous signs that are not specific develop, including dryness, pallor, petechiae, ecchymoses, jaundice, and alopecia. A characteristic change is a darkening of the skin of the hands, feet, abdomen, and face, a change that gave rise to the Indian name 'kala azar,' or black fever. Of patients who survive the acute phase of the disease, a variable number develop a post-kala azar dermal leishmaniasis. These cutaneous lesions may appear up to 2 years following treatment of the acute phase, and range from hypopigmented macules to large nodules resembling those seen in leprosy.

Leishmaniasis is associated with a number of cutaneous manifestations, including primary cutaneous inoculation lesions and secondary cutaneous lesions in visceral leishmaniasis. There are a number of nonspecific cutaneous changes associated with visceral disease, including pallor, darkening of the skin, petechiae, and alopecia.

Evaluation

Appropriate cultures in special media and serologic testing facilitate the diagnosis of the acute phase. Biopsy of the skin reveals the organism in specific cutaneous lesions.

Treatment

The drugs of choice are pentavalent antimonials. For localized cutaneous leishmaniasis a variety of local treatments, including cryotherapy, electrocautery destruction, and surgical excision, have been described.

Amebiasis

Amebae are spherical organisms that exist in two forms, a motile form called a trophozoite, and a nonmotile encysted form that is found when conditions are not favorable for the single-cell protozoan. *Entamoeba histolytica* is the most common member of the Amoeba group to be pathogenic in humans.

Clinical Manifestations

Amebiasis is primarily an intestinal disease, but may also present as cutaneous amebiasis. Usually, intestinal amebiasis is present concomitantly with cutaneous amebiasis, the skin being involved by direct extension from an internal viscus. Consequently, cutaneous amebiasis is most frequently seen in the groin and perineal regions, but can also be found on the face, abdomen, and buttocks, and around colostomy sites. The typical cutaneous lesion is a rapidly enlarging ulcer with a necrotic slough covered by exudate. Disseminated amebiasis with subcutaneous abscesses has been observed in AIDS.

Evaluation

Confirmation of the diagnosis depends on the demonstration of the trophozoite in fresh samples from the ulcer bed.

Treatment

Treatment includes an assortment of medications, depending on the site of involvement, because some medications may be active for luminal disease, whereas others are necessary for tissue involvement. The treatment of cutaneous amebiasis includes topical ulcer care and systemic medications.

SUGGESTED READINGS

Viral Infections

Arduino PG, Porter SR. Oral and perioral herpes simplex virus type 1 (HSV-1) infection: review of its management. Oral Dis 2006; 12: 254–270.

Bannister BA. Viral exanthems. In: Armstrong D, Cohen J, Berkley SF, et al., eds. Infectious diseases. Philadelphia: Mosby, 2000; 1–10.

Centers for Disease Control and Prevention. Achievements in public health: elimination of rubella and congenital rubella syndrome – US, 1969–2004. Ann Pharmacother 2005; 39: 1151–1152.

Centers for Disease Control and Prevention. Outbreak of measles – San Diego, California, January–February 2008. MMWR Morb Mortal Wkly Rep 2008; 57:203–206. CDC.gov/DiseasesConditions/

Fatahzadeh M, Schwartz RA. Human herpes simplex virus infections: epidemiology, pathogenesis, symptomatology, diagnosis and management. J Am Acad Dermatol 2007; 57: 737–763.

Hogan PA, Morelli JG, Weston WL. Viral exanthems. Curr Probl Dermatol 1992; 4: 1–95.

Hussey GD, Klein M. A randomized, controlled trial of vitamin A in children with severe measles. N Engl J Med 1990; 323: 160–164.

Madsen KM, Hviid A, Vestergaard M, et al. A population-based study of measles, mumps, and rubella vaccination and autism. N Engl J Med 2002; 347: 1477–1482.

Porras BH, Cockerell CJ. Dermatologic manifestations of HIV infection. In: Armstrong D, Cohen J, Berkley SF, et al., eds. Infectious diseases. Philadelphia: Mosby, 2000; 1–8.

Tyring S, ed. Mucocutaneous manifestations of viral disease. New York: Marcel Dekker, 2002.

Bacterial Infections

Advice for travelers. Med Lett Drugs Ther 1992; 34: 41–44.

Amagai M, Yamaguchi T, Hanakawa Y. Staphylococcal exfoliative toxin B specifically cleaves desmoglein 1. J Invest Dermatol 2002; 118: 845–850.

Buckingham SC, Marshall GS, Schutze GE, et al. Clinical and laboratory features, hospital course, and outcome of Rocky Mountain spotted fever in children. J Pediatr 2007; 150: 180–184.

CDC.gov/DiseasesConditions/

Cowan G. Rickettsial diseases: the typhus group of fevers – a review. Postgrad Med J 2000; 76: 269–272.

Elston D. Community acquired methicillin-resistant Staphylococcus aureus. J Am Acad Dermatol 2007; 56: 1–16.

Reynolds MG, Holman RC, Curns AT, et al. Epidemiology of cat-scratch disease hospitalizations among children in the United States. Pediatr Infect Dis J 2005; 24: 700–704.

Roggiani M, Schlievert PM. Streptococcal toxic shock syndrome, including necrotizing fasciitis and myositis. Curr Opin Infect Dis 1994; 7: 423–426.

Zangwill KM, Hamilton DH, Perkins BA, Regnery RL. Cat scratch disease in Connecticut. N Engl J Med 1993; 329: 8–13.

Fungal Infections

CDC.gov/DiseasesConditions/

Elewski BE, ed. Cutaneous fungal infections. New York: Igaku-Shoin, 1992.

Ellis D, Marriott D, Hajjeh RA, et al. Epidemiology: surveillance of fungal infections. Med Mycol 2000; 38: 173–182.

Friedman GD, Jeffrey Fessel W, Udaltsova NV, Hurley LB. Cryptococcosis: the 1981–2000 epidemic. Mycoses 2005; 48: 122–125.

Greenberg RN, Scott LJ, Vaughn HH, Ribes JA. Zygomycosis (mucormycosis): emerging clinical importance and new treatments. Curr Opin Infect Dis 2004; 17: 517–525.

Grossman MC, Silvers DN, Walther RR. Cutaneous manifestations of disseminated candidiasis. J Am Acad Dermatol 1980; 2: 111–116.

Herbrecht R. Posaconazole: a potent, extended-spectrum triazole anti-fungal for the treatment of serious fungal infections. Int J Clin Pract 2004; 58: 612–624.

Kuse ER, Chetchotisakd P, da Cunha CA, et al. Micafungin versus liposomal amphotericin B for candidaemia and invasive candidosis: a phase III randomised double-blind trial. Lancet 2007; 369: 1519–1527.

Krishnan-Natesan S, Chandrasekar PH. Current and future therapeutic options in the management of invasive aspergillosis. Drugs 2008; 68: 265–282.

Rico MJ, Penneys NS. Cutaneous cryptococcus resembling molluscum contagiosum in a patient with AIDS. Arch Dermatol 1985; 121: 901–902.

Protozoan Disease

Adams EB, MacLeod IN. Invasive amebiasis. I. Amebic liver abscess and its complications. Medicine 1977; 56: 325.

Berman J. Current treatment approaches to leishmaniasis. Curr Opin Infect Dis 2003; 16: 397–401.

Centers for Disease Control and Prevention. Cutaneous leishmaniasis in US military personnel – Southwest/Central Asia, 2002–2003. MMWR Morb Mortal Wkly Rep 2003; 52: 1009–1012.

Marsden PD, Nonata RR. Mucocutaneous leishmaniasis – a review of clinical aspects. Rev Soc Bras Med Trop 1975; 9: 309.

Most H, Lavietes PH. Kala-azar in American military personnel. Report of 30 cases. Medicine 1947; 26: 221.

Petri WA Jr, Singh U. Diagnosis and management of amebiasis. Clin Infect Dis 1999; 29: 1117–1125.

Schwartz E, Hatz C, Blum J. New world cutaneous leishmaniasis in travellers. Lancet Infect Dis 2006; 6: 342–349.

Chapter | 29 |

Jean L. Bolognia

Acquired Immunodeficiency Syndrome and Sexually Transmitted Infections

The focus of this chapter is diseases that are sexually transmitted, many of which have internal manifestations. A few disorders, e.g., mollusca contagiosa, condylomata acuminata, and scabies, are mentioned but not discussed in detail; for further information, the reader is referred to general textbooks of dermatology. Discussions of herpes simplex, herpes zoster, and reactive arthritis (the disorder formally referred to as Reiter's syndrome) are found in Chapters 28 and 5, respectively.

ACQUIRED IMMUNODEFICIENCY SYNDROME

The acquired immunodeficiency syndrome (AIDS) is due to infection with one of two retroviruses, HIV-1 (the majority of patients) or HIV-2. In the early 1980s, several of the initial descriptions of patients with AIDS came from dermatologists as they noted the appearance of cutaneous Kaposi's sarcoma (see Chapter 18) in a new patient population. The affected individuals were not elderly men of Mediterranean or Ashkenazi Jewish descent as expected, but rather young men who had had sex with other men, and who often had multiple partners. Over the years, additional high-risk populations were identified, including hemophiliacs who had received contaminated factor VIII concentrates, injection-drug users, and prostitutes and their sexual partners. In developing countries, where at least 90% of the individuals infected with HIV currently live, the predominant mode of transmission is heterosexual.

In the United States and western Europe, but not in other regions of the world such as sub-Saharan Africa, China and India, the annual incidence of AIDS has reached a plateau. Public education, routine testing of pregnant women followed by antiretroviral treatment of those who are HIV-positive, and highly active antiretroviral combination therapy (HAART) have all played a role in this stabilization. With HAART therapy, however, has come a novel set of cutaneous side effects, including redistribution of body fat. In this section, the cutaneous manifestations of HIV infection and AIDS will be divided into infectious, inflammatory, neoplastic, and miscellaneous.

Cutaneous Manifestations: Infectious

The cutaneous manifestations of HIV infection and AIDS that are infectious in nature can be categorized into four major groups: viral, bacterial, fungal, and parasitic/ectoparasitic.

Viral Infections

Acute HIV infection (acute retroviral syndrome) occurs approximately 2–4 weeks after exposure in up to 80% of patients. This process is a self-limiting clinical syndrome of varying severity. The symptoms are reminiscent of other viral infections and include fever, fatigue, weight loss, headache, myalgias, pharyngitis, and lymphadenopathy in addition to a morbilliform (measles-like) cutaneous eruption and mucosal ulcerations. Because the symptoms are rather nonspecific and anti-HIV antibodies are usually negative, the diagnosis is established by detecting plasma viral RNA (usually $>5 \times 10^4$ copies/mL, and as high as 1×10^6 copies/mL) and/or p24 antigen. The viremia is accompanied by a drop in the circulating CD4+ T-lymphocyte count and a rise in the CD8+ T-lymphocyte count.

Mucocutaneous infections due to herpes simplex virus (HSV)-1, HSV-2 and the varicella-zoster virus (VZV) are commonly seen in association with HIV infection and AIDS; the typical clinical presentations of these three viruses are reviewed in Chapter 28. Because herpes zoster (uni- or multi-dermatomal) can serve as one of the presenting signs of HIV infection (Fig. 29–1), this diagnosis should prompt a discussion of risk factors. In contrast to the self-limiting episodes of herpes zoster or orogenital herpes simplex that occur in immunocompetent hosts, patients with AIDS can have lesions that last for months until appropriate therapy is instituted. More recently, the development of herpes zoster or severe recurrent HSV infection has been described in patients whose immune system was reconstituted with HAART, i.e., in the setting of immune reconstitution inflammatory syndrome (IRIS).

Chronic perianal ulcers due to HSV are sometimes misdiagnosed as decubitus ulcers (Fig. 29–2) and chronic oral ulcers

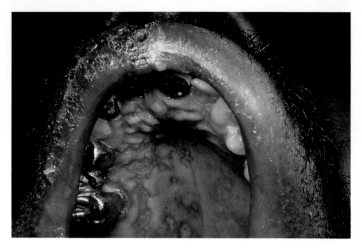

Figure 29–1 Herpes zoster involving the palate and lip in an HIV-infected patient.

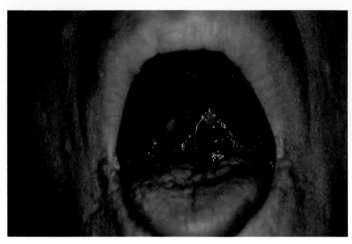

Figure 29–3 Multiple erosions on the hard and soft palate due to herpes simplex virus in an HIV-infected patient. (Courtesy of Yale Residents' Slide Collection.)

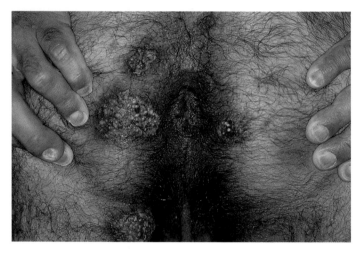

Figure 29–2 Chronic perianal ulcerations that represent herpes simplex infection in this HIV-infected man.

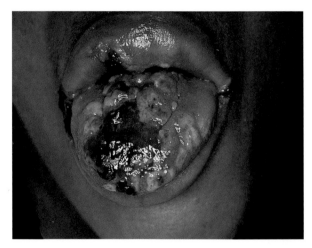

Figure 29–4 Multiple vesicles, some of which are hemorrhagic, on the tongue and upper lip of an HIV-infected patient. Note the scalloping of the border of the lesion on the lip that is characteristic of HSV infections. (Courtesy of Yale Residents' Slide Collection.)

as aphthous stomatitis (Fig. 29–3), until a direct immunofluorescence antibody assay or viral culture of scrapings from the ulcer edge points to the correct diagnosis. One clue to the diagnosis of HSV as the etiologic agent is scalloping of the border of the ulcer and preceding vesicles (Fig. 29–4). In patients with AIDS, chronic dermatomal and disseminated VZV lesions can become verrucous (Fig. 29–5) and the clinical diagnosis requires a high index of suspicion. For patients who are immunocompromised, including those with AIDS, antiviral therapy should be continued until there is complete clinical resolution (as opposed to a predetermined 5–10-day course of therapy).

When lesions of HSV or VZV fail to improve despite appropriate therapy (systemic acyclovir, famciclovir or valacyclovir), the possibility of an acyclovir-resistant strain needs to be excluded, especially when patients have been receiving chronic suppressive therapy with oral acyclovir. Intravenous foscarnet (which does not require phosphorylation to interact with viral DNA polymerase) is the recommended treatment for acyclovir-resistant strains. However, there are reports of patients developing foscarnet-resistant strains of HSV owing to muta-

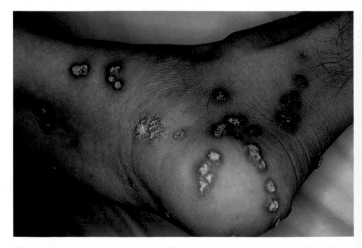

Figure 29–5 Verrucous papules of chronic VZV in a patient with AIDS. (Courtesy of Yale Residents' Slide Collection.)

tions in the DNA polymerase gene. An alternative treatment is topical (1% gel) or intravenous cidofovir. In patients with both HIV and HSV infection, antiherpetic suppressive therapy may lead to a better response to antiretroviral therapy, with a reduction in genital and plasma HIV-1 RNA levels.

Infections with two other members of the herpes family, cytomegalovirus (CMV) and Epstein–Barr virus (EBV), are seen in HIV-infected individuals. The most common EBV-induced mucocutaneous disorder is oral hairy leukoplakia, which is characterized by white plaques, primarily on the lateral aspects of the tongue (Fig. 29–6). These plaques may have a somewhat corrugated appearance, and improvement is seen in the setting of HAART therapy. Although the disorder most commonly associated with CMV is retinitis, this herpes virus can lead to gastrointestinal (GI) ulcers and, occasionally, orogenital or perianal ulcers as well as morbilliform eruptions. The detection (via specific immunohistochemical stains) of intranuclear CMV inclusions within dermal endothelial cells usually proves to be a more sensitive assay than viral cultures. In mucocutaneous ulcers, CMV often 'coexists' with other viruses such as HSV or VZV, and as a result its true pathogenicity has been questioned.

Because condylomata acuminata and mollusca contagiosa (MC) – cutaneous viral infections due to human papilloma viruses (HPV) and poxvirus, respectively – can be sexually transmitted, HIV-infected patients are at increased risk for both. Owing to the coexistent immunosuppression, their clinical manifestations frequently become quite exaggerated; for example, the individual lesions of MC often coalesce into broad-based plaques and may become so large as to be referred to as 'giant.' As expected, the condylomata involve the anogenital region, but the most common site of involvement for MC is the face (Fig. 29–7). Even banal warts (verrucae vulgares) can become widely distributed, as in organ transplant patients (Fig. 29–8; see Chapter 33), and often persist despite HAART.

In women, infections with certain subtypes of HPV, e.g., 16 and 18, are associated with the development of cervical cancer, and this risk increases in the setting of HIV infection. These same HPV strains also increase the risk of anal carcinoma (Fig. 29–9), more so in HIV-infected men than women. Serial anal examinations in combination with anal cytology have been advocated for screening such patients, as has histologic examination of any suspicious lesion. MC and HPV infections may prove recalcitrant to standard destructive therapies (e.g., curettage), but improvement of MC has been observed after the institution of HAART. Both MC and condylomata acuminata may respond to topical imiquimod or cidofovir; occasionally, intravenous cidofovir is administered for extensive confluent MC. In one study of HIV-positive men who had sex with men and had anal intraepithelial neoplasia (AIN), imiquimod cream (for perianal disease) and suppositories (for intra-anal disease) led to clinical and histologic clearing in 75% of those

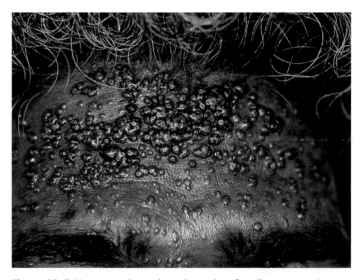

Figure 29–7 Numerous dome-shaped papules of mollusca contagiosa on the forehead of an HIV-infected patient. Note the central dell in several of the lesions. (Courtesy of Yale Residents' Slide Collection.)

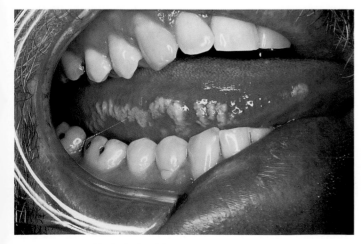

Figure 29–6 Oral hairy leukoplakia.

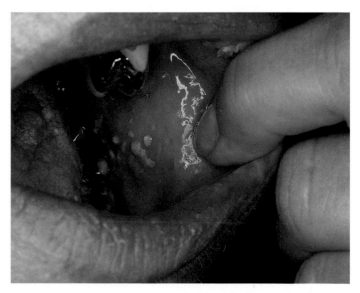

Figure 29–8 Verrucae vulgaris of the buccal mucosa in an HIV-infected patient. (Courtesy of Kalman Watsky, MD.)

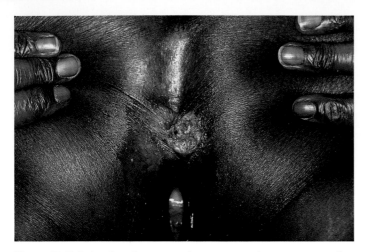

Figure 29–9 Perianal erythematous plaque representing squamous cell carcinoma developing within condylomata acuminata. (Courtesy of Yale Residents' Slide Collection.)

who used the medication as directed (three times per week for 16 weeks).

Bacterial Infections

Cutaneous bacterial infections that are seen in association with HIV infection and AIDS can be subdivided into a few major categories: soft tissue infections and folliculitis due primarily to Gram-positive cocci; bacillary angiomatosis; venereal diseases (see below); and mycobacterial and atypical mycobacterial infections. Because HIV is often acquired via sexual contact, patients who are HIV-positive need to be screened for other venereal diseases, and vice versa. In addition, the presence of erosions and ulcerations in the anogenital region due to bacterial diseases such as syphilis or viral diseases such as HSV can increase the transmission rate of HIV.

Soft tissue bacterial infections in patients with AIDS are often due to *Staphylococcus aureus* or *Streptococcus* spp., and their clinical presentations range from folliculitis and abscesses to cellulitis and necrotizing fasciitis (Fig. 29–10). When *S. aureus* is identified as the etiology of a cutaneous infection, the possibility of nasal carriage needs to be considered as well as the possibility of methicillin-resistant *S. aureus* (MRSA). The cutaneous manifestations of atypical mycobacterial infections are also protean and can vary from subtle areas of erythema to necrotic ulcers. Several species of atypical mycobacteria have been isolated from skin lesions in patients with AIDS, including *Mycobacterium haemophilum*, *M. fortuitum*, and *M. avium intracellulare*. HIV-infected patients are also at risk for developing cutaneous tuberculosis, including disseminated miliary tuberculosis. Multidrug treatment regimens for cutaneous mycobacterial infections are the same as for systemic disease.

Bacillary angiomatosis (BA) is a very interesting bacterial infection whose diagnosis warrants the exclusion of an underlying HIV infection or immunosuppression. Only occasionally is it seen in normal hosts. The microorganisms responsible for the appearance of discrete proliferations of cutaneous blood vessels are *Bartonella henselae* and *B. quintana*; the former is also the etiologic agent of cat scratch disease. The characteristic skin

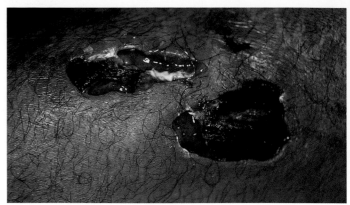

Figure 29–10 Necrotizing fasciitis due to *Staphylococcus aureus* on the thigh of a patient with AIDS; the infection began at the site of an injection of G-CSF. Note the undermining border.

lesion is a red to violet papule that resembles a 'hemangioma,' pyogenic granuloma, or lesion of Kaposi's sarcoma (Fig. 29–11). The diagnosis is established by identifying the bacteria in Warthin–Starry-stained histologic sections or by PCR-based analysis of biopsy specimens. Additional sites of involvement include the subcutis, with the formation of nodules, the liver (peliosis hepatitis), lymph nodes, bones, and heart (endocarditis). Treatment consists primarily of first- and second-generation macrolides.

Fungal Infections

Certain fungal infections, such as oral candidiasis (thrush), can serve as presenting signs of HIV infection (Fig. 29–12), whereas others, such as aspergillosis, are seen late in the course of the disease. HIV-infected patients are at increased risk for the development of mucocutaneous fungal infections due to *Candida* spp. and dermatophytes, as well as systemic infections due to *Cryptococcus neoformans*, *Candida* spp., and dimorphic fungi (e.g., *Histoplasma capsulatum*, *Coccidioides immitis*, *Penicillium marneffei*). The cutaneous lesions of cryptococcosis and dimorphic fungal infections are often nondescript papules or ulcers, and they sometimes resemble the dome-shaped papules of MC (Fig. 29–13). Examination of a KOH preparation of dermal scrapings or a PAS- or silver-stained histologic section allows a presumptive diagnosis, and a simultaneous tissue fungal culture provides a definitive diagnosis.

Infections with tinea (dermatophytoses) affect three keratin-containing structures, the skin, hair, and nails. HIV-infected patients are not only prone to the more common forms of tinea, e.g., tinea pedis, tinea manuum (hand), tinea unguium (nails) and tinea corporis, but they often have more severe or widespread lesions. These patients also develop an unusual form of tinea unguium known as proximal subungual onychomycosis (PSO). In the more common form of tinea unguium (distal subungual onychomycosis), the most pronounced dystrophic changes, e.g., thickening and yellow discoloration, are seen in the distal portions of the fingernails or toenails, whereas in PSO there is a white discoloration that first appears in the proximal portion of the nail (Fig. 29–14). PSO has also been observed in other immunocompromised patients, such as those who have received organ transplants.

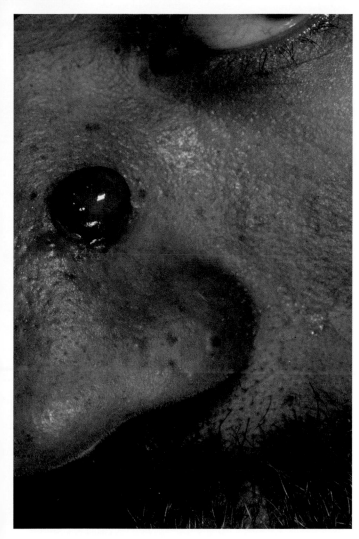

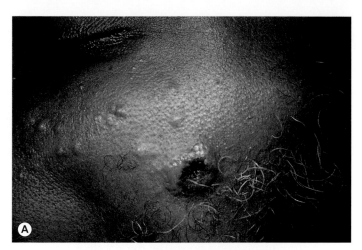

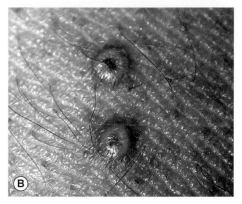

Figure 29–13 (A) Cutaneous cryptococcosis in a patient with AIDS manifesting as an annular plaque as well as multiple dome-shaped papules reminiscent of mollusca contagiosa. (B) Close-up of papules of cutaneous cryptococcosis, with rolled-borders and central erosion. (B, Courtesy of Yale Residents' Slide Collection.)

Figure 29–11 Red dome-shaped nodules of bacillary angiomatosis in an HIV-positive patient. The lesions have an appearance similar to pyogenic granulomas. (Courtesy of NYU Slide Collection.)

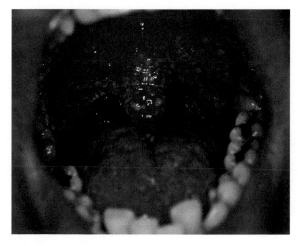

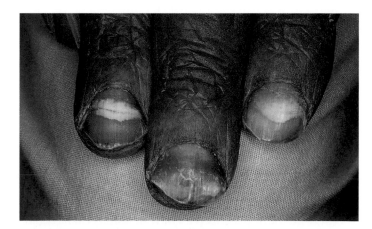

Figure 29–14 Proximal white subungual onychomycosis of the second and fourth fingernails in an HIV-infected patient. (Courtesy of Kalman Watsky, MD.)

Figure 29–12 White friable plaques of oral candidiasis in a patient with AIDS. (Courtesy of Yale Residents' Slide Collection.)

Recent DNA analyses have led to a reclassification of *Pneumocystis jiroveci* (*carinii*) as a fungal species. Pneumonia is the most common clinical presentation of *P. jiroveci* infection, but rarely cutaneous lesions do develop, especially in the external auditory canal and nares.

Parasitic/Ectoparasitic Infections

One of the more common ectoparasitic infections in patients who have AIDS is scabies, in particular a form characterized by thick scale-crusts and numerous mites of *Sarcoptes scabiei* var. *hominis*; this is sometimes referred to as crusted or Norwegian scabies. Unlike the form of scabies seen in immunocompetent hosts, in which each person is infested with a few dozen mites, these patients have hundreds to thousands of mites and are therefore highly contagious. The thick scale is one of the explanations for the difficulty in eradicating crusted scabies with topical scabicides such as 5% permethrin cream. One of the off-label uses of oral ivermectin is the treatment of such patients.

HIV-infected patients frequently develop folliculitis, and its etiology can vary from *S. aureus* and herpes simplex to *Malassezia* spp., dimorphic fungi and the *Demodex* mite. Although the latter ectoparasite is part of the normal flora and fauna of the hair follicle, its presumed pathogenetic role is based upon the numerous *Demodex* mites found in the expressed follicular contents from AIDS patients with folliculitis in whom there was no other explanation for the folliculitis. Patients with AIDS can also present with cutaneous lesions due to systemic infections with parasites such as *Toxoplasma gondii* (primarily CNS), *Acanthamoeba* spp. (primarily CNS and sinuses), *Strongyloides stercoralis* (primarily GI tract and lung), *Leishmania* spp. (primarily bone marrow), and microsporidia (primarily GI tract). Although these secondary cutaneous lesions are rather unusual and do not have unique clinical presentations, the diagnosis can be made fairly easily by identification of the responsible organisms in biopsy specimens.

Cutaneous Manifestations: Inflammatory

There are several inflammatory skin disorders that can serve as the initial clinical manifestation of HIV infection, in particular seborrheic dermatitis, psoriasis, and reactive arthritis (the disorder previously referred to as Reiter's syndrome – see Chapter 5) (Figs 29–15 to 29–17). For some patients, this represents new-onset disease, whereas in others there is a flare of a preexisting dermatosis. In this particular clinical setting, the seborrheic dermatitis, especially of the face, tends to be moderate to severe in intensity and the psoriasis rather extensive. Over two decades ago, an increased number of *Malassezia* organisms (yeast that are part of the normal flora) was observed in HIV-infected patients with seborrheic dermatitis, and this observation contributed to the subsequent use of antifungal creams and shampoos for the treatment of this disease, both in immunocompromised and immunocompetent hosts.

Less commonly, patients present with lesions characteristic of pityriasis rubra pilaris (PRP), a papulosquamous disorder that can resemble psoriasis, but which often has a follicular accentuation and spreads in a cephalocaudal direction. In

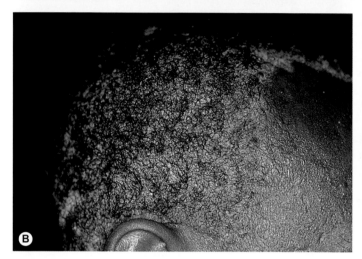

Figure 29–15 Seborrheic dermatitis characterized by scaling in (A) the nasolabial groove and (B) the scalp in two patients with AIDS. (Courtesy of Yale Residents' Slide Collection.)

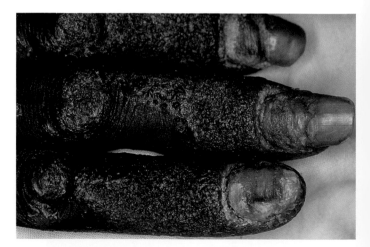

Figure 29–16 Psoriasis of the digits in an HIV-infected patient. Note the accompanying nail dystrophy. (Courtesy of Yale Residents' Slide Collection.)

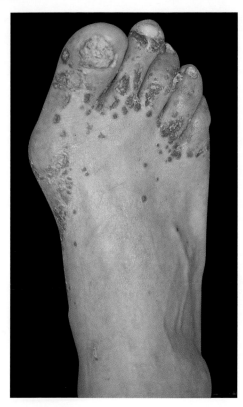

Figure 29–17 Psoriasiform lesions of reactive arthritis (the disorder formerly referred to as Reiter's syndrome) in an HIV-infected patient.

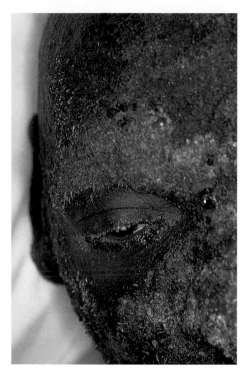

Figure 29–18 Keratotic spines in a patient with pityriasis rubra pilaris in the setting of AIDS; the patient also had a recent history of cystic acne requiring retinoid therapy.

addition, characteristic 'islands' of normal skin are frequently found within larger areas of involved skin. The unusual aspect of PRP in HIV-infected patients is its association with hidradenitis suppurativa, elongated follicular spines (Fig. 29–18), and the severe form of nodulocystic acne known as acne conglobata. This constellation of cutaneous findings is not seen in immunocompetent hosts with PRP.

Pruritus is a frequent complaint in patients with AIDS, and secondary lesions that simply represent chronic rubbing, e.g., lichen simplex chronicus and prurigo nodularis, can be seen admixed with more specific primary lesions. Once scabies, drug eruptions, specific dermatoses such as psoriasis, arthropod bite reactions, and 'systemic' causes of pruritus (e.g., cholestasis, renal failure, lymphoma, parasitic infections) are excluded, the differential diagnosis includes xerosis (see below), itching folliculitis, eosinophilic folliculitis, and the pruritic papular eruption of HIV/AIDS. Eosinophilic folliculitis is characterized by pruritic edematous perifollicular papules, primarily on the upper trunk and in the head and neck region (Fig. 29–19), and it is usually associated with advanced disease. In biopsy specimens, eosinophils are found within hair follicles and these same cells are seen in a Wright's stain of follicular contents. An aberrant Th2-type immune response to *Malassezia* or an as yet unidentified follicular antigen may be involved in its pathogenesis. The skin-colored papules of the pruritic papular eruption of HIV/AIDS tend to favor the extremities, but can also involve the trunk; one hypothesis is that the eruption represents an exaggerated response to arthropod bites. Both disorders may improve following UVB phototherapy.

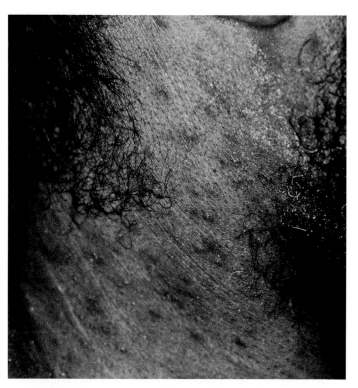

Figure 29–19 Pruritic lesions of eosinophilic folliculitis on the neck of a man with AIDS. (Courtesy of Yale Residents' Slide Collection.)

Patients who are HIV-positive have an increased incidence of cutaneous drug eruptions, usually morbilliform or urticarial, but occasionally photolichenoid, erythrodermic, or within the spectrum of Stevens–Johnson syndrome/toxic epidermal necrolysis. This proclivity for developing allergic drug reactions (approximately 10 times greater than in the general population) became apparent when antibiotic prophylaxis became commonplace, especially the use of oral trimethoprim–sulfamethoxazole against *Pneumocystis jiroveci* (*carinii*) pneumonia. Possible explanations for this phenomenon include the immune dysregulation that accompanies HIV infection, or a predisposition due to coexisting viral infections, e.g., CMV or EBV. As the name implies, photolichenoid eruptions favor sun-exposed areas, are often associated with sulfa-containing medications, and may present as areas of hyperpigmentation. However, idiopathic photosensitivity is also seen in patients with AIDS.

Lastly, cutaneous small-vessel vasculitis and erythema elevatum diutinum (see Chapter 4), a form of chronic vasculitis often associated with streptococcal infections, are also thought to be more prevalent in HIV-infected patients, as is localized lichen myxedematosus (also referred to as acral persistent papular mucinosis). The latter is characterized by skin-colored to pink papules that represent discrete dermal deposits of mucopolysaccharides, but in the absence of thyroid dysfunction. HIV-infected individuals may or may not have an associated paraproteinemia. An idiopathic disorder that also presents with skin-colored papules is granuloma annulare (Fig. 29–20), and in HIV-infected patients the generalized form is seen more often than the localized form (the opposite is true in immu-nocompetent hosts); occasionally, even oral lesions are noted.

Cutaneous Manifestations: Neoplastic

Individuals who are HIV-positive are at increased risk for the development of several neoplasms, including Kaposi's sarcoma (KS; see Chapter 18; Figs 29–21 and 29–22), lymphoma (usually non-Hodgkin's), and cervical and anal squamous cell carcinomas (see above). The non-Hodgkin's lymphomas seen in this setting are often extranodal, EBV-related, and involve the brain, gastrointestinal tract and/or skin. As a result, cutaneous lesions of lymphoma may occasionally be the initial clinical presentation. An HAART-associated reduction in the incidence of lymphoma has been observed.

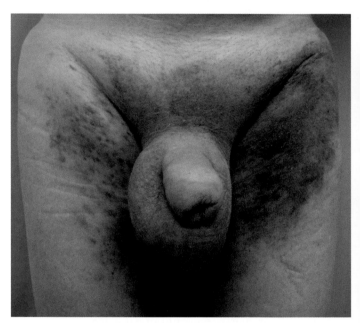

Figure 29–21 Kaposi's sarcoma with secondary lymphedema in a patient with AIDS. Administration of liposomal doxorubicin led to improvement.

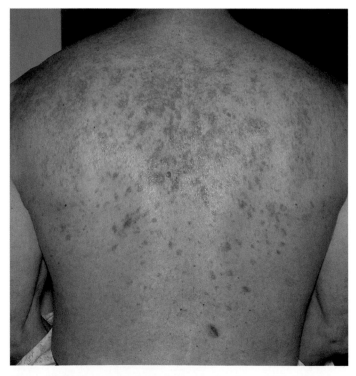

Figure 29–20 Disseminated granuloma annulare in an HIV-infected patient. The distribution pattern is atypical. (Courtesy of Kalman Watsky, MD.)

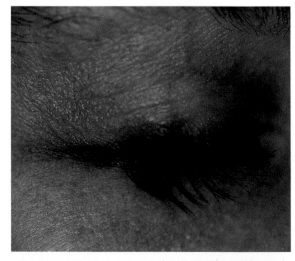

Figure 29–22 Trichomegaly of the eyelashes plus Kaposi's sarcoma of the upper eyelid in a patient with AIDS. (Courtesy of Yale Residents' Slide Collection.)

Co-infection with human herpesvirus 8 is associated with the development of KS as well as body cavity lymphoma and multicentric Castleman's disease. Improvement of KS has been noted after the institution of HAART, as have flares as part of the immune reconstitution inflammatory syndrome (IRIS). An atypical cutaneous lymphoproliferative disorder also has been described which is characterized clinically by a generalized eruption of pruritic papules, and histologically by dermal infiltrates of atypical CD8+ T lymphocytes. In HIV-positive patients with cutaneous T-cell lymphoma characterized by atypical CD4+ T lymphocytes, the possibility of HTLV-1 co-infection needs to be excluded.

Cutaneous Manifestations: Miscellaneous

There are several cutaneous manifestations of HIV infection that do not fit neatly into one of the previous categories of infectious, inflammatory, or neoplastic. These include dry skin (xerosis), which can become so pronounced as to resemble ichthyosis vulgaris; facial hyperpigmentation in the absence of systemic drugs or adrenal insufficiency; linear telangiectasias of the chest; trichomegaly of the eyelashes (Fig. 29–22); and changes in hair texture, e.g., thick curly hair can become fine and straight. Major aphthae, especially of the oral mucosa, can be a therapeutic challenge in patients who are HIV-positive. The ulcerations are similar in appearance to those seen in Behçet's disease, and once infectious etiologies have been excluded, systemic therapies are usually required. One of the off-label uses of oral thalidomide is the treatment of major aphthae in HIV-infected patients.

How changes in the skin such as xerosis and straightening of hair relate to the underlying HIV infection is completely unknown. However, the connection between HIV and hepatitis C-associated porphyria cutanea tarda (Chapter 24; Fig. 29–23) is rather more obvious. There is a significant overlap in the risk factors involved in the acquisition of both of these viruses. In an HIV-infected patient already receiving a nucleoside reverse transcriptase inhibitor, the addition of ribavirin (a

nucleoside analog) for the treatment of hepatitis C requires close monitoring for mitochondrial toxicity.

Lastly, lipodystrophy or the fat redistribution syndrome can be seen in patients receiving HAART. Clinical findings include a decrease of subcutaneous fat (lipoatrophy) in the face (especially of the cheeks; Fig. 29–24), extremities and buttocks, as well as a 'buffalo hump,' central obesity, hypertriglyceridemia, and insulin resistance. Nucleoside reverse transcriptase inhibitors such as stavudine (a thymidine analog) are associated with an increased risk of developing lipoatrophy, and protease inhibitors have been associated with abnormal fat accumulation.

SEXUALLY TRANSMITTED INFECTIONS

Syphilis

Syphilis, also known as lues, is an infectious disease that is most commonly transmitted via intimate contact, including sexual intercourse. Less often the transmission is vertical, from mother to unborn child. The causative agent is the spirochete *Treponema pallidum*. Since World War II and the introduction of penicillin, there has been an overall decline in the incidence of syphilis in the United States. However, a resurgence of the disease did accompany the HIV epidemic, and the behaviors that put individuals at risk for HIV infection also put them at risk for contracting syphilis. More recently – i.e., since 2000 – there has been an upturn in incidence, especially among men.

The clinical manifestations of syphilis are protean and can involve the cardiovascular, skeletal and central nervous systems as well as the skin and mucosal surfaces. Classically, syphilis is divided into four stages: primary, secondary, latent, and tertiary. Except for the latent phase, specific cutaneous lesions that aid in the clinical diagnosis of this disease are often present. Although compared to recurrent genital herpes simplex infection and pityriasis rosea, primary and secondary syphilis are relatively unusual diseases, failure to consider the diagnosis of syphilis can have more dire consequences.

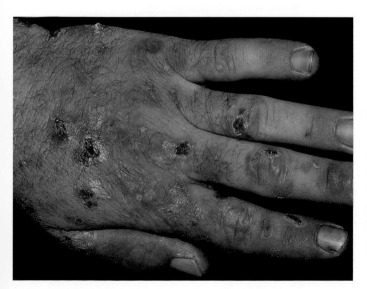

Figure 29–23 Porphyria cutanea tarda in an HIV-infected man.

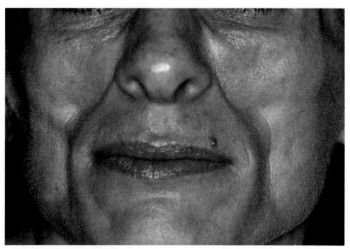

Figure 29–24 HAART-associated lipoatrophy of the cheeks. (Courtesy of Kalman Watsky, MD.)

Primary Syphilis

The characteristic lesion of primary syphilis is the chancre, an ulcer that is usually 1–1.5 cm in diameter. An average of 3 weeks after exposure, a chancre can appear at the site of penetration of the spirochetes (either via mucosa or abraded skin). The most common locations are the penis, labia, and cervix, followed by other urogenital sites, the lips, oral cavity, anus, breasts, and fingers. The majority of patients have a single ulcer (Fig. 29–25A), with multiple lesions seen in approximately one-quarter of patients (Fig. 29–25B). The base of the chancre is often moist, but not purulent, and the edges are more sharply defined than in ulcers due to *Haemophilus ducreyi*. Also, there is no scalloping of the border as is so often seen in orogenital ulcers due to herpes simplex (see Chapter 28).

Palpation with a gloved hand should follow visual inspection of any mucocutaneous ulcer. Unless there is a secondary bacterial infection, a chancre is not very tender to palpation. More importantly, the base of the ulcer is characteristically quite firm due to the infiltration of the underlying dermis with lymphocytes, macrophages, and plasma cells. There may be regional lymphadenopathy, and because the lesions of secondary syphilis can appear prior to the spontaneous resolution of the chancre, a complete skin and oral examination is recommended. Without antibiotic therapy, the lifespan of a chancre

is usually 4 weeks; with therapy (Table 29–1), the ulcer resolves within 2 weeks.

A dark-field examination of a chancre's serous exudate will demonstrate the motile corkscrew-shaped treponemes. However, if the lesion is located within the oral or anal cavity, then *T. pallidum* spirochetes must be distinguished from the similar-appearing, nonpathogenic, saprophytic treponemes that reside in these areas. This requires consultation with a microbiologist and the use of species-specific immunofluorescent stains.

In general, serologic assays are less sensitive in primary syphilis than in secondary syphilis, as the VDRL may be negative in up to 20% of patients. However, the FTA-ABS is negative in <5% of patients with primary disease, and the treponemal-specific antibodies begin to appear during the third week of infection. Occasionally, in difficult-to-diagnose cases, a skin biopsy specimen of the ulcer's edge may be obtained and a silver or immunoperoxidase stain performed to detect the spirochetes. Simultaneously, a search for the epidermal multinucleated giant cells indicative of a herpes simplex infection can be conducted.

Secondary Syphilis

The secondary lesions of syphilis are a reflection of a spirochetemia, and as a result, have a widespread distribution pattern. On the trunk and extremities the cutaneous lesions are usually papulosquamous, i.e., elevated with scale (Fig. 29–26), and less commonly macular. The papules and plaques vary in size from 2 mm to 2 cm and are pink to red-brown in color. The color is influenced by both the degree of inflammation and the melanin content of the skin. Similar-appearing lesions are seen on the palms and soles and are sometimes referred to as

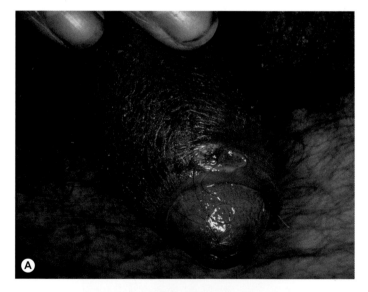
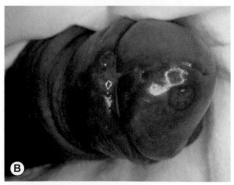

Figure 29–25 Penile chancres: (A) single and (B) multiple, with characteristic clean moist bases. (Courtesy of Yale Residents' Slide Collection.)

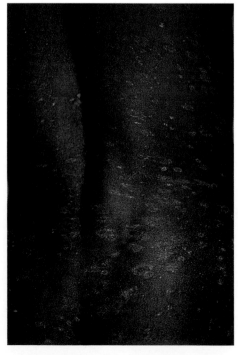

Figure 29–26 Multiple scaly plaques similar to pityriasis rosea in a patient with secondary syphilis.

Table 29–1 CDC recommendations for treatment of various stages of syphilis (2006)

		First-line	Second-line (if penicillin allergic)
Primary		benzathine penicillin G 2.4×10^6U IM	doxycycline 100 mg po BID $\times$ 2 wk[†]
Secondary*		benzathine penicillin G 2.4×10^6U IM	doxycycline 100 mg po BID $\times$ 2 wk[†]
Latent:	early	benzathine penicillin G 2.4×10^6U IM	doxycycline 100 mg po BID $\times$ 2 wk[†]
	late	benzathine penicillin G 2.4×10^6U IM qweek $\times$ 3	doxycycline 100 mg po BID $\times$ 4 wk[†]
Tertiary:	CV, skin	benzathine penicillin G 2.4×10^6U IM qweek $\times$ 3	doxycycline 100 mg po BID $\times$ 4 wk[††,†††]
	neuro	aqueous crystalline penicillin G 18–24 $\times 10^6$U IV in divided doses (q4h) $\times$ 10–14d or procaine penicillin 2.4 $\times 10^6$U IM qd plus probenecid 500 mg po q6h $\times$ 10–14d	desensitize; ceftriaxone 1 g IV qd $\times$14d not as effective
Primary, secondary, or latent			
During pregnancy		benzathine penicillin G 2.4×10^6U IM $\times$1 or qweek $\times$3 (depending upon stage)	desensitize
In association with HIV infection**		benzathine penicillin G 2.4×10^6U IM $\times$1 or qweek $\times$3 (depending upon stage) versus qweek $\times$3 (all stages except neuro)	for primary & secondary, same as HIV-negative; for latent, desensitize

[†]or tetracycline 500 mg po QID $\times$ 2 wk.
[††]or tetracycline 500 mg po QID $\times$ 4 wk.
[†††]HIV-negative and neurosyphilis excluded.
*without ophthalmologic or neurologic involvement.
**neurosyphilis excluded.
Detailed recommendations for treatment of syphilis can be found at the cdc website: www.cdc.gov/std

'copper pennies' (Fig. 29–27). Characteristically, the scale is concentrated at the edges of the thin palmoplantar papules. Rarely, pustules or ulcers develop within the lesions of secondary syphilis.

Additional mucocutaneous lesions of secondary syphilis include nonscarring 'moth-eaten' alopecia (primarily of the scalp), mucous patches (primarily of the oral mucosa), split papules at the oral commissures, annular plaques with central hyperpigmentation (primarily of the face), granulomatous nodules, and condyloma lata, primarily in the anogenital region (Fig. 29–28). Although skin involvement is the most common manifestation of secondary syphilis, the patient may be systemically ill with symptoms such as fevers, fatigue, headache and bone pain, as well as signs such as generalized lymphadenopathy and pharyngitis. This is in contrast to the patient with pityriasis rosea, who may have had a URI 6–10 weeks earlier, but at the time of eruption rarely has associated systemic complaints.

Serologic evaluation is quite helpful in patients with secondary syphilis as the VDRL and FTA-ABS are positive in >99% of patients. Once the prozone phenomenon is excluded, a negative VDRL would draw the diagnosis of cutaneous syphilis into question. Following appropriate treatment (Table 29–1), the titer of the VDRL should decline fourfold (e.g., 1:32–1:4) over a period of 6 months and gradually become negative (nonreactive). The FTA-ABS was once said to remain positive 'for life,' even in treated patients, and its titer is not measured serially to monitor therapeutic response; more recently, however, a nonreactive FTA-ABS was observed in 24% of patients (n = 882) 3 years after treatment of primary, secondary, or early latent syphilis. Occasionally, in patients with unusual presentations, histologic examination of the papulosquamous lesions is performed and dermal infiltrates of

lymphocytes and plasma cells are seen; a silver or immunohistochemical stain is required to detect the spirochetes. A dark-field examination of the serous exudate of condyloma lata can be performed, but requires exclusion of saprophytic treponemes (see above).

The mucocutaneous manifestations of secondary syphilis follow the appearance of the chancre by approximately 3–12 weeks; however, as stated previously, there may be a temporal overlap, such that both are present in a particular patient. As with chancres, the lesions of secondary syphilis resolve spontaneously, i.e., even in the absence of appropriate therapy, after 2–4 months. In a minority (25%) of patients, the cutaneous eruption recurs a second or third time, but always in a transient manner. Those patients who fail to receive appropriate therapy (Table 29–1) then enter the next phase of the disease, which is referred to as latent syphilis. Although there are no clinical signs or symptoms, latent syphilis is divided into early (<1 year) and late (>1 year) stages, and treatment recommendations do differ (Table 29–1).

Tertiary Syphilis

Only about a third of patients with latent syphilis eventually develop tertiary disease. In order of frequency, the most common sites of clinically apparent involvement are the skin (15% of untreated patients), cardiovascular system (10%), and central nervous system (5%). Given the number of untreated patients and the percentage of those who develop symptomatic disease of the skin, one can see why cutaneous tertiary syphilis is quite rare, especially in developed countries. There are two major types of cutaneous disease: granulomatous (nodular or psoriasiform) and gummatous. Thick, dusky, red plaques and nodules are seen in the former and often resemble

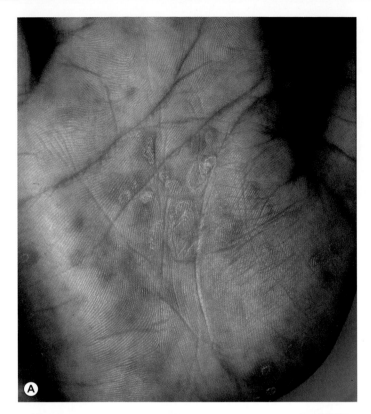

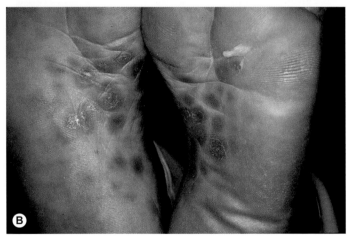

Figure 29–27 Pink-brown to dark brown (A) palmar and (B) plantar lesions of secondary syphilis. Note the peripheral collarette of scale (Courtesy of Yale Residents' Slide Collection.)

other granulomatous diseases, such as sarcoidosis. The combination of expansion plus central scar formation leads to the characteristic figurate lesions. There is more necrosis within gummas and, as a result, destruction of adjacent tissues can occur, including cartilage and bone. The VDRL may be negative during tertiary syphilis.

Congenital Syphilis

Congenital syphilis is classically divided into an early phase (<2 years of age) and a late phase (>2 years of age). However, it is equally important to distinguish between clinical signs and symptoms due to active infection as opposed to stigmata

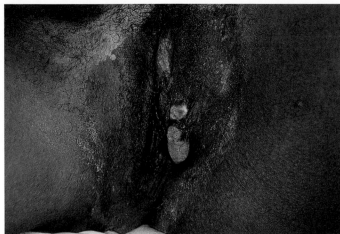

Figure 29–28 Condyloma lata – genital lesions of secondary syphilis.

that are sequelae of an in utero infection. Because congenital syphilis represents a bloodborne infection with *T. pallidum*, there is no primary phase. Many of the cutaneous manifestations of early congenital syphilis are reminiscent of secondary syphilis, except that the 'papulosquamous' lesions can be bullous and tend to be more erosive. Additional clinical manifestations include 'snuffles' (bloody or purulent mucinous nasal discharge), perioral and perianal fissures, hepatosplenomegaly, and osteochondritis. Manifestations of the late phase include gummas, interstitial keratitis, and neurosyphilis (usually asymptomatic). Because of their size, IgM antibodies cannot pass from the mother to the fetus via the placenta. Therefore, detection of IgM anti-*T. pallidum* antibodies in a neonate confirms the diagnosis of congenital syphilis; the Captia (IgM) enzyme-linked immunosorbent assay is said to have a sensitivity of 100% in this setting.

The later in pregnancy treatment is begun, the more likely it is that the infant, although cured, may have the stigmata of an in utero infection. The most common stigmata (>50% of patients) involve either the facial bones or the dentition: frontal bossing, short maxillae, high palatal arch, saddle nose, Hutchinson's teeth (permanent upper central incisors that are widely spaced and broader at the base), and mulberry molars (multiple small cusps rather than four well-formed cusps in the first lower molar). Some of the 'classic' stigmata are seen much less commonly, e.g., the complete Hutchinson's triad (Hutchinson's teeth, interstitial keratitis, and eighth-nerve deafness), rhagades (periorificial linear scars from previous fissures), saber shins, and Higouménakis' sign (unilateral thickening of the sternoclavicular portion of the clavicle).

Syphilis in Association with HIV Infection and AIDS

Because HIV and *T. pallidum* share a primary mode of transmission – sexual intercourse – the presence of one of these infectious diseases mandates screening for the other. In addition, the ulcerated surface of a chancre provides a portal of entry for the HIV; in men who have sex with men, syphilis is more common in those who are HIV-positive than in those who are

HIV-negative. The clinical course of early syphilis in patients with AIDS is often as described above; however, there are reports of more aggressive disease (lues maligna), an increased frequency of serologically defined treatment failures, an increased risk for the development of neurosyphilis, and a higher relapse rate of neurosyphilis following penicillin therapy. Rarely, a nonreactive VDRL has been observed at the onset of the secondary phase in HIV-infected patients. Lastly, HIV infection is one of the causes of a chronic false-positive VDRL.

Chancroid

As with syphilis, the primary mode of transmission for chancroid is intimate contact. Therefore, those with multiple sexual partners are at highest risk for developing this infectious disease. The etiologic agent is the Gram-negative bacterium *Haemophilus ducreyi*. Cutaneous ulcers of chancroid appear in the genital region (primarily on the penis and vulva) approximately 3–7 days following exposure. In contrast to syphilis, there are usually multiple lesions (Fig. 29–29), including kissing lesions. The ulcers range in size from 2 mm to 3 cm and have irregular, overhanging borders that are sometimes referred to as 'shaggy;' the ulcers are painful and tender to palpation, but soft. Tender prominent lymphadenopathy is frequently seen.

Confirmation of the clinical diagnosis of chancroid requires a bacterial culture and Gram stain of material obtained by swabbing the base of the ulcer and undersurface of the edges. Parallel linear arrays of Gram-negative rods can be seen on Gram stain which have been likened to a school of fish. This organism is fastidious and requires culture on specialized media supplemented with serum and hemoglobin. The appropriate therapy is outlined in Table 29–2. As with syphilis, the differential diagnosis includes the two most common causes of genital ulcers: herpes simplex and trauma. However, when the ulcers are chronic and nonhealing, then more unusual etiologies need to be excluded, such as squamous cell carcinoma, lymphoma, granuloma inguinale, and Behçet's disease (in the latter, the ulcers are often on the scrotum).

Granuloma Inguinale

Granuloma inguinale (GI) is an unusual venereal disease caused by the Gram-negative bacterium *Calymmatobacterium granulomatis*. The lesions are seen primarily in the genital region, and although they begin as papules, over time friable granulomatous plaques and ulcerations often attain a rather large size (Fig. 29–30). As a result, there is frequently destruction of normal tissues. The incubation period probably ranges from 2 weeks to 3 months, and the disease is much more prevalent in developing countries.

The diagnosis of GI is established via crush preparations or biopsy specimens in which the responsible organisms (Donovan bodies) are seen within dermal macrophages. The term 'parasitized macrophages' is often used to describe this histologic finding, and it is also seen in histoplasmosis, penicilliosis, rhinoscleroma, and leishmaniasis. The distinguishing features in GI are the clear haloes (representing nonstaining capsules) that surround the Donovan bodies in Giemsa-stained sections and the bipolar staining of the organisms such that they resemble safety pins. Treatment options are outlined in Table 29–2.

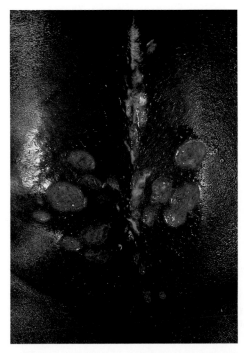

Figure 29–29 Multiple punched-out ulcerations of chancroid. (Courtesy of N.S. Penneys, MD.)

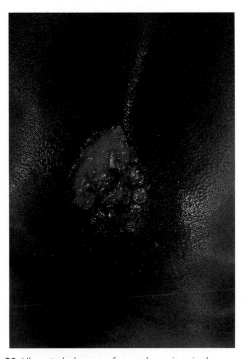

Figure 29–30 Ulcerated plaques of granuloma inguinale.

Table 29–2 Therapy of chancroid, granuloma inguinale, lymphogranuloma venereum, and gonorrhea as recommended by the CDC (2006; April 2007 update; www.cdc.gov/std/treatment). Fluoroquinolones are no longer recommended by the CDC for treatment of gonococcal infections, but may represent an alternative treatment if antimicrobial susceptibility can be documented by culture.

	Recommended	Alternative
Chancroid	**Azithromycin** 1 g orally in a single dose – or – **Ceftriaxone** 250 mg intramuscularly (IM) in a single dose – or – **Ciprofloxacin** 500 mg orally twice a day for 3 days*,** – or – **Erythromycin base** 500 mg orally three times a day for 7 days**	
Granuloma inguinale	**Doxycycline** 100 mg orally twice a day for a minimum of 3 weeks***,+	**Azithromycin** 1 g orally once per week for a minimum of 3 weeks***,+ – or – **Ciprofloxacin** 750 mg orally twice a day for a minimum of 3 weeks***,+ – or – **Erythromycin base** 500 mg orally four times a day for a minimum of 3 weeks***,+,++ – or – **Trimethoprim-sulfamethoxazole** one double-strength tablet orally twice a day for a minimum of 3 weeks***,+
Lymphogranuloma venereum	**Doxycycline** 100 mg orally twice a day for 21 days	**Erythromycin base** 500 mg orally four times a day for 21 days+++
Gonorrhea Uncomplicated gonococcal infections of the urethra, cervix, and rectum	**Ceftriaxone** 125 mg IM in a single dose – or – **Cefixime** 400 mg orally in a single dose (tablet) – or – **Cefixime** 400 mg orally in a single dose (suspension; 200 mg/5 ml) *PLUS, if chlamydial infection not excluded* **Azithromycin** 1 g orally in a single dose – or – **Doxycycline** 100 mg orally twice a day for 7 days	**Spectinomycin** 2 g IM in a single dose – or – **Ceftizoxime** 500 mg IM in a single dose# – or – **Cefotaxime** 500 mg IM in a single dose# – or – **Cefoxitin** 2 g IM with probenecid 1 g orally# – or – Desensitization to cephalosporin – or – **Azithromycin** 2 g orally only if desensitization not possible##
Uncomplicated gonococcal infection of the pharynx	**Ceftriaxone** 125 mg IM in a single dose *PLUS, if chlamydial infection not excluded* **Azithromycin** 1 g orally in a single dose – or – **Doxycycline** 100 mg orally twice a day for 7 days	Desensitization to cephalosporin – or – **Azithromycin** 2 g orally only if desensitization not possible##
Disseminated gonococcal infection (DGI)	**Ceftriaxone** 1 g IM or IV every 24 hours	**Cefotaxime** 1 g IV every 8 hours – or – **Ceftizoxime** 1 g IV every 8 hours – or – **Spectinomycin** 2 g IM every 12 hours – or – Desensitization to cephalosporin
	All regimens should be continued for 24–48 hours after clinical improvement, at which time therapy may be switched to one of the following regimens to complete at least 1 week of antimicrobial therapy: **Cefixime** 400 mg orally twice a day (tablet) – or – **Cefixime** 400 mg orally twice a day (suspension; 200 mg/5 mL) – or – **Cefpodoxime** 400 mg orally twice a day	

*Ciprofloxacin is contraindicated for pregnant and lactating women.
**Worldwide, several isolates with intermediate resistance to either ciprofloxacin or erythromycin have been reported.
***Therapy should be continued until all lesions have healed completely; however, relapse can occur 6–18 months later despite effective initial therapy.
+For any of the regimens, the addition of an aminoglycoside (gentamicin 1 mg/kg IV every 8 hours) should be considered if lesions do not respond within the first few days of therapy.
++Both pregnant and lactating women should be treated with the erythromycin regimen; the addition of a parenteral aminoglycoside (e.g., gentamicin) should be strongly considered.
+++Pregnant women should be treated with the erythromycin regimen.
#Perhaps cefpodoxime 400 mg or cefuroxime axetil 1 g may be oral alternatives as a single dose.
##Concern regarding emerging resistance.

Lymphogranuloma Venereum

Lymphogranuloma venereum (LGV) is also an unusual sexually transmitted disease, the etiologic agents of which are the invasive serovars L1, L2 or L3 of *Chlamydia trachomatis*. The initial lesion is a small (<1 cm) ulcer or 'button-like' papule that resolves spontaneously. This is followed by the development of inguinal and/or femoral lymphadenopathy that is often unilateral. When the enlarged coalescing lymph nodes are found both above and below Poupart's ligament, a central indentation can form, and this is commonly referred to as the 'groove sign.' LGV is associated with fistula formation (secondary to draining lymph nodes), lymphedema of the genitalia, and symptomatic rectal involvement. Additional manifestations include fever, conjunctivitis, arthralgias, and a papular photoeruption. Although a definitive diagnosis requires isolation of the organism via tissue culture, the clinician must often rely on less specific serologic assays. A high IgG titer (>1:64) and/or a fourfold increase supports the clinical diagnosis. Treatment options are outlined in Table 29–2.

Disseminated Gonococcal Infection

Bacteremia with *Neisseria gonorrhoeae* can lead to fever, tenosynovitis, arthralgias, arthritis, and a few scattered cutaneous lesions. The latter are usually in an acral location and have an erythematous to purpuric base (Fig. 29–31); a central pustule is often seen. Disseminated gonococcal infection (DGI) is seen more frequently in women (often in association with menstruation) as well as in men who have sex with men, presumably because both groups have a higher incidence of occult primary infections that remain untreated. Disseminated gonococcal infection is also referred to as the arthritis–dermatitis syndrome. Unusual manifestations of DGI include perihepatitis, endocarditis, and meningitis. Sites of primary infection include the cervix, urethra, rectum, and pharynx. Treatment requires a more aggressive approach than does treatment of primary sites of infection (Table 29–2). As of 2006, the CDC

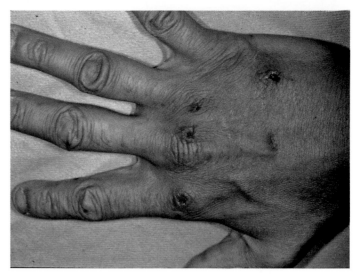

Figure 29–31 Multiple crusted papulopustules in a patient with disseminated gonococcemia. (Courtesy of Dr Neil A Fenske, Tampa, FL.)

no longer recommends the use of fluoroquinolones because of increasing resistance to this group of antibiotics in the United States. They may represent an alternative treatment, but only if antimicrobial susceptibility can be documented by culture.

SUGGESTED READINGS

Brown TJ, Yen-Moore A, Tyring SK. An overview of sexually transmitted diseases. Part I. J Am Acad Dermatol 1999; 41: 511–532.

Brown TJ, Yen-Moore A, Tyring SK. An overview of sexually transmitted diseases. Part II. J Am Acad Dermatol 1999; 41: 661–677. [erratum J Am Acad Dermatol 2000; 42: 148]

Centers for Disease Control and Prevention. Sexually transmitted diseases treatment guidelines 2006. MMWR Recomm Rep 2006; 55 (No. RR-11); 1–94. www.cdc.gov/std/treatment

Centers for Disease Control and Prevention. Update to CDC's Sexually transmitted diseases treatment guidelines, 2006: fluoroquinolones no longer recommended for treatment of gonococcal infections. MMWR Morb Mortal Wkly Rep 2007; 56: 332–336.

Czelusta A, Yen-Moore A, Van der Straten M, et al. An overview of sexually transmitted diseases. Part III. Sexually transmitted diseases in HIV-infected patients. J Am Acad Dermatol 2000; 43: 409–432.

Dlova NC, Mosam A. Inflammatory noninfectious dermatoses of HIV. Dermatol Clin 2006; 24: 439–448.

Hogan MT. Cutaneous infections associated with HIV/AIDS. Dermatol Clin 2006; 24: 473–495.

Majors MJ, Berger TG, Blauvelt A, et al. HIV-related eosinophilic folliculitis: a panel discussion. Semin Cutan Med Surg 1997; 16: 219–223.

Nagot N, Ouédrago A, Foulongne V, et al. Reduction of HIV-1 RNA levels with therapy to suppress herpes simplex virus. N Engl J Med 2007; 356: 790–799.

Paltiel M, Powell E, Lynch J, et al. Disseminated cutaneous acanthamebiasis: a case report and review of the literature. Cutis 2004; 73: 241–247.

Resneck Jr JS, Van Beek M, Furmanski L, et al. Etiology of pruritic papular eruption with HIV infection in Uganda. JAMA 2004; 292: 2614–2621.

Romanowski B, Sutherland R, Fick GH, et al. Serologic response to treatment of infectious syphilis. Ann Intern Med 1991; 114: 1005–1009.

Snoeck R, Andrei G, De Clercq E. Current pharmacological approaches to the therapy of varicella zoster virus infections: a guide to treatment. Drugs 1999; 57: 187–206.

Schmit I, Boivin G. Characterization of the DNA polymerase and thymidine kinase genes of herpes simplex virus isolates from AIDS patients in whom aciclovir and foscarnet therapy sequentially failed. J Infect Dis 1999; 180: 487–490.

Todd G. Adverse cutaneous drug eruptions and HIV: a clinician's global perspective. Dermatol Clin 2006; 24: 459–472.

Wieland U, Brockmeyer NH, Weissenborn SJ, et al., for the Competence Network HIV/AIDS. Imiquimod treatment of anal intraepithelial neoplasia in HIV-positive men. Arch Dermatol 2006; 142: 1438–1444.

Zabawski EJ Jr, Cockerell CJ. Topical and intralesional cidofovir: a review of pharmacology and effects. J Am Acad Dermatol 1998; 39: 741–745.

Chapter | **30** | *Joseph C. English III and Jeffrey P. Callen*

Sarcoidosis

Sarcoidosis is a multisystem disorder of unknown cause characterized by the accumulation of CD4+ T-cell and CD8+ T-cell lymphocytes, monocytes, and epithelioid macrophages from an unknown antigen(s) that induce the formation of noncaseating sarcoidal granulomas, leading to abnormal tissue and organ function. It most commonly involves the lungs, lymph nodes, liver, spleen, skin, eyes, glandular tissue, and bone; however, it can involve any organ system in the body. There are no consistent laboratory findings that permit the diagnosis of sarcoidosis. The diagnosis is dependent on the demonstration of a characteristic, albeit nonspecific, histopathologic finding. When this histopathologic change is present in tissue samples from multiple organ systems, and when appropriate tests exclude other causes of sarcoidal granulomas, the diagnosis of sarcoidosis can be confirmed.

The course of sarcoidosis is highly variable. It ranges from an acute self-healing process, to a chronic disease that exclusively affects the skin, to a debilitating systemic disease that can result in blindness and/or progressive respiratory insufficiency. Persistent evidence of disease for more than 2 years constitutes chronic sarcoidosis. Although associated with morbidity, sarcoidosis is rarely a primary cause of death.

CAUSE AND PATHOGENESIS

The cause of sarcoidosis is unknown. Over the years many causes have been postulated, including viruses (hepatitis C, HIV, HHV-8), bacteria (*Mycobacterium*, *Propionibacterium*, *Borrelia*, *Rickettsia*, cell wall-deficient bacteria), and foreign materials (pine pollen, beryllium). Coexistent 'autoimmune' diseases, such as autoimmune thyroiditis, have been reported, and patients with various collagen–vascular diseases (scleroderma, lupus, or dermatomyositis) may be more prone to develop sarcoidosis. Genetic factors have been implicated by histocompatibility antigen testing. Linkage with the MHC on the short arm of chromosome 6 revealed that alleles HLA DR 11, 12, 14, 15, and 17 confer susceptibility, whereas HLA DR1 and DR4 offer protection. Recently, linkage disequilibrium has been investigated with the BTLN2, TAP and TNFA1/A2 genes. Therefore, the disease is a multifactorial combination of possible immunologic (T-cell receptor), genetic (HLA), infectious, or environmental factors (antigen(s)), and to date no single component can explain all cases of sarcoidosis.

Owing to the lack of a consistent identifiable antigen(s), the polymorphic nature of the disease, and the lack of an animal model, a definitive pathogenesis is speculative at present and scientists are still searching for answers. Sarcoidosis is believed to be a disorder of the lymphoreticular system characterized by the depression of cell-mediated immunity (delayed-type hypersensitivity), an imbalance of CD4/CD8 cells (helper-to-suppressor T-cell ratio), a hyperreactivity of B cells, and increased production of circulating immune complexes. It is believed that the interaction between T cells and antigens, antigen-presenting cells and cytokines in the correct genetic milieu affects T-cell function, which results in a secondary increase in B-cell activity. Prolonged antigenic stimulation may affect macrophages. As sarcoidal granulomas develop, enzyme secretion (in particular, secretion of angiotensin-converting enzyme – ACE) may occur. Elevation of ACE is probably the result of granuloma formation. The precise reasons for the effects of the presumptive causative antigen(s) on patients with sarcoidosis are not understood. However, the result appears to be anergy to recall antigens, such as purified protein derivative, candida, and mumps, and the inability to sensitize an individual with sarcoidosis to an antigen such as dinitrochlorobenzene. Elevated levels of γ-globulin and nonspecific elevation of antibody titers to various viruses and fungal elements may also occur.

CLINICAL MANIFESTATIONS

Cutaneous Manifestations

Cutaneous manifestations of sarcoidosis are either specific or nonspecific, based on the histopathologic examination. Those cutaneous lesions represented histopathologically by noncaseating granulomas are termed specific cutaneous lesions of sarcoidosis. Those lesions that do not show noncaseating granulomas are termed nonspecific. The nonspecific cutaneous lesions consist mainly of erythema nodosum, pruritus, erythema multiforme, and clubbing. The specific cutaneous lesions include papules, plaques, nodules, subcutaneous nodules, infiltrative scars, and lupus pernio. In addition, there are multiple atypical presentations of specific cutaneous lesions such as acquired ichthyosis, erythrodermic, ulcerative, verrucous, scarring alopecia, morpheaform, palmar, photodistributed, and angiolupoid sarcoidosis. Interestingly, nail disease has been reported both as specific and nonspecific.

The most common nonspecific manifestation of sarcoidosis is erythema nodosum (EN; see Chapter 8). These lesions are firm, slightly erythematous, subcutaneous nodules, most commonly occurring on the anterior tibial surface. They are often tender to palpation. In some areas, sarcoidosis is the cause of roughly 20–25% of all cases of erythema nodosum. When erythema nodosum is associated with sarcoidosis, the symptom complex is often characterized by asymptomatic bilateral hilar lymphadenopathy, uveitis, fever, and arthritis. This four-symptom complex is referred to as Löfgren's syndrome. It is an acute form of sarcoidosis that resolves without treatment in 90% or more of affected individuals. It is postulated that these patients have circulating immune complexes that cause erythema nodosum. Biopsies of the lungs and lymph nodes in these patients reveal sarcoidal granulomas. Lung biopsy is not indicated in patients who have the typical tetrad. Recently, dermatologists have observed that patients with EN associated with sarcoidosis will have a higher frequency of papular sarcoidosis of the knees. This will be a location to look for and biopsy to help confirm the diagnosis. Several other sarcoidosis syndromes have been described, including Darier–Roussy sarcoidosis (multiple subcutaneous nodules of the trunk and extremity); Heerfordt–Waldenström syndrome (fever, parotid gland enlargement, anterior uveitis, and facial nerve palsy); Mikulicz's syndrome (bilateral sarcoidosis of the lacrimal, sublingual, submandibular, and parotid glands); and sarcoidosis–lymphoma syndrome (Hodgkin's or non-Hodgkin's lymphoma developing in patients with chronic active sarcoidosis). Spiegler–Fendt sarcoid is not a sarcoidosis syndrome and is a term for lymphocytoma cutis.

The 'specific' cutaneous lesions of sarcoidosis occur in roughly 10–35% of patients with documented systemic sarcoidosis. The diagnosis of a cutaneous sarcoidal granuloma is made by skin biopsy. Diascopy (Fig. 30–1) may help the dermatologist consider a granulomatous disease process, but is not exclusive to sarcoidosis. Certain cutaneous lesions may be highly suggestive of sarcoidosis, but none are clinically diagnostic. The cutaneous lesions of sarcoidosis can mimic many dermatoses and should frequently be included in differential diagnoses, especially the other noninfectious granulomatous diseases granuloma annulare, necrobiosis lipoidica, necrobiotic xanthogranuloma, actinic elastolytic granuloma, interstitial granulomatous dermatitis, palisaded neutrophilic granulomatous dermatitis, metastatic Crohn's disease, cheilitis granulomatosis, foreign-body reactions, and the granulomatous facial dermatides, as well as infectious granulomatous diseases such as deep fungal infections, atypical mycobacteria, leprosy, syphilis, and cutaneous tuberculosis. The most common cutaneous presentation of sarcoidosis is a papular lesion: small papules, 3–5 mm in diameter, with little epidermal change are frequently noted on the head and neck (Fig. 30–2). The periorbital region is commonly involved. The papules may be flesh colored, red, violaceous, or slightly

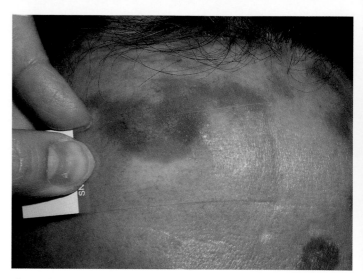

Figure 30–1 Diascopy in a patient with sarcoidosis may aid in the clinical diagnosis.

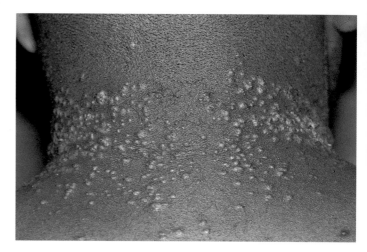

Figure 30–2 Small papular sarcoidosis lesions on the neck.

hyperpigmented. In blacks, they may be hypopigmented. At times the papules enlarge or coalesce to form either annular lesions or plaques (Figs 30–3 to 30–5). Papular disease at the corners of mouth may often coalesce and split, being indistinguishable from the classic split papule of secondary syphilis (Fig. 30–6).

Indurated plaque-type lesions (historically noted as Hutchinson's papillary psoriasis) represent a deeper cutaneous infiltration of sarcoidal granulomas than is seen in the papular lesions. The plaques can involve any area of the body. When they involve the scalp, scarring alopecia may result (Fig. 30–7). Infiltrated lesions involving the face, specifically the nose, with no epidermal change are classically referred to as lupus pernio (Fig. 30–8). If extensive telangiectatic lesions are evident, this is termed angiolupoid sarcoidosis. Chronic longstanding lupus pernio and angiolupoid sarcoidosis can ulcerate, and have an increased incidence of sarcoidosis of the upper respiratory tract (i.e., the sinuses), pulmonary fibrosis, and bone cysts. Patients with lupus pernio or angiolupoid sarcoidosis frequently have

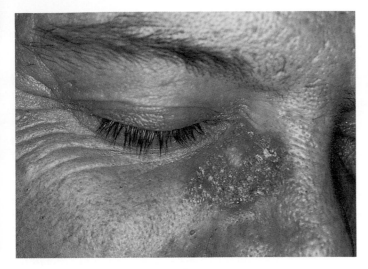

Figure 30–3 Violaceous plaque on the nose.

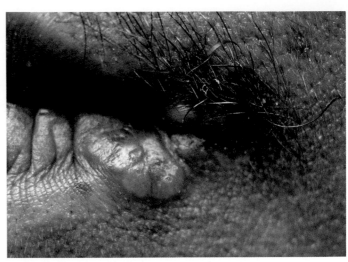

Figure 30–6 Split papule of sarcoidosis.

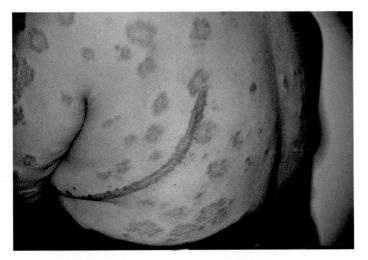

Figure 30–4 Multiple annular plaques in a woman with sarcoidosis.

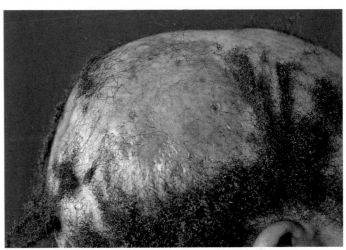

Figure 30–7 Scarring alopecia due to chronic cutaneous sarcoidosis.

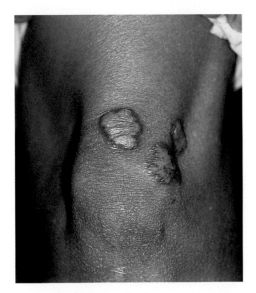

Figure 30–5 Infiltrative plaques on the knee.

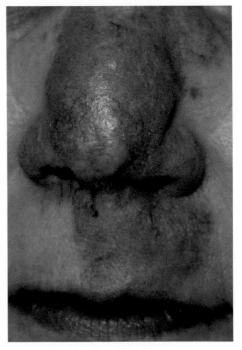

Figure 30–8 Lupus pernio of the central face.

pulmonary manifestations that are persistent and progressive. Patients with papular, nodular, or plaque-like lesions on the face have been misrepresented innumerable times as having lupus pernio, and are not associated with a greater risk of pulmonary disease. In fact, all cutaneous disease manifestations other than EN have yet to be convincingly proven as having prognostic implications.

Sarcoidosis often occurs in scars (Fig. 30–9) or on areas of skin chronically damaged by infection, radiation, or mechanical trauma. Sometimes it becomes difficult to determine whether these lesions are indeed cutaneous sarcoidosis, or whether they are local sarcoidal reactions to a foreign substance. Recent studies of patients with bona fide systemic sarcoidosis have demonstrated that foreign material is often present in the skin biopsy specimens. In the absence of systemic disease, a diagnosis of sarcoidosis cannot be made with confidence, particularly when only one area of the body is involved. However, if multiple areas, including or excluding scars, are involved with cutaneous sarcoidal granulomas, even in the absence of systemic disease, a diagnosis of sarcoidosis is reasonable. The subcutaneous nodular lesions are often asymptomatic, and they frequently occur on the trunk and extremities. These lesions are rarely tender. A review of Mayo Clinic patients with subcutaneous sarcoidosis noted that such

patients were more likely to be women in their fourth decade, and for there to be a strong association with bilateral hilar adenopathy.

There are many unusual forms of sarcoidosis, as previously mentioned. Ulceration of sarcoid lesions is unusual, except in lupus pernio, but can be seen on the lower extremities (Fig. 30–10). Verrucous lesions, although rare, occur most commonly in black females. They are reported most frequently on the lower extremities but may occur at any site (Fig. 30–11). Pustular lesions in a follicular pattern have been described, as well as macular hypopigmentation. Ichthyosis-like lesions occur in many patients with sarcoidosis. The lesions have the appearance of ichthyosis vulgaris, and an association of these lesions with systemic disease has been reported. Therefore, sarcoidosis must be included with HIV and lymphoma in the differential diagnosis of acquired ichthyosis. Sarcoidosis may also affect the orogenital mucosa.

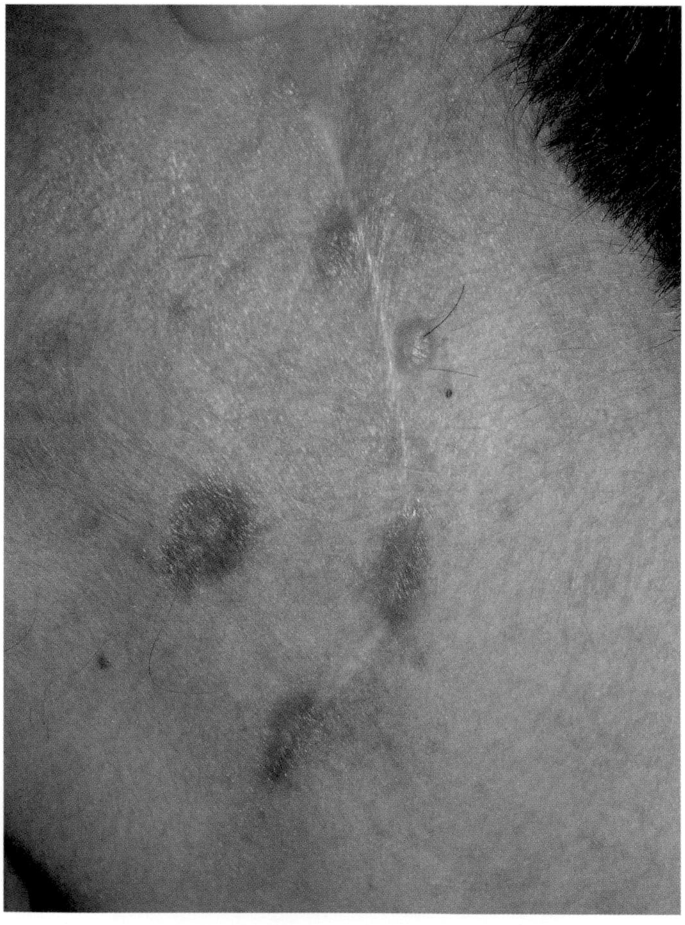

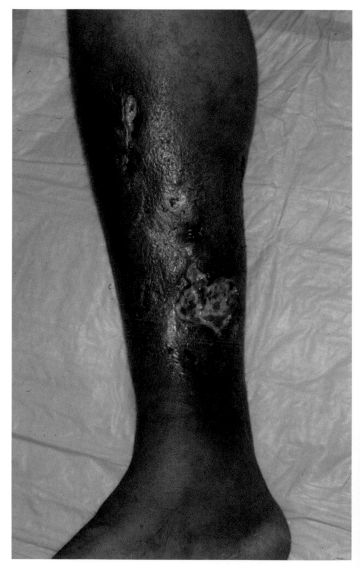

Figure 30–10 Ulcerative lesions on the legs due to sarcoidosis mimicking pyoderma gangrenosum.

Figure 30–9 Sarcoidal granulomas in a scar.

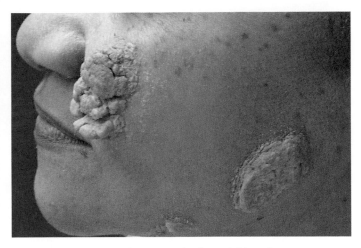

Figure 30–11 Verrucous lesions on the face of this patient are an unusual manifestation of sarcoidosis.

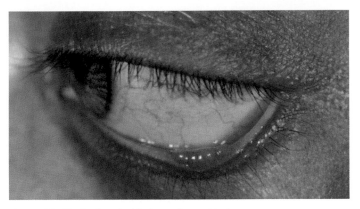

Figure 30–12 Conjunctival lesions of sarcoidosis.

Intrathoracic Disease

Intrathoracic disease, including hilar adenopathy and pulmonary parenchymal disease, is the most common manifestation of systemic sarcoidosis. Pulmonary sarcoidosis can be staged, according to chest X-ray findings, from 0 to III. Stage 0 disease consists of no changes seen on chest X-ray studies. Stage I includes bilateral hilar adenopathy in the absence of parenchymal disease recognized by chest X-ray studies. Stage II consists of hilar adenopathy with the presence of pulmonary fibrosis. Stage III consists of extensive pulmonary fibrosis in the absence of hilar adenopathy. The stages of radiographic findings do not represent chronological development. A diagnosis of sarcoidosis is often made on a 'routine' chest X-ray in an entirely asymptomatic patient. Patients who have bilateral hilar adenopathy without evidence of symptoms require monitoring; often the disease resolves spontaneously in all stages of pulmonary sarcoidosis. Abnormalities may be found by careful testing with pulmonary function tests and/or with bronchoalveolar lavage. Techniques such as gallium-67 and high-resolution CT scanning are also used.

Bilateral hilar adenopathy is the earliest and most common intrathoracic manifestation of sarcoidosis. Patients with this finding are often asymptomatic, although erythema nodosum, uveitis, arthritis, and fever may accompany the hilar lymphadenopathy, as previously mentioned. These patients with stage I disease rarely develop progressive parenchymal disease. Biopsy is not necessary in most patients with bilateral hilar adenopathy with symptoms of Löfgren's syndrome, or in those who are asymptomatic. However, only a small proportion of patients who have either unilateral hilar adenopathy or dyspnea have sarcoidosis. The differential diagnosis of bilateral hilar adenopathy includes deep fungal infection, tuberculosis, lymphoma, and bronchogenic carcinoma. Patients with these manifestations should undergo a lung biopsy and, possibly, mediastinal nodal biopsies. Stages II and III pulmonary sarcoidosis are associated with a much higher incidence of chronic progressive disease, and resolution of the X-ray findings becomes less likely. Symptoms may be present or absent.

However, abnormal pulmonary function testing correlates with more severe disease seen on chest X-ray studies.

Ocular Manifestations

Sarcoidosis may affect any portion of the eye; this occurs in one-quarter to half of patients with systemic sarcoidosis. Acute ocular sarcoidosis generally runs a course of 2 years or less, during which time active therapy may be needed. Chronic eye disease is less common. Early aggressive intervention can prevent scarring and blindness.

The most common ocular manifestation of sarcoidosis is uveitis, which usually affects the anterior segment of the eye. Patients may be entirely asymptomatic, or they may present with a red eye, photophobia, or increased tear production. The diagnosis is made by slit lamp examination, which reveals 'mutton fat' keratic precipitates in the anterior chamber. Less commonly, the posterior segment of the eye is involved, and its appearance correlates well with chorioretinitis and neurosarcoidosis. Uveitis must be aggressively treated to prevent adhesions, with resulting glaucoma, cataract development, or blindness.

Another common ocular finding in patients with sarcoidosis is conjunctival and lacrimal gland involvement. This may or may not produce symptoms of ocular irritation. Conjunctival granulomas (Fig. 30–12) occur in about one-third of patients with sarcoidosis. Conjunctival biopsy specimens may be positive even when the patient lacks clinical evidence of conjunctival involvement.

Lymph Nodes

Sarcoidal granulomas commonly infiltrate the lymph nodes. The incidence of peripheral lymphadenopathy is roughly 30% in patients with systemic sarcoidosis. Lymphadenopathy is associated with both acute and chronic disease patterns. The lymph node involvement is detected by palpation, is usually nontender, and is often not noticed by the patient. Because of the sarcoidosis–lymphoma syndrome, extensive adenopathy should be evaluated with FNA or biopsy of lymph nodes, as histologically they can be easily distinguished.

Splenic involvement in sarcoidosis is detected in approximately 20–25% of patients. It is manifested by splenomegaly, but functional abnormalities are rare.

Musculoskeletal Manifestations

Symptomatic muscle involvement in sarcoidosis is rare, although biopsy-based detection of a sarcoidal infiltrate is not uncommon. Clinical series of large numbers of patients with sarcoidosis reveal that approximately 1% have symptoms of muscle involvement. However, when patients with sarcoidosis undergo random muscle biopsies, more than 50% have histologic evidence of granulomatous disease. At times, muscle involvement may appear as subcutaneous nodules (Fig. 30–13).

Bone lesions occur in 10–15% of patients, usually correlating with chronic progressive disease. The X-ray changes are cystic lesions that usually occur in the terminal phalanges of the hands (Fig. 30–14). These may be accompanied by soft tissue swelling. Arthralgias are commonly experienced in acute sarcoidosis, particularly in patients with Löfgren's syndrome, and may be accompanied by arthritis. The wrists, knees, and ankles are the most commonly affected joints. Although chronic granulomatous arthritis has been reported, it is a rare complication of systemic sarcoidosis.

Neurosarcoidosis

Neurosarcoidosis affects 5–15% of patients with systemic sarcoidosis. Central nervous system involvement occurs in 50% of patients with neurosarcoidosis. The presence of neurosarcoidosis correlates with the presence of posterior uveitis and chronic cutaneous disease. The most common neurologic manifestations of sarcoidosis include optic nerve disease, facial nerve palsy, meningitis, and cerebral granulomas, which can lead to encephalopathy and seizures. Heerfordt–Waldenström syndrome is also frequently associated with central nervous system involvement. The detection of neurosarcoidosis can be difficult because affected tissue is not readily available for microscopic evaluation. The evaluation of a patient with suspected neurosarcoidosis can include skull X-ray studies, electroencephalography, a computed tomography (CT) scan, and/or magnetic resonance imaging of the head. Lumbar puncture may also be useful in patients with meningeal involvement.

Hepatic Sarcoidosis

Hepatic involvement in sarcoidosis is common. In a large study, hepatomegaly was detected in 20% of patients with sarcoidosis. Abnormal liver function tests are present in approximately half of the patients with hepatic involvement. Liver biopsy may be useful to obtain tissue to establish a diagnosis of sarcoidosis, although care must be taken to exclude other causes of granulomatous disease of the liver, and the findings must be correlated with evidence of sarcoidal disease elsewhere in the body. Hepatic involvement rarely progresses to functional abnormalities or cirrhosis. Combined hepatosplenomegaly is associated with a poorer outcome owing to the higher overall body granuloma and fibrosis burden.

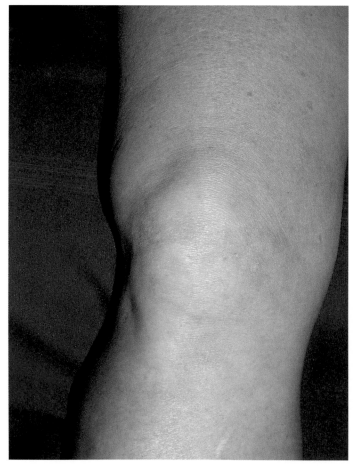

Figure 30–13 Distal vastus lateralis muscle enlargement due to sarcoidosis.

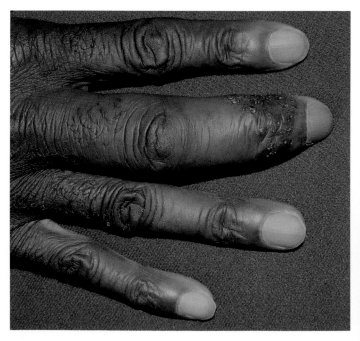

Figure 30–14 Sarcoid arthritis. This man also has papular cutaneous lesions.

Endocrine, Metabolic, and Laboratory Abnormalities

Endocrine glands may be infiltrated by sarcoidal granulomas. Functional abnormalities are not common, although pituitary or hypothalamic infiltration can cause diabetes insipidus or, on rare occasions, panhypopituitarism. An elevated prolactin level is a useful indicator of hypothalamic sarcoidal involvement. Other endocrine organs, such as the thyroid, parathyroid and adrenal glands and the pancreas, may be involved. However, functional impairment of these organs is unusual.

Hypercalcemia occurs in a small percentage of patients with systemic sarcoidosis. The serum calcium level elevation is often transient and seems to be responsive to therapy with systemic corticosteroids. In occasional patients with widespread sarcoidosis, the serum calcium level elevation can be persistent, and can lead to urinary tract stones, nephrocalcinosis, and even renal failure. Hypercalciuria is more common than hypercalcemia and may be used as a correlate with disease activity. The mechanism by which hypercalcemia is produced in sarcoidosis may be overproduction of 1,25-dihydroxyvitamin D by alveolar macrophages.

The serum ACE level is raised in approximately 60% of patients with systemic sarcoidosis. ACE is produced by epithelioid cells and may reflect the granuloma load in the body. Thus, the level of this enzyme may be useful in monitoring both disease activity and response to therapy in some patients with pulmonary sarcoidosis. However, the diagnostic accuracy of this enzyme level is limited because false-negative and false-positive tests may occur, limiting its use in determining disease progression or therapeutic response. Other blood levels, such as cytokines (e.g., IL-2), are investigational and are not clinically practical in evaluating patients with systemic sarcoidosis.

Cardiac Disease

The true incidence of cardiac involvement in sarcoidosis is not known. However, autopsy studies suggest that it is common and frequently asymptomatic. Cardiac sarcoidosis can result in symptoms of congestive heart failure, arrhythmia, or conduction defects. Sudden death in patients with sarcoidosis has been linked to cardiac involvement. Electrocardiography, 24-hour Holter monitoring, myocardial scintigraphy with thallium-201, echocardiography, gallium-67 scan, cardiac PET scan or MRI (PET-Positron Emission Tomography, MRI-magnetic resonance imaging) may be used to help define cardiac involvement.

Other Clinical Manifestations of Sarcoidosis

Almost any area of the body can be affected by sarcoidosis. Granulomatous renal disease has been reported on several occasions. Gastric granulomas, bone marrow granulomas, spinal cord lesions, and gonadal granulomas have also been reported. Difficulty arises in the white population with unilateral testicular disease, because testicular cancer is higher in this population than in blacks. Compounding the issue is that testicular cancer occurs at higher rates in sarcoidosis patients than in the general population.

Relationship of Cutaneous Disease to Systemic Disease

Many studies detail the cutaneous disease in patients with sarcoidosis. Unfortunately, none of these studies used the same methods, and many did not define the cutaneous lesions adequately. However, a few generalizations can be made. Patients with lupus pernio more frequently have sarcoidosis of the upper respiratory tract and lungs, as well as more frequent bone involvement than do patients without this combination of problems. Those patients with EN and bilateral hilar lymphadenopathy (Löfgren's syndrome) have a self-limiting course and a good prognosis. Patients with EN may have papular sarcoidal lesions on the knees to help aid in diagnosis. Patients with subcutaneous sarcoidosis have an increased association with bilateral hilar adenopathy. In all cases of cutaneous sarcoidosis, patients require evaluation for systemic involvement.

HISTOPATHOLOGIC FINDINGS

Sarcoidosis is characterized by granulomas composed principally of epithelioid cells with an occasional giant cell and little or no caseation necrosis. Inclusion bodies (Schaumann, Hamazalki–Wasserman, and asteroid bodies) are frequently observed, but these are not specific for sarcoidosis and may occur in other granulomatous conditions. The granulomas may remain seemingly unchanged for months or years, may resolve completely, or may undergo a fibrotic change. Although this is classically a dermal disease, epidermal change has been demonstrated histologically

The histopathologic differential diagnosis includes other granulomatous diseases, which may be excluded by special stains (infectious granulomas) and/or examination for foreign material (foreign body granulomas). Because noncaseating granulomas are not specific for sarcoidosis, other conditions must be vigorously excluded before a diagnosis of sarcoidosis can be confirmed. Thus, the diagnosis is one of exclusion. Special stains of the histopathologic specimens should include Fite stain, stains for mycobacteria, and periodic acid–Schiff stain for fungal elements. In addition, examination for a foreign body reaction with at least polarized light should be undertaken, although the presence of foreign material does not exclude the diagnosis. Various neoplasms should be excluded, particularly lymphomas, because there are occasional reports of sarcoidal tissue reactions occurring in nodes adjacent to neoplastic change. Immunologic testing (e.g., T-cell subset determination) of specimens has not been shown to be of diagnostic value.

DIAGNOSIS AND DIFFERENTIAL DIAGNOSIS

Sarcoidosis is diagnosed by a combination of clinical, radiologic, and laboratory findings plus the demonstration of noncaseating granulomas in the tissue. The differential diagnosis varies according to the organs involved. The differential mainly revolves around infectious and noninfectious granulomatous disease processes for each organ system, and has been discussed above. The only exception is the diagnosis in patients with asymptomatic bilateral hilar lymphadenopathy or in patients who have Löfgren's syndrome. These two clinical presentations are characteristic enough not to require histopathologic confirmation, but require appropriate follow-up to ensure resolution of the disease process. Tissue diagnosis through biopsies of various sites remains the main procedure to confirm the diagnosis of sarcoidosis. A prime tissue for biopsy is the skin, because it is an accessible, high-yield organ. Particular attention should be paid to changes in scars, or to any papular, nodular, or plaque-type lesion of recent onset. In addition, conjunctival biopsy, even in the absence of conjunctival nodules, may be positive in up to one-third of patients with sarcoidosis. Palpable lymph nodes may be biopsied when feasible. Lung biopsy through a fiberoptic bronchoscope and/or bronchial alveolar lavage is also helpful in establishing a diagnosis. Blind biopsy of the minor salivary glands on the lower lip is said to be positive in up to 60% of patients with sarcoidosis. Liver biopsy is a high-yield procedure, but its morbidity and mortality rates make it less useful than the previously mentioned techniques. Muscle biopsy may reveal sarcoidal granulomas in up to 50% of patients, particularly when a needle is used. Other sites for biopsy, although less valuable, include mediastinum, bone marrow, and spleen.

EVALUATION

After a diagnosis of sarcoidosis is made, the patient should be thoroughly evaluated to define the organ systems involved and to aid in prognostic predictions and therapeutic decisions. A team approach with the internist, ophthalmologist, pulmonologist, and dermatologist is required. A careful history and physical examination should be performed, focusing on all organ systems, but with preference given to the lungs, eyes, nervous system, and skin. Laboratory blood testing for chemistries, renal function, liver-derived enzymes, and calcium level monitoring should be done. An electrocardiogram is required. Chest imaging studies and pulmonary function tests with diffusion studies should be ordered. Additional testing could consist of skin tests to detect anergy, using multiple antigens, PPD, creatine kinase/aldolase for suspected muscle disease, urinalysis, and protein electrophoresis. The measurement of serum ACE levels is occasionally helpful in following patients with pulmonary sarcoidosis, but not routinely for skin disease.

PROGNOSIS

Mortality rates in sarcoidosis vary from 3% to 6%. Cardiac disease (the most common cause in Japan), progressive pulmonary disease (the most common cause in the United States), and neurosarcoidosis have been the cause of death in some patients.

The morbidity in sarcoidosis can be severe. Blindness can result from untreated ocular disease, and pulmonary disease can cause debilitating fatigue and shortness of breath. Renal failure has been reported from granulomatous involvement of the kidney, calcium deposits, and chronic urinary tract stones. Cosmetic deformities may occur in patients with cutaneous sarcoidosis, particularly in those with lupus pernio. Although many patients with pulmonary sarcoidosis may have resolution of their disease, the rates vary with the stage of pulmonary disease. Stage I sarcoidosis resolves in roughly 60% of patients; stage II resolves in 40% of patients; and stage III resolves in only 12%.

Despite the aberrations noted in tests of cell-mediated immunity, untreated sarcoidosis is not associated with an increased number of infections. However, it has been linked to an increase in the frequency of malignancy. Several studies have reported an increased incidence of hematologic malignancy – i.e., lymphoma, leukemia, and solid tumors (i.e., lung, testes, skin). Of note is that smoking has been associated with a reduced risk of developing pulmonary sarcoidosis owing to its ability to impair the pulmonary immune function, but for obvious reasons (increased risk of lung cancer in sarcoidosis) patients should not be encouraged to smoke. Some use the term 'paraneoplastic sarcoidosis' to describe the onset of sarcoidosis within 1 year of a diagnosis of malignancy, or vice versa. It is not clear, however, from these studies whether sarcoidosis is the primary disease, or whether a local sarcoidal reaction is a response to the malignancy in this group of patients. Of interest is the induction of new-onset sarcoidosis with antineoplastic agents used to treat oncology patients with Hodgkin's and non-Hodgkin's lymphoma, and the biologic modifier α-interferon (IFN) in leukemia. This has also been reported in noncancer patients who have received IFN-α for chronic hepatitis C.

TREATMENT

Acute sarcoidosis in which bilateral hilar adenopathy exists alone or in combination with erythema nodosum, uveitis, or arthritis is usually a self-limited disease and does not require specific therapy. Symptomatic therapy for the erythema nodosum or arthritis could include nonsteroidal anti-inflammatory drugs (NSAIDs), such as aspirin or indometacin. In addition, oral potassium iodide 325 mg t.i.d. is also useful for the treatment of EN. Acute uveitis can be treated with corticosteroid eyedrops.

Chronic cutaneous lesions, particularly lupus pernio and indurated plaques, which can cause scarring and disfigurement, should be treated more aggressively. Topical corticosteroids and topical immunomodulators are rarely effective because of the lack of penetration into the dermis. Intralesional corticosteroids are generally more effective but still not dramatically so. Antimalarials, particularly hydroxychloroquine sulfate (200–400 mg/day) or chloroquine phosphate (250–500 mg/day), are useful in treating patients with cutaneous sarcoidosis. Antimalarial therapy requires careful ophthalmologic monitoring. In addition, progressive systemic disease may occur despite antimalarial therapy. Methotrexate (10–15 mg/week) is the next-line therapy to supplement or replace the use of antimalarials. Cutaneous disease that has not responded to these measures and is significantly disfiguring may respond to systemic corticosteroids. Care must be taken not to induce flares of systemic disease when tapering the corticosteroids given for cutaneous manifestations. In addition, tetracyclines, pentoxyfylline, azathioprine, cyclophosphamide, cyclosporine, chlorambucil, thalidomide, leflunomide, adalimumab, infliximab, isotretinoin, melatonin, and allopurinol are reported to be valuable (in anecdotal reports or small case series) for treating cutaneous sarcoidosis. Nonmedical therapies have include surgical procedures such as the use of lasers, dermabrasion, surgical excision with grafting, plastic surgery, and phototherapy (narrowband ultraviolet B phototherapy, ultraviolet A-1 phototherapy, and photodynamic therapy), but there is not enough evidence to recommend any of these as the standard of care.

Ocular sarcoidosis, which can lead to scarring and blindness, must be aggressively treated. Corticosteroid eyedrops may be effective; however, patients who do not respond or who respond only partially may require intraocular corticosteroid injections or systemic corticosteroid therapy.

Progressive pulmonary disease is considered to be an indication for systemic corticosteroid therapy. Documented changes in pulmonary function tests as a result of therapy have been reported. In addition, changes in the serum ACE level and in abnormalities seen on bronchial alveolar lavage have been reported in patients treated with systemic corticosteroids. Alternative therapies that may be effective or that reduce the corticosteroid dosage include antimalarials, oxyphenbutazone, various antibiotics, various immunosuppressive agents, particularly methotrexate and cyclophosphamide, and TNF inhibitors such as thalidomide and infliximab. However, too few studies are available to reliably evaluate the effects of any agent other than systemic corticosteroids.

In addition to chronic disfiguring cutaneous lesions, ocular lesions, and progressive pulmonary disease, the indications for systemic corticosteroid therapy include hypercalcemia, neurosarcoidosis, symptomatic cardiac sarcoidosis, and functional endocrinologic abnormalities.

SUGGESTED READINGS

Ahmed H, Harsdad SR. Subcutaneous sarcoidosis: is it a specific subset of cutaneous sarcoidosis frequently associated with systemic disease? J Am Acad Dermatol 2006: 54: 55–60.

Bagwell C, Rosen T. Cutaneous sarcoidosis therapy updated. J Am Acad Dermatol 2007; 56: 69–83.

Baughman RP, Lower EE. A clinical approach to the use of methotrexate for sarcoidosis. Thorax 1999; 54: 742–746.

Callen JP. The presence of foreign bodies does not exclude the diagnosis of sarcoidosis. Arch Dermatol 2001; 137: 485–486.

Cohen PR, Kurzrock R. Sarcoidosis and malignancy. Clin Dermatol 2007; 25: 326–333.

Costabel U, Guzman J, Baughman RP. Systemic evaluation of a potential cutaneous sarcoidosis patient. Clin Dermatol 2007; 25: 303–311.

English JC 3rd, Patel PJ, Greer KE. Sarcoidosis. J Am Acad Dermatol 2001; 44: 725–743.

Izikson L, English JC 3rd. Cutaneous sarcoidosis. In: Williams HC, Bigby M, Diepgen T, Herxheimer A, Naldi L, Rzany B, eds. Evidence-based dermatology. London: BMJ Books; 2008: pp. 595–607.

James DG. Sarcoidosis 2001. Postgrad Med J 2001; 77: 177–180.

Marcoval J, Mana J, Moreno A, et al. Foreign bodies in granulomatous cutaneous lesions of patients with systemic sarcoidosis. Arch Dermatol 2001; 137: 427–430.

Marcoval J, Moreno A, Mana J. Papular sarcoidosis of the knees: a clue for the diagnosis of erythema nodosum-associated sarcoidosis. J Am Acad Dermatol 2003; 49: 75–78.

Nooer A, Knox KS. Immunopathogenesis of sarcoidosis. Clin Dermatol 2007; 25: 250–258.

Rossman MD, Kreider E. Lessons learned from ACCESS (A Case Controlled Etiologic Study of Sarcoidosis). Proc Am Thorac Soc 2007; 4: 453–456.

Sharma OP. Sarcoidosis: a historical perspective. Clin Dermatol 2007; 25: 232–241.

Spagnolo P, du Bois RM. Genetics of sarcoidosis. Clin Dermatol 2007; 25: 242–249.

Young RJ 3rd, Gilson RT, Yanase D, Elston DM. Cutaneous sarcoidosis. Int J Dermatol 2001; 40: 249–253.

Chapter | 31 |

Kathryn Schwarzenberger and Jeffrey P. Callen

Cardiovascular Diseases and the Skin

Cardiology and dermatology are two fields that generally are considered distinct, and rarely are they seen as overlapping. However, the heart can be affected in a variety of diseases that also affect the skin, some of which will be managed primarily by the dermatologist. It is essential that dermatologists be aware of potential cardiac manifestations of otherwise primarily dermatologic diseases to ensure that they are appropriately diagnosed and managed, and the converse is true for cardiologists. Furthermore, new drugs and therapies for cardiac diseases are recognized with increasing frequency as having cutaneous implications.

Several regions of the heart can be affected by disease, including the cardiac muscle, pericardium, valves, conduction system, and coronary vasculature, which supplies oxygen to the cardiac muscle. Therapies directed at improvement of muscle function (e.g., digoxin) rarely result in cutaneous disease, but therapies seeking to achieve fluid reduction (diuretics), afterload reduction, and control of rhythmic disturbances can affect the skin. With increasingly frequent use of potent immunosuppressive agents and the possibility of cardiac transplantation, resultant dermatological manifestations have also begun to be recognized.

Many of the multisystem disorders discussed in this text may have associated cardiovascular abnormalities. Table 31–1 lists cardiac abnormalities that occur with these multisystem disorders. Table 31–2 lists common dermatological findings that may be observed in association with primary cardiovascular disorders. Common cutaneous side effects of cardiac drugs are described in Table 31–3.

ANTIPHOSPHOLIPID ANTIBODY SYNDROME

Antiphospholipid antibodies, either anticardiolipin or the lupus anticoagulant, can occur in patients with or without systemic lupus erythematosus. Patients with these antibodies may have multisystem disease that can affect the skin and/or the heart. The disease is characterized by thrombotic disease of the arteries and/or veins, recurrent fetal loss, and/or cerebrovascular accidents. Patients with such antibodies who have

lupus erythematosus frequently have cardiac valvular vegetations, particularly on the mitral valve. Similarly, patients with primary antiphospholipid antibody syndrome also may have vegetations. These lesions may be clinically silent, but they can be detected with echocardiographic studies. The presence of these lesions may predispose the patient to bacterial endocarditis, and appropriate antibiotic prophylaxis is necessary for procedures that may result in bacteremia. Therapy for the antiphospholipid antibody syndrome includes the use of anticoagulants and platelet inhibitors, and approaches aimed at lowering the antibody level. It is not known whether these therapies have an effect on cardiac lesions.

CARCINOID SYNDROME

Paroxysmal flushing of the face and anterior chest occurs in association with carcinoid tumors that have metastasized to the liver or that begin in the lung. The symptoms are caused by the release of vasoactive substances – primarily serotonin – by the tumor. With continued disease, telangiectases and sclerodermoid changes may develop on affected areas. Asthma attacks may accompany the flushing episodes. Right-sided heart failure, tricuspid insufficiency, and pulmonic stenosis are the most common cardiac manifestations. In addition to the carcinoid syndrome, flushing may occur with pheochromocytoma, with systemic mast cell disease, as a feature of the dermatologic disease rosacea, or as an idiopathic phenomenon.

DEGOS DISEASE (MALIGNANT ATROPHIC PAPULOSIS)

Degos disease is an arteriopathy characterized by small areas of cutaneous necrosis that heal with an ivory porcelain white scar. Similar lesions may be present in the gastrointestinal tract or central nervous system and may result in death from uncontrolled hemorrhage. Cardiac involvement is rare, but when it does occur it is manifested by pericarditis and/or pericardial effusions.

Table 31–1 Cardiac manifestations in multisystem disorders with prominent cutaneous features

Disease	Cardiac manifestation	Cutaneous features	Comments
Primary systemic amyloidosis	Congestive heart failure, conduction disturbances, cardiomegaly	Pinch purpura, waxy skin	Proteinuria, association with myeloma
Behçet's disease	Pericarditis	Oral and genital aphthae, pathergy, pustular vasculitis, pyoderma gangrenosum-like lesions	Ocular involvement, CNS disease, colitis should be excluded
Carcinoid syndrome	Endocardial plaque – tricuspid insufficiency, conduction defects	Flushing, sclerodermoid features may occur as a late manifestation	Serotonin-producing tumor of the intestine. Usually metastatic to the liver at the time that symptoms develop
Cutis laxa	Aortic dilation and rupture, pulmonary artery stenosis, right-sided heart failure, asthmatic attacks	Looseness of the skin	Dominant (OMIM #123700), recessive (OMIM #219100) and X-linked (OMIM #304150) forms exist
Dermatomyositis	Cardiac arrhythmias, including atrial fibrillation/flutter, congestive heart failure, coronary artery disease	Gottron's papules, heliotrope rash, photodistributed poikiloderma	Clinically evident cardiac involvement is a poor prognostic sign
Diabetes mellitus	Coronary artery and peripheral vascular disease	See Chapter 20	—
Ehlers–Danlos syndrome	Aortic, pulmonary artery dilation, mitral, tricuspid valve prolapse, arterial rupture	Hyperelasticity of the skin, 'cigarette paper' scars, ecchymoses	Cardiac diseases is limited to classic (OMIM #130000), hypermobility (OMIM #130020) and vascular (OMIM #130050) types
Endocarditis – bacterial or fungal	Vegetations and dysfunction of the valves	Purpura, nailfold infarction, Janeway lesions, Osler's nodules	Fever. May simulate vasculitis or cryoglobulinemia
Exfoliative erythroderma	High-output cardiac failure	Exfoliative dermatitis	The eruption may be due to dermatitis, psoriasis, cutaneous T-cell lymphoma, drug eruption or other causes
Fabry disease	Mitral valve prolapse, conduction defects, congestive heart failure, myocardial infarction, cerebrovascular accidents	Angiokeratoma corporis diffusum	Alpha-galactosidase A deficiency, X-linked (OMIM #301500), gene map locus Xq22. Renal failure is the usual cause of death
Hemochromatosis	Congestive heart failure, supraventricular arrhythmias	Generalized bronze hyperpigmentation	Diabetes, cirrhosis
Kawasaki disease (mucocutaneous lymph node syndrome)	Coronary arteritis, coronary artery aneurysms	Glossitis, cheilitis, acral erythema, edema and desquamation, morbilliform eruption, conjunctival injection	High fever, lymphadenopathy, treatment with intravenous immune globulin is beneficial
Neonatal lupus erythematosus	Congenital heart block	Transient nonscarring lesions of LE (SCLE-like)	Presumed to be due to transplacental passage of autoantibodies, most commonly Ro (SS-A). May have transient cytopenia, hepatitis. Rash and cardiac disease rarely occur in the same patient, subsequent pregnancies may manifest either. Mothers often have or develop a connective tissue disease
Systemic lupus erythematosus	Verrucous endocarditis, pericarditis, coronary artery disease	Malar erythema, photosensitivity, lupus skin lesions	Anticardiolipin antibody may play a role. Therapy for LE with corticosteroids may predispose to coronary artery disease
Hyperlipidemias	Coronary artery disease	Xanthomas of all types	—

Table 31–1 Cardiac manifestations in multisystem disorders with prominent cutaneous features—cont'd

Disease	Cardiac manifestation	Cutaneous features	Comments
LEOPARD and Noonan syndromes	EKG abnormalities, hypertrophic cardiomyopathy	Multiple lentigines	L = lentigines, E = EKG abnormality, O = ocular hypertelorism, P = pulmonary stenosis, A = abnormalities of the genitalia, R = retardation of growth, D = deafness (OMIM #151100)
Multicentric reticulohistiocytosis	Pericarditis, congestive heart failure, coronary artery disease, cardiomegaly	Erythematous nodules of the hands and occasionally the face	Deforming arthritis is frequent
Carney complex (including NAME and LAMB syndromes)	Atrial myxoma	Cutaneous myxomas and lentigines	Carney's includes endocrine neoplasia of the adrenal, pituitary and/or testes
Neurofibromatosis	Hypertension due to pheochromocytoma	Café-au-lait macules, neurofibromas, axillary freckling	—
Pseudoxanthoma elasticum	Premature atherosclerotic vascular disease, aortic aneurysm, hypertension	Yellow papules on intertriginous surfaces, redundant lax skin	Upper or lower GI hemorrhage. Angioid streaks in the eye, uterine hemorrhage. Autosomal dominant and recessive variants have been described (OMIM #264800 and #177850). No known treatment is effective
Relapsing polychondritis	Aortic insufficiency, dissecting aortic aneurysm	Beefy, red ears or other tissue with cartilage. Late floppy ears and other areas where the cartilage was affected	Arthritis, tracheal collapse. Dapsone may be helpful. Corticosteroids and/or immunosuppressives are also used
Rheumatic fever	Pancarditis in the acute phase. Late manifestations include mitral and/or aortic valve dysfunction	Erythema marginatum, subcutaneous nodules	Rare in US. Follows pharyngitis due to group A β-hemolytic streptococcal infection. Polyarthritis, chorea, fever
Sarcoidosis	Conduction defects, congestive heart failure	Papules, nodules, plaques and/or lesions in scars	Pulmonary disease, lymphadenopathy, hepatic involvement, hypercalcemia. Cardiac involvement denotes a poor prognosis
Scleroderma	Conduction defects, pulmonary hypertension, pericarditis, visceral Raynaud's phenomenon	Cutaneous sclerosis, Raynaud's phenomenon	Cardiac involvement denotes a poor prognosis
Tuberous sclerosis	Cardiac rhabdomyomas	Adenoma sebaceum, periungual and subungual fibromas, ash leaf macule, shagreen patch	Renal hamartomas, CNS tumors, mental retardation, seizures
Vasculitis	Coronary artery vasculitis	Palpable purpura, nodules, livedo reticularis, ulcerations	Arthritis, GI colic or bleeding, cardiac involvement is uncommon
Werner's syndrome	Premature atherosclerosis	Premature graying, alopecia, sclerodermoid changes, loss of subcutaneous fat, ankle ulcerations	Myocardial infarction is usually responsible for death by the fifth decade. Autosomal recessive (OMIM #277700, gene map locus 8p12-p11.2). Other features include cataracts, malignancy
Loeys–Dietz syndrome	Arterial tortuosity and aneurysm	Velvety or translucent skin in some patients	Caused by heterozygous mutations in genes encoding TGF-β receptors 1 and 2; other features include hypertelorism, and bifid uvula or cleft palate
Psoriasis	Increased risk of myocardial infarction and coronary artery disease	Classic psoriasiform plaques on variable parts of body, often knees, elbows, umbilicus, gluteal cleft, scalp	Associated with metabolic syndrome, obesity, diabetes mellitus, hyperlipidemia, smoking

Table 31–2 Cutaneous findings observed in association with primary cardiac abnormalities

Cutaneous changes	Cardiac disorders
Xanthomas, cutaneous changes of diabetes, changes of premature aging, presence of an earlobe crease, male pattern baldness (early onset)	Coronary artery disease
Neurofibromas, café-au-lait spots, axillary freckling	Hypertension – pheochromocytoma
Features of scleroderma	Hypertension – renovascular
Palpable purpura, livedo reticularis, ulcerations	Embolic phenomenon – cholesterol emboli (often follows an invasive procedure, such as catheterization or angiography), left atrial myxoma (see Table 31.1), subacute bacterial endocarditis
Osler's nodes, Janeway's lesions, petechiae, purpuric pustules, splinter hemorrhages	Endocarditis – bacterial, fungal or vegetative
Changes of syndromes with myxomata, embolic phenomena, as in cholesterol emboli	Left atrial myxoma
Clubbing	Cyanotic heart disease, pulmonary disease may also be associated with clubbing

Table 31–3 Common cutaneous side effects of cardiac medications

Cutaneous changes	Medication
Photosensitivity, resultant slate blue-gray pigmentation	Amiodarone
Flare of psoriasis	β-Adrenergic blockers
Hypertrichosis	Minoxidil
Petechiae (thrombocytopenia), photosensitivity	Quinidine
Drug-induced lupus erythematosus	Procainamide HCl
Photosensitivity, drug-induced subacute cutaneous lupus erythematosus	Thiazide diuretics
Pedal edema	Calcium channel blockers

EARLOBE CREASES

An increased prevalence of a diagonal earlobe crease occurs with age. In some studies this finding has been correlated with increased cardiac morbidity and mortality rates from coronary artery disease, whereas in others it has not been shown to be an independent risk factor. It has been suggested that patients with a diagonal earlobe crease be evaluated for other cardiac risk factors. The cutaneous change is characterized by a visible crease that extends from the tragus to the posterior pinna and involves at least one-third of the distance. The depth of the crease seems to be unimportant. Two hypotheses link the earlobe crease to coronary artery disease: (1) both are sites supplied by end arteries with little collateral circulation; and (2) a generalized loss of elastin and elastic fibers occurs in these patients, producing both conditions.

MALE PATTERN BALDNESS

Male pattern baldness at an early age has been linked to insulin resistance and indirectly to an increased risk for coronary artery disease. Baldness, thoracic hairiness, and a diagonal earlobe crease have been linked to a slight increase in risk for coronary artery disease in men under 60 years of age.

HEMOCHROMATOSIS

Hemochromatosis is a common inherited disorder of iron metabolism that results in excessive iron deposition in the skin, heart, liver, and pancreas. The skin becomes darkened, with a bronze hue, from which the term 'bronze diabetes' was derived. Adult-onset diabetes mellitus is common, and hepatic dysfunction with eventual cirrhosis is another feature. Cardiac disease, of which congestive heart failure is the most common problem, is the presenting manifestation in about 15% of patients. Cardiac arrhythmias, including supraventricular tachycardias, atrial fibrillation and flutter, and heart blocks, are also seen. The treatment of choice is to remove excess iron stores by repeated phlebotomies.

RELAPSING POLYCHONDRITIS

Relapsing polychondritis is a rare disease characterized by recurrent episodes of inflammation affecting cartilaginous tissue. It has been linked in some patients to autoantibodies directed against type II collagen. The disease affects only cartilaginous tissue. The most common manifestation is the sudden onset of a tender, erythematous, warm, swollen external ear (Fig. 31–1). The inflammation subsides spontaneously over a 1–2-week period, and then recurs. Eventually the cartilage may be damaged, with resultant permanent deformity. Other tissues that contain cartilage may also be affected, including the joints and trachea. Biopsy specimens of ear cartilage support the clinical diagnosis. The heart may be involved, with aortic insufficiency or aortic aneurysms. Other valves, including the mitral valve, are rarely involved. The most dangerous development in this disorder is asphyxia as a result of tracheal collapse, which may be fatal. Therapy is directed at blocking the neutrophilic inflammatory reaction in the cartilage. Systemic corticosteroids, immunosuppressive agents, and dapsone have been used.

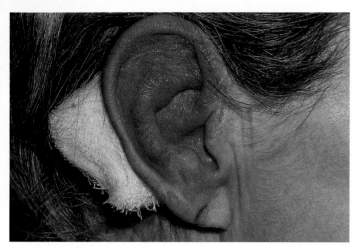

Figure 31–1 Erythematous eruption of the earlobe representative of relapsing polychondritis.

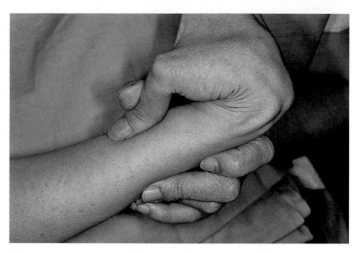

Figure 31–2 Hyperextensible skin and joints seen in Ehlers–Danlos syndrome.

EMBOLIC PHENOMENA

Emboli may occur from atrial myxomas, cholesterol deposits, or infections. The cutaneous lesions that result are caused by an 'upstream' blockage of medium-sized to small vessels with distal infarction and/or occlusion of the small vessels in the skin. Thus, splinter hemorrhages, petechiae, purpura, multiple sites of digital gangrene, and livedo reticularis are the most common findings. Cholesterol emboli or atheroemboli are not uncommon, and are often the result of the dislodging of atheromatous plaques during angiography. Not only is the skin affected, but also the central nervous system, eye, and kidney may be involved. Treatment is supportive.

EHLERS–DANLOS SYNDROME

The Ehlers–Danlos syndromes (EDS) are a heterogeneous group of genetic disorders that are characterized clinically by joint hypermobility, hyperextensible skin, and variable involvement of other organs (Fig. 31–2). The different syndromes were recently divided into seven subtypes, based on shared clinical and pathogenetic findings. Easy bruising is a frequent feature in patients with some forms of EDS. In addition, 'cigarette paper' scars form as a result of poor wound healing. Cardiac manifestations may include mitral valve prolapse, tricuspid valve prolapse, aortic dilatation with insufficiency, and arterial rupture. Cardiac abnormalities occur most commonly in the classic (type I), the hypermobility type (type III), and the vascular type (type IV).

LOEYS–DIETZ SYNDROME

Although not primarily a dermatologic disease, this recently described autosomal dominant disease may be considered in the differential diagnosis of patients who present with velvety or translucent skin and vascular disease. The syndrome, caused by heterozygous mutations in the genes encoding transforming growth factor-β receptors 1 and 2, is characterized primarily by arterial tortuosity and aneurysms, hypertelorism, and bifid uvula or cleft palate. Patients are at high risk of aortic dissection or rupture at an early age. Although the vascular abnormalities are similar to those seen in the vascular type of EDS, these patients lack joint hypermobility and can often be successfully treated with vascular surgery.

LEOPARD AND NOONAN SYNDROMES

LEOPARD syndrome is an autosomal dominant disorder manifested by lentigines, electrocardiographic abnormalities, ocular hypertelorism, pulmonary stenosis, abnormalities of the genitalia, retardation of growth, and deafness (sensorineural). The lentigines are concentrated on the trunk and are present at birth or in early childhood; they darken with age (Fig. 31–3). The electrocardiographic abnormalities include axis deviation, prolonged P–R intervals, left anterior hemiblock, bundle branch block, and/or complete heart block. Hypertrophic cardiomyopathy is the most common cardiac problem other than pulmonary stenosis. LEOPARD syndrome is an allelic variant of Noonan syndrome. Mutations in the PTPN11 gene have been identified in some patients with both syndromes.

CARNEY COMPLEX

The term 'Carney complex' is now used to describe patients with myxomas (skin, heart, and/or breast), endocrine disorders, and lentigines. Myxomas, which are the most common cardiac tumor, may involve the atrium or, less frequently, the ventricle. LAMB (lentigines, atrial myxoma, mucocutaneous myxoma, and blue nevi) and NAME (nevi, atrial myxoma, myxoid neurofibromata, and ephelides) syndromes are now considered to be variants of Carney complex. Mutations in the PRKRA1A gene have been identified in many patients with familial cardiac myxomas.

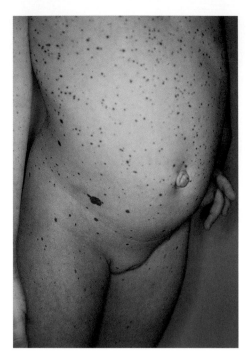

Figure 31–3 Multiple lentigines in a patient with the LEOPARD syndrome. (Courtesy of Paul Lucky, MD, Cincinnati, Ohio. Reprinted with permission from Color Atlas of Dermatology. Philadelphia: WB Saunders, 2000.)

WERNER'S SYNDROME

Werner's syndrome results in findings that resemble premature aging. The skin becomes atrophic, weathered, and sclerotic. The nose may appear beak-like, and the voice takes on a high-pitched, nasal quality. Coronary artery disease with myocardial infarction occurs at an early age and is often the cause of death.

PSEUDOXANTHOMA ELASTICUM

Pseudoxanthoma elasticum (see Chapter 25) is a group of inherited disorders with autosomal dominant or recessive inheritance patterns. The disease is associated with an abnormal calcification of elastic fibers. Cutaneous lesions are frequently seen on intertriginous surfaces (including the neck) as yellow papules that resemble the skin of a plucked chicken. The patients usually have angioid streaks, which are seen on

ophthalmologic examination, and widespread premature vascular disease. Hypertension is common. Cardiac manifestations include ischemic disease, manifested by angina pectoris, myocardial infarction, and eventual congestive heart failure. Similar disease affects other vasculatures; thus, peripheral vascular disease with intermittent claudication, stroke, and/or abdominal angina may occur. In many of these patients, life expectancy is shortened.

PSORIASIS AND HEART DISEASE

An increased risk of cardiovascular disease, with an accompanying increased risk of death, has been associated with moderate to severe psoriasis. Several large observational studies have identified an association of psoriasis with known cardiac risk factors, including obesity, hypertriglyceridemia, diabetes, and hypertension. The prevalence of metabolic syndrome, with its associated insulin resistance, has been shown to be increased in patients with moderate to severe psoriasis. Although some of these may be a side effect of common systemic medications used to treat severe psoriasis (cyclosporine: hypertension and hyperlipidemia; acitretin: hyperlipidemia; methotrexate: hyperhomocysteinemia), the disease itself appears to convey an increased relative risk of heart disease and, specifically, myocardial infarction. The precise mechanisms responsible for this increased cardiac disease are still being evaluated, but a contributory role for chronic inflammation has been proposed. It is not yet known whether or not aggressive treatment of the skin, particularly with drugs that lower the levels of C-reactive protein, will minimize the cardiac risk of psoriasis.

MYOSITIS

The exact incidence of cardiac involvement in the idiopathic inflammatory myopathies dermatomyositis and polymyositis is not known. It is thought that whereas clinically evident disease is probably fairly rare, subclinical disease, primarily in the form of conduction abnormalities and arrhythmias, may be more common. Conduction abnormalities, ranging from atrial fibrillation/flutter, and bundle branch blocks, to A-V heart block, have been reported in many myopathies, including dermatomyositis. Congestive heart failure, possibly from myocarditis, is recognized, as is coronary artery disease; an increased death rate from myocardial infarction has been identified in these patients. Overt cardiac disease in dermatomyositis patients portends a poor prognosis.

SUGGESTED READING

Abdelmalek NF, Gerber TL, Menter A. Cardiocutaneous syndromes and associations. J Am Acad Dermatol 2002; 46: 161–183.

Christophers E. Comorbidities in psoriasis. Clin Dermatol 2007; 25: 529–534.

Gelfand JM, Neimann, AL, Shin DB, et al. Risk of myocardial infarction in patients with psoriasis. JAMA 2006; 296: 1735–1741.

Kremers HM, McEvoy MT, Dann FJ, et al. Heart disease in psoriasis. J Am Acad Dermatol 2007; 57: 347–354.

Lundberg IE. The heart in dermatomyositis and polymyositis. Rheumatology 2006; 45: iv18–iv21.

Matilainen V, Koskela P, Keinänen-Kiukaanniemi S. Early androgenetic alopecia as a marker of insulin resistance. Lancet 2000; 356: 1165–1166.

Miric D, Fabijanic D, Giunio L, et al. Dermatological indicators of coronary risk: a case-control study. Int J Cardiol 1998; 67: 251–255.

Motamed M, Pelekoudas N. The predictive value of diagonal ear-lobe crease sign. Int J Clin Pract 1998; 52: 305–306.

Pupo RA, Wiss K, Solomon AR. Disorders affecting the skin and the heart. Dermatol Clin 1989; 7: 517–529.

Wakkee M, Thio HB, Prens EP. Unfavorable cardiovascular risk profiles in untreated and treated psoriasis patients. Atherosclerosis 2007; 190: 1–9.

Renal Disease and the Skin

INTRODUCTION

Acute and chronic kidney diseases are common and reflect an ongoing rise in the prevalence of diabetes and hypertension, the two most common causes of renal failure. Cutaneous manifestations of renal disease occur frequently, particularly in the setting of chronic renal failure. These skin disorders have many origins. Some cutaneous problems, such as renal pruritus and uremic frost, appear to relate to failure of renal function per se. Others occur as a consequence of the secondary sequelae of renal failure (e.g., calciphylaxis due to hyperparathyroidism). In addition, dermatologic findings may be important clues to the diagnosis of heritable syndromes with important renal manifestations or other systemic disease that may involve the kidneys, such as vasculitis. Lastly, other skin changes, such as seen in nephrogenic systemic fibrosis, can occur iatrogenically in patients with kidney disease.

Advances in the treatment of chronic renal failure (CRF) have resulted in an improved life expectancy for these patients, but with their increased longevity comes an increased opportunity for the development of cutaneous complications. Thus, one can predict that the incidence and prevalence of skin disease related to CRF and/or its treatment will continue to increase.

HERITABLE DISORDERS WITH RENAL AND CUTANEOUS FEATURES

A number of heritable disorders have both cutaneous and renal manifestations. The most important of these are summarized in Table 32–1.

SKIN DISORDERS ASSOCIATED WITH ACUTE AND CHRONIC RENAL FAILURE

Renal Pruritus

Itching, often of a severe and maddening intensity, is the most common dermatologic manifestation of CRF. A recent epidemiologic study of 18 801 hemodialysis patients found moderate to severe pruritus in 42%. Anecdotally, the prevalence of renal itch seems to be falling, perhaps reflecting changes in hemodialysis technology, earlier transplantation, or other factors. Pruritus may predate the initiation of dialysis, suggesting that CRF is itself associated with itching, but the most severe and intractable cases are hemodialysis associated. Severe pruritus is associated with significantly increased mortality in hemodialysis patients, although the mechanism of this is unclear.

Many etiologies have been proposed for renal pruritus, and no single cause has been identified. Logically, it has been supposed that impaired clearance of pruritogenic molecules is fundamentally the cause, but no candidate molecule has been found. Also, pruritus does not appear to correlate with the efficiency of dialysis (Kt/V), although this index only measures the clearance of small molecules such as urea. Renal itch is very probably multifactorial, requiring the interplay of two or more of the following: impaired clearance of pruritogens, the type of dialysis membrane or dialysis tubing employed, dry skin, and environmental heat. There is some evidence suggesting a role for dialysis-associated neuropathy of type C unmyelinated nociceptive nerve fibers in the skin; endogenous opioids; parathyroid hormone itself; or disturbance of calcium–phosphate metabolism in secondary hyperparathyroidism. Surprisingly, there is very little evidence that medications play any important role in causing renal pruritus.

Not surprisingly, given our poor understanding of the pathomechanisms of renal pruritus, treatment is far from satisfactory. Xerosis should always be treated with emollient or humectant moisturizers. Patients should be advised that maintaining a cool environment is helpful. Secondary lichenification and dermatitis may be treated in the usual fashion. Broadband UVB phototherapy is often beneficial, but must be used sparingly in patients who may subsequently undergo renal transplantation, because of the risk of skin cancer. Topical menthol relieves itch well; topical capsaicin does not. Systemic antipruritics are notoriously ineffective, and H_1 blockers such as diphenhydramine and hydroxyzine are poorly cleared in CRF. The oral opioid receptor antagonist naltrexone has been reported helpful, although the authors have not found it so. Similarly, gabapentin or pregabalin may have a role, particu-

Table 32–1 Heritable disorders with renal and cutaneous features

Syndrome	OMIM number	Skin features	Renal features	Other features
Fabry's disease	301500	Generalized angiokeratomas (Fig. 32–1)	Proteinuria, CRF; neuropathic pain; sensorineural deafness	X-linked recessive; α-galactosidase-A deficiency
Birt–Hogg–Dubé	135150	Trichodiscomas, fibrofolliculomas, acrochordons (see Chapter 13)	Renal carcinoma	Spontaneous pneumothorax; autosomal dominant; folliculin gene FLCN mutation
Tuberous sclerosis	191100	Angiofibromas, connective tissue nevi, hypopigmented macules (see Chapter 13)	Angiomyolipomas, simple renal cysts, polycystic kidneys, renal carcinoma; CRF due to compression of renal parenchyma by angiomyolipomas or cysts	Seizures, learning difficulty, behavioral problems; genetically heterogeneous; autosomal dominant transmission with high spontaneous mutation rate
Nail–patella syndrome	161200	Nail 'dysplasia': triangular lunulae, hypoplastic nails (Fig. 32–2)	Characteristic nephropathy causing proteinuria, edema; may progress to CRF	Hypoplasia of patellae; iliac horns; elbow abnormality limiting pronation/supination; autosomal dominant transmission; mutation in LIM-homeodomain protein LMX1B
Hereditary multiple leiomyomas of skin	150800	Multiple cutaneous leiomyomas, typically regionally grouped; 'school of fish' appearance (see Chapter 13)	Renal carcinoma	Autosomal dominant, mutation in gene encoding fumarate hydratase; uterine leiomyomas occur as well

Figure 32–1 Fabry's disease.

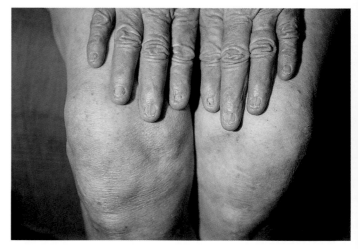

Figure 32–2 Nail–patella syndrome. Note the hypoplasia of the nails. Also, in this particular individual the patellae are missing. (Courtesy of Dr Neil. A. Fenske, Tampa, Florida.)

larly in individuals whose pruritus symptoms have a 'neuropathic' quality (burning or painful itch).

Calciphylaxis

Calciphylaxis is a poorly understood, rare, often fatal disease. Synonyms include calcific uremic arteriolopathy, calcifying panniculitis, and uremic gangrene syndrome. Calciphylaxis has most often occurred in the setting of renal failure; however, there are many reports of patients without renal failure who have developed calciphylaxis, particularly in association with malignancy, hyperparathyroidism, alcoholic liver disease, and autoimmune connective tissue diseases.

Clinically, calciphylaxis is characterized by painful, symmetric, violaceous lesions that often evolve into areas of ulceration and ischemic necrosis (Fig. 32–3), and it is considered to be a specific form of metastatic calcification. It frequently occurs in anatomic regions that contain large amounts of subcutaneous fat, and it generally spares the face. Calciphylaxis is more common in women, obese patients, and Caucasians. The main differential diagnoses include dystrophic calcification, vasculitis, occlusive vasculopathy, embolic phenomena, anticoagulant necrosis, and panniculitis.

The key histologic features include medial calcification and intimal proliferation of subcutaneous arteries and arterioles, which ultimately manifests as ischemic, cutaneous necrosis (Fig. 32–4). Thrombosis is often found as well, but is an inconstant feature. Although nonspecific tissue calcification may also be seen, the defining feature of calciphylaxis is calcification of the vessels, which is detected with the use of the von Kossa stain. It is important to note that vessel calcification can often be found in patients with chronic renal disease; however,

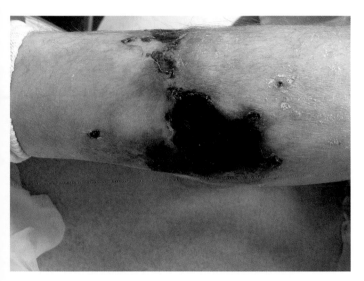

Figure 32–3 Calciphylaxis: necrosis and livedo reticularis. (Courtesy of Jeffrey Callen, MD.)

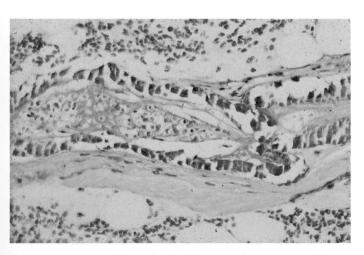

Figure 32–4 Histopathology of calciphylaxis: calcification in a small artery. (Courtesy of James W. Patterson, MD.)

those vessel abnormalities do not usually lead to ischemic necrosis.

Proposed risk factors for calciphylaxis include hyperparathyroidism, hyperphosphatemia, elevated calcium–phosphate product, diabetes, obesity (which may reduce local blood flow), female gender, protein C or S deficiency, systemic corticosteroid use, immunosuppression, and trauma. In the setting of CRF there is impaired excretion of phosphate as well as a decrease in activation of vitamin D_3, which leads to reduced absorption of calcium and subsequent hyperparathyroidism. Through the increased production of parathyroid hormone the calcium level normalizes, but extreme hyperphosphatemia may result, which leads to a high calcium–phosphate product. However, it has been well documented that an elevated calcium–phosphate product does not have to be present for calciphylaxis to occur, and in fact was found in one series to be present in fewer than 50% of patients.

The diagnosis of calciphylaxis is made by correlation of clinical findings and characteristic biopsy findings with histopathological examination of the skin and subcutaneous fat in the affected area. Laboratory abnormalities may include an abnormally elevated intact parathyroid hormone (iPTH) level, or an elevated calcium–phosphate product, but the latter is not pathognomonic and may be absent altogether.

Treatment options for calciphylaxis are limited and are usually directed at correcting metabolic abnormalities and minimizing other controllable disease risk factors. Proposed therapies include local wound care, calcium-free phosphate binders, cinacalcet, sodium thiosulfate, subtotal or total parathyroidectomy, and hyperbaric oxygen. Although controversial, some investigators feel that there is evidence for improved outcomes with surgical debridement, and it has been suggested that parathyroidectomy should not be performed in patients without well-documented hyperparathyroidism. Future therapies may include recombinant osteoprotegerin and thrombolytic therapy (such as low-dose tissue plasminogen activator). The prognosis for patients with calciphylaxis is poor, with mortality rates reaching approximately 46% at 1 year. Death is most commonly due to overwhelming sepsis.

Nephrogenic Systemic Fibrosis

Originally described by Cowper and colleagues in 1997, nephrogenic systemic fibrosis (NSF) is a disease that primarily involves the skin and subcutaneous tissues and mimics scleroderma and scleredema. It was originally described as a scleromyxedema-like dermatosis in hemodialysis patients, but eventually it was called nephrogenic fibrosing dermopathy until cases with systemic involvement were documented. Although the exact etiology remains unclear, it is a process that has thus far only been detected in patients with renal disease. However, the likelihood of developing NSF has not been associated with the duration or cause of renal insufficiency in affected patients. NSF has occurred in patients of all races and has no gender predilection. Middle-aged patients constitute the majority of cases, but NSF has been documented in both children and the elderly. In addition to renal disease, other associated conditions include hypercoagulability, deep venous thrombosis, hepatic disease, and systemic lupus erythematosus. Cardiomyopathy and idiopathic pulmonary fibrosis also occur in these patients, but are probably due to the disease process rather than being causally associated with NSF.

Clinically, NSF presents with symmetric thickening of the skin of the extremities and occasionally the trunk, but generally spares the face. The most frequently involved site is the area from the ankles to the mid-thighs, and it may initially be confused clinically with cellulitis. Initially, involved areas appear erythematous and then become 'woody' with a peau d'orange surface change (Fig. 32–5). Over time, involved sites may even become papular or nodular, and rarely blisters have been reported in association with edema of the hands and feet. The progressive thickening of the skin over joints often limits mobility owing to contractures, which leads to significant morbidity. Approximately 5% of patients will have a rapidly fulminant course, and there are reports of patients with involvement of skeletal muscle, fascia, heart, lung, diaphragm, and kidney which can lead to death.

Much effort has been made to elucidate the etiology and pathogenesis of this disease process, but it remains unclear. Although the great majority of patients who develop NSF are on dialysis, it is not felt that any component of dialysis is responsible for the disease. Temporally, it appears that patients who undergo vascular surgical procedures or experience thrombotic events may be at increased risk for developing NSF in the weeks that follow those events. In this context, vascular injury has been proposed to be an inciting risk factor for an inflammatory cascade that may lead to an aberrant wound healing response which manifests as NSF. The extensive fibrosis may be related to the recruitment of bone marrow-derived CD34/procollagen I+ circulating fibrocytes. In response to a trigger, these fibrocytes apparently leave the circulation and enter the tissues, where they differentiate into cells that mimic fibroblasts. Recently, NSF has been found to occur primarily in patients who have undergone magnetic resonance imaging (MRI) using gadolinium contrast. It has been proposed that dissociated free gadolinium in the tissues of a subset of patients

with renal insufficiency may be a target for circulating fibrocytes.

Treatment is largely aimed at improving renal function, and there is no single treatment that has consistently been shown to improve outcomes in patients with NSF. Treatments that have been shown anecdotally to have varying degrees of benefit include topical calcipotriol under occlusion, oral prednisone, extracorporeal photophoresis, plasmapheresis, thalidomide, RePUVA, pentoxifylline, and renal transplantation. Physical therapy is recommended whenever possible. Patients with NSF should not undergo MRI with gadolinium contrast, and coagulopathy should be ruled out prior to transplantation or other surgical procedures. Spontaneous clearance of this disease has not yet been reported, and the overall prognosis for patients with NSF is poor.

Uremic Frost

Severe azotemia in the setting of CRF uncommonly leads to white, crystalline deposits on the skin known as uremic frost. This occurs when urea and other nitrogenous waste products accumulate in the sweat and crystallize onto the skin, and it is considered a grave prognostic sign.

Acquired Perforating Disorder (APD)

Various perforating skin diseases occur with increased frequency in CRF, and these have been lumped together under the term 'acquired perforating disorder of chronic renal failure.' Acquired perforating disorder is associated with renal pruritus and diabetes mellitus. Presumably, in the setting of azotemia, diabetes, or both, some chemical alteration occurs in the dermis which, when combined with skin injury due to scratching, results in extrusion of dermal protein fibers. Clinically, acquired perforating disorder manifests as intensely pruritic papules or nodules (Fig. 32–6). In most cases a hard plug of proteinaceous material, which can be pried loose with forceps, is present in the center of the lesion. Histologically, lesions of acquired perforating disorder most commonly demonstrate the patterns of reactive perforating collagenosis or Kyrle's disease. Perforating folliculitis and elastosis perforans serpiginosa are only rarely seen in CRF.

Bullous Disease (Porphyria and Pseudoporphyria)

The blistering dermatoses porphyria cutanea tarda (PCT) and pseudoporphyria (sometimes referred to together as bullous disease of chronic renal failure) are relatively rare in renal patients. PCT is related to a defect in heme biosynthesis secondary to a deficiency in uroporphyrinogen decarboxylase. In renal patients, azotemia may result in reduced activity of uroporphyrinogen decarboxylase. Additionally, renal failure may lead to relatively slower than normal clearance of porphyrins, with their accumulation in the skin. This in turn may result in PCT-like skin fragility and blistering (Fig. 32–7), despite normal or nearly normal blood porphyrin levels. This paradoxical situation of PCT without elevated porphyrin levels has been dubbed pseudoporphyria. Pseudoporphyria may also

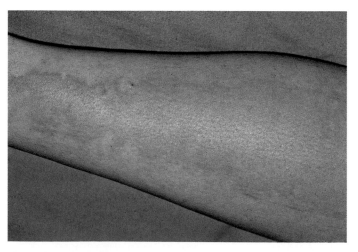

Figure 32–5 Nephrogenic systemic fibrosis: sclerotic dermal and subcutaneous plaque resembling scleromyxedema. (Courtesy of Kenneth E. Greer, MD.)

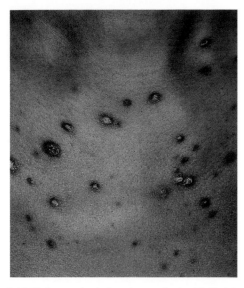

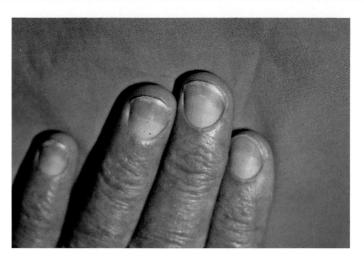

Figure 32–8 'Half-and-half' nails in a patient with chronic renal failure – Lindsay's nails. (Courtesy of Kenneth E. Greer, MD.)

Figure 32–6 Multiple papular lesions in a patient with Kyrle's disease. The patient has diabetes and is undergoing hemodialysis.

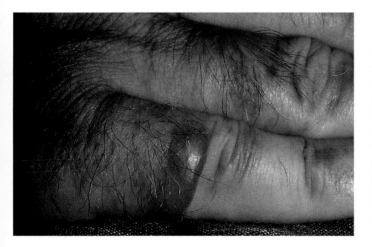

Figure 32–7 Bullous dermatosis of hemodialysis with an appearance similar to porphyria cutanea tarda.

result from decreased clearance of photoactive drugs such as furosemide and tetracycline in CRF patients.

Skin Color Changes

Skin color is often altered in CRF. In patients who are normally lightly pigmented, the skin may have a grayish-brown 'putty'

hue. In those with a darker constitutive skin color, the skin may exhibit brown hypermelanosis or slate-gray dermal pigmentation. These color changes result from the interplay of several chromophores. Pallor, due to anemia, reduces the impact of hemoglobin on skin color, while yellowish urochromes and carotenoids deposit in the dermis and subcutaneous fat. These deeply deposited chromophores may create a grayish hue due to the Tyndall effect. In addition, melanin production is increased as a result of impaired clearance of α-melanocyte-stimulating hormone, and some drugs used in CRF, particularly diltiazem, cause photosensitivity and dermal hyperpigmentation.

Nail Changes

The most common nail changes associated with renal disease are half-and-half nails, also called Lindsay's nails. Each nail is characterized by a pink/brown color distally and a white proximal portion (Fig. 32–8). The white color change is attributed to nailbed edema, and the nail plate itself remains unaffected. Nonspecific nail changes such as Beau's lines and onycholysis also occur commonly in patients with chronic renal disease.

SUGGESTED READINGS

Galan A, Cowper S, Bucala R. Nephrogenic systemic fibrosis (nephrogenic fibrosing dermopathy). Curr Opin Rheumatol 2006; 18: 614–617.
Nigwekar SU, Wolf M, Sterns RH, Hix JK. Calciphylaxis from nonuremic causes: a systematic review. Clin J Am Soc Nephrol 2008; 3: 1139–1143.

Robinson-Bostom L, DiGiovanna JJ. Cutaneous manifestations of end-stage renal disease. J Am Acad Dermatol 2000; 43: 975–986.
Weenig RH, Sewell LD, Davis MD, et al. Calciphylaxis: natural history, risk factor analysis, and outcome. J Am Acad Dermatol 2007; 56, 569–579.

Dennis L. Cooper
and Jean L. Bolognia

Chapter | **33** |

Manifestations in Transplant Recipients

Because of the progress that has occurred over the past 40–50 years in the field of transplantation, an increasing number of patients have undergone solid organ and hematopoietic (bone marrow and peripheral blood) stem cell transplants with long-term graft survival. Complications of these procedures are now well recognized, and the associated cutaneous manifestations are commonly observed in this patient population. As a direct result of the required immunosuppression, there is an increase in the incidence and prevalence of both skin infections and neoplasms. Beyond the skin signs of graft-versus-host disease (GVHD), the immunosuppressive agents themselves can produce a wide range of cutaneous side effects.

The clinical diagnosis of cutaneous disorders in transplant recipients can prove challenging because the clinical presentation, including the morphology of the lesions, is often altered by the ongoing immunosuppression. This immunosuppression can also lead to an exaggeration of clinical findings, as in the case of verrucae vulgares, or more aggressive behavior, as in the case of cutaneous squamous cell carcinoma.

INFECTIONS

The early years of renal transplantation, for example, were marked by frequent life-threatening infections, with over half of patients dying of infections during the first 3 years after transplantation. Although much progress has been made in the past decade with regard to prophylaxis (antibacterial, antifungal, and antiviral), early diagnosis and effective treatment, infections remain a major cause of morbidity and mortality in transplant recipients.

Infections during the first month after transplantation are usually caused by nosocomial pathogens or reactivation of latent disease. Up to 6 months after transplantation, reactivation of latent disease or opportunistic infections predominate. Continuation or initiation of moderate- to high-dose corticosteroids increases the risk of developing the latter. Late infections may be caused by opportunistic or conventional pathogens, with the former seen more commonly in those with heightened immunosuppression because of the need to treat graft rejection or active GVHD.

Viral

Infections with herpesviruses (in particular herpes simplex virus-1 [HSV-1], HSV-2, varicella-zoster virus [VZV], and cytomegalovirus [CMV]) were once a common cause of morbidity and mortality during the first year following transplantation. For example, in one series, 97% of patients had one or more herpesvirus infections. However, with the routine use of prophylactic acyclovir and the pre-emptive use of valganciclovir or ganciclovir (e.g., based on weekly blood CMV antigen or PCR assays in allogeneic hematopoietic stem cell transplant patients), this situation has improved dramatically. Chronic human papillomavirus infections, however, still remain a significant problem in patients who have received solid organ transplants, because of their need for lifelong immunosuppression. In contrast, an attempt is made to taper and then discontinue immunosuppressive therapy in allogeneic hematopoietic stem cell transplant patients over 12–18 months – that is, unless there is active GVHD.

Herpes Simplex Virus (HSV-1, HSV-2)

Herpes simplex virus (HSV) was a common cause of infection in transplant recipients until the use of prophylactic acyclovir became commonplace. Although active infections with this virus can occur at any time, they were observed most frequently during the first month after transplantation. In the absence of antiviral therapy, viral shedding rates were found to be as high as 70% in renal transplant patients, 20% in heart–lung recipients, and 60% in bone marrow recipients. The vast majority of HSV infections represent reactivation of a latent infection; occasionally, transplant patients can develop primary disease, and rarely, HSV transmission via transplanted organs has been reported. Reactivation of HSV appears to be a consequence of impaired cellular immunity, as it occurs despite high titers of antibodies directed against the virus.

In mucocutaneous sites, the initial primary lesions of HSV are similar to those seen in immunocompetent hosts, i.e., grouped vesicles, crusts or erosions on an erythematous base. However, in addition to sites such as the nasal mucosa, vermilion border of the lip, oral mucosa that overlies bone, fingers, buttocks, and genitalia, HSV infections in immunocompromised hosts often involve the 'soft' oral mucosa, the perianal region, and the esophagus. In addition, rather than being self-limited infections that last for 7–10 days even in the absence of antiviral therapy (as in immunocompetent hosts), these herpetic ulcers tend to be chronic and expansive (Fig. 33–1).

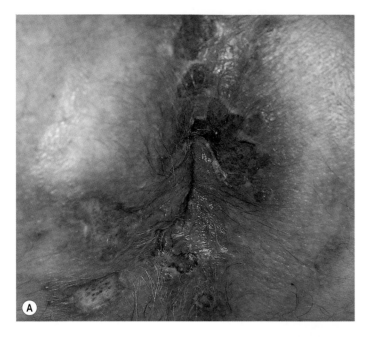

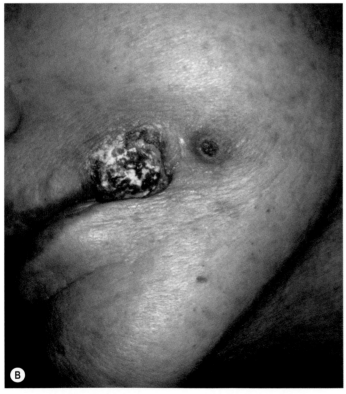

Figure 33–1 Chronic and expansive herpes simplex virus infections of the perianal and perioral regions in a bone marrow transplant patient (A) and a renal transplant patient (B), respectively. The lesions can appear as ulcerations (A) or thick hemorrhagic crusts (B). (B, Courtesy of Yale Residents' Slide Collection.)

In transplant patients, systemic HSV infections are rather uncommon and are often not accompanied by cutaneous lesions. As a result, the clinical diagnosis requires a high index of suspicion. Reported sites of systemic involvement include the central nervous system (CNS), lungs and liver, as well as the gastrointestinal tract. Occasionally, in the setting of immunosuppression, cutaneous lesions of HSV are 'disseminated' on the trunk or extremities.

Because of its accuracy and rapid turnaround time of a few hours, the most helpful diagnostic procedure for HSV infections is the direct immunofluorescent antibody (DFA) assay. In the case of mucocutaneous lesions, it is important to provide the laboratory with an ample supply of keratinocytes. A viral culture should also be done on any tissue sample, including skin, submitted for the DFA assay. Dermatologists still do an office-based test known as a Tzanck preparation (Fig. 33–2) to look for virally infected multinucleated giant cells (seen in HSV-1, HSV-2, VZV, and occasionally CMV infections), but this test is less sensitive than the DFA assay and requires more expertise to interpret. Rapid detection of HSV is also possible via PCR-based assays, which are very sensitive but less widely available.

Depending on the severity, treatment options for active HSV infection in an immunocompromised host include oral agents with enhanced bioavailability (e.g., famciclovir, valacyclovir), or intravenous acyclovir. The antivirals should be continued until there is complete clinical clearing (rather than for a preset number of days), and treatment is usually successful if the diagnosis is made promptly. As in patients with HIV infection who have received multiple or prolonged courses of acyclovir, acyclovir-resistant strains of HSV have been reported, and in these patients intravenous foscarnet (and less often intravenous cidofovir) is employed; topical cidofovir (1% gel) may be tried in milder cases.

Varicella-Zoster Virus

Herpes zoster is a common infection in transplant recipients, occurring in up to 15% of cases. As in immunocompetent hosts, it is a result of the reactivation of the varicella-zoster

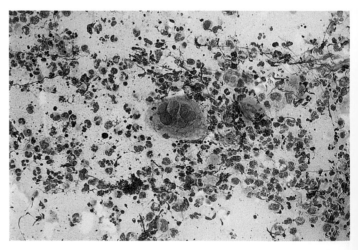

Figure 33–2 Tzanck smear demonstrating a multinucleated giant cell centrally.

virus (VZV) that resides in dorsal root or cranial nerve ganglia. Clinical disease is usually characterized by a unilateral distribution of grouped vesicles or crusts on an erythematous base, with lesions usually being confined to one or a few adjacent dermatomes. However, both chronic VZV and cutaneous dissemination of VZV can occur in this patient population (Fig. 33–3A,B); in the latter situation, at least 20 lesions reminiscent of varicella are widely scattered on the trunk and extremities (Fig. 33–3C). Less often there is associated meningoencephalitis, pneumonitis, or hepatitis. Prolonged infection is associated with reduced specific cellular immune responsiveness.

As is the case with HSV infections, the diagnosis of herpes zoster is established via the DFA assay, Tzanck smears, and/or PCR; viral cultures of VZV require a longer incubation period than those of HSV. In patients with severe disease, cutaneous dissemination, or suspected systemic involvement, the treatment of choice is intravenous acyclovir. If the disease is mild and there is no evidence of cutaneous dissemination, then oral agents with greater bioavailability (e.g., famciclovir, valacyclovir) can be prescribed.

Cytomegalovirus

Cytomegalovirus (CMV) is one of the more common opportunistic infections in transplant recipients and is potentially a major source of morbidity and mortality. Until the develop-

ment of more effective anti-CMV medications, this virus accounted for up to 25% of deaths, 20% of graft failures, 30% of febrile episodes, and 35% of leukopenic episodes in renal transplant patients. One of the major advances, especially in allogeneic hematopoietic stem cell transplant patients, has been the use of weekly antibody staining of circulating neutrophils or weekly PCR-based assays of peripheral blood as means of detecting CMV antigen or CMV DNA, respectively, and hence early infections. The latter assays are particularly helpful in neutropenic patients. In the setting of positive results, 'pre-emptive' oral valganciclovir or intravenous ganciclovir therapy can be instituted prior to the development of clinical symptoms such as fever, pneumonitis or enterocolitis.

Infections in transplant recipients may be primary, i.e., due to the presence of CMV in the transplanted organ or cells, or they may represent reactivation of a latent infection. In the past, clinical infections were most common during the first 6 months after transplantation; e.g., in one series of kidney transplant patients the median time of onset was 46 days after transplantation. However, with more solid organ transplant patients receiving prophylactic therapy during the first 3 months after transplantation, the time of onset is often delayed until after discontinuation of antiviral therapy.

Clinical manifestations of CMV infection include leukopenia, pneumonitis, gastroenteritis, retinitis, hepatitis, and

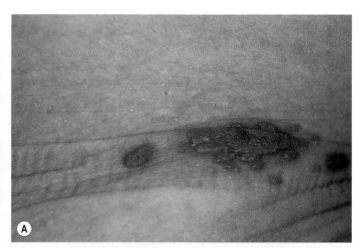

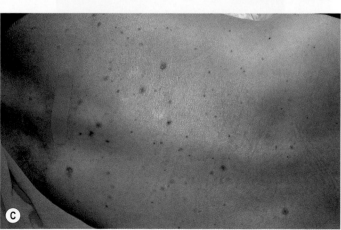

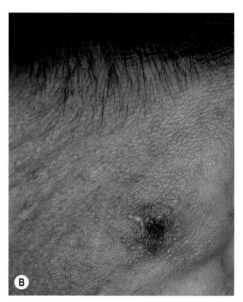

Figure 33–3 Dermatomal (T10) distribution of herpes zoster (A) in association with cutaneous dissemination (B; neck) in a liver transplant patient. Multiple crusted papules that resemble varicella in an immunocompromised patient with disseminated zoster (C). (C, Courtesy of Yale Residents' Slide Collection.)

encephalitis, as well as a mononucleosis-type syndrome. Skin involvement is present in a small percentage of patients with systemic CMV infection; cutaneous presentations include morbilliform eruptions, verrucous plaques, petechiae and purpura, and ulcerations. In mucocutaneous ulcers CMV often coexists with other viruses such as HSV or VZV, and as a result its true pathogenicity has been questioned.

The diagnosis of CMV infection is suggested histopathologically by the presence of intranuclear inclusions surrounded by a halo within endothelial cells. Viral culture or a PCR-based assay of involved tissues, including the skin, is required for confirmation. It is important not to confuse active infection with viral shedding, as is commonly seen in the urine or throat washings of transplant patients.

Human Herpesvirus 6

In addition to causing exanthema subitum (roseola infantum) in healthy young children, human herpesvirus 6 (HHV-6) has been associated with fever, pancytopenia, pneumonitis, gastroenteritis, and encephalitis in transplant patients. There are also a few scattered reports of an associated morbilliform eruption at the time of reactivation. Viral DNA can be detected in the skin as well as peripheral blood mononuclear cells.

Epstein–Barr Virus and Human Herpesvirus 8

Infections with two other herpesviruses, Epstein–Barr virus (EBV) and human herpesvirus 8 (HHV-8), are associated with the development of neoplasms in transplant patients: post-transplant lymphoproliferative disorder and Kaposi's sarcoma (KS), respectively. The term post-transplant lymphoproliferative disorder is used rather than lymphoma because the histologic findings range from a polyclonal B-cell infiltrate to a monoclonal B-cell lymphoma. Rarely, T-cell lymphomas are seen.

Because this lymphoproliferative disorder is reflective of 'over'-immunosuppression, a reduction in immunosuppressive therapy is a component of the initial therapy. Clearly, the extent to which the immunosuppressive agents can be reduced depends on the type of transplant. Renal transplant patients have the option of being placed back on dialysis, but patients with heart or liver transplants cannot afford graft rejection. For localized disease, surgical excision or radiation therapy combined with a reduction in immunosuppression may prove sufficient. However, extensive or rapidly progressive disease requires systemic therapy with rituximab, often in combination with multidrug chemotherapy. Discontinuation of standard immunosuppression in conjunction with administration of chemotherapy usually does not lead to graft rejection, given the immunosuppressive effects of the chemotherapy.

The association between HHV-8 and KS is seen in both immunocompetent and immunosuppressed patients (see Chapters 18 and 29). In solid organ transplant recipients, the prevalence of KS is 50 times that of the general population in endemic areas, and increases to 400–500 times in nonendemic areas. Regression of the mucocutaneous lesions of KS has been observed in transplant patients following a reduction in the level of immunosuppression or a switch from a systemic calcineurin inhibitor to sirolimus (rapamycin).

Human Papillomavirus

Verrucae vulgares (viral warts) are very common in patients who have received solid organ transplants and reflect their requirement for lifelong immunosuppression. The prevalence of warts increases with the duration of graft survival, such that the majority of renal transplant recipients with graft durations of more than 5 years have verrucae. There are over 90 different types of human papillomavirus (HPV), and specific types or groupings are associated with particular clinical forms of the disease. For example, HPV types 1, 2, and 4 are associated with banal warts, often on the hands and feet (Fig. 33–4); HPV types 3 and 10 are associated with flat warts (verruca plana); and HPV types 6 and 11 (nononcogenic) as well as 16 and 18 (oncogenic) are associated with condylomata acuminata (venereal warts) (Fig. 33–5).

Not only can transplant patients have all of the HPV types just mentioned, but they have been found to harbor unusual types that were once thought to be uniquely associated with a rare disease known as epidermodysplasia verruciformis (e.g.,

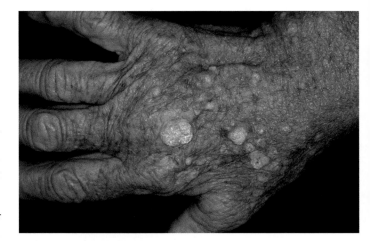

Figure 33–4 Multiple verrucae vulgares in a patient who had received a renal transplant 25 years previously.

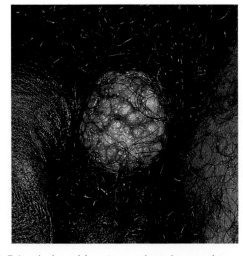

Figure 33–5 Inguinal condylomata acuminata in a renal transplant patient. (Courtesy of Yale Residents' Slide Collection.)

HPV 5, 8, 19–25). In addition, the warts are frequently extensive and even more difficult to treat than in the general population. The oncogenic potential of some of these HPV types combined with the chronic immunosuppression creates a difficult situation in a number of patients. The potential for developing squamous cell carcinomas of the cervix, vulva and anus in addition to the skin (see below) represents a real threat to these patients, and an ongoing screening program that includes close inspection and biopsy of any suspicious lesion is required. Treatment of HPV infections is discussed in Chapter 29.

Molluscum Contagiosum

Mollusca contagiosa (MC) are 2–10-mm dome-shaped skin-colored to pink papules that have a central umbilication. They are caused by a poxvirus. Infections with MC are more common in patients with atopic dermatitis and in immunocompromised hosts (see Chapter 29). In the latter group, lesions can prove difficult to treat. Cutaneous lesions of cryptococcosis and systemic dimorphic fungal infections can resemble MC, and therefore dermal scrapings or a skin biopsy specimen should be examined if the diagnosis is uncertain.

Bacterial

Pyogenic Bacteria

Staphylococcus aureus and *Streptococcus pyogenes* cause the majority of cutaneous bacterial infections in transplant patients. Folliculitis, abscesses, furuncles, wound infections, cellulitis and septicemia all occur with increased frequency. Their clinical presentations may be atypical owing to the concomitant immunosuppression (Fig. 33–6); in the case of cellulitis, there may be less erythema than is observed in normal hosts. Methicillin-resistant *S. aureus* is a problem in transplant patients as it is in immunocompetent hosts. Incision and drainage of abscesses is a key component of treatment, and for severe infections empiric intravenous vancomycin is recommended until antimicrobial susceptibility results become available.

A condition dubbed 'transplant elbow,' consisting of recurrent staphylococcal infections in the skin overlying the extensor elbows, has been described in transplant recipients. The cause is related to skin atrophy secondary to the use of systemic corticosteroids, and is linked to repeated trauma produced when the patients use their elbows to rise from sitting because of the corticosteroid-induced myopathy affecting the hip girdle.

In transplant patients the cause of cutaneous infections cannot be assumed to be Gram-positive cocci: additional organisms need to be considered, such as Gram-negative rods (Fig. 33–7), Gram-positive rods (e.g., *Bacillus cereus*), atypical mycobacteria, herpesviruses, and opportunistic fungi and parasites. In immunocompromised hosts there are multiple infectious etiologies for lesions that resemble ecthyma gangrenosum (see below), i.e., the list extends beyond *Pseudomonas aeruginosa*. Pseudomonal infection is, of course, still high in the differential diagnosis when the lesions involve the groin (Fig. 33–8).

Nocardia

Both cutaneous and systemic nocardiosis have been reported in transplant patients. The cutaneous form can present as a localized soft tissue infection at a site of trauma or in a lymphocutaneous pattern (see below). Hematogenous dissemination from a pulmonary focus can lead to secondary sites of infection in the skin, as well as other organs such as the brain. These cutaneous lesions range from erythematous papules and abscesses to subcutaneous nodules.

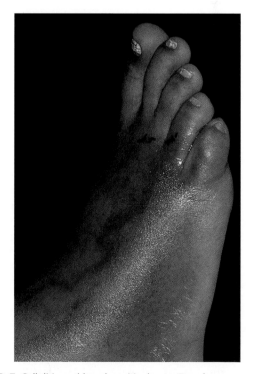

Figure 33–7 Cellulitis and lymphangitis due to *Pseudomonas aeruginosa* in an allogeneic bone marrow transplant patient; the primary focus was an interdigital toe web infection.

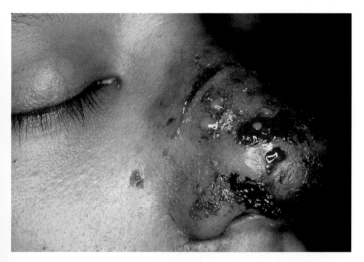

Figure 33–6 Soft tissue infection of the nose due to *Staphylococcus aureus* in a patient with leukemia and neutropenia prior to allogeneic hematopoietic stem cell transplant. (Courtesy of Yale Residents' Slide Collection.)

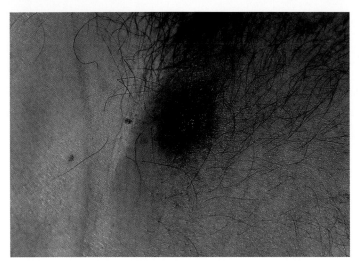

Figure 33–8 Necrotic ulcer of ecthyma gangrenosum in the inguinal region due to *Pseudomonas aeruginosa*. (Courtesy of Yale Residents' Slide Collection.)

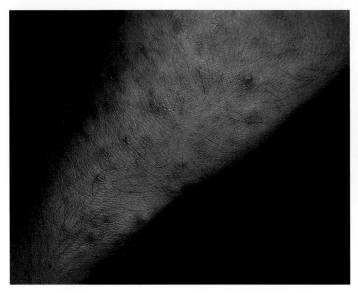

Figure 33–9 Papules and pustules of Majocchi's granuloma on the distal upper extremity due to follicular involvement with *Trichophyton rubrum* in a renal transplant patient. (Courtesy of Yale Residents' Slide Collection.)

A presumptive diagnosis can be made by identifying fine-branching filaments in a Gram stain of dermal scrapings or a biopsy specimen; a modified acid-fast stain can also be used to identify the organisms. Both *Nocardia asteroides* and *N. brasiliensis* are slow-growing bacteria and culture plates need to be held for longer periods than in the case of other more common bacteria. For isolated lesions, surgical excision is an option, but treatment with antibiotics, in particular trimethoprim–sulfamethoxazole, is usually successful.

Mycobacteria

In endemic areas the incidence of tuberculosis is significantly greater in renal transplant patients than in the general population. Infection may represent reactivation of latent disease, community-acquired disease, or very rarely transmission by the donor kidney. Cutaneous lesions due to *Mycobacterium tuberculosis* range from scrofuloderma and lupus vulgaris as manifestations of reactivation to periorificial ulcers and widespread papulovesicles in patients with overwhelming disease.

Atypical mycobacterial infections of the skin can either be primary, e.g., due to inoculation of organisms at a site of trauma, or secondary as a reflection of systemic disease. The former are seen in both immunocompetent and immunocompromised hosts, and a classic example of an associated organism would be *M. marinum*. A lymphocutaneous pattern, also referred to as sporotrichoid, is commonly observed with the initial papule or nodule at the site of inoculation and the subsequent development of nodules along the path of lymphatic drainage. In immunocompromised hosts, the clinical appearance of atypical mycobacterial infections can be muted due to the suppression of inflammation, or exaggerated due to the suppression of host defenses, i.e., they can vary from subtle erythema to large, nonhealing ulcers.

The diagnosis of cutaneous mycobacterial infections depends on the identification of acid-fast bacilli in biopsy specimens and isolation of the responsible organisms by specialized culture techniques. If available, PCR can also be performed for more rapid results. In the case of tuberculosis, the QuantiFERON-TB Gold test, in which the amount of interferon (IFN)-γ is measured following incubation of the patient's blood with two synthetic peptides from *M. tuberculosis* (but absent in BCG vaccine strains), is increasingly being utilized. However, indeterminate results (i.e., failure of the internal positive control) are more common in immunocompromised individuals. Lastly, a search should be undertaken for additional sites of involvement, e.g., pulmonary. Specific multidrug treatment regimens are dictated by the species isolated and the antibiotic sensitivities (www.cdc.gov/mmwr/preview/mmwrhtml/rr5211a1.htm).

Fungal

Superficial Fungi

Superficial fungal infections are due primarily to yeasts, in particular *Candida* spp., and dermatophytes, especially *Trichophyton rubrum* and *T. mentagrophytes*. Cutaneous candidiasis is exacerbated by oral corticosteroids and broad-spectrum antibiotics as well as hyperglycemia, a confounding problem in many renal transplant patients. The clinical presentations include oral thrush, perlèche, onycholysis, chronic paronychia, onychomycosis of the fingernails, intertrigo, balanitis, and vulvovaginitis. Another yeast that can cause clinical disease in transplant patients is *Malassezia furfur* (previously known as *Pityrosporum*). The primary manifestations are pityriasis (tinea) versicolor and 'Pityrosporum' folliculitis. Diagnoses of these yeast infections can be accomplished by examination of a potassium hydroxide (KOH) preparation and, in the case of candidiasis, fungal culture.

In addition to the very common dermatophyte infections such as tinea pedis (feet), tinea manuum (hands), and tinea unguium (nails), transplant patients can develop extensive lesions of tinea corporis. The immunosuppression also increases the risk of developing Majocchi's granuloma (a tinea infection of the hair follicles which is characterized by follicular papules and papulopustules; Fig. 33–9) as well as a particular type of nail infection known as proximal subungual onychomycosis (see Chapter 29). Deep or invasive dermatophytosis, where the fungi are actually found in the dermis, is quite rare but is usually seen in immunocompromised hosts. Diagnosis rests on the KOH examination and fungal culture. Cutaneous infections due to *Candida* and *Malassezia* spp. are best treated with topical imidazoles or oral fluconazole, whereas cutaneous dermatophyte infections are best treated with topical or oral allylamines (e.g., terbinafine).

Deep Fungal Infections

In patients who require more profound immunosuppression, systemic infections due to opportunistic pathogens such as *Cryptococcus*, *Candida*, *Aspergillus*, and saprophytes can occur. Systemic infections due to dimorphic fungi can also become widely disseminated in transplant patients.

Candida

Disseminated candidiasis was classically the most common systemic mycosis, but a significant reduction in incidence and mortality has occurred with the use of prophylactic fluconazole. The replacement of bone marrow transplants (average time to engraftment, 21 days) with peripheral blood stem cell transplants (average time to engraftment, 14 days) has also reduced the incidence of disseminated candidiasis in the immediate post-transplant period.

Neutropenia, systemic corticosteroids, hyperglycemia, placement of central intravenous catheters, and the use of broad-spectrum antibiotics are predisposing factors. Fever, myalgias, and cutaneous lesions are the classic triad, but cutaneous lesions are present in only 10–15% of patients. Most commonly, multiple firm pink papules with central pallor are observed (Fig. 33–10A); additional skin findings include purpuric macules and papules (Fig. 33–10B), pustules and subcutaneous nodules. The pustules may initially be misdiagnosed as simple folliculitis. Whereas myalgias are classically associated with systemic candidiasis, muscle pain and tenderness due to septic emboli can be seen with other opportunistic infections (see below).

Although disseminated candidiasis is associated with positive blood cultures more often than are other systemic fungal infections, blood cultures may be negative. However, a biopsy specimen from a purpuric lesion is usually diagnostic, with yeast forms and pseudohyphae present in the dermis (Fig. 33–10C) and vascular spaces. A tissue fungal culture should be performed using sterile technique, i.e., the culture should be representative of organisms growing in the dermis, not the surface stratum corneum. *Candida* spp. that have been isolated from patients with disseminated candidiasis include *C. albicans*, *C. tropicalis*, *C. krusei*, *C. parapsilosis*, and *C. glabrata*.

Treatment of disseminated candidiasis depends on the severity of the illness as well as the specific isolate and its sensitivities. The use of prophylactic fluconazole has led to a greater incidence of non-*C. albicans* species which may be resistant to fluconazole: e.g., *C. krusei* is well known to be resistant

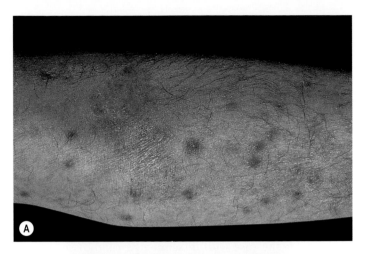

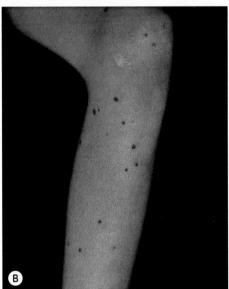

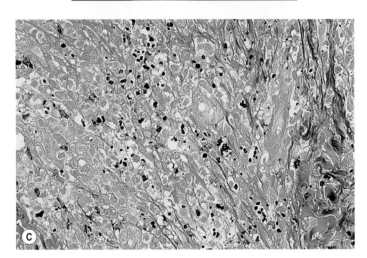

Figure 33–10 Disseminated candidiasis in two patients with leukemia and neutropenia due to the preparative regimen prior to transplant (A, B). A silver stain of the skin biopsy specimen demonstrates the numerous yeast forms and pseudohyphae in the dermis (C). (Courtesy of Yale Residents' Slide Collection.)

to fluconazole. Therapeutic options include intravenous and oral azoles/triazoles (e.g., fluconazole [unless disease developed while on this drug], voriconazole) or echinocandins (e.g., caspofungin, micafungin, anidulafungin), which inhibit glycan synthase. Intravenous amphotericin (including the liposomal forms) is also effective, but its use has declined owing to its toxicity, as well as the availability of other equally effective drugs with fewer side effects.

Aspergillus

Immunocompromised hosts are also at risk for the development of infections with the opportunistic fungus *Aspergillus*, in particular *A. flavus* and *A. fumigatus*. The major risk factors remain systemic corticosteroid therapy and prolonged neutropenia. As is the case with disseminated candidiasis, shorter engraftment times after peripheral blood stem cell transplants (compared to bone marrow transplants) have reduced the number of early *Aspergillus* infections. Later infections in hematopoietic stem cell transplant patients are usually associated with the use of corticosteroid therapy for GVHD. Voriconazole is increasingly being used as prophylaxis in high-risk patients.

Primary cutaneous infections develop at sites of trauma, including those from intravenous catheter use. Both occlusive adhesive tape and arm boards have been associated with primary *Aspergillus* infections, but fortunately their use has decreased as the use of indwelling central venous catheters has increased. Secondary cutaneous lesions of *Aspergillus* represent septic emboli due to systemic infection. The primary source is often pulmonary, and the cutaneous lesions vary from erythematous papules to ecthyma gangrenosum-like lesions (Fig. 33–11A). Biopsy specimens demonstrate septate, acute-branching fungi in the dermis and invading the walls of blood vessels (Fig. 33–11B).

If the primary lesions of aspergillosis are fairly well circumscribed, treatment consists of surgical excision and oral voriconazole. Currently, systemic disease is treated with voriconazole, which has been shown to be more effective than amphotericin for documented *Aspergillus* infections. Echinocandins represent second-line therapy. An attempt is also made to reduce the dose of oral corticosteroids, but despite all these measures the mortality rate for systemic aspergillosis remains quite high.

Cryptococcus

Immunocompromised hosts, from those with AIDS to those who have undergone renal transplantation, are prone to infections with the yeast *Cryptococcus neoformans*. Both primary and secondary skin lesions are seen in transplant patients, and the latter represent systemic dissemination, usually from a primary focus in the lungs. In addition, a very common site of involvement is the central nervous system (CNS). Cutaneous manifestations vary from nondescript papules and ulcers to cellulitis and lesions that resemble molluscum contagiosum (see Chapter 29). Biopsy specimens of involved skin demonstrate multiple yeast forms within the dermis, and in the majority of patients the characteristic capsules are also seen. Depending

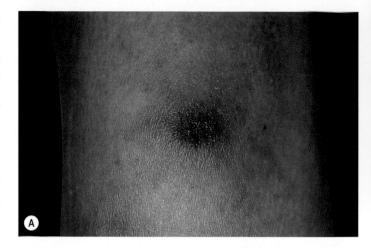

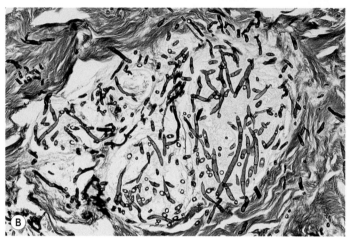

Figure 33–11 Septic embolus due to *Aspergillus* in a neutropenic patient with leukemia (A). As demonstrated in this silver stain of a biopsy specimen, there is invasion of dermal blood vessels by the fungus; this leads to ischemic necrosis of the skin (B). (A, Courtesy of Yale Residents' Slide Collection.)

on the severity of the infection and the sites of involvement, treatment consists of fluconazole, and if necessary, amphotericin B; in the setting of CNS infection, flucytosine is added to amphotericin B.

Dimorphic Fungi

In the United States, the three major dimorphic fungi are *Histoplasma capsulatum*, *Coccidioides immitis*, and *Blastomyces dermatitidis*. Each is associated with a particular region of the country: the Ohio Valley (histoplasmosis), the southwest and California (coccidiomycosis), and the southeast and midwest river valleys (blastomycosis). The primary route of infection is inhalation, and individuals in endemic regions often have asymptomatic infections or flu-like syndromes. With immunosuppression, reactivation and dissemination can occur.

All three dimorphic fungi can produce a wide range of mucocutaneous lesions, including papulonodules, pustules, expanding plaques with peripheral pustules, abscesses, and ulcerations; in the case of histoplasmosis, oral ulcers are characteristic. Biopsy specimens demonstrate both granulomatous and neutrophilic infiltrates, and yeast forms of *H. capsulatum* and *B. dermatitidis* can be found within macrophages and giant cells. In the case of coccidiomycosis, large spherules full of endospores are seen rather than yeast forms.

Additional sites of involvement vary depending on the specific fungus, with *H. capsulatum* favoring the reticuloendothelial system (liver, spleen and bone marrow), *C. immitis* favoring the bones, joints and CNS, and *B. dermatitidis* favoring the skin and bones. For all three fungal infections, treatment options include itraconazole and amphotericin B, and in the case of coccidiomycosis, fluconazole is an additional option.

Other Opportunistic Mycoses and Parasites

Immunocompromised hosts develop infections secondary to saprophytic fungi which in normal hosts are often disregarded as contaminants. The genera include *Alternaria*, *Dreschlera*, *Fusarium*, *Mucor*, *Rhizopus*, and *Absidia*. The cutaneous lesions often represent septic emboli, and their clinical appearances are similar to emboli due to Gram-negative rods or other fungi such as *Aspergillus* (Fig. 33–11). In addition, cutaneous extension of underlying fungal sinus infections can present initially as unilateral facial edema. Recognition of this subtle presentation allows earlier diagnosis and treatment. Soft tissue extension and systemic spread can also occur in immunocompromised hosts with saprophytic onychomycosis (Fig. 33–12). Unfortunately, even with proper therapy consisting of surgical debridement (if possible) and institution of systemic medications such as voriconazole (*Fusarium*) or amphotericin B, treatment failure is common (Fig. 33–13).

In addition to saprophytic fungi, immunocompromised patients can also develop folliculitis due to *Demodex* mites (demodicidosis; see Chapter 29) as well as systemic infections with parasites such as *Strongyloides stercoralis* and *Acanthamoeba* spp. In disseminated strongyloidiasis purpuric macules and patches are seen, especially on the abdomen, in addition to pulmonary and gastrointestinal involvement; the mortality rate is quite high. Infections with *Acanthamoeba* spp. often originate in the paranasal sinuses or lungs, and systemic dissemination can involve the CNS as well as the skin (Fig. 33–14).

NEOPLASMS

Patients who have received transplants are at increased risk for the development of several different neoplasms, including Kaposi's sarcoma (see Chapter 18) and nonmelanoma skin cancers. This is particularly true of solid organ transplant patients, because they require lifelong immunosuppression, and the incidence of cutaneous tumors increases with the duration of immunosuppression.

Squamous Cell and Basal Cell Carcinoma

The two major forms of nonmelanoma skin cancer (NMSC) are basal cell carcinoma (BCC) and squamous cell carcinoma

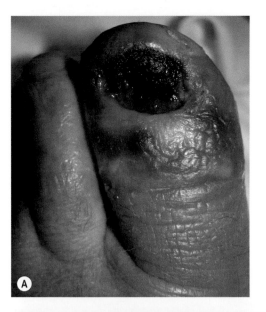
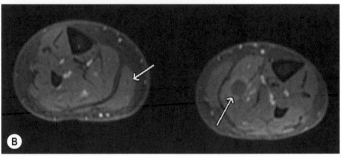

Figure 33-12 Soft tissue infection with necrosis in a patient who had received an allogeneic hematopoietic stem cell transplant and in whom the primary focus was saprophytic onychomycosis due to *Fusarium* (A). MRI scan of the lower extremities demonstrating multiple septic emboli of *Fusarium* within muscles (white arrows; B). (A, Courtesy of Yale Residents' Slide Collection.)

(SCC). In the general population, the usual ratio of BCC to SCC is approximately 4:1, but this ratio is nearly reversed in solid organ transplant patients. Compared to the general population, there is a 65-fold and a 10-fold increase in the incidence of cutaneous SCCs and BCCs, respectively, in solid organ transplant recipients. In two studies from the United States and Australia, the incidence of NMSCs was 35% 10 years post transplant (heart transplant recipients) and 44% 9 years post transplant (renal transplant recipients), respectively. A striking statistic derived from an investigation of Australian heart transplant recipients was that metastatic NMSC accounted for 27% of the deaths that occurred more than 4 years post transplant.

The clinical appearance of these tumors is the same as in normal hosts. The BCCs are pearly to pink-colored papules that often have telangiectasias within them; some of the lesions develop a central hemorrhagic crust (scab), and others have pinpoint areas of pigmentation. The SCCs are usually pink to red papules, nodules, or plaques that have associated scale, such that they may resemble a common wart, psoriasis, or

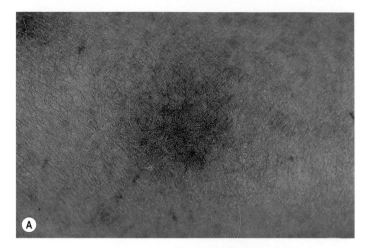

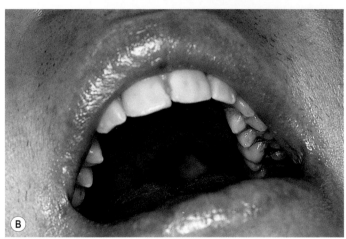

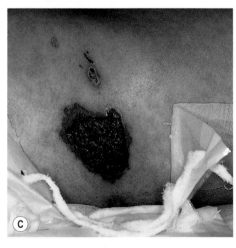

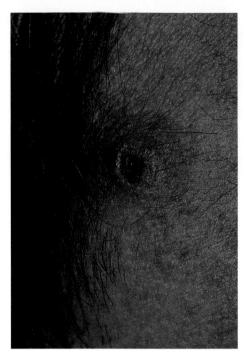

Figure 33–14 Septic embolus due to *Acanthamoeba* in a patient who received a haploidentical stem cell transplant and subsequently died of this amebic infection. (Courtesy of Yale Residents' Slide Collection.)

Figure 33–13 Septic emboli due to *Fusarium* (A) and *Dreschlera* (B, C) in two allogeneic bone marrow transplant patients. Note the similarity of the clinical appearance of these lesions to those seen in Figs 33–8 and 33–11. (A, Courtesy of Yale Residents' Slide Collection.)

eczema. This is especially true of the in situ form of SCC known as Bowen's disease.

In general, these tumors develop in sun-exposed sites as in normal hosts, and are seen most commonly in fair-skinned individuals who have received a significant amount of cumulative sun exposure. Clues to the latter include wrinkles, yellow

discoloration of the posterior neck and lateral forehead (solar elastosis), mottled pigmentation, and actinic (solar) keratoses. Actinic keratoses (AKs) are often referred to as precancers because they can develop into SCCs (but not BCCs); they have a characteristic hard scale and are best appreciated by palpation.

Sun exposure is not the only factor involved in pathogenesis. Infection with HPV also plays a role, especially in SCCs that develop in association with condylomata acuminata due to oncogenic types of HPV. However, the degree to which HPV plays a role in the development of cutaneous SCCs is still controversial. This is because data are conflicting as to the percentage of specimens of cutaneous SCCs from renal transplant patients that contain HPV DNA. Although the frequency and spectrum of HPV types detected in cutaneous SCCs depend on the type of PCR assay used, these differences are not sufficient to explain the discrepancies described in the literature to date.

The frequency of total body skin examinations is determined according to the degree and duration of immunosuppression, skin pigmentation, amount of cumulative sun exposure, presence or absence of condylomata acuminata, and number of previous actinic keratoses and nonmelanoma skin cancers. At one end of the spectrum are those individuals who develop multiple tumors every few months, and in this group reduction of immunosuppression as well as prophylactic therapies such as oral retinoids need to be considered. Acitretin has been shown to reduce the number of new SCCs that develop in transplant patients, but only as long as the patient is on the medication. The side effects of the oral retinoids, e.g., birth defects, hypertriglyceridemia, must of course be weighed against the benefits.

Prompt diagnosis and treatment of cutaneous SCCs is indicated in transplant patients, given the aggressive nature that some of these tumors may display. Therapeutic options include electrodessication and curettage for in situ lesions, routine surgical excision, microscopically controlled excision (Mohs' technique) for large, rapidly growing, ill-defined or recurrent lesions, and, occasionally, adjuvant radiation therapy (e.g., if there is neurotropism). Topical 5-fluorouracil or imiquimod and photodynamic therapy have been used in individuals with numerous AKs and significant actinic damage. In solid organ transplant recipients who continue to develop multiple NMSCs, immunosuppression with sirolimus (rapamycin), rather than cyclosporine or tacrolimus, can be considered.

Miscellaneous

Follicular dystrophy of immunosuppression (trichodysplasia spinulosa) is an entity that has been described over the past decade in patients (including transplant recipients) who are immunocompromised. Various theories have been proposed with regard to etiology, from being virally induced ('viral-associated trichodysplasia of immunosuppression') to a side effect of cyclosporine ('cyclosporine-induced follicular dystrophy'). Patients develop follicular papules, especially on the central face, as well as loss of the eyebrows and eyelashes.

GRAFT-VERSUS-HOST DISEASE

Graft-versus-host disease (GVHD) is the most common cause of morbidity and mortality in allogeneic hematopoietic stem cell transplant recipients. It is caused by an immunologic reaction of immunocompetent donor T lymphocytes in a recipient who is incapable of rejecting the graft. T-cell depletion of the allograft reduces the risk of GVHD but is associated with a higher incidence of tumor recurrence and graft failure. The reason for the higher risk of recurrence is the lack of a graft-versus-tumor effect. As a result, most transplants are still carried out with unmodified (i.e., T-cell replete) grafts and are associated with a significant risk of acute and chronic GVHD.

Treatment of recurrent lymphomas and leukemias after allogeneic transplant includes a rapid reduction in immunosuppression and infusions of donor T lymphocytes. The major risk of these strategies is GVHD, and as a result the clinician is constantly trying to balance tumor control on the one hand with GVHD on the other.

Acute GVHD

GVHD is classically divided into acute (<100 days post transplant) and chronic (>100 days post transplant), but this division has become less distinct with currently employed protocols. Significant acute GVHD occurs in 25–40% of allogeneic hematopoietic stem cell transplant patients. Risk factors include an unrelated (but matched) donor, a related donor but with a mismatch at one or more HLA antigens, an unmodified graft, an older age of the donor or the recipient, and a female donor with a male recipient.

In acute GVHD the major sites of involvement are the skin, liver (hepatitis), and GI tract (diarrhea). The cutaneous eruption is reminiscent of the common maculopapular (morbilliform) drug eruption. The initial lesions often appear on the hands and feet (Fig. 33–15). There is a grading system for acute cutaneous GVHD which takes into account the percentage of body surface area (BSA) involved when the eruption is maculopapular (stage I, <25%; stage II, 25–50%; stage III, >50%). Erythroderma with bulla formation (Fig. 33–16) and/or desquamation represents stage IV. Additional sites of involvement include mucosal surfaces such as the conjunctivae (Fig. 33–17).

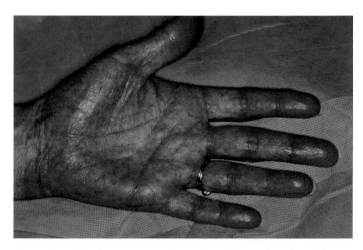

Figure 33–15 Erythematous macules and papules on the palm of a patient 30 days post allogeneic bone marrow transplant.

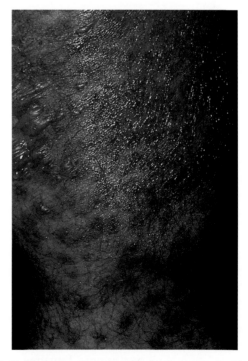

Figure 33–16 Edematous plaques and bullae in a patient with acute GVHD following an allogeneic bone marrow transplant. (Courtesy of Yale Residents' Slide Collection.)

321

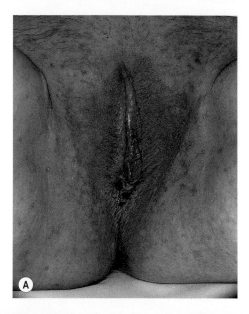

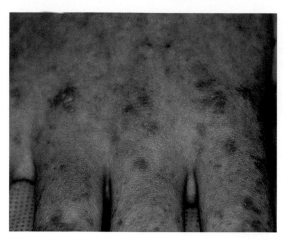

Figure 33–18 Flat-topped pink scaly papules of chronic GVHD on the dorsal aspect of the hand. (Courtesy of Yale Residents' Slide Collection.)

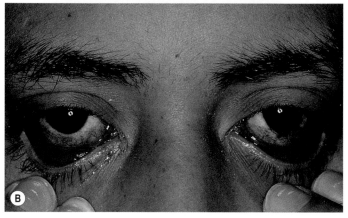

Figure 33–17 Acute GVHD involving the mucous membranes of the genitalia (A) and the conjunctivae (B) in two patients following allogeneic bone marrow transplants. (B, Courtesy of Yale Residents' Slide Collection.)

Histologic features of acute cutaneous GVHD include necrotic keratinocytes and lymphocytes within the epidermis as well as in the upper papillary dermis. When the lymphocytes are adjacent to necrotic keratinocytes, this is termed satellite cell necrosis. Unfortunately, the histologic findings in early GVHD may be rather nonspecific, and the differential diagnosis includes drug eruptions and viral exanthems, the same as the clinical differential diagnosis of the morbilliform eruption. One study suggested that the decision to treat suspected acute GVHD depended not on skin biopsy findings, but rather on the clinical severity of the presumed acute GVHD (at the time of the biopsy). However, this study did not address the subsequent taper of immunosuppressants, which could be influenced by the biopsy findings.

Classically, prophylactic treatment for acute GVHD consists of cyclosporine (CSA) or tacrolimus in conjunction with methotrexate. However, methotrexate is increasingly being replaced by mycophenolate mofetil or sirolimus (rapamycin), because these two drugs result in a reduced incidence of mucositis. The CSA or tacrolimus is continued for approximately 180 days post transplant and then tapered. Treatment of acute GVHD which develops during prophylactic therapy consists initially of systemic corticosteroids. In patients who do not respond to the addition of corticosteroids, there is no standard treatment protocol, but options include infliximab, daclizumab and mycophenolate mofetil, with most unresponsive patients developing chronic GVHD.

Chronic GVHD

Chronic GVHD is more common in allogeneic hematopoietic stem cell transplant patients who have had acute GVHD. It may occur as a progression of acute GVHD, as a recurrence following a disease-free interval, or in the absence of a history of acute GVHD (i.e., de novo). Chronic GVHD occurs in approximately 50–80% of patients who have received such transplants. In addition to the skin, gut and liver, chronic GVHD can affect the eyes and salivary glands (a Sjögren's-like syndrome), the lung (bronchiolitis obliterans), and the esophagus (a scleroderma-like process). Chronic cutaneous GVHD is classically divided into two major forms, lichenoid and sclerodermoid.

Lichenoid GVHD shares clinical and histologic features with lichen planus and is characterized by flat-topped, pink to violet scaly papules (Fig. 33–18) and white lacy plaques on the oral mucosa. Occasionally, there is scalp involvement that results in scarring alopecia. Biopsy specimens demonstrate a lichenoid infiltrate (lymphocytes abutting the dermoepidermal junction) with vacuolar degeneration of the basal layer and necrotic keratinocytes, similar to the histologic findings of lichen planus.

The name sclerodermoid GVHD comes from the more diffuse cutaneous sclerosis that is seen in late-stage, severe chronic GVHD. However, the early and potentially reversible form of this disease would more appropriately be termed morpheaform. This is because these earlier lesions are circumscribed firm plaques measuring several centimeters in diameter and thus have a clinical appearance very similar to that of morphea. Early lesions frequently involve the girdle area as well as the extensor aspects of the extremities. In addition, patients often have plaques – especially on the neck, upper trunk, and previous intravenous catheter sites – that resemble lichen sclerosus, i.e., shiny, hypopigmented plaques with scale and/or follicular plugging. With progression, the morphea-form plaques coalesce and may encase the trunk circumferen-tially; the clinical picture is then more reminiscent of diffuse scleroderma. Histologically, there is thickening and sclerosis of the dermis, with replacement of subcutaneous fat and entrapment of eccrine glands (similar findings are seen in morphea and scleroderma).

In addition to the morpheaform and sclerodermoid forms of chronic GVHD, an occasional patient will have a clinical presentation that resembles eosinophilic fasciitis. This should come as no surprise, given the overlap between deep morphea and eosinophilic fasciitis. Similarities between several autoim-mune connective tissue diseases and chronic GVHD may reflect a failure to either delete autoreactive T cells or produce immu-noregulatory T cells.

Treatment of chronic GVHD is similar to that of acute GVHD and includes prednisone, CSA, tacrolimus, and myco-phenolate mofetil. For chronic GVHD limited to the skin, topical corticosteroids, hydroxychloroquine, psoralens plus UVA (PUVA), or extracorporeal photopheresis can be employed. Recently, rituximab was shown to be effective for the cutaneous and musculoskeletal manifestations of chronic GVHD and imatinib mesylate improved cutaneous sclerosis, but the mechanisms of action of these agents are unclear. None of these modalities, however, are predictably effective.

DRUG EFFECTS

The cutaneous side effects of the primary medications pre-scribed for transplant patients are outlined in Table 33–1. In recent years there has been a movement away from CSA and towards tacrolimus, as well as a movement away from azathio-prine and towards mycophenolate mofetil and sirolimus (rapamycin). In the future, agents that have specific anti-inflammatory effects will probably play a larger role in the treatment of GVHD and organ rejection.

Table 33–1 Characteristic mucocutaneous side effects

Medication	Mucocutaneous side effects*
Corticosteroids	Folliculitis, acne, abnormal fat distribution, atrophy, striae, purpura, acanthosis nigricans
Cyclosporine	Hypertrichosis, gingival hyperplasia, sebaceous hyperplasia, epidermal cysts, folliculitis, alopecia
Tacrolimus	Pruritus, peripheral edema, ecchymoses, alopecia, photosensitivity, folliculitis
Azathioprine	Morbilliform eruption, urticaria, hypersensitivity reaction
Mycophenolate mofetil	Peripheral edema, acne, thrombophlebitis, hypersensitivity reaction
Sirolimus (rapamycin)	Acne, peripheral and facial edema, aphthae, gingival hyperplasia

*In addition to cutaneous infections and neoplasms.

SUGGESTED READINGS

Bavinck JN, Tieben LM, Van der Woude FJ, et al. Prevention of skin cancer and reduction of keratotic skin lesions during acitretin therapy in renal transplant recipients: a double-blind, placebo-controlled study. J Clin Oncol 1995; 13: 1933–1938.

Chakrabarti S, Pillay D, Ratcliffe D, et al. Resistance to antiviral drugs in herpes simplex virus infections among allogeneic stem cell transplant recipients: risk factors and prognostic significance. J Infect Dis 2000; 181: 2055–2058.

Herbrecht R, Denning DW, Patterson TF, et al., for the Invasive Fungal Infections Group of the European Organisation for Research and Treatment of Cancer and the Global Aspergillus Study Group. Voriconazole versus amphotericin B for primary therapy of invasive aspergillosis. N Engl J Med 2002; 347: 408–415.

Horn TD, Zahurak ML, Atkins D, et al. Lichen planus-like histopathologic characteristics in the cutaneous graft-vs-host reaction. Prognostic significance independent of time course after allogeneic bone marrow transplantation. Arch Dermatol 1997; 133: 961–965.

Lugo-Janer G, Sanchez JL, Santiago-Dephin E. Prevalence and clinical spectrum of skin diseases in kidney transplant recipients. J Am Acad Dermatol 1980; 24: 410–414.

Meyer T, Arndt R, Christophers E, Stockfleth E. Frequency and spectrum of HPV types detected in cutaneous squamous-cell carcinomas

depend on the HPV detection system: a comparison of four PCR assays. Dermatology 2000; 201: 204–211.

Nichols WG. Management of infectious complications in the hematopoietic stem cell transplant recipient. J Intens Care Med 2003; 18: 295–312.

Novick NL, Tapia L, Bottone EJ. Invasive Trichophyton rubrum infection in an immunocompromised host. Case report and review of the literature. Am J Med 1987; 82: 321–325.

Sable CA, Strohmaier KM, Chodakewitz JA. Advances in antifungal therapy. Ann Rev Med 2008; 59: 361–379.

Schaffer JV, McNiff JM, Seropian S, et al. Lichen sclerosus and eosinophilic fasciitis as manifestations of chronic graft-versus-host disease: expanding the sclerodermoid spectrum. J Am Acad Dermatol 2005; 53: 591–601.

Shamanin V, zur Hausen H, Lavergne D, et al. Human papillomavirus infections in nonmelanoma skin cancers from renal transplant recipients and nonimmunosuppressed patients. J Natl Cancer Inst 1996; 88: 802–811.

Traywick C, O'Reilly FM. Management of skin cancer in solid organ transplant recipients. Dermatol Ther 2005; 18: 12–18.

Valks R, Fernandez-Herrera J, Bartolome B, et al. Late appearance of acute graft-vs-host disease after suspending or tapering immunosuppressive drugs. Arch Dermatol 2001; 137: 61–65.

Venkatesan P, Perfect JR, Myers SA. Evaluation and management of fungal infections in immunocompromised patients. Dermatol Ther 2005; 18: 44–57.

Wolfson JS, Sober AJ, Rubin RH. Dermatologic manifestations of infections in immunocompromised patients. Medicine 1985; 64: 115–133.

Yoshikawa T. Human herpesvirus 6 infection in hematopoietic stem cell transplant patients. Br J Haematol 2004; 124: 421–432.

Zhou Y, Barnett MJ, Rivers JK. Clinical significance of skin biopsies in the diagnosis and management of graft-vs-host disease in early postallogeneic bone marrow transplantation. Arch Dermatol 2000; 136: 717–721.

Neurocutaneous Disease

Discussions of neurocutaneous disease are frequently limited to descriptions of the four 'phakomatoses.' These conditions were grouped together because they all involved central nervous system and retinal tumors (phakomas). They include the developmental disorders neurofibromatosis, tuberous sclerosis, Sturge–Weber syndrome, and von Hippel–Lindau syndrome, the first three of which have striking cutaneous manifestations. Knowledge of the pathogenesis of these disorders had been static for many years. However, advances in gene identification have led to characterization of the genes responsible for specific disorders such as neurofibromatosis. Subsequent analysis of the gene products should allow significant advances in knowledge of the pathogenesis and potentially offer gene therapy for these disorders.

This discussion includes a variety of other developmental disorders as well as metabolic and infectious diseases in which cutaneous and nervous system findings are shared.

The term 'phakomatosis' is derived from the Greek word *phakos*, meaning 'mother spot or mole.' Although originally used to describe the retinal lesions of tuberous sclerosis, it has come to refer to a group of disorders, including tuberous sclerosis, neurofibromatosis, Sturge–Weber disease, and von Hippel–Lindau syndrome. These disorders, as well as other vascular abnormalities, will be discussed in detail. The remainder of the developmental disorders are disorders of epidermal cells and their appendages that share an ectodermal origin with the nervous system. The syndromes mentioned in Table 34–1 are rare, but represent examples of probable neural crest abnormalities as well as poorly understood but well-documented disorders involving both the skin and the nervous system. Metabolic, infectious, and immune disorders that involve both the nervous system and the skin are discussed in less detail because many of them are reviewed in other chapters.

CLASSIFICATION

The relationship between the skin and the nervous system may be based on: (1) a developmental abnormality, frequently a result of a shared embryogenesis; or (2) the systemic effect on both organ systems of a metabolic disorder, infection, or immune response. The developmental and metabolic disorders are primarily genetic in origin, whereas the infectious and immune abnormalities represent the response of the skin and nervous system to a common insult. The neural crest is a transient embryonic structure that gives rise to dorsal root ganglion cells, Schwann cells, and autonomic ganglion cells, as well as melanocytes. Abnormalities of the neural crest cells lead to myriad clinical findings. Unfortunately, the resulting disease entities can seldom be distilled to a pattern that can be totally explained by deductive reasoning. Disorders involving both the skin and the nervous system can be briefly categorized if one includes only the phakomatoses, but the list becomes very extensive if less common syndromes and systemic diseases involving both organ systems are included. The classifications in Table 34–1 include the classic neurocutaneous disorders, representative examples of various syndromes, and pertinent systemic disorders.

NEUROFIBROMATOSIS (VON RECKLINGHAUSEN'S DISEASE)

Neurofibromas may occur in several clinical settings. Sporadic solitary cutaneous tumors can arise in adulthood and are not associated with café-au-lait spots. Classic neurofibromatosis (type 1 or NF1 – OMIM *162200) as described by von Recklinghausen is characterized by multiple café-au-lait spots, cutaneous neurofibromas, and systemic involvement with marked variability of expression. Acoustic neurofibromatosis (type 2 or NF2 – OMIM *101000) presents with bilateral acoustic neuromas as well as café-au-lait spots and cutaneous neurofibromas. The gene for NF2 is localized on chromosome 22 and encodes a negative growth regulator called MERLIN. Segmental (dermatomal) neurofibromatosis is a fascinating syndrome where café-au-lait spots, cutaneous neurofibromas, and sometimes visceral neurofibromas are limited to a sharply defined unilateral body segment. Watson's syndrome, a variant of neurofibromatosis type 1, has multiple café-au-lait spots, short stature, and pulmonary valvular stenosis, but only a small number of neurofibromas. This discussion will be limited to classic neurofibromatosis, and the term 'neurofibromatosis' is used to refer to only that disorder.

Table 34–1 Classification of neurocutaneous disease

A. Developmental disorders
  1. Dysplasia of neural crest cells
    a) Neurofibromatosis
    b) Tuberous sclerosis
  2. Vascular malformations
    a) Sturge–Weber disease
    b) Cobb's syndrome
    c) Ataxia–telangiectasia
    d) von Hippel–Lindau syndrome
  3. Pigmentary abnormalities
    a) LEOPARD syndrome
    b) Waardenburg's syndrome
    c) Incontinentia pigmenti
    d) Hypomelanosis of Ito
    e) Vogt–Koyanagi–Harada syndrome
  4. Epidermal nevus
  5. Ectodermal dysplasia
  6. Ichthyosis-associated syndromes

B. Metabolic disorders
  1. Angiokeratoma corporis diffusum
  2. Congenital hypothyroidism
  3. Amino acid abnormalities

C. Infectious disorders
  1. Viral
    a) Herpes simplex
    b) Herpes zoster
    c) Viral exanthem
  2. Bacterial: meningococcemia
  3. Rickettsial: Rocky Mountain spotted fever
  4. Spirochetes: syphilis

D. Immune disorders
  1. Cutaneous small-vessel vasculitis (including Henoch-Schönlein purpura)
  2. Behçet's syndrome
  3. Lupus erythematosus

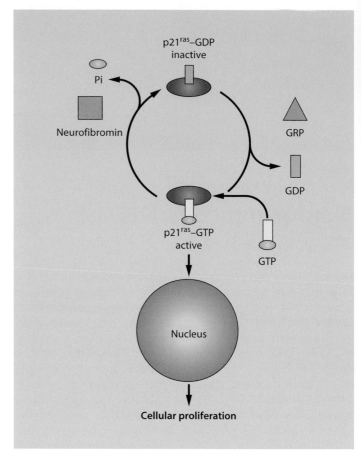

Figure 34–1 Neurofibromin is involved in inactivating the p21^{ras}–GTP complex.

Pathogenesis

The incidence of neurofibromatosis is estimated at around 1 per 3000 live births. It is inherited as an autosomal dominant trait, with almost complete penetrance by age 5. De novo mutations represent around 30–50% of patients with neurofibromatosis. With an estimated mutation rate of 1 in 10 000 per gamete per generation, the neurofibromatosis gene has one of the highest mutation rates of any genetic disorder. Currently over 800 different mutations have been identified. About 90% of new mutations occur on the paternally derived chromosome, with 80% of these showing truncation mutations.

The NF1 gene has been localized to chromosome 17q11.2. It has 60 exons, spans 350 kb, and encodes an mRNA of 11–13 kb. In addition, three embedded genes located on the NF1 gene are transcribed in the opposite direction. The basic defect lies in the abnormal expression of a tumor suppressor gene called neurofibromin. This gene product has functional and structural homology with a guanosine triphosphatase-activation protein (GTPase) that downregulates p21^{ras} proto-oncogene activity. In its active (GTP) state, the p21^{ras} protein binds guanine nucleotides with high affinity, acting as a signal trans-

ducer for cellular proliferation. Neurofibromin switches off this signaling by hydrolyzing GTP to GDP (Fig. 34–1). A defect in neurofibromin would result in a constitutively active p21^{ras} protein, leading to cell growth and possible tumor formation. Interestingly, neurofibromin is found in the skin, brain, spleen, liver, and muscle, not just in the neural crest cells. The abnormal proliferation seen in neurofibromatosis is focused on the neural crest for reasons that are not yet clear at the molecular level.

It is generally believed that a somatic 'second-hit' mutation with loss of heterozygosity results in the progression of malignant tumors, and possibly in the formation of benign neurofibromas. However, given the wide clinical phenotypes found even among close relatives, a defect in the neurofibromin protein cannot in itself explain this variability. Other studies point to evidence that modifying genes (genes which are unlinked to the NF1 gene but play a phenotypical role in neurofibromatosis) may be behind these differences. Clinical outcomes would depend on where the second mutation at another gene occurs. Finally, the environment, especially trauma, may lead to the formation of benign neurofibromas. Because neurofibromin is involved in the healing process, defective neurofibromin in conjunction with a traumatic event may lead to abnormal cellular proliferation and tumor formation.

Clinical Manifestations

Café-au-Lait Spots

Present in more than 90% of patients, these are the earliest clinical features found in neurofibromatosis (Table 34-2). The current criterion for the disease is the presence of six or more café-au-lait spots >1.5 cm for adults, and >0.5 cm for prepubertal individuals (Fig. 34-2). Café-au-lait spots are usually present at birth and progressively increase in number and size. The macular hyperpigmentation is usually homogeneous, with sharply defined edges. Distribution of larger café-au-lait spots is random. They usually spare the face. Intertriginous areas are involved in 20% of cases, with freckle-like pathognomonic lesions (Crowe's sign) (Fig. 34-2). Other involved areas include the neck, under the chin, and the submammary region in women. Hyperpigmentation may occur over plexiform neurofibromas. When such pigmentation extends to the midline, it often indicates that a tumor involves the spinal cord.

Neurofibromas

These occur in 60–90% of patients. There are three types: plexiform, cutaneous, and subcutaneous. All are composed of various combinations of neurons, Schwann cells, fibroblasts, vascular elements, and mast cells. They become diffuse, are somewhat vascular, and may be associated with overlying hyperpigmentation. Cutaneous neurofibromas are rarely present in infancy: more often they begin to appear in late childhood and adolescence, and gradually increase in size and number. Clinically, they are at first sessile, then become pedunculated, fleshy tumors that can be invaginated (buttonholing) (Fig. 34-3). Subcutaneous neurofibromas tend to become apparent in late childhood or early adulthood; they are tender, and may lead to neurological symptoms. Subcutaneous neurofibromas occur either as discrete nodules on a peripheral nerve or as highly vascular diffuse plexiform neuromas (16% of cases) which involve a nerve trunk and may account for segmental hypertrophy and obstruction of neighboring vital structures. Both pregnancy and puberty are known to increase the number and size of neurofibromas. In addition, there have been isolated cases where cutaneous neurofibromas presented initially as clitoromegaly. Endocrine work-up is usually normal. Malignant degeneration of neurofibromas into malignant peripheral neural sheath tumors occurs in 2–3% of cases. Malignancy is most common within a plexiform neuroma, and often carries a poor prognosis, although limb lesions may have a better outcome.

Lisch Nodules

These pigmented iris hamartomas are present in more than 90% of patients aged 6 years or over. However, fewer patients younger than 6 years of age have them. They are asymptomatic and are not correlated with other manifestations or with disease severity. Clinically they appear as randomly distributed cream-colored to brownish nodules on the iris. Although most are easy to visualize, a slit lamp evaluation by an experienced

Table 34-2 Order of appearance of the clinical features listed in the NIH criteria for neurofibromatosis

Café-au-lait macules
Axillary freckling
Lisch nodules
Neurofibromas

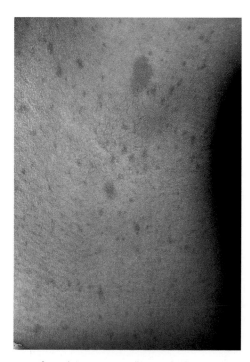

Figure 34-2 A café-au-lait spot as well as multiple freckles (Crowe's sign) in the axillary vault is seen in this patient with neurofibromatosis.

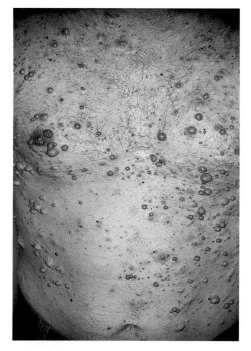

Figure 34-3 Multiple neurofibromas are present in this individual.

ophthalmologist is often needed to rule out the presence of single 'salt grain' lesions. Histologically, they represent melanocytic hamartomas.

Central Nervous System Involvement

Central nervous system (CNS) tumors develop in 3–10% of patients and include benign neoplasms such as optic nerve gliomas, acoustic neuromas, neurolemmomas, meningiomas, ependymomas, astrocytomas, and neurofibromas. Such growths present clinically with signs and symptoms of CNS mass lesions. Spinal tumors often present with localizing peripheral signs. Optic nerve gliomas, the most common of these tumors, may result in papilledema, retrobulbar neuritis, and eventually optic atrophy. Most develop within the first 6 years of life; the majority of cases run a benign course and do not require intervention. For those whose tumors do progress, treatment options include surgery or radiation. Malignant tumors, most commonly low-grade astrocytomas, may also occur. They affect the brainstem and may present with symptoms of mass effect, such as cranial neuropathies and hydrocephaly. However, these lesions tend to have a less aggressive course than pontine tumors, which are not associated with neurofibromatosis.

A more recent issue is the presence of high-intensity signals on T_2-weighted MRI. These findings, called 'unidentified bright objects' (UBO), are found within the basal ganglia, cerebellum, and brainstem in up to 70% of people with neurofibromatosis, but what they represent remains unclear. Current speculation includes harmatomas, dysplasia, demyelination, vacuolar changes, or low-grade tumors. The clinical significance of these findings is also in dispute. Some studies have shown that the presence of UBO is associated with lower IQ scores, but this conclusion has remained controversial. Some practitioners believe that the findings of UBO should be included as a criterion for the diagnosis of neurofibromatosis, and may be diagnostic in 30% of children who do not meet the current criteria. However, children may need anesthesia to have the procedure performed.

Intellectual handicap affects about 40% of patients, although obvious retardation occurs in less than 5%. It does not worsen with time and does not correlate with the degree of skin involvement. Headaches occur with increased frequency even in the absence of CNS tumors. Mild speech impediments are present in 30–40% of cases, and cerebrovascular compromise as a result of involvement of cerebral arteries with neurofibromas does occur. Major and minor motor seizures occur in less than 5% of cases in the absence of identifiable mass lesions or cerebral vascular involvement. An additional 26% of patients will have abnormal or borderline findings on electroencephalography.

Macrocephaly is present in at least 27% of patients, and is more common after 6 years of age. There is no correlation between macrocephaly and impaired intellectual performance, seizures, or electroencephalographic abnormalities.

Musculoskeletal Disorders

Pseudoarthrosis occurs in less than 1% of cases and clinically becomes evident in the first year of life. There appears to

be a male preponderance. The tibia or the radius is most frequently involved. It is characterized by congenital bowing of the involved bone with subsequent variable displacement of the joint (varying from a minimal radiologic abnormality to severe displacement with total loss of function). Radiographic bone abnormalities may also result from pressure by intraosseous or paraosseous neurofibromas. There is no consensus on treatment, and severe cases have led to amputation.

Kyphoscoliosis occurs in at least 2% of patients, often associated with paravertebral neurofibromas; however, it is not certain whether there is a cause-and-effect relationship between the two. Kyphoscoliosis usually has its onset in childhood and may progress rapidly to produce severe cardiorespiratory and neurologic compromise.

Short stature is another feature that is more prominent in those with neurofibromatosis. Growth curves comparing unaffected with affected children show similar growth profiles until preadolescence, at which point the growth rate for children with neurofibromatosis decreases significantly. They are also at increase risk of osteoporosis and osteopenia later in life.

Gastrointestinal Disorders

Visceral tumors arise from intra-abdominal neural tissue and include neurofibromas, leiomyomas, and miscellaneous tumors. The most common complications are obstruction, intussusception, and hemorrhage caused by erosions or necrosis of pedunculated tumors. Persistent constipation occurs in 10% of cases, due to disorganization of the tunica muscularis and Auerbach's plexus of the colon.

Endocrine Disorders

Aberrant endocrine function is not a regular finding in neurofibromatosis, and although frequently mentioned is probably present in less than 1% of cases. Pheochromocytoma, often benign and unilateral, is the most common endocrine abnormality. It mainly produces norepinephrine (noradrenaline). Medullary carcinoma of the thyroid and hyperparathyroidism are even less common. In addition, it has been reported that optic tumors in children are associated with precocious puberty, possibly due to hypothalamic involvement. Other reported endocrine associations probably occur only coincidentally.

Miscellaneous Disorders

Other findings that may be associated with neurofibromatosis are significant because of their systemic implications. These include congenital pulmonary stenosis, idiopathic interstitial pulmonary fibrosis, and an extramural or intramural involvement of the renal arteries producing renal artery stenosis and hypertension. Pregnant women and adolescents are more likely to develop hypertension, but, regardless of age, all patients should have their blood pressure checked regularly.

Miscellaneous malignancies, including Wilms' tumor, rhabdomyosarcoma, and juvenile myelomonocytic leukemia (especially in patients with juvenile xanthogranulomas), are more common in patients with neurofibromatosis than in the population at large. It is felt that the loss of the tumor suppression function of the NF1 gene predisposes those with neurofibromatosis to myeloid disorders.

Differential Diagnosis

The diagnostic criteria for type 1 neurofibromatosis were summarized by Riccardi and Eichner. Two or more of the following criteria are needed:

1. Six or more café-au-lait spots > 1.5 cm in adults and >0.5 cm in prepubertal children.
2. Two or more neurofibromas of any type, or one plexiform neurofibroma.
3. Axillary or inguinal freckling.
4. Optic glioma.
5. Two or more Lisch nodules.
6. A distinctive bony lesion, such as pseudoarthrosis or thinning of a long bone cortex.
7. A first-degree relative with neurofibromatosis type 1.

Other minor features that may assist in the diagnosis include macrocephaly, hypertelorism, short stature, and thorax abnormalities.

McCune–Albright syndrome (OMIM #174800) consists of polyostotic fibrous dysplasia, endocrine dysfunction, melanotic macules, and precocious puberty in females. The melanotic macules of McCune–Albright syndrome are also present at birth, but tend to be unilateral, segmental, and frequently linear in arrangement. The border of the pigmented lesions in Albright syndrome has been said to be serrated (likened to the coast of Maine), as opposed to the smooth borders of café-au-lait spots in neurofibromatosis. Further evaluation of this finding has found it to be of questionable diagnostic importance. Macromelanosomes are common in neurofibromatosis but are rare in Albright syndrome. However, they have been found not to be specific for the café-au-lait spots of neurofibromatosis.

Patient Evaluation

Given the myriad clinical features in neurofibromatosis, the utility of extensive screening tests remains controversial. Riccardi and Eichner have published recommendations for extensive patient evaluation aimed at confirming the diagnosis, identifying complications, and monitoring progression. They include intelligence testing, psychologic evaluation, electroencephalography, audiography, slit lamp examination, skeletal survey (with attention to the skull, optic foramina, and spine), cranial imaging (MRI or CT) to include the orbits and optic chiasm, and measurement of 24-hour excretion levels of norepinephrine (noradrenaline) and epinephrine (adrenaline). This detailed evaluation has been felt to be justified because 5–10% of patients will have significant findings and the remainder will benefit significantly from the reassurance of a negative evaluation. However, in a study of 152 patients by Wolkenstein et al. only two cases were found in which these evaluations altered the treatment, whereas there were 22 com-

plications from these investigations. They recommend annual clinical examinations and more focused screenings based on the physician's clinical evaluation.

Several important points concerning natural history should be kept in mind:

1. Progression in the number and size of all lesions is relentless throughout life.
2. The presence of one feature of the disease in no way correlates with the other features.
3. One cannot predict the course of neurofibromatosis based on the current severity of the disease.

Genetic Testing

Molecular genetic diagnosis has made tremendous advances during these past few years. With current methodologies, approximately 85–95% of known mutations can be identified. In familial cases of neurofibromatosis, linkage studies can be performed. Genes are said to be linked when markers close to the NF1 locus congregate together during recombination. Through extensive evaluation of multiple family members, analysis of the markers associated with the abnormal NF1 gene can be identified and used for genetic counseling. In addition, in utero diagnosis studies are currently available. However, genetic testing in neurofibromatitis remains problematic. The large variability in phenotypic expression of neurofibromatosis does not currently allow any correlation with the specific genetic mutation. Positive genetic results do not predict the presence, age of onset, or the severity of disease. In addition, a negative result does not exclude the disease. As a result the demand for prenatal testing remains limited, but it may offer benefit as a diagnostic tool in suspected patients who do not meet the criteria. As the interpretation of genetic test results may be difficult, referral to a genetic counselor for interpretation is recommended.

Treatment

Patients with NF1 have an estimated lifespan that is 15 years shorter than that of the general population, malignant degeneration being the major cause. Close evaluations and surgical removal of rapidly enlarging lesions should be undertaken. In addition, removal of disfiguring or functionally compromising lesions is recommended. Anticonvulsants, analgesics, and H_1 antihistamines are useful for symptomatic therapy of appropriate manifestations.

The disease presents serious psychosocial problems. The various complications may involve sight, hearing, and learning, as well as growth and development. Awareness of these problems and methods of coping with them are essential to reduce long-term morbidity.

TUBEROUS SCLEROSIS (BOURNEVILLE'S DISEASE)

Tuberous sclerosis (OMIM #191100 and *191092) is a disorder that classically consists of the triad of epilepsy, adenoma sebaceum, and mental retardation. However, about half of these patients will have normal intelligence, and up to a quarter do not have epilepsy. In addition, a variety of other lesions may affect the skin, nervous system, heart, kidney, and other organs.

Pathogenesis

Tuberous sclerosis shows no racial, ethnic, or sexual predilection. The incidence is estimated at 1 in 10 000 live births. It is inherited in an autosomal dominant pattern, with almost complete penetrance, but the majority of cases are attributed to sporadic new mutations. Fertility is reduced by the frequent severe mental retardation. The phenotype of tuberous sclerosis is highly variable.

Two genes, TSC1 and TSC2, are identified as the genetic defects in tuberous sclerosis, each accounting for half of all cases, although patients with TSC2 are felt to have a more severe disease process. Currently there are over 1200 allelic variants of both genes. TSC1 is found on chromosome 9q34. It is a 900-kb region containing at least 30 genes and encodes a 130-kDa protein called hamartin. TSC2 is found on chromosome 16p13. It spans 43 kb and encodes a 180-kDa protein called tuberin. It is believed that loss of heterozygosity through a somatic 'second-hit' mutation leads to the unmasking of the disease process.

Only recently has the function of these two gene products become better elucidated. Current evidence supports the belief that tuberin and hamartin form an intracellular heterodimer that functions as a tumor suppressor and senses various intra- and extracellular signals, including growth factor stimulation and hypoxia. This complex also targets a Ras homolog enriched in the brain (Rheb), which in turn inhibits mamillian target of rapamycin (mTOR), a serine/threonine kinase involved in cell growth and proliferation. This tuberin–hamartin complex contains a region with homology to the catalytic domain of rap1 guanosine triphosphatase-activation protein. This heterodimer protein induces the inactive state by stimulating GTPase activation protein (GAP) and functions by downregulating Rheb. Rheb in its active states induces mTOR, which in turn phosphorylates 4E binding protein (4e-BP1), ribosomal protein S6 kinase b (S6K1), and eukaryotic translation factor 2; all are involved in ribosomal biosynthesis recruitment and translation initiation. It is a mutation within the GAP domain of the protein that results in most cases of tuberous sclerosis. With better understanding of the tuberin–hamartin complex, Rheb, and mTOR, there is hope for the development of new targets for future therapies.

Clinical Manifestations

Facial Angiofibroma (Adenoma Sebaceum)

The hamartomas known as adenoma sebaceum are actually angiofibromas, and the sebaceous glands are generally atrophic. The lesions are erythematous, smooth papules involving the nasolabial folds, cheeks, and chin in a symmetrical distribution (Fig. 34–4). On close examination they are found in 70–90% of patients with tuberous sclerosis older than 5 years, and progressively increase in size and number, particularly during puberty. They are commonly associated with facial tel-

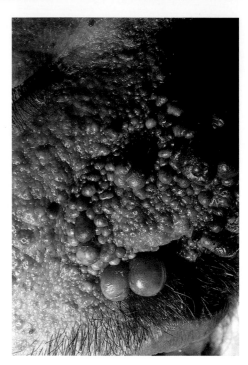

Figure 34–4 Multiple lesions of adenoma sebaceum in a patient with tuberous sclerosis.

angiectasia and facial flushing. When found, they are virtually pathognomonic of tuberous sclerosis. The main histologic findings are those of a fibrovascular hamartomatous proliferation with concomitant atrophy and compression of adnexal structures in the skin.

Hypomelanotic Macules (Ash Leaf Macules)

These consist of asymmetrically distributed, hypopigmented macules that are most common over the trunk and buttocks and rare over the face (Fig. 34–5). They vary in size from a few millimeters to 3 cm in diameter, and range in number from three to 100. Their configuration is usually leaf-like ('ash leaf macule') or oval. They have been reported in 75–80% of cases of tuberous sclerosis. However, ash leaf macules are probably present at birth in the vast majority of patients with tuberous sclerosis (based on studies in which neonates were closely examined using a Wood's light). They persist throughout life and constitute the earliest cutaneous sign of tuberous sclerosis. A Wood's light, by accentuating areas of depigmentation, may assist in detecting subtle macules on light-skinned individuals. Examination of biopsy specimens reveals a normal number of melanocytes but a reduced intensity of melanization, with a reduction in the size and degree of melanization of the melanosomes on electron microscopy.

Ungual Fibromas (Koenen's Tumors)

These are pink to flesh-colored papules ranging in size from 1 mm to 1 cm that arise from the nail bed (Fig. 34–6). They can be located in the lateral nail groove, under the nail plate, or along the proximal nail groove. They usually appear at puberty and are present in about 50% of cases. They may cause pain, and have a tendency to recur after surgical removal. His-

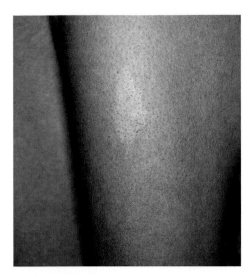

Figure 34–5 A hypopigmented spot on the thigh in the shape of an ash leaf is present in this patient with tuberous sclerosis.

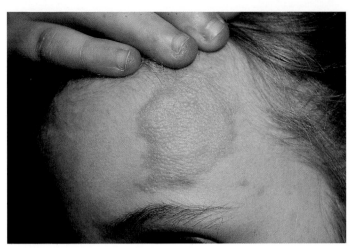

Figure 34–7 An erythematous plaque representative of a connective tissue nevus is present in this patient with tuberous sclerosis.

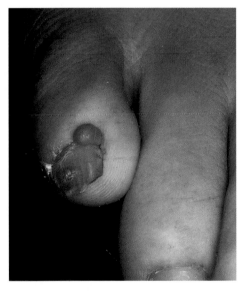

Figure 34–6 A periungual fibroma is present in this patient with tuberous sclerosis.

tologically, they resemble facial angiofibromas, with fibrosis and capillary dilatation. Older lesions may contain large, stellate fibroblasts with a 'glial appearance.'

Shagreen Patch

These connective tissue hamartomas are plaques (Fig. 34–7) that are usually found on the trunk, particularly in the lumbosacral area. They vary in size from a few millimeters to >10 cm. They are yellowish-brown to pink in color and have a firm consistency. The lesions are rarely found in infancy and become more common after puberty, reaching a peak prevalence of 70–80% of cases of tuberous sclerosis. The Shagreen patch, however, differs neither clinically nor histopathologically in any way from other connective tissue nevi that may occur as isolated developmental defects in otherwise normal individuals.

Miscellaneous Nevoid Lesions

Café-au-lait spots may occur as an isolated finding in 10–20% of tuberous sclerosis patients. Interestingly, Crowe found that 10% of the general population has one or more café-au-lait spots. Patches of gray or white have also been noted in up to 20% of patients with tuberous sclerosis.

Fibromas of various sizes and shapes may occur in other locations. These include: (1) large, asymmetrical fibromas of the face and scalp; (2) soft, pedunculated growths on the neck, trunk, or extremities (molluscum fibrosum pendulum); (3) grouped, firm papules of the neck, trunk, and extremities; and (4) pedunculated or sessile nodules of the buccal or gingival mucosa.

Central Nervous System Involvement

Focal or generalized seizures occur in over 80% of patients with tuberous sclerosis and may be the first symptom to suggest the diagnosis. These are largely related to 'tuberous' tumors of the cerebral cortex. Cerebral tumors up to 3 cm in size represent hamartomas of glioblasts and neuroblasts. Most lesions are multiple and involve the frontal or parietal lobe. In about 50% of patients these tumors calcify and produce characteristic roentgenographic changes. In addition, certain subependymal lesions called subependymal giant cell astrocytomas may enlarge and obstruct the flow of CSF and result in hydrocephalus. These lesions, found in 5–10% of all cases, differ from the typical intracranial nodules of tuberous sclerosis and can lead to significant mortality. Neoplastic transformation to astrocytomas, glioblastomas, and meningiomas may be seen. The number of tubers correlates with the degree of learning disability, with mental function gradually deteriorating with time: 60–70% of patients demonstrate both seizures and mental retardation by 3 years of age.

Retinal and optic nerve involvement is the most frequent ophthalmic manifestation of tuberous sclerosis, occurring in 50% of patients. Retinal gliomas may appear as peripheral, noncalcified lesions that are flat, white to salmon-colored, and circular (phakoma – 'white spot'). On funduscopic examination they can be difficult to identify before calcification has occurred, but after calcification they are easily identified as pearly white tumors near the disc margin. They are frequently located superficial to a retinal vessel. The second type of retinal lesion is the classic nodular lesion resembling a mulberry, with clusters of small, glistening granules. Generally, the retinal lesions do not grow significantly and blindness is rare. Treatment is not necessary. Hypopigmented macules of the iris, white eyelashes, and hamartomatous tumors of the eyelids and conjunctivae may also occur.

Renal Involvement

Two characteristic renal lesions occur in tuberous sclerosis: angiomyolipomas and renal cysts. The prevalence of angiomyolipomas increases with age (being present in more than 90% of patients over the age of 10). They can be the sole manifestation of the tuberous sclerosis complex. Angiomyolipomas are usually multiple, bilateral, and innocuous. When they are symptomatic, the patient may manifest pain and/or hematuria. They range in size from a few millimeters to 20 cm, and the mass effect of the tumor is usually responsible for symptoms. Tumors larger than 4 cm are at an increased risk for bleeding. Renal failure is very rare. There are many reports of malignant transformation of angiomyolipomas, but in none of these has the tumor metastasized.

Renal cysts may be small and asymptomatic or large and result in renal impairment. Interestingly, the TSC2 gene is located next to the gene responsible for autosomal dominant polycystic kidney disease (PKD1). Mutation involving both TSC2 and PKD1 has been associated with severe forms of renal cysts. Smaller cysts are found in those with mutations involving only the TSC2 or TSC1 gene. Rare cases of renal cell carcinoma have been seen.

Cardiac and Pulmonary Involvement

Cardiac involvement in tuberous sclerosis includes multiple discrete rhabdomyomas, which occur in 30% of patients. These lesions are usually benign and regress over time. However, the deaths that do occur are related to outflow obstruction or conduction defects. In addition, there may be an association with Wolff–Parkinson–White syndrome, especially in those with rhabdomyomas. Up to 80% of children with rhabdomyomas of the heart have tuberous sclerosis.

Pulmonary involvement is rare and usually consists of diffuse leiomyomatosis. This produces a pattern on chest X-ray that may range from a fine reticular pattern to multiple cysts. Pneumothorax, progressive exertional dyspnea, and cor pulmonale may occur.

Miscellaneous Systemic Findings

A number of variable and nonspecific findings have been reported. These include goiter, hypothyroidism, Cushing's syndrome, abnormal glucose tolerance tests, precocious puberty, adrenal hyperplasia, cystic radiographic lesions of the metacarpals and phalanges, sclerotic lesions of the skull, pitted defects of dental enamel, and splenic hamartomas.

Differential Diagnosis

The characteristic ash leaf macules in children with seizures and/or mental retardation are sufficient to establish the diagnosis. However, the early stages of the disease and the forme fruste may give trouble in diagnosis. There is also a poor correlation of severity among the individual components of the disease. For example, young adults with normal intelligence may have angiofibromas and various systemic lesions. In such situations, the search for individual cutaneous or noncutaneous components of the syndrome in a patient with an isolated finding confirms the diagnosis.

Patient Evaluation

A detailed family history with examination of family members is required. However, 85% of cases represent de novo mutations, and a negative family history should not be used to rule out tuberous sclerosis. Studies that may support the diagnosis include the biopsy of appropriate skin lesions. Computed tomographic (CT) scanning should be performed for the radiographic evaluation of the central nervous system in tuberous sclerosis. A National Institute of Health Consensus Conference has revised the diagnostic criteria for tuberous sclerosis (Table 34–3).

Patients with established cases should have a detailed ophthalmologic examination, looking for gliomas; CT scan of the brain to evaluate the severity of CNS involvement; chest X-ray to detect pulmonary involvement; echocardiogram to evaluate intracardiac tumors; and radiographic evaluation for renal masses. During the NIH Consensus Conference, the panel recommended that cranial imaging (MRI or CT) and renal ultrasonography be performed every 1–3 years for evaluation of interval changes. In addition, women should have a chest CT at least once during adulthood to evaluate the rare risk of developing lymphangioleiomyomatosis. Other periodic studies should be based on any clinical changes.

Treatment

Genetic counseling is essential for adults with even minimal involvement from tuberous sclerosis, as their children may be severely affected. There is a 50% risk of an affected parent transmitting the disorder to the offspring.

Molecular genetic testing is currently available for detection of 75–80% of the mutations found in TSC1 or TSC2. However, at present the use of genetic testing remains limited owing to the cost. Prenatal testing can be performed in families where the mutation is known. Testing can best be used to confirm a diagnosis when TS is suspected in a patient who does not currently meet the established criteria. It can also be helpful in unaffected parents with an affected child in determining who might carry the gene. However, testing does not rule out

Table 34–3 Revised diagnostic criteria for tuberous sclerosis complex (TSC)

Major features

Facial angiofibromas or forehead plaque
Nontraumatic ungual or periungual fibroma
Hypomelanotic macules (>3)
Shagreen patch (connective tissue nevus)
Multiple retinal nodular hamartomas
Cortical tuber*
Subependymal nodules
Subependymal giant cell astrocytoma
Cardiac rhabdomyoma, single or multiple
Lymphangiomyomatosis†
Renal angiomyolipoma†

Minor features

Multiple randomly distributed pits in dental enamel
Hamartomatous rectal polyps§
Bone cysts
Cerebral white matter migration lines*‡
Gingival fibromas
Nonrenal hamartoma
Retinal achromic patch
'Confetti' skin lesions
Multiple renal cysts§

Definite TSC: either 2 major features or 1 major feature with 2 minor features.
Probable TSC: 1 major feature and 1 minor feature.
Possible TSC: either 1 major feature or 2 or more minor features.
*When cerebral cortical dysplasia and cerebral white matter migration tracts occur together, they should be counted as 1 rather than 2 features of TSC.
†When both lymphangiomyomatosis and renal angiomyolipomas are present, other features of TSC should be present before a definitive diagnosis is assigned.
§Histologic confirmation is suggested.
‡Radiographic confirmation is sufficient.
Adapted from Roach ES, Gomez MR, Northrup H. Tuberous sclerosis complex consensus conference: revised clinical diagnostic criteria. J Child Neurol 1998; 13: 624–628.

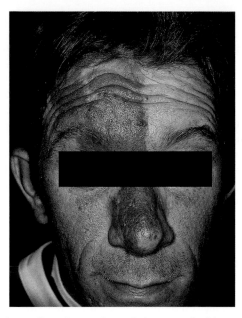

Figure 34–8 A unilateral port-wine stain is present in this man with Sturge–Weber syndrome.

the possiblity of a mosaicism within the parental gonadal cells.

Symptomatic treatment with anticonvulsants is valuable. Surgical removal of extracutaneous hamartomas is indicated if symptoms become evident or if such lesions enlarge rapidly, indicating possible malignant degeneration. Removal of cutaneous lesions is for cosmetic reasons only. Adenoma sebaceum responds to electrocautery and laser ablation with excellent cosmetic results, but regrowth is common.

With progress in our understanding of the mechanism of tuberous sclerosis, there is excitement at the development of a nonsurgical intervention. Rapamycin, also known as sirolimus, is an antibiotic derived from *Streptomyces hygroscopicus* and is commonly used in organ transplantations. In cells lacking functional TSC1 or TSC2, sirolimus has been shown to normalize the dysfunctional mTOR pathway. Clinical trials are currently under way evaluating the efficacy of sirolimus in various aspects of tuberous sclerosis. In one open-label 24-month study, 25 patients with angiomyolipomas were treated with a 12-month course of sirolimus. The angiomyolipomas tended to regress during treatment, but the improvement was not maintained after cessation of therapy. Some patients had

persistent improvement of spirometric measurements even after cessation. In another study, five patients with astrocytoma had regression, and in one case necrosis of the tumor, after initiation of treatment. Recent mouse studies have shown increased efficacy of sirolimus when combined with interferon-γ. These and possible other new advances have raised the prospect of a new era in the treatment of tuberous sclerosis.

STURGE–WEBER DISEASE

Sturge–Weber disease is characterized by a nevus flammeus, or port-wine stain, in the area of the ophthalmic branch of the trigeminal nerve (Fig. 34–8). Cutaneous lesions are present at birth. In addition, there are ipsilateral leptomeningeal angiomas that lead to progressive calcification and degeneration of the underlying cerebral cortex. This degeneration may lead to seizure disorders, contralateral hemiparesis, and ipsilateral ocular involvement with angiomatosis of the choroid and glaucoma.

Pathogenesis

Sturge–Weber disease is not believed to be genetically transmitted, as almost all cases are sporadic. Rare familial occurrences have been reported and may suggest an autosomal dominant form of inheritance. The incidence is not reliably known, but it is probably around 1 : 10 000 births. Trisomy 22 has been reported in isolated patients, but no genetic or metabolic defect has yet been identified.

The vascular abnormalities of Sturge–Weber disease probably represent a mesodermal defect that occurs in the fourth to eighth weeks of embryonic development. At this point, the ectoderm, which will form the skin, overlies the tissue that will eventually become the ipsilateral cerebrum. Subsequently, the leptomeningeal vessels develop into venous angiomas with a network of thin-walled ectatic venules filling the subarachnoid space. At birth, the port-wine stain is flat and grows in proportion to the growth of the child. The cerebral angiomas develop progressive loss of venous drainage, with subsequent venous stasis and calcification. Calcification is believed to be the result of deposition of colloid fibers on a matrix of reticulin fibers, and precipitation of calcium salts on reticulin fibers. This calcification increases throughout life. The combination of vascular ectasia and calcification then produces ischemia of the underlying cerebral tissue, with resultant diffuse cortical atrophy and nervous system abnormalities.

It has been proposed that the trigeminal distribution of the nevus flammeus represents a co-migration of skin vasculature and the underlying trigeminal nerve during embryogenesis. Occasional angiomas in the trigeminal nerve ganglion support this theory, but the hypothesis fails to explain the frequent finding of port-wine stains that intrude on neighboring cervical and contralateral dermatomes. Others feel this relationship is merely coincidental.

Clinical Manifestations

The port-wine stains are flat, vascular lesions ranging in color from pink to deep purple. The area of involvement may range from a single eyelid to bilateral extensive angiomas. Eight percent of patients demonstrate unilateral involvement of the face, usually both above and below the palpebral fissure. When a nevus flammeus lies entirely below the ophthalmic branch of the trigeminal nerve (below the palpebral fissure and the upper eyelid), cranial involvement is rare and the clinical skin abnormality is best termed nevus flammeus, or port-wine stain, rather than Sturge–Weber disease. The lesion consists of dilated and excessively numerous but well-defined capillaries in the dermis. As port-wine stains age, the vessel walls become progressively more ectatic, producing exophytic blueberry-like ectasias in mid-adult life. The gingival hypertrophy may be greatly accentuated by pregnancy.

The facial angioma may not conform to the division of the trigeminal nerve and involvement of the face, scalp, trunk, and extremities is common. The term Klippel–Trenaunay–Weber syndrome is sometimes applied to cases with extensive lesions of the extremities.

In 5–14% of cases the characteristic cerebral angiomas, calcification, and atrophy may occur in the absence of skin lesions. Such cases are still termed Sturge–Weber disease, but obviously do not fulfill the traditional criteria for the syndrome.

Cutaneous involvement of the upper eyelid is associated with intraocular abnormalities. Intraocular abnormalities occur in half of the patients as angiomas of the conjunctiva, iris, or choroid. Angiomas of the choroid may produce glaucoma or retinal detachment, which may be congenital or may occur later in life. Glaucoma is the most serious ocular involvement and occurs in about one-third of cases. Involvement of both lids of the affected eye is usually associated with glaucoma. Angioid streaks of the retina and enlargement of the globe may occur. Oculocutaneous melanosis produced by ectopic dermal melanocytes presents as slate-blue discoloration of the sclera and of the periorbital skin, resembling nevus of Ota. This is not a common occurrence.

Seizures may begin shortly after birth, but usually occur in late infancy or early childhood. Up to 20% of patients never develop seizures. Seizures frequently begin with febrile episodes that precipitate contralateral focal motor seizures. Generalized seizures develop later. Hemiparesis, hemiplegia, hemisensory defects, homonymous hemianopsia, and limb atrophy also occur.

Mental retardation may be minimal in early childhood, but is progressive after the onset of seizures. Some evidence points to the possibility that seizures may inhibit blood flow, resulting in increased neurological impairment. Control of seizures by medical or surgical means may slow the progression of the mental defect.

Radiologic calcifications are seldom present at birth, but develop in early childhood. The X-ray findings of intracranial calcification are highly characteristic, showing double lines of curvilinear densities that parallel the cerebral convolutions to produce the characteristic railroad-track pattern. Electroencephalographic evidence of brain involvement usually occurs in early childhood.

Patient Evaluation and Treatment

The appearance of cutaneous lesions is best improved with cosmetics (e.g., Covermark or Dermablend). Electrodesiccation usually produces unacceptable scarring. New laser technology has improved the cosmetic results of therapy. The pulsed dye laser is specifically designed for cutaneous vascular lesions. These lasers function by taking advantage of the fact that red blood vessels selectively absorb the laser energy, thereby selectively destroying the hemangioma. These modalities have proved particularly effective in the treatment of port-wine stains in young children. More than 75% lightening may eventually be achieved, although recurrence of lesions with time is common. Laser treatments are also effective for shrinking oral lesions, or for the papular ectatic lesions that develop later in life.

If the characteristic cutaneous lesion is present, the affected child should be aggressively evaluated and treated in the hope of averting brain damage. Calcification can be demonstrated by CT earlier and more consistently than with conventional X-ray studies, but is still often not detectable before the age of 2 years. MRI is less sensitive than CT for identifying calcification, but may provide for better documentation of intracranial vascular abnormalities that can confirm the diagnosis in younger children.

Medical prophylactic treatment of seizure disorders as well as surgical removal of leptomeningeal angiomas may then be justified. If seizures are resistant to medical therapy, surgical intervention including hemispherectomy may be required. When present, glaucoma should be controlled by medical or, if necessary, surgical means. Mental deterioration may not be severe in half of patients, and such people may then lead relatively normal lives.

COBB'S SYNDROME

Cobb's syndrome is the association of a port-wine stain or cavernous hemangioma in a dermatomal distribution with an angioma of the spinal cord that corresponds to the cutaneous distribution. Neurologic deficits of spinal cord compression may then occur.

ATAXIA–TELANGIECTASIA (LOUIS–BAR SYNDROME)

Ataxia-telangiectasia (OMIM #208900) is an autosomal recessive disorder consisting of progressive cerebellar ataxia, ocular and cutaneous telangiectasia, and variable immunodeficiency. The immunodeficiency predisposes the patient to recurrent sinopulmonary infections and to an increased incidence of neoplasia. Patients have a defect in cell growth and chromosomal integrity that is associated with an increased sensitivity to ionizing radiation. Recent advances in the understanding of diseases with similar radiosensitive phenotypes have led to the elucidation and better understanding of various ataxia–telangiectasia-like disorders (ATLD). The discussion here will be limited to the classic ataxia–telangiectasia phenotype.

Pathogenesis

The incidence is approximately 1 in 40000 births, with the incidence of asymptomatic heterozygotes being as high as 1 in 100. The gene responsible for ataxia–telangiectasia is located on chromosome 11q22–23. This ATM (ataxia–telangiectasia mutation) gene encompasses 150 kb of DNA with 66 exons and encodes a 370 kDa phosphoprotein. This protein has significant homology to a subunit of phosphatidylinositol 3-kinase, which is involved in cell cycle regulation, maintenance of genomic stability, and response to DNA damage.

Fibroblasts and lymphoblasts are extremely sensitive to X-rays and chemotherapeutic killing. These cells have defective DNA repair following radiation and fail to slow their rate of DNA synthesis. These defects are due to the inability to arrest the cell cycle at the G1 and G2 phase in response to DNA damage, instead progressing to the S phase and mitosis, respectively. It is believed that the ATM protein activates the p53 protein, triggering the p53 signaling pathway involved in checkpoint regulation in the DNA cell cycle.

In addition, there is evidence that ATM is involved in the activation of proteins involved in DNA strand repair and recombination regulation. The absence of this functional protein leads to higher rates of intrachromosomal recombination, rearrangement interruptions of the T-cell receptor and immunoglobulin heavy chain gene, and ultimately genetic instability. The ability to repair damaged DNA remains intact in patients with ataxia–telangiectasia, who appear to have defects in rejoining breaks in DNA strands. These breaks in double-stranded DNA may induce apoptosis, leading to cell death when exposed to ionizing radiation. The ATM gene is also involved in meiosis, possibly explaining the etiology behind gonadal atrophy and impaired fertility in ataxia–telangiectasia. It appears that these defects in DNA synthesis and repair lead to degenerative CNS changes and to premature senescence, in addition to failure of organ maturation, malignancy, and immunologic abnormalities.

Clinical Manifestations

Affected children have ataxia that becomes evident when they begin to walk. At the same time, problems with choreoathetosis, nystagmus, and difficulty in initiating voluntary eye movements develop. Telangiectasias develop between 2 and 8 years of age and occur first as wire-like vessels on the bulbar conjunctiva, and later on the exposed areas of the auricle, the neck, and the flexor folds of the extremities. Other skin abnormalities may include premature graying of hair, loss of subcutaneous fat, vitiligo, and café-au-lait spots. Endocrine abnormalities frequently develop with time, and include hyperinsulinism with insulin resistance, hypogonadism with delayed sexual development, and growth retardation. Recurrent sinopulmonary infections occur in most patients, with eventual bronchiectasis, respiratory failure, and death.

Defects in both cellular and humoral immunity are seen. Cellular defects are to be expected, in view of the consistent finding of an absent or hypoplastic thymus. They include impaired skin test responses to recall antigens, reduced lymphocyte numbers, and reduced percentages of T cells. Two-thirds of patients have a reduced in vitro proliferative response to mitogens and to specific antigens. Antigen challenge with foreign protein or with virus produces a poor antibody response related to abnormal antibody levels. Seventy percent of patients are IgA deficient, and 80% are IgE deficient. These defects are caused primarily by defective antibody synthesis. It is hypothesized that genetic recombination, required for normal humoral and cellular immune function, is impaired with deficiency of the ATM gene. There is persistent production of fetal proteins, as evidenced by the nearly constant finding of elevated serum α-fetoprotein levels.

Approximately 10% of patients develop malignancy, usually before the age of 15. Eighty percent of these neoplasms are lymphoproliferative disorders. In addition, those who are heterozygous for the ATM gene are at a three- to fivefold increased risk for malignancy, particularly breast cancer in women. These striking abnormalities are believed to be due to compromised immune surveillance, chromosomal instability, and possible tumor suppressor function of the ATM gene.

Treatment

Therapy is limited to treatment of infections, early detection of malignancy, and genetic counseling. Most patients die of infection or malignancy in childhood. Although genetic testing is available, its use is limited by the cost and the labor intensiveness of these tests. Currently over 400 known mutations have been found on the ATM gene, and genotype–phenotype relationships remain poorly understood. The diagnosis may be suspected antenatally by the in utero elevation of α-fetoprotein concentration. Although most treatments are symptomatic, some data show that iron chelators may increase the genetic stability of AT cells and hopefully may provide a treatment option for this disorder.

OTHER NEUROCUTANEOUS DISEASES

von Hippel–Lindau Syndrome

This condition is characterized by single or multiple benign cerebellar tumors of capillaries. These tumors gradually increase in size, producing cerebellar signs. The retina may also be involved, with vascular proliferation. A port-wine stain may occur over the head and neck in some patients, but most have no cutaneous lesions. The defect in von Hippel–Lindau syndrome is found on chromosome 3p26, which encodes a tumor suppressor gene.

Waardenburg's Syndrome (OMIM *193500)

This syndrome combines piebaldism, depigmented macules on the skin, congenital deafness, and ocular hypertelorism. In this disorder, melanocytes are totally absent from the depigmented areas. It is categorized into four types. Type I, which is most associated with dystopia canthorum and white forelock, is an autosomal dominant disorder with its defect located on the PAX 3 gene on chromosome 2q35. Type II (which is subdivided into two groups, A and B) is associated with increased frequency of deafness, but does not present with dystopia canthorum. Type IIA is linked to chromosome 3p14.1-p12.3, and type IIB is found on chromosome 1p21. Type III is a severe form due to the homozygous inheritance of the abnormal PAX 3 gene. Type IV, inherited in an autosomal recessive manner, has a defect in the endothelin receptor B gene on chromosome 13.

Incontinentia Pigmenti (OMIM #308300)

Incontinentia pigmenti is an X-linked dominant (localized in Xq28) disorder that is usually fatal in utero in affected males. It presents in the perinatal period as scattered vesicular inflammatory lesions and progresses over a matter of months to verrucous lesions that are eventually replaced by hyperpigmentation (Fig. 34–9). In about 80% of patients other congenital abnormalities of the CNS, bones, eyes, and teeth may occur. CNS involvement occurs in 25% of cases, and may include epilepsy, microcephaly, mental retardation, and slow motor development. The biologic effect of the genetic defect is unknown and represents an unusual combination of an inflammatory cutaneous disorder and congenital CNS abnormalities.

Hypomelanosis of Ito (Incontinentia Pigmenti Achromians OMIM #300337)

This disorder is characterized by depigmented macules that are not preceded by the inflammatory patches noted in incontinentia pigmenti. Pigmentary abnormalities may give a whorled or streaked appearance (Fig. 34–10) and may be present at birth, or may develop early in childhood. Nervous system

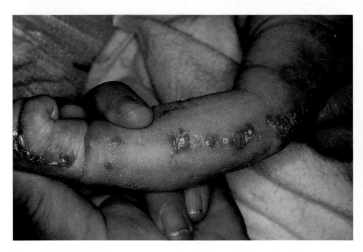

Figure 34–9 Multiple verrucous and vesiculated lesions in a linear distribution in this patient with incontinentia pigmenti.

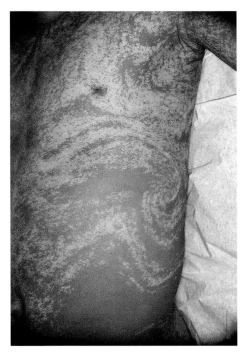

Figure 34–10 Hypopigmented swirls of skin in a patient with incontinentia pigmenti achromians.

abnormalities occur in about half of the patients and may include seizures, electroencephalogram abnormalities, strabismus, and language retardation. Hypopigmentation tends to fade with age. Most of the defects are due to unbalanced translocations or aneuploidy.

Vogt–Koyanagi–Harada Syndrome

This syndrome features depigmentation of the skin (especially of the eyebrows and eyelashes), headache, stiff neck, uveitis, and, occasionally, optic neuritis. Onset is associated with a febrile illness and is not known to be inherited or related to an existing neural crest defect.

Epidermal Nevus (Nevus Unius Lateris, Systematized Nevus)

This disorder is characterized by unilateral or occasionally bilateral verrucous papules or scaling plaques that are arranged in continuous or interrupted streaks (Fig. 34–11). The lesions vary in color from yellow to brown and are usually asymptomatic. A subset has a mosaic expression of epidermolytic hyperkeratosis with abnormal keratins 1 and 10. The offspring of affected patients are at increased risk for this autosomal dominant disorder. Otherwise, there is no known hereditary predisposition. Histologically, one sees benign hyperkeratosis, acanthosis, and papillomatosis of epidermal cells. Epidermal nevi may be associated with skeletal deformities and CNS disease, including arteriovenous malformations, epilepsy, mental retardation, and peripheral nerve disorders. Although the lesions frequently appear to have a dermatomal distribution, there is no pathogenetic link between the skin lesion and the peripheral nerve, as is seen in herpes zoster. Rather, this association represents the coexistence of unexplained abnormalities in structures that share an ectodermal origin. Sebaceous nevi have also been reported to be associated with similar CNS defects.

Ectodermal Dysplasia

Hidrotic ectodermal dysplasia is an autosomal dominant disorder characterized by dystrophic nails, hypotrichosis, palmoplantar keratosis, and dental abnormalities. Sweat glands are normal. Neural deafness, epilepsy, and mental retardation may occur.

Ichthyosis-Associated Syndromes

There have been many cases of congenital abnormalities of the nervous system associated with ichthyosis, usually lamellar ichthyosis. These include the following:

1. Sjögren–Larsson syndrome, which is an autosomal recessive disorder localized to chromosome 17p11.2, and is characterized by lamellar ichthyosis, thickened palms and soles, mental retardation, epilepsy, and spastic diplegia or quadriplegia.
2. Rud's syndrome, which is believed to be a sex-linked disorder characterized by generalized ichthyosis of uncertain type in association with epilepsy and mental retardation.
3. Cases described by Tay that were characterized by lamellar ichthyosis, thickening of the palms and soles, pili torti, mental retardation, dwarfism, and progeria-like facies.
4. Jorizzo and coworkers described two patients in whom lamellar ichthyosis was found in association with involvement of the palms, soles, nails, and trichothiodystrophy. Subsequent patients have been reported as having IBIDS (ichthyosis, brittle hair, intellectual impairment, decreased fertility, and short stature) syndrome or trichothiodystrophy. Associated defects included dwarfism, mental retardation, and defective teeth.

The remaining disorders listed in Table 34–1 include a variety of metabolic, infectious, and immune disorders in which both the skin and the nervous system are affected. For the most part, this occurs on the basis of circulating factors or pathogens that affect both organ systems. Many of these disorders are discussed in other parts of the text. The clinical findings of these disorders will be briefly described.

Metabolic Disorders

Angiokeratoma corporis diffusum (Fabry's disease) is caused by defective galactosidase A (ceramide trihexosidase) (see Chapter 37). The characteristic cutaneous finding is that of clusters of dark red to blue-black angiectases, especially in the scrotum or umbilical area. Neurologic findings frequently include extremity pain and paresthesias, which may be indicative of lipid infiltration of the vasa nervorum. Cerebral findings are multiple and result from multifocal small-vessel involvement of cerebral arteries.

Congenital as well as acquired hypothyroidism may produce dryness and laxity of the skin, with coarseness of the hair. If left uncorrected, congenital hypothyroidism may be associated with profound psychomotor maldevelopment.

Disorders of amino acid metabolism frequently cause abnormalities of hair and skin in combination with neurologic disease. The best known example is phenylketonuria, in which reduced pigmentation of hair and skin and frequently atopic dermatitis are associated with mental deficiency and epilepsy. Myriad other cutaneous findings may be found in various aminoacidurias, which will not be detailed here.

Infectious Disorders

Both herpes simplex and herpes zoster represent an intimate pathogenic association between skin and peripheral nerves. Migration of latent virus along sensory nerves causes the char-

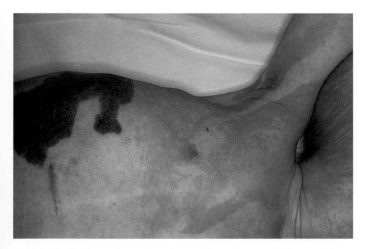

Figure 34–11 The patient shown has epidermal nevus syndrome with multiple anomalies, hemangiomas, and epidermal nevi, as represented by the fine, slightly pigmented skin.

acteristic lesions of cutaneous herpes infections. Clinically, pain and tingling precede the cutaneous eruption by hours to days. Viral exanthems may be of great help when searching for causes of encephalitis.

The remaining infectious disorders are self-explanatory. Bacterial sepsis may produce both meningitis and skin lesions of septic vasculitis, as typified by meningococcemia. Rocky Mountain spotted fever is characterized by a progression of erythematous papules of the extremities that subsequently become hemorrhagic. CNS findings include headache, occasionally meningeal symptoms, and even coma.

Immune Disorders

Immune disorders frequently affect both skin and nervous system, usually via inflammation of blood vessels. In such cases, neurologic symptoms may range from headaches to cerebral vascular accidents. Cutaneous findings include palpable purpuric papules (Henoch–Schönlein purpura). Behçet's syndrome may additionally show scattered, sterile pustules that progress to pyoderma gangrenosum-like lesions. Lupus erythematosus is discussed elsewhere in the text.

SUGGESTED READINGS

Bissler JJ, McCormack FX, Young LR, et al. Sirolimus for angiomyolipoma in tuberous sclerosis complex or lymphangioleiomyomatosis. N Engl J Med 2008; 358: 140–151.

DeBella K, Szudek J, Friedman JL. Use of the National Institutes of Health criteria for diagnosis of neurofibromatosis 1 in children. Pediatrics 2000; 105: 608–614.

Ferner RE. Neurofibromatosis 1 and neurofibromatosis 2: a twenty first century perspective. Lancet Neurol 2007; 6: 340–351.

Ferner RE, Huson SM, Thomas N, et al. Guidelines for the diagnosis and management of individuals with neurofibromatosis 1. J Med Genet 2007; 44: 81–88.

Hyman MH, Whittemore VH. National Institutes of Health consensus conference: tuberous sclerosis complex. Arch Neurol 2000; 57: 662–665.

Paul E, Thiele E. Efficacy of sirolimus in treating tuberous sclerosis and lymphangioleiomyomatosis. N Engl J Med 2008; 358: 190–192.

Riccardi VM. The potential role of trauma and mast cells in the pathogenesis of neurofibromas, tuberous sclerosis and neurofibromatosis: Epidemiology, pathophysiology, biology and management. Amsterdam, Elsevier Science, 1990, 167–190.

Thomas-Sohl KA, Vaslow DF, Maria B. Sturge–Weber syndrome: a review. Pediatr Neurol 2004; 30: 303–310.

Lisa M. Cohen and
George Kroumpouzos

Chapter | 35 |

Pregnancy

The skin may undergo adaptive physiologic changes in response to pregnancy or, at the other extreme, develop a true pathologic process. Pregnancy-related cutaneous changes are classified into the following categories: (1) physiologic changes; (2) pruritus in pregnancy; (3) changes to cutaneous tumors; (4) pre-existing skin disease or internal disease with skin manifestations affected by pregnancy; (5) dermatoses specific to pregnancy. This chapter reviews these categories, emphasizing correct classification of skin problems in pregnancy and prompt recognition of the associated maternal or fetal risks.

PHYSIOLOGIC SKIN CHANGES

The physiologic cutaneous changes of pregnancy are caused by endocrine, metabolic, mechanical, and blood flow alterations. The physiologic skin changes that are induced by pregnancy do not impair the health of the mother or fetus but can cause cosmetic complaints; these are expected to improve or resolve postpartum.

Pigmentary Changes

Hyperpigmentation

Up to 90% of pregnant women demonstrate some degree of hyperpigmentation, which is usually mild, generalized, and most noticeable in normally pigmented areas, such as the areolae, genital skin, and inner thighs. A familiar example of localized darkening is the linea nigra, a darkening of the linea alba (the tendinous median line on the anterior abdominal wall), which appears in the first trimester of pregnancy and is more pronounced in dark-complexioned women. Hyperpigmentation may also affect the skin adjoining the areolae. Pigmentary demarcation lines have been reported to darken or appear de novo. Uncommon pigmentary patterns that can be encountered in pregnancy include pseudoacanthosis nigricans, vulvar melanosis, dermal melanocytosis, and verrucous areolar hyperpigmentation.

Melasma (chloasma) or 'mask of pregnancy' has been reported in 50–75% of pregnant women. It usually appears in the second trimester, and is more prominent in dark-complexioned women. It refers to symmetric, irregular, poorly demar-

cated, hyperpigmented patches on the malar areas (malar pattern) or often on the entire central face (centrofacial pattern); hyperpigmentation of the ramus of the mandible (mandibular pattern) is encountered in less than 10% of cases. Melasma also occurs in up to one-third of women taking oral contraceptives, 87% of whom also experience melasma in pregnancy. Melasma is caused by melanin deposition in the epidermis (70%; enhancement under Wood's light), dermal macrophages (10–15%; no enhancement under Wood's light), or both (20%); a Wood's-inapparent form can be seen in dark-skinned patients. Although the etiology of melasma has not been fully clarified, the ultraviolet light and hormonal changes of gestation appear to play a role. Estrogens show melanogenic effects in vitro, and an increased expression of α-melanocyte-stimulating hormone has been shown in melasma.

Melasma usually resolves postpartum, although persistence has been reported in up to 30% of patients after 10 years. It may recur in subsequent pregnancies or with the use of oral contraceptives. Preventive measures include the use of a broad-spectrum sunscreen, avoidance of potentially irritating and sensitizing cosmetics, and use of nonhormonal methods of contraception. Recalcitrant melasma can be treated postpartum with hydroquinone (2–4%) with or without tretinoin (0.05–0.1%) and a low-potency topical corticosteroid. Challenging cases have been treated postpartum with combination therapies including laser treatment and chemical peels.

Jaundice

Severe hepatic dysfunction during pregnancy is rare; the most common cause of jaundice in pregnant women is viral hepatitis. The serum bilirubin level may increase in 2–6% of uncomplicated pregnancies but is almost always less than 2 mg/dL. Jaundice can develop in severe cases of intrahepatic cholestasis of pregnancy (discussed in the section on 'pruritus in pregnancy').

Vascular Changes

These result from a dramatic increase in blood flow to the skin, which is secondary to increased blood volume and rising estrogen levels.

Spider Nevus (Nevus Araneus, or Spider Angioma)

Spider angiomas have been reported in about two-thirds of white women and 11% of black women between the second and fifth months of pregnancy; these lesions increase slowly in number and size until term. Spider angiomas are small telangiectases radiating from a central 'feeding' arteriole; many show an anemic 3–4-mm halo. The spider angiomas of pregnancy develop most commonly in areas drained by the superior vena cava, such as the neck, throat, face, and arms, and may resolve spontaneously postpartum. Treatment modalities, such as electrodessication and pulsed dye laser, can be employed after delivery in women who find them cosmetically troublesome.

Palmar Erythema

Approximately 70% of white women and 30% of black women develop palmar erythema in pregnancy. The erythema is symmetric and blanching, but may occasionally be diffuse or mottled, and follows the same time course as the spider angiomas. It develops on hypothenar and thenar areas, the first phalanges, and the tips of terminal phalanges. It is indistinguishable from that seen in patients with hyperthyroidism or hepatic cirrhosis.

Edema

Nonpitting edema of the eyelids, face and lower extremities develops usually in late pregnancy and may be present in one-third of women by the 38th week. Edema of the eyelids occurs in approximately 50% of pregnant women, whereas edema of the lower extremities (unrelated to pregnancy-induced hypertension or pre-eclampsia) develops in about 70%. However, the presence of edema in a pregnant woman should alert the physician to the possibility of pregnancy-induced hypertension, which carries a significant risk to mother and fetus.

Varicosities

Varicosities of the lower extremities appear in 40% of pregnant women. Prolonged sitting and standing and use of elastic garters and panty girdles may be exacerbating factors. Gradient support hose, frequent elevation of the legs, sleeping in a Trendelenburg position, reclining in a lateral decubitus position, and avoiding clothing that interferes with venous return should be instituted. Varicosities may improve postpartum but do not usually regress completely, and are likely to recur in subsequent pregnancies.

Cutis Marmorata

This appears on the lower extremities as a transient, bluish, mottled discoloration upon exposure to cold. It has been attributed to vasomotor instability secondary to increased estrogen levels.

Striae Gravidarum

Striae gravidarum (striae distensae, or stretch marks) are seen in about 90% of white pregnant women during the last trimes-

ter. They are less common in Asians and blacks, and show a familial tendency. Apart from genetic susceptibility, other risk factors include younger maternal age, increased pregnancy weight gain, and concomitant use of topical steroids. These irregular, linear, atrophic, and finely wrinkled bands develop opposite the skin tension lines; their red color tends to become pale or white over time. They first appear on the abdomen and then on the breasts, upper arms, lower back, buttocks, thighs, and inguinal areas. They may become less apparent postpartum, but do not usually disappear. Cosmetically bothersome striae can be treated postpartum with tretinoin 0.1% cream with or without topical glycolic acid (up to 20%), with some success. The erythema of striae responds well to pulsed dye laser and intense pulsed light treatment.

Glandular Changes

Eccrine function has been reported to increase during pregnancy, which may explain the increased prevalence of miliaria, dyshidrosis, and hyperhidrosis. Reduced sweating, however, has been reported on the palms. Apocrine gland activity may decrease during pregnancy, contributing to the reduced prevalence of Fox–Fordyce disease in pregnancy. Nevertheless, the effect of pregnancy on hidradenitis suppurativa, another disease of the apocrine glands, seems to be less beneficial than previously thought. Variable changes in sebaceous gland activity have been reported, and the course of acne during gestation is unpredictable. One study showed that acne was affected by pregnancy in 70% of patients, with 41% experiencing improvement and 29% worsening with gestation. Sebaceous glands on the areolae enlarge in the first trimester and appear as small brown papules (Montgomery's glands or tubercles).

Hair Changes

Hirsutism occurs in most pregnant women, generally beginning in early pregnancy. It is more prominent in women with abundant body hair or dark hair at the outset. It is most pronounced on the face (upper lip, chin, and cheeks), but may also involve the arms, legs, back, and genital skin areas. Suprapubic midline hair growth may also be increased during pregnancy. Most of the new fine lanugo hair regresses within 6 months postpartum, although the coarse, bristly hair usually remains. If hirsutism is severe, androgen-secreting tumors of the ovary, luteomas, lutein cysts, and polycystic ovary disease should be excluded.

Postpartum hair shedding (telogen effluvium) refers to hair loss that results when a greater proportion of hairs enter the telogen phase in a synchronous fashion. In the later stages of pregnancy as much as 95% of scalp hair is in the anagen phase, which abruptly cycles into the telogen phase after delivery. Postpartum telogen hair counts of 24% at 6 weeks and 65% at 2 months have been reported. Causes of this shift can be the stress of delivery and changes in endocrine balance, including prolactin secretion with breastfeeding. Increased hair loss becomes apparent several months later; the severity of telogen effluvium varies considerably among patients. Hair regrowth occurs spontaneously within 6–12 months, but complete resolution may require up to 15 months; nevertheless, the hair may occasionally not be as thick as it was before pregnancy, especially in women with concomitant female pattern hair loss.

Frontoparietal hair recession reminiscent of male pattern alopecia has been reported in the later months of pregnancy. This usually reverts to normal hair growth pattern postpartum. Diffuse hair thinning during the later months of pregnancy has also been reported, and was thought to be secondary to inhibition of anagen hairs.

Nail Changes

Nail changes in pregnancy include transverse grooving, brittleness, softening, distal onycholysis, and subungual hyperkeratosis. These changes may occur as early as the sixth week of pregnancy and their etiology remains unclear. It seems, however, that some of these nail changes may also be seen in nonpregnant women taking oral contraceptives. Nail changes are expected to improve postpartum, and generally no specific treatment is required. External sensitizers (nail polish and polish removers) should be eliminated, and infections need to be ruled out. The nails should be kept short, especially if they are brittle or show onycholysis; the use of a rich nail moisturizer can be helpful.

Mucous Membrane Changes

Marginal gingivitis affects most pregnant women and is more noticeable about the lower front teeth. It appears in the first trimester of pregnancy and worsens until the ninth month, at which point the inflammation starts to improve. It is characterized by edematous, hyperemic gums that may bleed spontaneously or in response to minimal injury or tooth brushing. Enlargement and blunting of one or more dental papillae are seen, and the marginal gingiva becomes engorged, shiny and smooth. This gingivitis persists throughout pregnancy and may last for 1–2 months postpartum. The pyogenic granuloma of pregnancy develops in 2% of patients with gingivitis (discussed under 'cutaneous tumors affected by pregnancy'). Other mucous membrane changes in pregnancy include a bluish or purple discoloration of the vaginal mucosa (Chadwick's sign) and a bluish discoloration of the cervix (Goodell's sign).

PRURITUS IN PREGNANCY

Pruritus has been reported in 3–14% of pregnancies, and is the most common cutaneous symptom of gestation. Before pruritus can be attributed to pregnancy status, pruritic skin diseases (such as atopic dermatitis, drug eruption, pediculosis, and scabies) and systemic skin diseases complicated by pruritus (lymphoma, liver, renal, and thyroid disease) need to be ruled out. When the above etiologies have been ruled out and the pruritus is not associated with an eruption (primary skin lesions), the diagnosis of intrahepatic cholestasis of pregnancy (ICP) should be considered (discussed below).

Intrahepatic Cholestasis of Pregnancy

Intrahepatic cholestasis of pregnancy is the most common pregnancy-induced liver disorder. Hormonal, immunologic, genetic, environmental, and alimentary factors have been implicated in its etiopathogenesis. The prevalence of intrahepatic cholestasis of pregnancy varies dramatically worldwide, the highest being in Chile, Bolivia, and Scandinavia; in 50% of cases there is a family history. The spectrum of expression of intrahepatic cholestasis of pregnancy varies from mild pruritus without jaundice (pruritus gravidarum) to cholestatic jaundice (obstetric cholestasis). Excoriations due to scratching are typically seen, but there are no primary skin lesions. Pruritus typically develops after 30 weeks' gestation and may precede the laboratory abnormalities of the condition; it is occasionally accompanied by mild nausea and discomfort in the right upper quadrant. Mild jaundice (20%) may develop 2–4 weeks after the onset of itching, and is accompanied by subclinical steatorrhea and an increased risk of hemorrhage secondary to malabsorption of vitamin K. Half of the patients may notice darker urine and light-colored stools.

Laboratory abnormalities include mild abnormalities of liver function tests (transaminases, alkaline phosphatase, cholesterol, and triglycerides) that indicate a cholestatic pattern. Elevation of serum bile acids, especially postprandial levels, is the most sensitive biochemical marker of intrahepatic cholestasis of pregnancy and correlates with the severity of pruritus. Serum bilirubin is elevated in jaundiced patients. The symptoms and laboratory abnormalities of intrahepatic cholestasis of pregnancy resolve within 2–4 weeks postpartum. Intrahepatic cholestasis of pregnancy may recur in subsequent pregnancies (40–60%) or with oral contraceptives. The patient should be advised to avoid oral contraceptives because they can precipitate the pruritus. Fetal risks include distress, stillbirth, and prematurity. Malabsorption of vitamin K has been associated with an increased risk of intracranial hemorrhage; prophylactic administration of vitamin K has been advocated. The increased prevalence of fetal risks makes intensive fetal surveillance mandatory.

Symptomatic treatment with topical corticosteroids, antipruritics, emollients, and oral antihistamines may be effective only in mild cases of intrahepatic cholestasis of pregnancy. Ursodeoxycholic acid (450–1200 mg/day) is first-line treatment for moderate to severe cholestasis, and reduces bile acid levels in cord blood, colostrum, and amniotic fluid. Ursodeoxycholic acid works faster than any other oral medication, and is safe for both mother and fetus. There is substantial evidence that ursodeoxycholic acid reduces the fetal risks associated with intrahepatic cholestasis of pregnancy. Cholestyramine (up to 18 g/day) can be effective but does not improve the biochemical abnormalities of intrahepatic cholestasis of pregnancy, and may be associated with rebound of pruritus after the first week of treatment. It needs to be administered in conjunction with weekly vitamin K supplementation because it can precipitate vitamin K. Epomediol, silymarin, S-adenosyl-L-methionine, activated charcoal, and phenobarbital have met with limited results, and the initial promising results of dexamethasone treatment were not confirmed by a recent randomized placebo-controlled trial. Effective control of pruritus with ultraviolet B light has been reported in some cases.

CUTANEOUS TUMORS AFFECTED BY PREGNANCY

Various cutaneous tumors are affected by pregnancy (Table 35–1).

Granuloma Gravidarum, or Pregnancy Epulis (Pyogenic Granuloma of Pregnancy)

This occurs in about 2% of women and is a vascular proliferation arising from the interdental gingival papillae or the buccal or lingual mucosa, usually in the setting of pregnancy-induced gingivitis, but may also develop in extramucosal locations. Clinically, it is a dark red, oval or rounded, easily bleeding tumor that appears in pregnant women after the first trimester and continues to enlarge until delivery, after which it typically resolves spontaneously. It tends to recur in subsequent pregnancies. Interventions such as electrodesiccation or excision during pregnancy may not impede the tumor's growth.

Molluscum Fibrosum Gravidarum

These are soft tissue fibromas (acrochordons or skin tags) that may increase in number or enlarge during gestation, and may not regress postpartum. They are pedunculated, skin-colored or slightly pigmented papules or nodules that range from 1–5 mm to several centimeters in size, and appear usually on the sides of the neck, inframammary areas, chest, and axillae. Treatment consists of removal or destruction of the lesions by various methods, including snipping, cryotherapy, and electrocautery.

Pigmented Lesions

Melanocytic nevi and ephelides often darken and/or increase in size during pregnancy. New nevi may appear. A case of disseminated Spitz nevi that developed in pregnancy was reported. Recent studies using dermoscopic analysis of nevi showed that the pigment network becomes thicker and more evident and the globules darker during pregnancy, features that are accompanied by some architectural changes. Nevertheless, these features return to their original condition 1 year after delivery. A statistically significant increase in diameter in nevi on the front of the body between the first and third trimesters of pregnancy, reported in a recent dermoscopic study, was attributed to the expansion of the skin during pregnancy. No treatment is generally required, although some authors have suggested excision of fast-growing melanocytic lesions. The pregnant woman should be advised that there is no evidence that gestation induces malignant transformation of pre-existing nevi.

Neurofibromas

These often enlarge or develop in pregnancy, but may regress postpartum. They can be complicated by massive hemorrhage within the tumor. Pregnant women with neurofibromatosis are at high risk of vascular complications during pregnancy, such as hypertension and renal artery rupture. Fetal risks include spontaneous abortion, stillbirth, intrauterine growth retardation, and perinatal complications.

Melanoma

Women in their reproductive years account for 30–35% of patients with melanoma. Despite initial concerns about an adverse effect of pregnancy on malignant melanoma, several epidemiologic studies evaluating the effect of pregnancy status at diagnosis on the prognosis of melanoma showed that the 5-year survival rate was not affected after controlling for other factors. This has been attributed to the inhibitory effect of estrogens on melanoma cell lines through type II estrogen receptors, and the fact that melanoma cell lines lack type I estrogen receptors. The major prognostic factors in the largest study that included pregnant women with localized melanoma are tumor thickness (Breslow's level) and ulceration status, with level of invasion only significant in women with tumors <1 mm thick. Placental and fetal metastases are extraordinarily rare (27 cases), and even in the case of placental metastasis, fetal metastasis occurs in only 17% of cases. The presence of placental metastases is associated with a dismal maternal prognosis. For pregnant women with metastatic disease, the risks and benefits of adjuvant systemic therapy should be discussed; the option of termination of pregnancy should be considered early.

Table 35–1 Cutaneous tumors affected by pregnancy
Dermatofibroma
Dermatofibrosarcoma protuberans
Desmoid tumor
Granuloma gravidarum (pyogenic granuloma)
Hemangioma
Hemangioendothelioma
Glomangioma
Glomus tumor
Keloid
Leiomyoma
Melanocytic nevus
Melanoma
Molluscum fibrosum gravidarum (acrochordon)
Neurofibroma

PRE-EXISTING SKIN DISEASES AND INTERNAL DISEASES WITH SKIN MANIFESTATIONS AFFECTED BY PREGNANCY

Various diseases are often aggravated by pregnancy (Table 35-2). Diseases that may improve during gestation, however, include chronic plaque psoriasis, sarcoidosis, Fox–Fordyce disease, hidradenitis suppurativa, atopic dermatitis, acne vulgaris, autoimmune progesterone dermatitis, linear IgA disease, and rheumatoid arthritis.

Atopic Dermatitis

Atopic dermatitis is the most common dermatosis in pregnancy, accounting for 36–49% of total cases. Exacerbation of atopic dermatitis (52%) is more likely than remission (24%). A history of atopy has been reported in 27%, a family history of atopy in 50%, and a history of infantile eczema in offspring in 19% of all eczema cases in pregnancy. Atopic dermatitis can develop for the first time in pregnancy: the prevalence of 'new eczema' (diagnosis of eczema established for the first time in pregnancy) was high in the largest study on pruritic dermatoses. The clinical presentation of eczema in pregnancy is identical to that in the nonpregnant woman; less common presentations are follicular truncal eczema, facial eczema, and dyshidrosis. Bacterial or antiviral superinfection can develop during pregnancy.

The disease is not associated with an increased risk of adverse fetal outcomes. The influence of breastfeeding and maternal food antigen avoidance during pregnancy and lactation on atopic eczema in the offspring has been debated. Risk factors for development of infantile eczema include black and Asian race/ethnicity, male gender, higher gestational age at birth, a maternal history of eczema, and maternal smoking.

Impetigo Herpetiformis

Impetigo herpetiformis is a variant of generalized pustular psoriasis triggered by pregnancy, hypocalcemia, or infections during gestation in a genetically predisposed individual. Although familial clustering has been reported, a personal or family history of psoriasis is often absent. It usually develops in the third trimester, but has also been reported in earlier trimesters and postpartum. Impetigo herpetiformis typically resolves postpartum, but recalcitrant cases have been reported and were often associated with the use of oral contraceptives.

The primary lesion in impetigo herpetiformis is a sterile pustule. These pustules are pinhead sized, superficially seated in the epidermis, and arranged in groups or rings at the periphery of erythematous patches. As confluent pustules in the center of the lesions dry, they form large yellow crusted plaques. New pustules develop at the periphery of the primary lesion, forming polycyclic lesions. The eruption is often generalized and usually more pronounced in the intertriginous areas, flexures, scalp, and neck. The face, hands, and feet are usually spared. The itching is usually mild. The oral mucosa can be involved with painful erosions, and the nails with resultant onycholysis or nail shedding. The onset of the eruption is accompanied by a high fever, malaise, chills, diarrhea, and vomiting, with resultant dehydration. Complications secondary to hypocalcemia, such as tetany, convulsions, and delirium, are seen less often.

Skin histopathology shows features of pustular psoriasis and is characterized by the spongiform macropustule of Kogoj. Laboratory abnormalities include leukocytosis, elevated erythrocyte sedimentation rate, and occasionally hypocalcemia, reduced serum vitamin D levels, or hypoparathyroidism. Cultures of pustular lesions and macropustules are usually negative, except in cases of bacterial superinfection.

Occasional case reports that span decades indicate serious maternal risks, including increased perinatal mortality from cardiac or renal failure or septicemia. These risks are currently uncommon, and maternal prognosis has improved dramatically with early diagnosis, supportive care, and aggressive treatment. Fetal risks, such as stillbirth, premature birth, and fetal abnormalities secondary to placental insufficiency, have been reported even when the disease was well controlled, and make intensive fetal monitoring mandatory.

Table 35–2 Skin diseases and internal diseases with cutaneous manifestations aggravated by pregnancy

Infections

Candida vaginitis
Trichomoniasis
Condyloma acuminatum
Pityrosporum folliculitis
Herpes simplex
Varicella-zoster
Leprosy
Acquired immunodeficiency syndrome

Autoimmune diseases

Lupus erythematosus
Systemic sclerosis
Dermatomyositis
Pemphigus vulgaris/vegetans
Pemphigus foliaceus

Metabolic diseases

Porphyria cutanea tarda
Acrodermatitis enteropathica

Connective tissue diseases

Ehlers–Danlos syndrome
Pseudoxanthoma elasticum

Miscellaneous disorders

Acanthosis nigricans
Bowenoid papulosis
Erythema multiforme
Erythema nodosum
Erythrokeratoderma variabilis
Hereditary hemorrhagic telangiectasia
Mycosis fungoides
Tuberous sclerosis

Impetigo herpetiformis may dramatically improve with systemic steroids: 20–40 mg/day of prednisone is usually effective. Successful treatment with cyclosporine has also been reported. Calcium and vitamin D supplementation should be undertaken when necessary, and can lead to dramatic improvement of the eruption. Supportive care to prevent dehydration and to treat bacterial superinfection may contribute to the favorable maternal outcome reported in the recent literature. Recalcitrant impetigo herpetiformis has been treated in the postpartum period with systemic steroids, oral retinoids, or PUVA, either as single agents or in combination. Postpartum administration of PUVA was combined in some cases with clofazimine or methotrexate, with good results.

Infections

Pregnancy increases the prevalence and severity of a number of infections (Table 35–2), most characteristically that of candida vaginitis, *Trichomonas*, *Pityrosporum* folliculitis, and papillomavirus infections. Candida vaginitis is more frequent during pregnancy (reported in up to 50% of pregnant women), but among those women who become infected 10–40% are asymptomatic. Candida vaginitis has been associated with intra-amniotic infection: the organism can be cultured from almost half of neonates born to infected mothers. Neonatal candidiasis can develop from passage of the infant through an infected birth canal. It is characterized by an erythematous, erosive eruption with satellite pustules involving the diaper area and/or thrush appearing several days after delivery. Congenital candidiasis is characterized by generalized erythematous papules and pustules that appear within 12 hours of delivery, and results from an ascending infection in utero.

Condylomata acuminata (genital warts) are caused by the human papillomavirus (HPV, types 6 and 11 being the most common). Condylomata have been reported to grow more rapidly during pregnancy, and may become so large that they can interfere with vaginal delivery. Condylomata acuminata in pregnant women have been associated with laryngeal papillomas in infants; these papillomas are most commonly caused by HPV types 2, 5, and 11. Cesarean delivery for the prevention of HPV transmission to the newborn has been debated. It may, however, be indicated when the pelvic outlet is obstructed by genital warts, or when vaginal delivery would result in excessive bleeding. Ablative or destructive therapies for condylomata are acceptable, but podophyllin therapy is contraindicated during pregnancy.

Maternal herpes simplex virus (HSV) infections associated with fetal risks include: (1) disseminated mucocutaneous and/or visceral HSV infection; (2) localized primary or recurrent genital HSV infection. Disseminated HSV infection may occur during the third trimester. Sequelae from dissemination can be severe, and increase maternal and fetal mortality rates to approximately 40%. Localized maternal genital HSV infection occurs either as a primary or a recurrent infection. Although transmission of HSV to the fetus may occur in either form, primary maternal genital infection poses a much higher risk to the fetus. The fetus acquiring HSV in the second or third trimesters may sustain severe neonatal morbidity and death. Prematurity, spontaneous abortion, intrauterine growth retar-

dation, and neonatal herpes may occur in 40% of neonates born to women with primary HSV infection during pregnancy. Neonatal herpes is often a mild illness localized to skin, eyes, and mouth, but may occasionally progress to encephalitis (15% mortality rate) or disseminated disease (57% mortality rate). Nevertheless, neonates exposed to HSV at the time of vaginal delivery to mothers with a history of recurrent genital HSV infections rarely become infected.

Primary varicella, especially in the third trimester, is associated with serious maternal and fetal risks: 21% of women who develop varicella during pregnancy have medical or obstetric complications. Pneumonia occurs in 9% and can be fatal. Premature labor is observed in 10% of cases. Fetal morbidity includes congenital varicella syndrome (associated with first-trimester infections), herpes zoster in infancy, primary varicella occurring at birth (associated with maternal varicella 10–14 days prior to birth), and neonatal varicella (associated with maternal varicella less than 10 days prior to delivery).

Leprosy reactions are triggered by pregnancy: type 1 (reversal) reaction peaks postpartum and type 2 reaction (erythema nodosum leprosum) occurs throughout pregnancy and lactation; the latter has been associated with 'silent neuritis,' with resultant early loss of nerve function. These reactions should be treated with oral steroids because thalidomide is contraindicated in pregnancy. Fetal risks include increased fetal mortality and low birthweight. Twenty percent of children born to mothers with leprosy will develop the disease by adolescence.

Autoimmune Diseases

Chronic cutaneous lupus erythematosus is not affected by gestation. Pregnant women with systemic lupus erythematosus not complicated by renal or cardiac disease, or who has been in remission for at least 3 months prior to conception, do not experience worsening of their disease in pregnancy. Exacerbation during pregnancy occurs in less than 10% of patients with mild renal dysfunction. Half of patients with active disease at the time of conception will worsen during gestation; this rate of exacerbation, however, is similar to that in nonpregnant women with active disease. When systemic lupus presents initially during pregnancy, a high rate of severe manifestations, such as renal disease, cardiac disease, hepatic disease, pancreatitis, fever, and lymphadenopathy, is observed. The rate of spontaneous abortion in affected patients is increased about two or four times above that observed in controls, and premature delivery occurs in 16–37% of pregnancies.

Neonatal lupus can develop secondary to transplacental passage of maternal anti-Ro/SS-A, or occasionally anti-La/SS-B or anti-U$_1$RNP antibodies. It is characterized by a self-limited papulosquamous or annular–polycyclic eruption and serious systemic complications, including congenital heart block (15–30%), pericarditis/myocarditis, cytopenias, and hepatosplenomegaly. The risk of bearing a second child with congenital heart block is 25%. Although half of mothers are asymptomatic, many of these women eventually develop a connective tissue disease. Recurrent fetal loss has been reported in women with antiphospholipid antibody syndrome. These patients may also have thrombotic venous or arterial disease, thrombocytopenia, and/or cardiac valve disease.

Dermatomyositis often worsens during gestation, and may occur for the first time in pregnancy. An exacerbation of cutaneous manifestations and/or proximal muscle weakness has been reported in about half of the affected individuals. Spontaneous abortions, stillbirths, and neonatal deaths have been reported in more than half of cases of active disease.

The skin manifestations of scleroderma are not affected by pregnancy, and Raynaud's phenomenon may improve. Pregnant women with limited disease do much better than those with systemic scleroderma.

Pemphigus vulgaris, vegetans, or foliaceus may develop or worsen during pregnancy, whereas linear IgA disease may improve. In cases of pemphigus vulgaris, fetal and neonatal skin lesions can develop secondary to transplacental transfer of IgG antibody, but resolve spontaneously within 2–3 weeks postpartum. Pemphigus has been associated with preterm labor or stillbirth, often in those cases in which the fetus had typical bullous lesions.

Other Diseases

Porphyria cutanea tarda, acute intermittent porphyria, and variegate porphyria can worsen in pregnancy because they are adversely affected by estrogen; exacerbation due to oral contraceptives has been reported. Exacerbation of porphyria cutanea tarda has been reported during the first trimester, followed by improvement later in pregnancy. These changes parallel an increase in serum estrogen levels and urinary porphyrins in the first trimester, and a fall in levels later in gestation. Fetal prognosis is not usually affected. Acrodermatitis enteropathica may flare early in gestation as serum zinc levels decrease, but may also flare with the use of oral contraceptives. Erythema nodosum can develop in pregnancy; it commonly occurs in the second trimester and usually persists until delivery.

Pregnancy may worsen the vascular complications of pseudoxanthoma elasticum, and has been associated with an increased risk of first-trimester miscarriage and intrauterine growth retardation. Ehlers–Danlos syndromes type I and IV have been associated with serious maternal complications in gestation and an increased maternal mortality. The serious maternal risks associated with the vascular complications of tuberous sclerosis, Marfan's syndrome, and hereditary hemorrhagic telangiectasia should be promptly recognized.

Autoimmune Progesterone Dermatitis

Autoimmune progesterone dermatitis is caused by hypersensitivity to progesterone through autoimmune or nonimmune mechanisms, and presents with premenstrual lesions that can have clinical features of urticaria, eczema, erythema multiforme, dyshidrotic eczema, or dermatitis herpetiformis-like eruption. In some cases premenstrual exacerbations were associated with exacerbation of the eruption during pregnancy. Nevertheless, autoimmune progesterone dermatitis improved or resolved during pregnancy in three cases, which has been attributed to the increased cortisol levels and/or gradual increase in the sex hormone levels during pregnancy, with

subsequent hormonal desensitization in some patients. Autoimmune estrogen dermatitis (attributed to estrogen sensitivity) has been reported in a patient presenting with urticaria in early pregnancy.

SPECIFIC DERMATOSES OF PREGNANCY

The classification of specific dermatoses of pregnancy has been a matter of controversy. Pemphigoid (herpes) gestationis and polymorphic eruption of pregnancy are well-defined entities; the etiopathogenesis of other dermatoses, such as the prurigo of pregnancy and pruritic folliculitis of pregnancy, is not well understood. A recent attempt to classify prurigo of pregnancy and pruritic folliculitis of pregnancy under a broad category of 'atopic eruption of pregnancy' has been debated.

Pemphigoid (Herpes) Gestationis

Pemphigoid (herpes) gestationis is a rare, pruritic, autoimmune skin disease of pregnancy and the puerperium that occurs in approximately 1:50 000 pregnancies. It shares many features with bullous pemphigoid, and has also been associated with choriocarcinoma or hydatidiform mole. Pemphigoid gestationis affects predominantly white women and usually starts in the second trimester of pregnancy; the onset of lesions has been reported as early as the second week after conception. Ten to 16% of cases occur in the early postpartum period. The cutaneous lesions are invariably accompanied by intense pruritus, and may appear abruptly or gradually as vesicles and bullae arising on erythematous or urticarial papules and/or plaques (Figs 35–1 and 35–2). The disease usually starts on the abdomen and involves the umbilicus. The lesions then spread to involve the trunk and limbs. Mucous membrane involvement is rare, and the face is usually spared. There is a tendency for annular patterns of new vesicles to develop at the periphery of the polycyclic lesions. Healing occurs without scarring unless there is superinfection. Pemphigoid

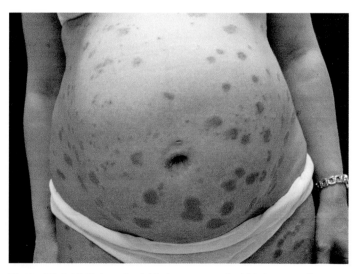

Figure 35–1 Multiple urticarial lesions, many of which have small vesicles at the periphery.

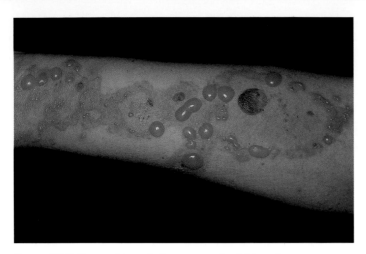

Figure 35–2 Grouped tense bullae on an urticarial base in a woman with herpes gestationis.

gestationis typically remits spontaneously just prior to delivery, only to flare at delivery or postpartum (75%). Oral contraceptive use has been implicated in postpartum flares. The duration of pemphigoid gestationis postpartum is highly variable, ranging from 5 weeks to 18 months. Patients who develop prolonged or chronic disease tend to be older, with higher parity, more generalized lesions, and a history of pemphigoid gestationis in previous pregnancies. Breastfeeding was associated with a significantly shorter duration of active lesions in a cohort of 25 patients. Pemphigoid gestationis recurs in 95% of future pregnancies; it may be more severe with each subsequent pregnancy, and usually starts earlier and persists longer postpartum. It may recur with menses in 12–64% of patients, and in 20–50% of women who use oral contraceptives.

Even though immunologic factors are crucial in the pathogenesis of pemphigoid gestationis, the mechanisms by which the disease is produced remain unknown. Although some authors have suggested that exposure to paternal antigens may play a role in disease initiation, 'skip pregnancies,' despite having the same partner, have been reported in 8% of cases. Direct immunofluorescence of perilesional skin shows linear C3 deposition along the basement membrane zone, with demonstrable IgG in only 25% of cases. Nevertheless, IgG is always positive when indirect complement-added immunofluorescence is performed. In salt-split testing, the antibody binds to the roof of the specimen. The antibody that incites the disease belongs to the IgG_1 subclass and targets an epitope (NC16A2 or MCW-1) in the noncollagenous domain of the bullous pemphigoid 180-kDa hemidesmosomal glycoprotein; it is believed to activate complement through the classic pathway. Linear deposition of C3 and IgG_1 has been shown also in the skin of neonates of affected mothers, and in the basement membrane zone of amniotic epithelium. A characteristic feature of pemphigoid gestationis is peripheral blood eosinophilia. Serum antibody levels and eosinophilia do not correlate with disease severity. Skin histopathology of urticarial lesions shows spongiotic epidermis, marked papillary dermal edema, and an eosinophilic infiltrate. Vacuolar degeneration of keratinocytes, occasionally accompanied by individual basal cell necrosis, and subepidermal blister formation

may be seen in early urticarial lesions, but is more prominent in fully developed bullae.

Pemphigoid gestationis has been associated with an increased maternal risk of Graves' disease. Several small cohorts have shown an association with low birthweight and premature delivery. The largest cohort of 74 women showed a 16% rate of delivery at less than 32 weeks in the pemphigoid (herpes) gestationis group versus 2% in the control group. The fetal complications are thought to be due to low-grade placental insufficiency. No increase in fetal mortality has been documented, with the exception of one case of fetal cerebral hemorrhage. Transient vesiculobullous lesions occur in 5–10% of neonates born to mothers with pemphigoid (herpes) gestationis secondary to passive transplacental transfer of pemphigoid gestationis antibody.

Oral steroids are the cornerstone of treatment. Dosages up to 180 mg/day of prednisone have been required to control the disease, although most patients respond promptly and rapidly to daily dosages of 20–40 mg. Prednisone should be tapered after control is achieved, but should be increased at the time of delivery in anticipation of the immediate postpartum exacerbation. Plasmapheresis is an alternative option when oral steroids are ineffective or contraindicated. Methotrexate, azathioprine, gold, cyclosporine, cyclophosphamide, high-dose intravenous immunoglobulin, and minocycline with niacinamide have been used postpartum in nonlactating mothers, with inconsistent results. Successful treatment of recalcitrant pemphigoid gestationis with goserelin-induced chemical oophorectomy or ritodrine has been reported.

Polymorphic Eruption of Pregnancy (Pruritic Urticarial Papules and Plaques of Pregnancy)

Polymorphic eruption of pregnancy is the most common specific dermatosis of pregnancy, occurring in about 1 : 240 pregnancies. Other terms used to describe this disorder include 'toxemic rash of pregnancy', 'late-onset prurigo of pregnancy', and 'toxic erythema of pregnancy'. Polymorphic eruption of pregnancy has not been traditionally associated with any fetal or maternal risks. An association with cesarean delivery and increased number of hospitalizations was recently reported. It occurs classically in primigravidae in the third trimester (80% of cases); onset of the disease in other trimesters or postpartum has been reported in the remainder. In two large studies it was associated with male fetuses in approximately 55% of cases. The disease resolves spontaneously within hours to days after delivery, and does not recur in subsequent pregnancies. The eruption begins with intensely pruritic, erythematous papules with edematous centers and surrounding blanched haloes. A typical feature is the onset of pruritic urticarial coalescing papules within abdominal striae in two-thirds of patients (Fig. 35–3). Nevertheless, the eruption is often polymorphous, including vesicular, purpuric, polycyclic, or targetoid lesions. Contrary to impetigo herpetiformis, the umbilicus and periumbilical area are usually spared. During the course of several days the lesions spread to involve the buttocks, proximal thighs, trunk, proximal arms, and breasts; the face, palms,

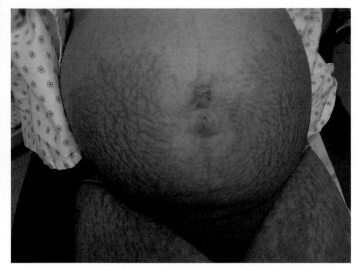

Figure 35–3 Polymorphic eruption of pregnancy typically starts with lesions along abdominal striae and shows sparing of the periumbilical area.

soles, and mucous membranes are usually spared. When generalized, polymorphic eruption of pregnancy may occasionally resemble atopic dermatitis or a toxic erythema.

The disease lacks pathognomonic histopathologic features and laboratory abnormalities. Skin histopathology shows variable epidermal changes, such as focal spongiosis, parakeratosis, mild acanthosis, and exocytosis, and a superficial and mid-dermal perivascular lymphohistiocytic infiltrate with variable numbers of eosinophils. Direct immunofluorescence studies are negative and help differentiate from the prebullous phase of pemphigoid gestationis.

The pathogenesis remains unclear. The immunohistologic profile of the skin lesions may imply a delayed hypersensitivity reaction to an unknown allergen. A significant increase in maternal and newborn birthweight and an association with multiple gestation pregnancy have been reported in patients with polymorphic eruption of pregnancy compared to age- and parity-matched controls. A recent meta-analysis of the authors revealed a 10-fold higher prevalence of multiple gestation pregnancy in women affected by polymorphic eruption of pregnancy. This lends support to the theory that rapid over-distension of the abdominal wall (or a reaction to it) may trigger an inflammatory process that starts polymorphic eruption of pregnancy. Interestingly, progesterone receptors were increased in lesions in one study, and progesterone has been shown to aggravate the inflammatory cutaneous process. Finally, fetal DNA was detected in polymorphic eruption of pregnancy lesions in one study, and it was suggested that migration of fetal cells to maternal skin can cause polymorphic eruption of pregnancy. Although pregnancy has been associated with peripheral blood chimerism, it remains speculative that the latter could be involved in the pathogenesis of polymorphic eruption of pregnancy, and has not been confirmed by any other studies.

Treatment is symptomatic, with antipruritic topical medications, topical steroids, and oral antihistamines. A short course of prednisone is rarely required and appears to have no adverse effect on pregnancy. Anecdotal reports show that UVB treat-

ment can be helpful. The pregnant woman should be reassured that the disease is not associated with any significant maternal or fetal risks, and that the perinatal outcome is favorable. The increased risk of cesarean delivery in women with polymorphic eruption of pregnancy that was shown in two recent large studies needs to be discussed with the patient. Nevertheless, induction of labor should be the last resort in every case, so that unnecessary cesarean section can be avoided. Induction of labor has not gained support even in the most refractory cases.

Prurigo of Pregnancy

Prurigo of pregnancy affects approximately 1:300–1:450 pregnancies. Many different names have been historically applied to this disease, including 'Besnier's prurigo gestationis,' 'Nurse's early prurigo of pregnancy' and 'papular dermatitis of Spangler.' It occurs predominantly in the second or third trimester of pregnancy. Prurigo of pregnancy was first described by Nurse as a pruritic, excoriated, papular eruption with occasional crusting, occurring mainly on the extensor surfaces of proximal extremities and trunk. The lesions may at times be nodular, reminiscent of prurigo nodularis. The disease runs a protracted course through gestation and typically resolves after delivery, although cases that persisted for up to 3 months postpartum have been reported. Recurrence with subsequent pregnancies is variable, and there is no increase in maternal or fetal morbidity or mortality. Early reports of a dismal fetal outcome by Spangler have not been confirmed.

The etiology of prurigo of pregnancy remains unknown. It has been associated with intrahepatic cholestasis of pregnancy, and some authors have suggested that the two disorders are closely associated and may represent different levels of severity of the same process. Nevertheless, the lack of liver function test abnormalities in prurigo of pregnancy would argue against this association. Other authors have recently classified prurigo of pregnancy under 'atopic eruption of pregnancy,' based on serum IgE elevation and a personal or family history of atopic dermatitis in a significant percentage of patients with prurigo of pregnancy. Nevertheless, many prurigo of pregnancy patients may fulfill only minor criteria of atopy, and IgE has not been measured in a control group of pregnant women without the eruption. Furthermore, the regulation of IgE in gestation seems to be affected by a number of factors that are not relevant to atopic disease, and warrants further investigation.

Treatment of prurigo of pregnancy is symptomatic, with topical antipruritic medications, moderately potent topical steroids, and oral antihistamines. The pregnant woman should be advised that the disease has not been associated with any fetal risks.

Pruritic Folliculitis of Pregnancy

Pruritic folliculitis of pregnancy is a rare sterile folliculitis that was first described by Zoberman and Farmer in six patients. Since the original report 26 cases have been reported. Nevertheless, it remains unclear whether some of the reported cases were true sterile folliculitis or, instead, microbial folliculitis.

The lesions usually develop between the fourth and ninth months of gestation and resolve spontaneously at delivery or in the early postpartum period; they may recur in subsequent pregnancies. Patients develop a generalized mildly pruritic eruption consisting of excoriated 3–5-mm erythematous papules and pustules. The lesions often show an acneiform appearance, although two patients had an urticarial component. Features of florid folliculitis, such as those seen in *Pityrosporum* folliculitis, are not observed. Skin histopathology is that of a sterile folliculitis, and stains for microorganisms are negative. Direct immunofluorescence and serologic tests are negative. Cultures from the pustules are negative and help exclude microbial folliculitis.

The etiology of pruritic folliculitis of pregnancy remains elusive, and some authors have suggested that it should not be included in specific dermatoses of pregnancy. Associations with increased serum androgens or intrahepatic cholestasis of pregnancy seem to have been coincidental. Clinical similarities with steroid acne prompted some authors to propose that pruritic folliculitis of pregnancy may be a form of hormonally induced acne. Nevertheless, there have been no studies that lend support to this theory, and pruritic folliculitis of pregnancy lacks a comedonal component that is typically seen in steroid acne. An effort to classify the disorder under polymorphic eruption of pregnancy based on reports of follicular lesions in some patients was unsuccessful because the clinical and histopathologic features of the two entities differ significantly. A recent study classified pruritic folliculitis of pregnancy under 'atopic eruption of pregnancy,' but this was based only on one case. Overall, data to support a revised classification of this entity have been insufficient.

Pruritic folliculitis of pregnancy has been treated with topical steroids, benzoyl peroxide, or narrowband UVB. Oral antihistamines are usually helpful in the relief of pruritus. The pregnant woman should be advised that the condition has not been associated with any fetal risks. A reduced birthweight and a male:female ratio of 2:1 that were reported in the largest series of patients may have been biased by the inclusion of cases of microbial folliculitis under pruritic folliculitis of pregnancy. Preterm delivery has been reported in one case.

SUGGESTED READINGS

Ambros-Rudolph CM, Müllegger RR, Vaughan-Jones SA, et al. The specific dermatoses of pregnancy revisited and reclassified: results of a retrospective two-center study on 505 pregnant patients. J Am Acad Dermatol 2006; 54: 395–404.

Cohen LM, Kroumpouzos G. Pruritic dermatoses of pregnancy: to lump or to split? J Am Acad Dermatol 2007; 56: 708–709.

Engineer L, Bhol K, Ahmed AR. Pemphigoid gestationis: a review. Am J Obstet Gynecol 2000; 183: 483–491.

Kroumpouzos G. Intrahepatic cholestasis of pregnancy: what's new. J Eur Acad Dermatol Venereol 2002; 16: 316–318.

Kroumpouzos G, Cohen LM. Dermatoses of pregnancy. J Am Acad Dermatol 2001; 45: 1–19.

Kroumpouzos G, Cohen LM. Specific dermatoses of pregnancy: an evidence-based systematic review. Am J Obstet Gynecol 2003; 188: 1083–1092.

Regnier S, Fermand V, Levy P, et al. A case–control study of polymorphic eruption of pregnancy. J Am Acad Dermatol 2008; 58: 63–67.

Winton GB. Skin diseases aggravated by pregnancy. J Am Acad Dermatol 1989; 20: 1–13.

Wong RC, Ellis CN. Physiologic skin changes in pregnancy. J Am Acad Dermatol 1984; 10: 929–940.

Zoberman E, Farmer ER. Pruritic folliculitis of pregnancy. Arch Dermatol 1981; 117: 20–22.

Mast Cell Disease

Mast cell disease (MCD), or mastocytosis, represents a spectrum of clinical disorders that results from an abnormal proliferation of mast cells. The onset ranges from the time of birth into late adulthood. Approximately 55% of patients develop mast cell disease by 2 years of age, and another 10% experience disease onset between the ages of 2 and 15 years. This disorder is equally distributed between males and females; it has been reported in all races, and most patients have no familial association; however, there have been over 40 cases of familial mast cell disease, some of which have involved several generations.

PATHOGENESIS

Mast cells (MCs) are derived from CD34+ precursor cells arising in the bone marrow and circulating as monocytic cells. Circulating mast cell precursors in the blood express CD34, the tyrosine kinase KIT (CD117), and FcγRII, but not high-affinity IgE receptors (FcεRI). KIT is a type III tyrosine kinase that is expressed on mast cells, melanocytes, primitive hematopoietic stem cells, primordial germ cells, and interstitial cells of Cajal. Activation of KIT induces cellular growth and differentiation. The ligand for KIT is stem cell factor (SCF), which is important for mast cell growth. SCF is produced by bone marrow stromal cells, fibroblasts, keratinocytes, endothelial cells, and reproductive Sertoli and granulosa cells. Under normal conditions, once mast cell precursors enter tissues they become KIT+/CD34–/FcγRII–/FcεRI+ and develop characteristic cytoplasmic granules.

Alterations in KIT structure have been implicated in the pathogenesis of adult-onset mast cell disease. Specifically, somatic point mutations in codon 816 (D816V, D816Y, D816F and D816H) of the c-kit proto-oncogene have been identified in adult mast cell disease patients without familial disease. This mutation causes constitutive activation of KIT, thereby leading to continued mast cell development. Additional mutations in c-kit (del419, K509I, F522C, V533D, A533D, V559A, V560G, R815K, I817V, D820G, E839K) also have been reported in mast cell disease, but appear to be rare and are less well characterized as a direct cause of mastocytosis. Although some children with mast cell disease have detectable c-kit mutations

(V533D, A533D, E539K, V559A, R815K, and D816F), most do not have demonstrable defects in this receptor. In fact, in some childhood-onset mastocytosis patients an inactivating c-kit mutation (E539K) has been described. In the extremely rare familial MCD, c-kit mutation detection has been variable, ranging from none to the expression of K509I and A533D mutations. Taken together, these observations suggest that there may be several different mechanisms responsible for mast cell disease in adults and children.

CLASSIFICATION OF MAST CELL DISEASE

The classification of mast cell disease has been recently redefined by the World Health Organization (WHO). As a result, seven disease categories are currently recognized: cutaneous mastocytosis (CM), indolent systemic mastocytosis (ISM), systemic mastocytosis with an associated clonal hematologic nonmast cell lineage disease (SM-AHNMD), aggressive systemic mastocytosis (ASM), mast cell leukemia (MCL), mast cell sarcoma, and extracutaneous mastocytoma (Table 36–1). Patients with cutaneous mastocytosis and indolent systemic mastocytosis represent the largest groups and include most children with cutaneous mastocytosis and many adults with indolent systemic mastocytosis. All cutaneous mastocytosis patients and many indolent systemic mastocytosis patients have cutaneous lesions. Cutaneous involvement in mast cell disease is defined by typical lesions of mastocytosis (see Clinical manifestations), and pathological changes that may demonstrate either monomorphic mast cells clusters (>15 MCs/cluster) or scattered MCs at more than 20 MCs/high-power field (hpf). Systemic mast cell disease is defined by major and minor criteria in which the major criteria are represented by multifocal dense MC infiltrates (15 MCs/aggregate) in the bone marrow or other extracutaneous organs, and the minor criteria include the presence of >25% spindle-shaped or atypical-appearing MCs in tissue sections or a bone marrow aspirate smear, the presence of a c-Kit point mutation at codon 816V, the expression of CD2 and/or CD25 by MCs and a persistent total serum tryptase level of >20 ng/mL (Table 36–2). The diagnosis of SM is established in patients having the major and one minor criteria or three minor criteria. Whereas most patients

Table 36-1 Classification of mast cell disease

Cutaneous mastocytosis (CM)
  Macular and papular CM
  Diffuse CM
  Mastocytoma

Indolent systemic mastocytosis (ISM)
  Smoldering systemic mastocytosis
  Isolated bone marrow mastocytosis

Systemic mastocytosis with an associated clonal hematologic non-mast cell lineage disease (SM-AHNMD)
  SM–myelodysplastic syndrome
  SM–myeloproliferative disorder
  SM–chronic eosinophilic leukemia
  SM–non-Hodgkin lymphoma

Aggressive systemic mastocytosis (ASM)
  With eosinophilia (SM-eo)

Mast cell leukemia (MCL)

Mast cell sarcoma

Extracutaneous mastocytoma

Table 36-2 Criteria for diagnosing systemic mast cell disease

Major
Multifocal dense MC infiltrates (>15 MCs/aggregate) in the bone marrow or extracutaneous organs

Minor
25% MCs are spindle shaped or atypical in a bone marrow aspirate smear or tissue sections
c-Kit point mutation at codon 816V
Expression of CD2 and/or CD25 by MCs
Total serum tryptase persistently >20 ng/mL (in the absence of another nonmast cell hematologic disorder)

Table 36-3 Mast cell mediators

Preformed mediators	Cytokines
Histamine	TNF-α
Heparin	IL-4
Chemotatic factors for PMNs and eosinophils	IL-5
Tryptase	IL-6
Chymase	IL-8
	SCF

Newly formed mediators	
PGD_2	
LTC_4, LTD_4, LTE_4	
PAF	

with SM have indolent disease, a smaller subset has an associated clonal hematologic nonmast cell disorder, aggressive mast cell disease without or with eosinophilia, or mast cell leukemia. Hematologic diseases associated with systemic mastocytosis having an associated clonal hematologic nonmast cell lineage disease include polycythemia rubra vera, myelodysplastic syndrome, chronic eosinophilic leukemia, chronic myeloid leukemia, chronic myelomonocytic leukemia, lymphocytic leukemia, acute erythroblastic leukemia, megaloblastic leukemia, and non-Hodgkin's lymphoma. Patients with systemic mastocytosis having an associated clonal hematologic nonmast cell lineage disease may or may not have skin lesions, but frequently have liver, spleen, and/or lymph node involvement. Patients with systemic mastocytosis having an associated clonal hematologic nonmast cell lineage disease are often older adults, and many have constitutional symptoms such as fever, anorexia, weight loss, and generalized malaise. Aggressive mast cell disease is characterized by lymphadenopathy with or without peripheral blood eosinophilia. Patients with this rare disorder often lack cutaneous lesions, but frequently have mast cells infiltrates involving the bone marrow, gastrointestinal tract, liver, spleen, and lymph nodes. Mast cell leukemia is an extremely rare condition, and the diagnosis is established by demonstrating MCs in the peripheral blood and/or >20% MCs in a bone marrow aspirate smear. Most mast cell leukemia patients do not have cutaneous lesions, but frequently experience fever, weight loss, abdominal pain, diarrhea, nausea, and vomiting. These patients also have detectable hepatosplenomegaly and lymphadenopathy resulting from extensive mast cell infiltration of these organs. Bone marrow biopsies from mast cell leukemia patients demonstrate increased MCs, which are often spindle shaped or morphologically atypical. Mast cell sarcomas and extracutaneous mastocytomas are extremely rare, with only a few isolated case reports.

CLINICAL MANIFESTATIONS

Symptoms

Symptoms associated with mast cell disease are attributable in great part to the release of mast cell mediators, such as histamine, eicosanoids, and cytokines (Table 36-3). These symptoms may range from pruritus and flushing to abdominal pain and diarrhea, to palpitations, dizziness, and syncope (Table 36-4). In many instances the symptoms can be reduced or suppressed by antihistamines, suggesting MC-derived histamine as a cause. Many patients with cutaneous mastocytosis or indolent systemic mastocytosis have few, if any, symptoms, and may experience only intermittent bouts of pruritus. Of interest is the relative lack of pulmonary symptoms in SM patients. Complaints of fever, night sweats, malaise, weight loss, bone pain, epigastric distress, and problems with mentation (cognitive disorganization) often signal the presence of SM. Symptoms of mast cell disease can be exacerbated by exercise, heat, local trauma to skin lesions, as well as the ingestion of alcohol, narcotics, salicylates, and anticholinergic agents.

Cutaneous Lesions

Most children have cutaneous mastocytosis, which is frequently manifest by either a solitary tan or yellow-tan plaque

Table 36–4 Symptoms and signs of mastocytosis

Cardiopulmonary	Gastrointestinal
Chest pain	Abdominal cramps
Dizziness	Diarrhea
Dyspnea	Epigastric pain*
Palpitations	Nausea
Syncope	Vomiting
Skin	**Neurologic**
Bullae	Cognitive disorganization*
Flushing	Headaches
Pruritus	
Urticaria	
Skeletal	**Constitutional**
Bone pain*	Fatigue*
	Fever*
	Malaise*
	Weight loss*

*Suggests the possibility of types II-IV mastocytosis.

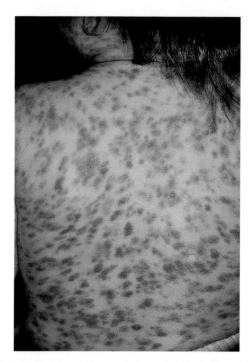

Figure 36–2 Multiple tan to brown lesions of urticaria pigmentosa.

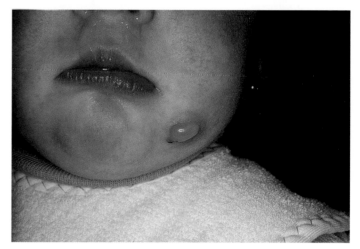

Figure 36–3 Bullous mastocytoma.

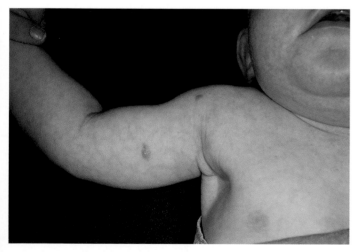

Figure 36–1 Solitary mastocytoma.

or nodule (mastocytoma) (Fig. 36–1) or variable numbers of tan to brown papules (urticaria pigmentosa, UP) (Fig. 36–2). Mastocytomas often occur on the distal extremities, but may arise in any anatomical location. Urticaria pigmentosa usually presents early in childhood and often spares the face, scalp, palms, and soles. Whereas telangiectatic macules (telangiectasia macularis eruptiva perstans, TMEP) are a rare manifestation of cutaneous mastocytosis in young patients, at least three children have been reported with TMEP. Some children will develop diffuse cutaneous mastocytosis which appears as numerous erythematous, yellow-tan papules and plaques.

Infants and children with UP and diffuse cutaneous mastocytosis also may experience nonscarring vesicles or bullae (Fig. 36–3). Blistering reactions in cutaneous mastocytosis lesions usually resolve by 3–5 years of age. The skin manifestations of adult mastocytosis differ significantly from those in children. The most common lesions of adult mast cell disease are reddish-brown macules and papules a centimeter or less in diameter (Fig. 36–4). These lesions are most numerous on the trunk and proximal extremities, and appear less frequently on the face, distal extremities, palms, or soles. Mastocytomas and diffuse cutaneous mastocytosis in adults are extremely rare.

The presence of increased mast cell numbers in the skin of patients with mast cell disease can be demonstrated clinically by firmly rubbing a characteristic lesion. The formation of an urticarial wheal (Darier's sign) (Fig. 36–5) at the lesion site is

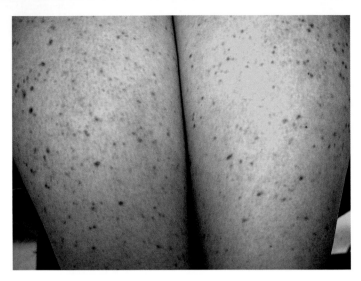

Figure 36–4 Telangiectasia macularis eruptiva perstans.

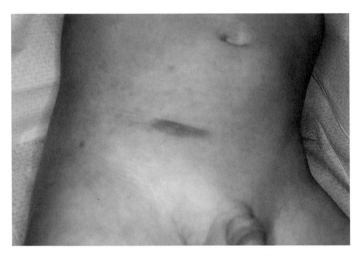

Figure 36–5 Mast cell mediators and their effects on different organs.

indicative of mast cell mediator release. Darier's sign is readily demonstrated in mastocytomas and childhood UP lesions, whereas it may be barely detectable in common adult mast cell disease lesions and TMEP. This can be explained by the fact that mast cell concentrations in mastocytomas and childhood UP are respectively approximately 150 and 40 times higher than in normal skin, whereas the mast cell content in adult mast cell disease lesions is only nine times greater than in normal skin.

Systemic Manifestations

Skeletal involvement is common in adult patients with SM, with a reported incidence of approximately 70%. On X-ray these changes appear as radio-opacities, radiolucencies, or a mixture of the two, with the skull, spine, and pelvis being most commonly involved. Osteoporosis is the most common change in patients with diffuse skeletal disease, followed by osteosclerosis and mixed lesions of osteosclerosis and osteoporosis. These bony changes are believed to result from the local release

of mast cell mediators. Children with mastocytosis rarely have bone involvement.

Bone marrow involvement frequently occurs in adult SM patients but is rarely seen in children. The diagnosis of mast cell disease in the bone marrow is established by identifying clusters of MCs (>15 tryptase-positive staining MCs/cluster) that express CD25 and/or CD2 which are not routinely detected on normal MCs. The diagnosis of SM on bone marrow biopsy may be difficult in patients with systemic mastocytosis with an associated clonal hematologic nonmast cell lineage disease because of the coexistence of the hematologic disorder. The presence of >5% MCs on a bone marrow aspirate smear in SM patients suggests an unfavorable prognosis, and the identification of >20% MCs on a bone marrow smear is diagnostic of MCL.

Splenomegaly has been reported in approximately 50% of adult SM patients and is most common in aggressive systemic mastocytosis and mast cell leukemia. Lymph node enlargement is uncommon in indolent systemic mastocytosis patients, but occurs in patients with aggressive systemic mastocytosis and mast cell leukemia. Patients with SM also may experience gastrointestinal symptoms such as abdominal pain, diarrhea, nausea, and vomiting. Diarrhea is usually episodic and can result from malabsorption, increased motility, and/or acid hypersecretion. Gastrointestinal hemorrhage has been reported in some patients with SM, and is often secondary to gastritis or peptic ulcers. Radiographic changes in the GI tract of SM patients include urticaria-like lesions, thickened gastric, duodenal or jejunal folds, as well as mucosal nodules and/or peptic ulcers. Biopsies of mucosal nodules often show numerous mast cells with varying numbers of eosinophils. Hepatomegaly also is detectable in approximately 40% of adult SM patients, but most of these have normal liver function tests.

A mixed organic brain syndrome manifested by irritability, fatigue, headache, poor attention span and motivation, limited short-term memory, inability to work effectively, and difficulty in interacting with other people has been described in SM patients. It has been hypothesized that these symptoms are secondary to released mast cell mediators. Electroencephalographic studies in these patients have ranged from normal to changes consistent with a toxic or metabolic process.

DIAGNOSIS

The diagnosis of mastocytosis is established by demonstrating increased mast cells in one or more organs (Table 36–5). In patients with skin lesions, increased mast cells can be established in a biopsy of lesional skin. Nodular, papular, and macular lesions of mast cell disease have been reported to have respectively 150-, 40- and ninefold increases in mast cell content compared to normal skin. The proposed pathological criteria for skin involvement in mastocytosis patients includes either the presence of >15 monomorphic MCs/cluster or >20 scattered MCs/hpf on microscopic evaluation of a lesional skin biopsy and on the presence of a KIT mutation at the 816 codon. Normal-appearing skin from patients with mast cell disease has normal numbers of mast cells, and skin biopsies of normal-appearing skin in patients with suspected mast cell

Table 36–5 Diagnostic tests for patients with mastocytosis

Direct tests
Biopsy of the skin
Biopsy of the GI tract
Biopsy of the bone marrow

Indirect tests
Serum tryptase (total or α) levels
24-hour urinary histamine metabolite levels (methylimidazole acetic acid)
Urinary PGD$_2$ levels
Bone X-rays or bone scan

disease are not helpful in establishing the diagnosis. Biopsies from either the bone marrow or the gastrointestinal tract may be indicated for patients in whom the diagnosis of mast cell disease is expected, but who lack skin lesions.

The detection of circulating mast cell mediators and/or their metabolites can offer indirect evidence of mast cell disease (Table 36–5). Two forms (α and β) of mast cell-derived tryptase have been identified. α-Tryptase is persistently elevated in patients with SM, and thus may be useful for assessing total body mast cell burden. β-Tryptase, on the other hand, is often detected in mast cell disease patients as well as in other hematologic disorders and normal patients experiencing anaphylactic symptoms. Mastocytosis patients with persistent total serum tryptase levels >20 ng/mL are likely to have SM. Elevations in urinary histamine metabolites also have been documented in some SM patients. In many instances, unmetabolized urinary histamine levels may be normal in asymptomatic SM patients, whereas the major metabolite of histamine, 1,4-methylimidazole acetic acid (MeImAA), is often persistently elevated. Certain foods with high histamine content, such as spinach, egg plant (aubergine), cheeses (Parmesan, blue, and Roquefort), and red wines, can artificially elevate the levels of urinary histamine and its metabolites. The major urinary metabolite of PGD$_2$, 9α,11β-dihydroxy-15-oxo-2,3,18,19-tetranorprost-5-ene-1,20-diolic acid (PGD$_2$M) has also been reported to be increased in some SM patients.

PROGNOSIS

Most children have cutaneous mastocytosis and thus an excellent prognosis with a limited disease course. Approximately 50% of these patients are expected to have their disease resolve by adolescence, with the remainder noting a marked reduction in lesion numbers. Activating c-KIT mutations have been reported in a few children with mast cell disease, and it has been postulated that this patient group may represent the 10–15% of children whose disease persists into adulthood. It is believed that these children have the same prognosis as adult-onset mast cell disease patients, with an increased potential for systemic involvement and more aggressive disease. The overall prognosis of patients having systemic mastocytosis with an associated clonal hematologic nonmast cell lineage disease appears to be directly related to the severity of the associated hematologic disorder. Patients with aggressive systemic mas-

tocytosis have an unfavorable prognosis, with a mean survival of only a few years, and the prognosis for mast cell leukemia is also extremely poor, with an expected survival of a year or less from the time of diagnosis.

TREATMENT

At present there is no cure for mast cell disease; treatment is therefore directed at alleviating symptoms. Patients with cutaneous mastocytosis and indolent systemic mastocytosis often have few, if any, symptoms, and therefore require little or no therapy. Patients should be cautioned to avoid potential mast cell-degranulating agents such as ingested alcohol, anticholinergic preparations, aspirin, nonsteroidal agents, narcotics, and polymyxin B sulfate. In addition, heat and friction can induce local or systemic symptoms, and therefore should be avoided whenever possible. A number of systemic anesthetic agents, including lidocaine (lignocaine), morphine, codeine, D-tubocurarine, metocurine, etomidate, thiopental, succinylcholine, enflurane, and isoflurane, have been directly or indirectly implicated in precipitating anaphylactoid reactions in mastocytosis patients. Although observations are limited, it appears that propofol, vecuronium, and fentanyl appear to be safe alternative systemic anesthetics for patients with mast cell disease. In addition, local injections of lidocaine can be used safely in these patients.

Histamine (H$_1$) or combined H$_1$ and H$_2$ antagonists are often helpful in controlling many of the symptoms associated with mast cell disease. The second-generation antihistamines, cetirizine, loratadine, and fexofenadine, have distinct advantages over first-generation antihistamines because they have longer half-lives and are more specific H$_1$ antagonists. In some instances the addition of an H$_2$ antagonist (cimetidine, ranitidine, famotidine, or nizatidine) may prove beneficial, especially in patients with gastric acid hypersecretion. Ketotifen, which has both antihistamine and mast cell-stabilizing properties, has been effective in combination with ranitidine in controlling symptoms of mast cell disease, as has the tricyclic antidepressant doxepin. Oral disodium cromoglycate (DSCG) (400–1000 mg/day) may alleviate gastrointestinal, cutaneous, and central nervous system symptoms associated with mast cell disease.

PUVA therapy given four times a week is helpful in controlling the pruritus and cutaneous whealing in MCD patients. However, it does not alter other symptoms associated with this disorder, and does not permanently eliminate cutaneous mast cell infiltrates. In contrast to oral PUVA, bath PUVA is not beneficial for symptomatic mast cell disease patients.

Topical corticosteroids under occlusion for 6 weeks or more can greatly reduce the skin mast cell content as well as symptoms associated with mast cell disease. Intralesional injections of triamcinolone acetonide also have been successful in clearing mast cell infiltrates in the skin of mast cell disease patients. Systemic corticosteroids are usually of little benefit in most patients with mast cell disease, but may provide relief of cutaneous and GI symptoms in patients with more advanced disease. Cyclosporine A has been used in combination with systemic corticosteroids in a patient with advanced mast cell disease, resulting not only in relief of symptoms but also in a decline in serum tryptase and urinary histamine metabolite levels.

The subcutaneous administration of interferon-α_{2b} (IFN-α_{2b}) also has been used with variable success in patients with more aggressive forms of SM. In a prospective study, six patients with indolent systemic mastocytosis were treated with IFN-α_{2b}; however, only a modest decline in bone marrow mast cells and urinary MeImAA levels was noted, and no change in serum tryptase levels was observed. Potential side effects of the IFN therapy include anaphylaxis, hypothyroidism, thrombocytopenia, and depression.

Some mast cell disease patients experience recurrent life-threatening episodes of hypotension resulting from mast cell mediator release. These patients should be supplied with a premeasured epinephrine (adrenaline) preparation (EpiPen). In some instances they may experience recurrent similar attacks within hours of the initial event. The administration of prednisone (20–40 mg/day for 2–4 days) can often abort or eliminate these recurring episodes.

Numerous chemotherapeutic agents have been used unsuccessfully in the treatment of advanced MCD. Recently, however, 2-chlorodeoxyadenosine has been reported effective in eliminating skin lesions and markedly reducing the numbers of bone marrow mast cells in patients with widespread systemic disease. Chemotherapeutic approaches, on the other hand, are important, and can be effective for the treatment of associated hematologic disorders seen in systemic mastocytosis with an associated clonal hematologic nonmast cell lineage disease. Local radiation therapy (approximately 2000–30,000 cGy) may provide relief of bone pain. In some instances pain relief can be achieved during treatment or shortly thereafter, thereby reducing the frequency and amount of oral analgesics required for pain control. Splenectomy may be indicated for mast cell disease patients who experience hypersplenism leading to significant cytopenia, and it appears to improve survival in patients with more aggressive disease.

The identification of activating KIT mutations as a possible cause of SM has led to the use of tyrosine kinase (TK) inhibitors for the treatment of these patients. Although the TK inhibitor imatinib mesylate inactivates normal KIT and c-kit mutations in the juxtamembrane region, it has been proved ineffective in treating SM patients with 816V KIT mutations. However, imatinib may be useful in the treatment of SM patients who express the V560G KIT mutation. Newer TK inhibitors capable of inhibiting 816V autoactivated KIT are under development and offer promise as more effective therapeutic agents for patients with mast cell disease.

SUGGESTED READING

Andrew SM, Freemont AJ. Skeletal mastocytosis. J Clin Pathol 1993; 46: 1033–1035.

Barton J, Lavker RM, Schechter NM, et al. Treatment of urticaria pigmentosa with corticosteroids. Arch Dermatol 1985; 121: 1516–1523.

Borgeat A, Ruetsch YA. Anesthesia in a patient with malignant systemic mastocytosis using a total intravenous anesthetic technique. Anesth Analg 1998; 86: 442–444.

Butterfield JH. Response of severe systemic mastocytosis to interferon-alpha. Br J Dermatol 1998; 138: 489–495.

Caplan RM. The natural course of urticaria pigmentosa. Arch Dermatol 1963; 87: 146–157.

Kasper C, Freeman RG, Tharp MD. Diagnosis of mastocytosis subsets using a morphometric point counting technique. Arch Dermatol 1987; 123: 1017–1021.

Keyzer JL, DeMonchy JGR, vanDoormaal JJ, et al. Improved diagnosis of mastocytosis by measurement of urinary histamine metabolites. N Engl J Med 1983; 309: 1603–1605.

Kolde G, Frosch P, Czarnetzki B. Response of cutaneous mast cells to PUVA in patients with urticaria pigmentosa: histomorphometric,

ultrastructural, and biochemical investigations. J Invest Dermatol 1984; 83: 175–178.

Longley BJ, Metcalfe DD, Tharp MD, et al. Activating and dominant inactivating c-kit catalytic domain mutations in distinct forms of human mastocytosis. Proc Natl Acad Sci USA 1999; 96: 1609–1614.

Patnaik MM, Tefferi A, Pardanani A. Kit: molecule of interest for the diagnosis and treatment of mastocytosis and other neoplastic disorders. Curr Cancer Drug Targets 2007; 7: 492–503.

Rogers M, Bloomingdale K, Murawski B, et al. Mixed organic brain syndrome as a manifestation of systemic mastocytosis. Psychosom Med 1986; 48: 437–447.

Sagher F, Even-Paz Z. Mastocytosis and the mast cell. Chicago: Yearbook Medical Publishers, 1967; 10–291.

Valent P, Akin C, Escribano L, et al. Standards and standardization in mastocytosis: consensus statement on diagnostics, treatment recommendations and response criteria. Eur J Clin Invest 2007; 37: 435–453.

Valent P. Systemic mastocytosis. Cancer Treat Res 2008; 142: 399–419.

Chapter | **37** | *Raechele C. Gathers and Amy J. McMichael*

Hair Disorders in Systemic Disease

Disorders of hair growth are commonly encountered by clinicians, and can be one of the manifestations of a multitude of systemic diseases. Although clinicians must be astute at recognizing patterned disorders of hair growth and their associations with disease, it is also important that they be sensitive to the unique emotional and psychosocial implications of hair. In addition to its obvious relationship to appearance and ideas of physical attractiveness, hair may play a significant role in defining identity, ethnicity, and even social status. Hair loss has been associated with depression, anxiety, and a reduced quality of life. Likewise, Americans have been estimated to spend over $2 billion annually on the removal of unwanted hair. In diagnosing and treating diseases that are associated with hair disorders, it is imperative that clinicians are mindful of the unique needs and sensitivities inherent to this group of patients.

FOLLICULAR BIOLOGY

In order to understand the behavior of the hair follicle in the setting of systemic disease, it is first important to appreciate normal follicular biology. At the time of birth, there are approximately 150 000 hair follicles on the scalp. Each undergoes a continuous cyclic pattern of changes (the follicular lifecycle) during the person's lifetime. The first cycle of hair growth actually occurs in utero, resulting in the fine, nonpigmented, soft lanugo hair that covers much of the fetus. Lanugo hair is shed before birth in a single molt. A second wave of hair growth then occurs, and this hair is shed as a second molt shortly after birth. Unlike many mammals, in which hair follicles remain in synchrony with one another, this second molt is the last time that human hair follicles are in synchrony. After that, each follicle seems to have a growth cycle independent of those around it. The duration of hair growth cycles is dependent on varying factors, including location of the hair, the individual's age, nutritional habits, hormonal factors, and health status.

It is widely accepted that in healthy individuals scalp hair grows approximately 0.35 mm/day (1 cm per month). It should be noted, however, that recent data suggest that African textured hair grows more slowly, at approximately 0.77 cm per month. Vellus hairs, rooted in the upper dermis, are 0.03 mm or less in diameter and less than 1 cm long. They lack melanin and medulla. Terminal hairs exceed the diameter and length of vellus hairs, are typically pigmented and medullated, and are rooted in subcutaneous tissue or deep dermis. Each hair follicle passes through three cycles: anagen (growth), catagen (involution), and telogen (rest). A latency or exogen phase is noted in up to 80% of hair cycles. In exogen, the hair shaft is shed without regrowth and a new anagen phase is turned on. For scalp hair, where the majority are long, thick terminal hairs, the anagen cycle may last from 2 to 7 years, and at any given time about 85% of hairs are in anagen. At other body sites, such as the eyelids, arms, and legs, where hair is much shorter and finer than scalp hair, anagen has duration of only weeks to months. Hair length is determined by the rate and duration of the anagen phase, which is terminated by an internal biologic 'clock' built into every follicle. The biochemical mechanisms that regulate this clock are as yet unknown, but are probably related to hormones, growth factors, and cytokines. The catagen phase marks the termination of the growing phase.

Catagen, a transitional phase of acute follicular regression, is irreversible and of relatively short duration, lasting only 2–3 weeks. In catagen, the bulb of the hair moves towards the skin surface, and the previously elongated anagen follicle is shortened and reduced in volume. The completion of catagen is marked by formation of the keratinized and depigmented club hair. Only 1–2% of scalp hairs are in catagen at any one time.

Telogen, the resting phase, begins when catagen is complete. With an average duration of 3 months, about 15% of the scalp hairs are in telogen at any given time. Telogen hairs account for the 50–100 scalp hairs normally shed each day. The percentage of hairs in the telogen phase, called the telogen count, normally varies from person to person and even between parts of the scalp. In men, the telogen count is higher in the frontal and vertex areas than in the occiput. Likewise, telogen counts may be higher in those with African hair type. Metabolically, the telogen hair follicle is relatively inactive, and is therefore uninfluenced by factors that affect rapidly growing tissues. Telogen follicles are located high in the dermis, with an angiofibrotic tract ('streamer') extending down to the subcutaneous tissue and marking the position of the former anagen follicle. The telogen hair (club hair) is shed during the exogen phase, which may or may not coincide with the new anagen phase. The next anagen phase begins anew from the reservoir of follicular stem cells residing in the so-called bulge area, near where the arrector pili muscle inserts into the hair follicle. These stem cells proliferate rapidly downwards to form a new anagen hair.

HAIR DISORDERS AND SYSTEMIC DISEASE

Hair loss, or alopecia, has traditionally been subdivided into three main categories: scarring (cicatricial), nonscarring (non-cicatricial), and hair shaft disorders. This classification is highly controversial, however, as not all disorders classified under the term 'scarring' alopecia have histological evidence of true scar formation. For example, in scleroderma, which is classified as causing a type of scarring alopecia, collagen fibers are thickened, but true scars are not formed. Because of this, the terms 'permanent' and 'nonpermanent' alopecia have been proposed instead. For purposes of our discussion, however, we will continue to use the terms scarring and nonscarring, as they are widely accepted and firmly entrenched in the literature.

Hair loss in the setting of systemic disease may occur through one of five mechanisms (Table 37–1): telogen effluvium, anagen arrest, and hair miniaturization (all forms of nonscarring alopecia); scarring alopecia; and hair shaft disorders. Further, two mechanisms for increases in hair density may be seen: hypertrichosis and hirsutism. An important concept in the evaluation and diagnosis of hair disorders is that more than one mechanism may be operating at a given time. This can amplify the degree of hair loss, modify its pattern, and complicate the clinical picture.

ALOPECIA

Telogen Effluvium

Telogen effluvium is the most common cause of hair loss, and is probably the most common form of hair loss associated with systemic disease, especially serious debilitating illness. It is the result of a perturbation of the hair cycle that is manifest by the increased loss of normal telogen club hairs. A follicle can be suddenly thrust into catagen and the succeeding telogen phase by a variety of external factors. In addition to systemic diseases, telogen effluvium may be associated with a severely restricted diet, endocrine disorders, surgical procedures and anesthesia, androgenetic alopecia, and drugs. In fact, most

drugs that have been associated with hair loss, with the exception of chemotherapeutics, cause hair loss via telogen effluvium. The etiologic factors that lead to telogen effluvium fall into two main categories: stress to the follicle in the form of metabolic disturbance or mild injury; and a primarily physiologic means, without real injury or insult to the follicle. About 3–4 months after a precipitating event (the time it takes for a hair to move through catagen and the early stages of telogen) normal-appearing club hairs begin to fall out in large numbers. Often, the patient may admit to one of the precipitating events listed in Table 37–2.

Telogen Effluvium and Drugs

A number of drugs have been associated with telogen effluvium (Table 37–3). A few (i.e., captopril, quinacrine, nadolol, sulfasalazine) have been associated with a histologically inflammatory telogen effluvium.

Telogen Effluvium and Androgenetic Alopecia

Early-onset androgenetic alopecia is often accompanied by a brisk and episodic telogen effluvium. Androgenetic telogen effluvium is related to shortened cycle times as large scalp terminal hairs are miniaturized and shortened secondary to decreased matrix volume and reduced duration of anagen, respectively. Hair shedding is obvious only when large terminal hairs are being shed. With ensuing hair cycles, the involved

---

Table 37–1 Five mechanisms for alopecia in systemic disease

Telogen effluvium
Anagen arrest
Androgenetic alopecia/hair miniaturization
Scarring alopecia (cicatricial alopecia)
Hair shaft disorders

Table 37–2 Causes of telogen effluvium

Injury or physiologic stress
Post-febrile state (extremely high fevers, e.g., malaria)
Severe infection, including HIV infection
Severe chronic illness
After general surgical procedure
Hypothyroidism and other endocrinopathies
Extreme dieting and/or weight loss
Drugs
Heavy metals
Physiologic effluvium of the newborn
Postpartum state
Early stages of androgenetic alopecia

Table 37–3 Drugs associated with telogen effluvium

Retinoids (etretinate, isotretinoin)
Anticoagulants (coumadin, heparin)
Antithyroid (propylthiouracil, methimazole)
Anticonvulsants (phenytoin, valproic acid, carbamazepine)
Heavy metals
β-Adrenergic blockers
Amphetamine
Bromocriptine
Captopril
Enalapril
Danazol
Levodopa
Lithium
Pyridostigmine

follicles produced progressively miniaturized (vellus) hairs, whose loss is inapparent.

Chronic Telogen Effluvium

Another category that merits mention is chronic telogen effluvium. Most common in middle-aged women, this is a diffuse, chronic, fluctuating form of hair loss that affects the entire scalp. Sometimes confused with androgenetic alopecia, chronic telogen effluvium may cause diffuse thinning and bitemporal recession, but severe and obvious balding is rare.

Recently, Headington has proposed five different functional types of telogen effluvium based on changes in different phases of the follicular cycle. These are: 1) immediate anagen release; 2) delayed anagen release; 3) short anagen syndrome; 4) immediate telogen release; and 5) delayed telogen release.

Immediate anagen release

Immediate anagen release is a very common form of telogen effluvium. Follicles that would normally complete a longer cycle by remaining in anagen enter telogen prematurely. Immediate anagen release has a relatively short onset – typically 3–5 weeks – and is probably the mechanism by which many drugs and physiological stressors (such as episodes of high fever) induce shedding.

Delayed anagen release

In delayed anagen release some follicles remain in prolonged anagen rather than cycling into telogen. When they are finally released from this prolonged anagen, if sufficient follicles were involved, increased shedding will be noted. Postpartum hair loss is a classic example. The percentage of follicles in telogen progressively decreases during pregnancy, particularly during the last trimester. The physiologic basis for this is unknown, but metabolic and endocrine changes are suspected. After parturition, hormonal restraint is lost and numerous follicles suddenly enter the catagen and telogen phases. The onset of hair loss usually becomes apparent by the second or third postpartum month.

Short anagen

Idiopathic shortening of the anagen cycle may result in a mild but persistent increased shedding and inability to grow long hair. Shedding is typically not noticed until anagen is reduced by 50%.

Immediate telogen release

Immediate telogen release results from a shortening of the normal telogen cycle. There is good evidence that drugs such as minoxidil exert their effect via immediate telogen release, with affected follicles promptly stimulated to enter anagen.

Delayed telogen release

Delayed telogen release is the mechanism by which some mammals synchronously shed their winter coats at the onset of spring. The operative signal is to end prolonged telogen and to initiate anagen. This same mechanism may cause the slight degrees of telogen effluvium in some humans who complain of seasonal hair shedding.

Diagnosis and Treatment

In telogen effluvium, patients typically report increased hair in the shower drain, on bathroom floors, or on clothing. Reduced hair volume is typically apparent to the patient after the loss of about 20% of the hair. However, normal hair density may be reduced by up to 50% before thinning is apparent to clinicians. If alopecia is clinically obvious, the loss appears diffuse (Fig. 37–1). In the typical patient with telogen effluvium the telogen count seldom exceeds 50%. However, in some documented cases telogen counts can reach up to 80%. Patients with more than 80% telogen hair counts probably do not represent a simple case of telogen effluvium. A detailed medical, dietary, and drug history is essential in establishing a diagnosis of telogen effluvium. Physical examination should include the scalp surface, hair shafts, and a pull test of 25–50 hairs. A gentle pull will dislodge more than four hair shafts in telogen effluvium, the roots of which show the depigmented, keratinized, clubbed morphology of telogen hairs (Fig. 37–2). A forcible hair pluck extracts a mixture of normal anagen and telogen hairs and an occasional catagen hair. The percentage of telogen hairs is increased, a criterion without which the diagnosis of telogen effluvium cannot be established with certainty (Fig. 37–3). On biopsy, a 4-mm scalp punch specimen should contain 25–50 terminal follicles. More than 12–15% of hairs in telogen is probably an indication of telogen effluvium. To treat telogen effluvium, the cause or causes must be identified. Because most cases of telogen effluvium, particularly those associated with drugs and acute-onset physiologic events, are self-limiting, management should involve psychological support to limit patient anxiety, and reassurance that shed hair is being replaced.

Anagen Arrest

Anagen arrest represents a diffuse loss of anagen hairs from growing follicles. Inhibition of cell division in the hair bulb

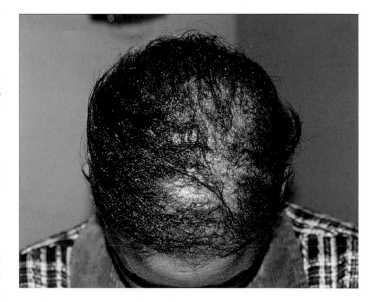

Figure 37–1 Young woman with diffusely thin hair from telogen effluvium secondary to diffuse irritant reaction to hair-straightening chemicals.

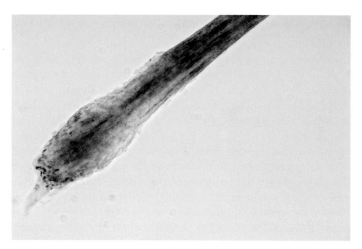

Figure 37–2 Spontaneously shed telogen hair. These are increased in number in patients with telogen effluvium.

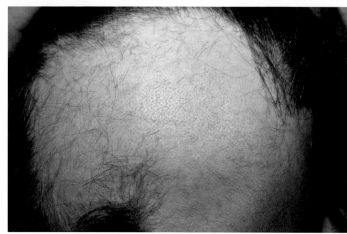

Figure 37–4 Anagen arrest secondary to radiotherapy for an intracranial malignancy. Although eventual hair regrowth is expected in such cases, high enough doses of radiation can result in permanent hair loss.

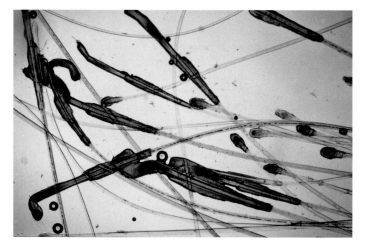

Figure 37–3 Forcible hair pluck in a patient with telogen effluvium. A mixture of normal-appearing telogen hairs and anagen hairs is found, but in this case the percentage of telogen hairs exceeds 30%.

Table 37–4 Systemic causes of anagen arrest
Noninflammatory
Anticancer chemotherapy
Drugs (colchicine, levodopa, cyclosporine, bismuth)
Radiation therapy
Endocrine diseases
Cicatrizing diseases
Trauma/pressure
Toxins (poisons, e.g., thallium, boron, arsenic)
Inflammatory
Alopecia areata, totalis, or universalis
Systemic lupus erythematosus (patchy)
Secondary syphilis (patchy or diffuse)

matrix leads to a progressive narrowing of the hair shaft and sometimes failure of hair formation. When the metabolic and mitotic activity of the follicular epithelium is rapidly halted, the hair shaft markedly thins and tapers to a point, like the tip of a sharpened pencil. At this stage, the most trivial external force, such as gentle combing or pressure from a pillow, causes the distal portion of the shaft to break off and fall out of the follicle. Although anagen arrest is sometimes referred to as anagen effluvium, this is a misnomer because only tapered shafts and not entire anagen hairs are shed. Thinning of the shaft with resulting breakage occurs within days to a few weeks of the metabolic insult, unlike telogen effluvium, in which shedding takes 3 months to occur. Because 85% of scalp hairs are in anagen at any one time, anagen arrest causes severe baldness.

All therapeutic measures intended to inhibit the proliferation of actively dividing cells can cause the dramatic hair loss seen in anagen arrest. The classic example of noninflammatory anagen arrest occurs in the setting of a chemotherapeutic drug given systemically to treat a malignancy. The various agents

may act in different ways (e.g., as antimetabolites or alkylating agents), but they all inhibit metabolism of rapidly dividing anagen matrix cells. Anagen arrest is more common and severe with combination chemotherapy than with the use of a single drug, and the severity is usually dose dependent. The most severe hair loss occurs with doxorubicin, the nitrosoureas, and cyclophosphamide. Anticancer doses of radiation therapy have a similar effect on hair follicles (Fig. 37–4). Other agents causing anagen arrest include bleomycin, fluorouracil, methotrexate, bismuth, levodopa, colchicine, and cyclosporine. Exposure to toxic substances such as thallium, boron, and arsenic may precipitate anagen arrest, as may anticancer doses of radiation therapy (Table 37–4). Of note, both thallium and X-irradiation have been used with the intention of causing total hair depilation for therapeutic purposes. Anagen arrest may also be caused by endocrine diseases, trauma or pressure, and pemphigus vulgaris.

Anagen arrest may also have an inflammatory etiology. The classic example is alopecia totalis, in which the rapid onset and progression can resemble the hair loss associated with chemotherapy. Presumably, the inflammatory infiltrate surrounding the anagen hair bulb is related to the metabolic shutdown. Although the exact mechanism is unknown, perhaps there is a release of cytokines that inhibit epithelial growth. The patchy hair loss seen in some systemic lupus erythematosus patients, and the patchy or diffuse hair loss seen in secondary syphilis is another example of inflammatory anagen arrest. However, it should be noted that anagen arrest is only one of several mechanisms leading to hair loss in systemic lupus erythematosus and syphilis patients.

Diagnosis and Treatment

The diagnosis of anagen arrest is easily made by history, the observation of extensive hair loss, and hair pull tests that yield easily broken hairs with proximal tapering and pigmentation loss (Fig. 37–5). On horizontal punch biopsy sections, a normal anagen-to-telogen ratio in a patient with hair loss is characteristic of anagen arrest. Because hairs are rapidly shed over the course of only a few weeks in anagen arrest, late in the course of the shedding, if a cluster of hairs is forcibly plucked, virtually all of them will be telogen, as most of the anagen hairs have already shed (Fig. 37–6). This is in contrast to telogen effluvium, where the telogen count rarely exceeds 50% and the remaining hairs are all normal anagen hairs. Identification and treatment of the underlying cause of hair loss is key to the treatment of anagen arrest. Chemotherapy-induced anagen arrest may be retarded by the application of a pressure cuff around the scalp and local hypothermia during the infusion of the medication. However, it should be noted that because the scalp may act as a safe house for circulating malignant cells, patients with hematologic malignancies are usually not candidates for these procedures. Whereas topical minoxidil will not prevent chemotherapy-induced anagen arrest, it may significantly shorten the period before hair regrowth occurs. Although anagen arrest is typically reversible, on occasion the color and texture of the hair that regrows after chemotherapy-induced arrest may be different from those of the original hair. Also, sufficiently high doses of chemotherapy or radiation could conceivably injure the follicular stem cells, resulting in permanent hair loss.

Androgenetic Alopecia/Hair Miniaturization

Androgenetic alopecia is the third nonscarring mechanism by which alopecia can be associated with systemic disease. In androgenetic alopecia a complex interplay of genetic and hormonal influences combine to result in changes in follicular architecture and deviations in the hair growth cycle. There is shortening of the anagen phase and a reduction in the volume of the hair matrix cells. These two forces in combination result in the conversion of terminal hairs into the short and fine vellus hairs characteristically seen in patterned baldness. In addition, whereas the telogen phase remains stable, the latency between telogen and new anagen is found to increase in androgenetic alopecia.

Androgenetic alopecia is an autosomal dominant disorder with variable penetrance that affects both men and women. One-third of individuals with a strong family history of androgenetic alopecia can expect to be affected, irrespective of gender. Alopecia takes the form of male (Hamilton) or female (Ludwig) patterns. Androgens such as testosterone, dihydrotestosterone (DHT), and sulfonated dehydroepiandrosterone all influence hair loss. The most potent of these, DHT (formed from testosterone by the type II 5α-reductase enzyme), reduces the amount of scalp hair and increases the amount of body and genital hair. One manifestation of hyperandrogenism in women is androgenetic alopecia. Under the influence of excessive androgens, certain hair follicles become progressively miniaturized, producing ever shorter and finer hairs. Clinically, the loss of hair mass appears as diffuse thinning of the scalp crown with maintenance of the frontal hairline.

The cause of hyperandrogenism can be excessive androgen production, hereditary hypersensitivity to androgen action, or a combination of the two. Excessive androgen production may be associated with acne, hirsutism, and irregular menstrual periods. Syndromes of androgen excess include polycystic ovarian disease, late-onset congenital adrenal hyperplasia (Fig. 37–7), Cushing's syndrome, and the HAIR-AN syndrome

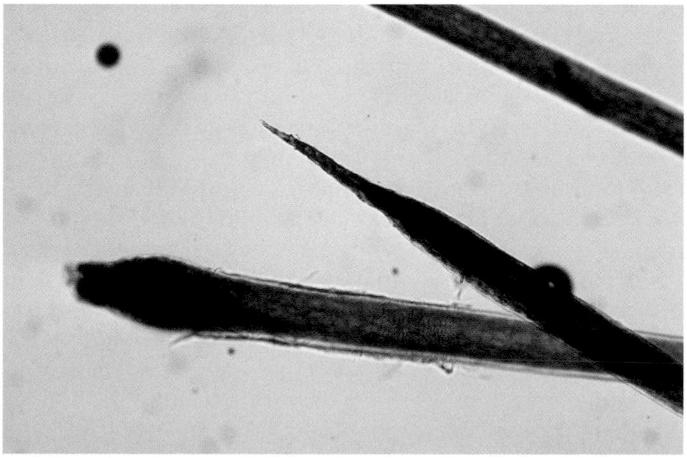

Figure 37–5 Spontaneously shed 'pencil point' hairs in a patient who received systemic chemotherapy. Hair shafts taper abruptly to a point and are shed.

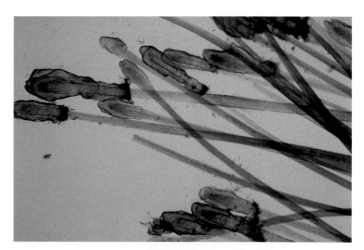

Figure 37–6 Forcible hair pluck in a patient who had already experienced massive hair loss from systemic chemotherapy. Only the shafts of telogen hair remain in the scalp, and so the hair count is 100% telogen hairs.

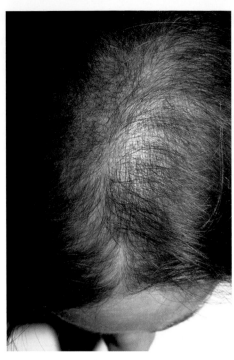

Figure 37–7 Severe thinning of the hair on the crown (androgenetic alopecia) in a 14-year-old girl with late-onset congenital adrenal hyperplasia. This patient's hair loss prompted an endocrinologic evaluation.

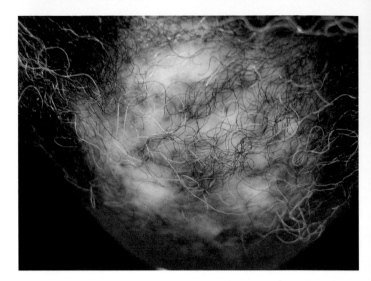

Figure 37–8 Frontal thinning in a patient with scarring from discoid lesions of lupus.

(i.e., hyperandrogenism, insulin resistance, and acanthosis nigricans).

In males, a number of epidemiologic studies have linked androgenetic alopecia to increased risk for ischemic heart disease. More recently, an association between prostate cancer and vertex balding has been proposed.

Diagnosis and Treatment

The diagnosis of androgenetic alopecia is based on clinical presentation and a strong family history. If hyperandrogenism is suspected, the appropriate work-up should be pursued. Hair pull tests may demonstrate an excessive proportion of telogen hairs and a reduced hair shaft diameter. On scalp biopsy, the characteristic miniaturization of follicles will be noted. Currently available treatments for androgenetic alopecia include topical minoxidil, oral finasteride (approved only for men), and surgical hair restoration. Minoxidil, an arterial vasodilator, enhances DNA synthesis in follicular keratinocytes, though its mechanism of action is poorly understood. Finasteride, an inhibitor of type II 5α-reductase, exerts its effect by significantly reducing scalp follicle DHT. In surgical hair restoration, hairs are taken from the less androgen-sensitive occipital scalp and redistributed to the affected vertex or frontal scalp. In women, off-label systemic treatments have included spironolactone and flutamide, which block androgen uptake by the follicles. Similarly, contraceptive pills and hormone replacement therapy have been used adjunctively.

Scarring Alopecia (Cicatricial Alopecia)

Scarring alopecia represents the destruction of hair follicles and can be associated with several diseases. Also termed cicatricial alopecia, it presents clinically as areas of hair loss in which the underlying scalp is scarred, sclerosed, or atrophic, with loss of follicular orifices. The unifying concept in all scarring alopecias is the disruption of follicular anatomy and injury to follicular stem cells that is so severe that the ability to regrow hair in affected areas is forever lost. Scarring alopecia can be classified into two subtypes: primary and secondary. In primary scarring alopecia the hair follicle itself is the target for destruction, with relative sparing of the interfollicular dermis. Chronic cutaneous lupus erythematosus and alopecia mucinosa are classic examples of systemic diseases that may cause a primary scarring alopecia (Fig. 37–8). Secondary scarring alopecia results from nonfollicular processes that impinge upon the follicle by circumstance, eventually destroying it. The follicle is, in effect, an innocent bystander. Most scarring alopecias associated with systemic diseases fall into the secondary category (Fig. 37–9). Sarcoidosis, scleroderma (Fig. 37–10), lupus erythematosus with discoid lesions, graft-versus-host disease, and primary systemic amyloidosis all cause secondary scarring alopecias. The destructive force may be physical compression, altered blood supply, or the release of detrimental cytokines. Infectious diseases such as lupus vulgaris (cutaneous tuberculosis), leprosy, tertiary syphilis, and leishmaniasis may also be associated with secondary scarring alopecia. Malignancies metastatic to the scalp, such as those seen in breast carcinoma, may cause alopecia via physical compression, or by releasing chemical mediators that facilitate the hair loss. Likewise, sufficient ischemia or pressure, radiation, and chemotherapy can lead to secondary scarring alopecia. Bullous disorders such as cicatricial pemphigoid and epidermolysis bullosa may lead to secondary scarring. Finally, hereditary disorders such as incontinentia pigmenti or KID syndrome have been associated with secondary scarring alopecia (Table 37–5).

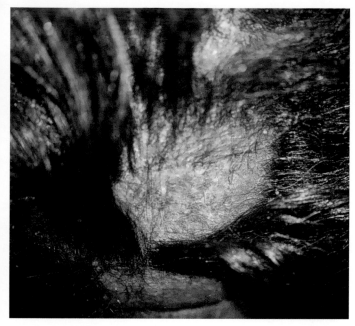

Figure 37–9 Patient with hairless plaque due to scleroderma involving the scalp.

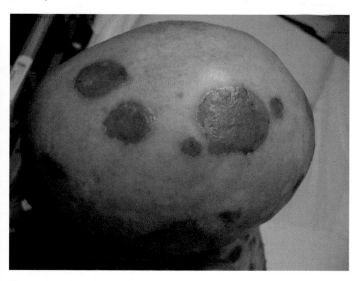

Figure 37–10 Patient with active lesions of cutaneous T-cell lymphoma causing scarring hair loss in multifocal manner across the scalp.

Diagnosis and Treatment

In making the diagnosis of scarring alopecia, a comprehensive history and careful physical examination are key. Scalp biopsy for both horizontal and vertical sectioning is recommended. Horizontal (transverse) sections allow for assessment of follicular distribution, number and type, and for visualization of all follicles at different levels. Vertical sections allow for visualization of the dermoepidermal junction and any alterations associated with the infundibular epidermis and the adjacent dermis. Additional tests such as direct immunofluorescence, elastin, PAS, and mucin stains may also be helpful if the primary diagnosis is not clear. The treatment of scarring alopecias associated with systemic disease hinges on establishing an accurate diagnosis for the systemic illness and instituting appropriate treatment protocols to slow the process of hair loss.

Table 37–5 Causes of scarring alopecia

Primary
Chronic cutaneous lupus erythematosus
Lichen planopilaris
Frontal fibrosing alopecia
Central centrifugal cicatricial alopecia
Pseudopalade
Folliculitis decalvans
Dissecting cellulitis
Acne keloidalis nuchae
Alopecia mucinosa

Secondary
Infectious
Bacterial
Viral
Fungal
Leprosy
Leishmaniasis
Tertiary syphilis
Inflammatory/autoimmune
Cicatricial bullous pemphigoid
Scleroderma
Graft-versus-host disease
Sarcoidosis
Physical/chemical destruction
Ischemia
Thermal injury
Radiation therapy
Drugs (e.g., high-dose chemotherapy)
Neoplastic
Hereditary (e.g., KID syndrome, incontinentia pigmenti)

Hair Shaft Disorders

Hair shaft disorders, also called trichodystrophies, are associated with numerous systemic diseases (Table 37–6). Hair density may be nearly normal or markedly reduced, depending on the condition. Often, a congenital reduction in hair density is coupled with hair fragility, making the alopecia appear particularly severe. There are several dermatologic syndromes that have hair shaft defects as a prominent feature. In some cases the hair shaft may change in diameter or shape, resulting in an alteration of hair texture. In other cases the hair shafts become excessively fragile and fracture, resulting in alopecia.

In trichothiodystrophy the hairs are excessively brittle and subject to transverse fractures (trichoschisis) (Fig. 37–11) secondary to reduced sulfur content. With polarizing microscopy the hair shows alternating bright and dark regions (tiger tail hair). Other features of trichothiodystrophy may include ichthyosis, short stature, mental deficiency, photosensitivity, nail dystrophy, seizures, and infertility. Various names have been associated with differing combinations of these physical findings, including Tay syndrome and PIBIDS (photosensitivity, ichthyosis, brittle hair, impaired intelligence, decreased fertility, and short stature). The defect resides in genes encoding helicases of the transcription/repair factor TFIIH. Different mutations in the ERCC2 DNA repair gene may lead to the varied phenotypic expressions of the disease. Marinesco–

Table 37–6 Systemic diseases with hair shaft disorders

Menkes' kinky hair syndrome
Argininosuccinic aminoaciduria
Trichothiodystrophy
Pohl–Pinkus sign
Bjornstad's syndrome
Crandall's syndrome
Beare's syndrome
HIV disease
Scurvy

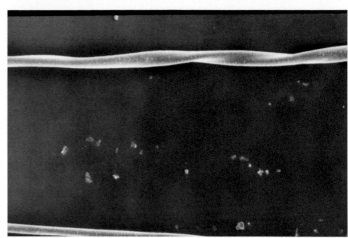

Figure 37–12 Pili torti in a patient with Menkes' kinky hair syndrome.

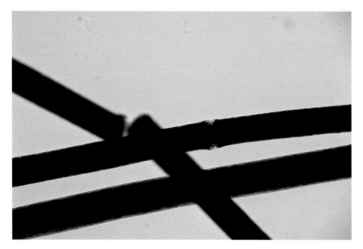

Figure 37–11 Trichoschisis in a patient with trichothiodystrophy.

Sjögren syndrome, inherited in an autosomal recessive manner, is characterized by cerebellar ataxia, mental retardation, and sparse hairs that lack the normal layers and have narrow bands of abnormal incomplete keratinization. Pili torti, a malformation in which the hair is twisted on its own axis, leads to brittle and easily broken hairs. Classic pili torti, which follows a dominant inheritance pattern, usually starts in early childhood and improves by puberty. However, pili torti has also been associated with anorexia nervosa, Bjornstad's syndrome, Crandall's syndrome, isotretinoin and etretinate therapy, and trichothiodystrophy. In Menkes' kinky hair syndrome, a disorder of copper transport results in abnormal neurodevelopment, connective tissue problems such as skin laxity, and premature death. Psychomotor retardation is noted in the first few months of life, with drowsiness, impaired temperature regulation, and convulsions. The defective gene is located on the X chromosome (Xq13), and encodes a highly evolutionary conserved, copper-transporting P-type ATPase. This gene is expressed in nearly every human tissue, explaining the multisystem nature of the disorder. The hair is pale, brittle, and demonstrates pili torti (Fig. 37–12).

Trichorrhexis nodosa, the most common hair shaft abnormality, is characterized by nodular swellings of the hair shaft accompanied by frayed fibers and cuticular loss. Albeit often associated with physical or chemical trauma, trichorrhexis nodosa can also be seen in argininosuccinicaciduria, a disorder of the urea cycle. Owing to the lack of the enzyme argininosuccinase, these patients are unable to excrete waste nitrogen as urea. In addition to hair fragility, argininosuccinicaciduria may be associated with hepatomegaly and mental retardation. HIV-

positive patients with normally kinky or curly hair may notice a straightening of hair in late-stage disease. Hair shaft dystrophy with variation in hair shaft diameter, longitudinal ridging, cuticular loss, and trichoschisis has also been observed, and may help explain textural changes and hair fragility.

Diagnosis and Treatment

The diagnosis of hair shaft disorders can be made through a comprehensive family history and a detailed physical examination. A genetics consultation may be helpful if the diagnosis is not clear, especially in children. Microscopic examination of hair shafts is often useful. Treatment of hair shaft disorders is aimed at treatment of the primary disorder if applicable (i.e., arginine supplements and protein restriction in argininosuccinicaciduria) and the minimization of hair shaft trauma by limiting manipulation of the hair and avoiding excessive heat or other chemical trauma.

EXCESSIVE HAIR

Hypertrichosis

Hypertrichosis is the excessive growth of nonandrogen-dependent hair. In hypertrichosis, the hair growth is abnormal for the age, sex or race of an individual, or for a particular body area. Hypertrichosis may be localized or generalized, congenital or acquired. Hypertrichosis may occur via one of two major mechanisms: the conversion of vellus to terminal hairs; or via changes in the hair growth cycle. A less well understood mechanism for hypertrichosis is an increase in hair follicle density.

Many congenital causes of hypertrichosis can be described. Large congenital melanocytic nevi, which may place the patient at increased risk for developing a malignant melanoma, may be hypertrichotic. Brachmann de Lange syndrome (also known as Cornelia de Lange syndrome) is a congenital disorder in which patients suffer from physical and mental retardation, a characteristic facies, and irregular teeth. These patients also exhibit hypertrichotic eyelashes, extensive vellus hypertrichosis on the trunk, posterior neck and elbows, and thick and convergent eyebrows (synophrys). Fetuses exposed to hydantoin during the first 9 weeks of gestation may develop the fetal hydantoin syndrome, characterized by hypertrichosis, nail hypoplasia, cleft lip, and low birthweight. Hypertrichosis may also be a feature of fetal alcohol syndrome. Hypertrichosis may be seen in the mucopolysaccharidoses, including Hunter's, Sanfilippo, and Hurler's syndromes. Hypertrichosis may also be noted in the sun-exposed skin of patients with porphyria cutanea tarda, erythropoietic protoporphyria, erythropoietic porphyria, and variegate porphyria. The area lateral to the eyebrows is most prominently affected.

Acquired localized hypertrichosis may be associated with chemically induced dermatitis. Localized hypertrichosis may also be seen overlying areas of thrombophlebitis or chronic osteomyelitis. Hypertrichosis of the eyelashes (trichomegaly) may be associated with HIV, and is also rarely seen in systemic lupus erythematosus. Generalized hypertrichosis may be seen in acrodynia, a reaction to chronic mercury exposure, and in children with hypothyroidism. Juvenile dermatomyositis has been associated with hypertrichosis, most prominent on the face and limbs. Generalized hypertrichosis has also been reported in 36% of patients with bulimia nervosa and 77% or patients with anorexia nervosa. Acquired hypertrichosis lanuginosa, also known as 'malignant down', is a well-documented cutaneous manifestation of internal malignancy, most commonly cancer of the lung or colon. Systemic therapy with minoxidil and cyclosporine frequently results in generalized hypertrichosis. The topical glaucoma medication latanoprost has been shown to cause regional hypertrichosis of the eyelids and eyelashes. Psoralens have been reported to cause temporary hypertrichosis in light-exposed areas. Other drugs associated with hypertrichosis are listed in Table 37–7.

Diagnosis and Treatment

If hypertrichosis is secondary to an underlying condition, management of that condition will often result in the resolution of the hypertrichosis. However, when hypertrichosis is congenital, or if it is a significant cosmetic concern, a number of treatment modalities exist. Albeit temporary, several mechanical and chemical depilatory methods may be used. Electrolysis involves the destruction of the follicle by a direct electric current. Thermolysis involves destruction of the follicle by the heat produced by an alternating electric current. The efficacy of both of these methods is operator dependent, but considered permanent when performed correctly. Laser hair removal has gained tremendous popularity and can be very effective for dark, coarse hair. Topical eflornithine hydrochloride, an inhibitor of ornithine decarboxylase, is approved for increased facial hair in women but is used off-label by many patients. It slows hair growth, probably by inhibiting cell synthetic or mitotic function.

Hirsutism

Hirsutism is the excessive growth of androgen-dependent terminal body hair. Affected patients grow hair in places in which terminal hair is not typically found, such as the face, chest, abdomen, and back of a woman (Fig. 37–13). Hirsutism, acne, and androgenic alopecia are the cutaneous manifestations of hyperandrogenic states. Hirsutism may be secondary to adrenal, ovarian, or mixed adrenal and ovarian etiologies (Table 37–8). Polycystic ovarian disease is the most common cause of abnormal androgen production, and in addition to

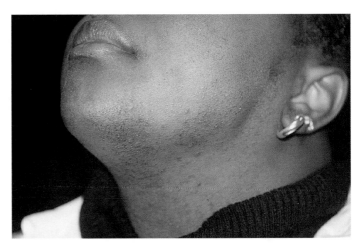

Figure 37–13 Hirsutism in the beard area of a woman with polycystic ovarian syndrome.

Table 37–7 Drugs associated with hypertrichosis
Dilantin
Streptomycin
Latanoprost
Cyclosporine
Psoralens
Diazoxide
Minoxidil
Acetazolamide

Table 37–8 Etiologies of hirsutism
Adrenal
Congenital adrenal hyperplasia
Cushing's syndrome
Androgen-secreting adrenal tumors
Severe insulin resistance
Ovarian
Androgen-secreting adrenal tumors
Combined adrenal/ovarian
Polycystic ovarian disease
Idiopathic (including increased skin sensitivity to androgens)
Other
Androgen therapy
Anabolic steroids
Androgenic progestins
Glucocorticoids
Hyperprolactinemia
Thyroid dysfunction
Acromegaly

the cutaneous signs of hyperandrogenism may also be characterized by irregular menstrual periods, insulin resistance, hypertension, and dyslipidemia. Hirsutism may also be associated with acromegaly and thyroid dysfunction. Anabolic steroids, androgenic progestins, and glucocorticoids are iatrogenic causes of hirsutism.

Diagnosis and Treatment

Serious underlying disorders must be ruled out in the hirsute patient. The medical treatment of hirsutism consists of suppressing ovarian or adrenal androgen secretion, or of blocking androgen action in the skin. Oral contraceptives and antiandrogens such as spironolactone, cyproterone acetate, and flutamide have been used therapeutically. Glucocorticoids, gonadotropin-releasing hormone agonists such as leuprolide, and insulin sensitizing agents have also been used. Although the endocrinologic evaluation and treatment of hirsutism is beyond the scope of this chapter, excellent references are available. Cosmetic improvement of hirsutism may be achieved via previously mentioned modalities.

SUGGESTED READING

Bernard BA. Hair shape of curly hair. J Am Acad Dermatol 2003; 48: S120–S126.

Drake L, Hordinsky M, Fiedler V, et al. The effects of finasteride on scalp skin and serum androgen levels in men with androgenetic alopecia. J Am Acad Dermatol 1999; 41: 550–554.

Giles GG, Severi G, Sinclair R, et al. Androgenetic alopecia and prostate cancer: findings from an Australian case-control study. Cancer Epidemiol Biomark Prev 2002; 11: 549–553.

Glorio R, Allevato M, De Pablo A, et al. Prevalence of cutaneous manifestations in 200 patients with eating disorders. Int J Dermatol 2000; 39: 348–353.

Headington JT. Telogen effluvium. Arch Dermatol 1993; 129: 356–363.

Khumalo NP. African hair length: the picture is clearer. J Am Acad Dermatol 2006; 54: 886–888.

Kuster W, Happle R. The inheritance of common baldness: two b or not two b? J Am Acad Dermatol 1984; 5: 921–926.

McMichael AJ. Hair and scalp disorders in ethnic populations. Dermatol Clin 2003; 21: 629–644.

Molnar JA. Laser hair removal. Emedicine 21 February 2007. http://www.emedicine.com/plastic/topic438.htm.

Rittmaster RS. Hirsutism. Lancet 1997; 349: 191–195.

Schwartz RA. Anagen effluvium. Emedicine 30 May 2007. http://www.emedicine.com/derm/topic894.htm.

Sellheyer K, Bergfeld WF. Histopathologic evaluation of alopecias. Am J Dermatopathol 2006; 28: 236–259.

Sinclair R, Jolley J, Mallari R, et al. Morphological approach to hair disorders. J Investig Dermatol Symp Proc 2003; 8: 56–64.

Trevisan M, Farinaro E, Krogh V, et al. Baldness and coronary heart disease risk factors. J Clin Epidemiol 1993; 46: 1213–1218.

van der Donk J, Hunfeld JAM, Passchier J, et al. Quality of life and maladjustment associated with hair loss in women with alopecia androgentica. Soc Sci Med 1994; 33: 159–163.

Wendelin DS, Pope DN, Mallory SB. Hypertrichosis. J Am Acad Dermatol 2003; 48: 161–179.

Whiting DA. Chronic telogen effluvium. Dermatol Clin 1996; 14: 723–731.

Whiting DA. Cicatricial alopecia: clinico-pathological findings and treatment. Clin Dermatol 2001; 18: 211–225.

Wolfram LJ. Human hair: a unique physiochemical composite. J Am Acad Dermatol 2003; 48: S106–S114.

Chapter | **38** | *Christopher B. Yelverton and Joseph L. Jorizzo*

Nail Signs of Systemic Disease

Few elements of the surface anatomy offer a glimpse into as much pathology as the nails. Anatomically, the bony hard nail plate covers the nail bed and the distal portion of the nail matrix, which is seen distally as the white 'half-moon' area called the lunula. The rest of the matrix extends about 5 mm proximally. The undersurface of the proximal nailfold forms the eponychium (cuticle), its horny end product. The nail bed lies beneath the nail plate. The proximal and lateral nailfolds border the nail plate. The blood supply to the nail arises from the superficial and deep palmar branches of the digital arteries. The hyponychium is the area under the free edge and the distal portion of the nail plate (Fig. 38–1).

Its high sulfur content, in the form of cysteine, contributes to the hardness of the nail plate. The mitotically active nail matrix forms the keratin of the nail plate. The proximal third of the matrix provides keratin to the upper third of the nail plate; the middle part of the matrix forms the midportion; and the distal third of the matrix forms the lower third of the plate.

A complete and detailed history and physical examination are essential in evaluating patients with suspected ungual changes due to systemic disease. All 20 nails should be examined. Generally, toenails provide less information than do fingernails because trauma, which may confuse the evaluation, occurs more frequently on the toenails and because their growth rate is much slower. The matrix is often the site where changes in nail pigmentation related to systemic disease begin. If the pigmentation is carried over to the nail plate, the change in pigmentation progresses as the nail plate grows out. The clinician can approximate when the specific disease began by measuring the distance from the cuticle to the most advanced border of color change, and using the knowledge that the fingernail grows 0.1–0.15 mm/day.

ANATOMIC CHANGES OF THE NAIL APPARATUS (Table 38–1)

Nail Matrix and Plate Abnormalities

Beau's Lines

Beau's lines are transverse depressions in the nail plate that occur after a stressful event that temporarily interrupts nail for-

mation within the proximal matrix. The precipitating event may be local trauma, chemotherapeutic agents that interrupt cell division, or the abrupt onset of systemic disease. The most common systemic precipitant is an infectious disease, but drug reactions, toxin ingestion, surgery, renal failure, and myocardial infarction have all been implicated. Unilateral Beau's lines have been reported with reflex sympathetic dystrophy (RSD) and brachial plexopathy. The clinician can estimate the date of this stressful event by measuring the distance from the cuticle to the Beau's line and comparing this to the rate of nail growth.

Mees' Lines

Transverse white bands in the nail plate are frequently caused by trauma to the proximal or mid matrix, such as from manicuring (striate leukonychia). However, other types of transverse white bands may be seen with systemic disease. The clinician can differentiate between these two causes because lines resulting from systemic disease more frequently occur on several nails at once. In addition, these lines tend to have smoother borders, are more homogeneous, and may spread across the entire breadth of the nail plate. The lines associated with systemic disease have the same configuration as the distal lunula. The major cause of Mees' lines is arsenic poisoning, but many different systemic diseases are associated with them, as are some chemotherapeutic drugs, and exposure to other heavy metals.

Pitting

Pitting is due to aberrant keratinization within the proximal nail matrix, which detaches from the nail plate, leaving a depression. This nonspecific finding is associated with many diseases involving the proximal matrix, including psoriasis, psoriatic arthritis, and Reiter's syndrome. It has been reported in many other diseases, including alopecia areata, atopic dermatitis, Langerhans' cell histiocytosis, and junctional epidermolysis bullosa.

Longitudinal Pigmented Bands (Melanonychia)

Most single longitudinal pigmented bands are not associated with internal disorders. They may be caused by trauma, drugs,

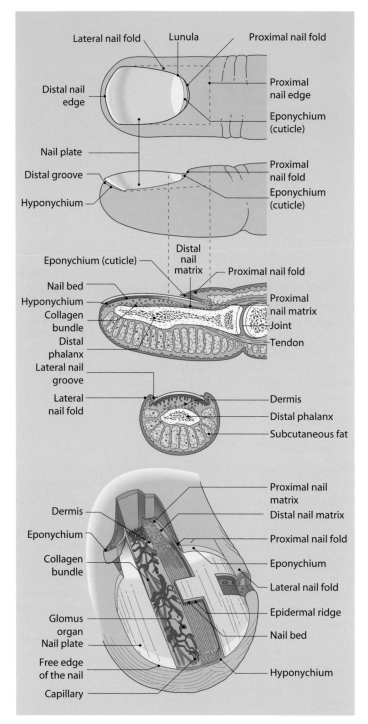

Figure 38–1 Anatomic structure of the nail apparatus. (Reproduced with permission from Bologna JL, Jorizzo, JL, Rapini RP, eds. Dermatology, 2nd edn. Chicago: Mosby, 2007.

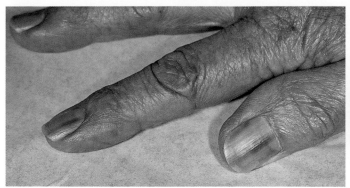

Figure 38–2 Longitudinal pigmented bands caused by zidovudine administration in a patient with HIV infection.

The clinician should be more suspicious of the possibility of a melanoma, or a pigmented nonmelanoma skin cancer, when the longitudinal band is seen on a single nail, is darkening or widening, and occurs in a patient of at least middle age, especially if the pigment is found on the surrounding nailfold (Hutchinson's sign). Longitudinal pigmented bands may be caused by many medications, including bleomycin, fluoride, melphalan, cyclophosphamide, doxorubicin, antimalarials, and zidovudine (Fig. 38–2). Dark transverse bands may be associated with quinacrine, doxorubicin, and cyclophosphamide. Nitrogen mustard and methotrexate produce diffuse hyperpigmentation of the nail plate.

Brittle Nails

Brittle fingernails, thought to be caused by dehydration of the nail plate and loss of adhesion, may be caused by trauma or by chemicals and, in some instances, by systemic disease. Arterial insufficiency, Raynaud's phenomenon, iron deficiency, bronchiectasis, diabetes mellitus, osteoporosis, amyloidosis, hyper- and hypothyroidism, gout, tuberculosis, hypopituitarism, and sarcoidosis have all been associated with brittle nails.

Koilonychia

There are many hypotheses concerning the cause of koilonychia (spoon nails). One is that spooning occurs when the distal matrix is angled downward in relation to the proximal matrix. The reverse anatomic association would produce clubbing. Another hypothesis relates this dystrophy to softening and thinning of the nail plate.

Spooning of the nails is a frequent, but temporary, finding in infants. Iron deficiency anemia (Plummer–Vinson syndrome) is classically thought to be the most frequent cause (Fig. 38–3). Replacement therapy usually corrects the disorder. There are three major types of koilonychia: hereditary (autosomal dominant), acquired, and idiopathic. The acquired type is the largest group, most commonly seen in psoriasis, fungal infection, distal ischemia (e.g., Raynaud's phenomenon), and trauma. It may occur in porphyria and hemochromatosis, and occupationally (secondary to softening with oils or soaps). Koilonychia has also been reported in association with carcinoma of the upper gastrointestinal tract.

fungi, nevi, PUVA phototherapy, and many other conditions. They have been seen in Addison's disease following adrenalectomy, in scleroderma, and in leprosy. There seems to be a direct correlation between the depth of skin pigmentation and the likelihood of development of melanonychia: a light-complexioned individual is more likely to have melanoma or nevi as the cause of longitudinal pigmented bands. Bands related to systemic disease are usually in multiple nails.

Table 38–1 Abnormalities and associations

Nail condition	Description	Causes/Associated disease states
Beau's lines	Transverse grooves in nail plate	Nonspecific; acute infection or other metabolic insult; renal failure; myocardial infarction; epilepsy; reflex sympathetic dystrophy or brachial plexopathy (unilateral); deep sea diving/ mountain climbing; Heimler syndrome; Guillain–Barré syndrome
Brittle nails (fragilitas unguium)	Abnormal brittleness of the nails	Nonspecific; nutritional deficiency; thyroid dysfunction; glucagonoma; diabetes; trichothiodystrophy; drugs; trauma; arterial insufficiency; renal failure; ectodermal dysplasias; deposition disorders (gout, amyloidosis, etc.); osteoporosis; tuberculosis; bronchiectasis; hypopituitarism; sarcoidosis
Bywater's lesions	Hemorrhage/infarct of the nailfolds	Rheumatologic-associated vasculitis & arthritis
Clubbing	Loss of Lovibond (~165–180°) angle between nail plate and proximal nailfold	Nonspecific; idiopathic; cardiac; pulmonary; vascular abnormality (aneurysm, fistula, shunt); renal failure; cirrhosis; reflex sympathetic dystrophy (unilateral); erythromelalgia
Koilonychia	Spoon-shaped nails	Nonspecific; hereditary; iron deficiency anemia; fungal infection; psoriasis; high altitude; trichothiodystrophy; Raynaud's phenomenon/ischemia; trauma; liver disease; gastrointestinal malignancies
Leukonychia	White discoloration of nails (true or apparent)	True leukonychia (nail plate): zinc deficiency; trauma; RSD; chemotherapy; congestive heart failure; altitude changes (increase); infection; diabetes; lymphoma; Heimler's syndrome; see Beau's lines Apparent leukonychia (nail bed): see Lindsay's nails (half-and-half nails), Terry's nails; Muercke's nails; renal; hypoalbuminemia
Lindsay's nails/half-and-half nails	White discoloration of proximal half of nail bed, with reddish brown band distally; blanches with pressure	Renal failure; Crohn's disease
Lunular discoloration		Blue/gray/silver – Wilson's disease (copper); argyria (silver); cyanosis Red – congestive heart failure; carbon monoxide poisoning; systemic lupus erythematosus; alopecia areata; vitiligo; lichen sclerosus; rheumatoid arthritis; psoriasis (absent lunulae – normal variant with aging; nail patella syndrome; syphilis; leprosy)
Mees' lines (Aldrich–Mees' lines)	Transverse white bands (usually multiple nails) that grow out with nail plate; nonblanching	Arsenic, thallium or other heavy metal poisoning; infection; renal failure/hemodialysis
Melanonychia (longitudinal pigment bands)	Black or brown pigmentation of nails	Normal variant; nevus; Laugier–Hunziner syndrome; infection; pregnancy; PUVA therapy; Addison's disease (following adrenalectomy for Cushing's); drugs; scleroderma; leprosy; tumors – squamous cell carcinoma, melanoma (Hutchinson's sign = pigment involvement of proximal nailfold, worrisome for melanoma)
Micronychia	Abnormal small appearance of nails	Folliculitis decalvans; congenital onychodysplasia of the index finger (COIF, Iso-Kikuchi syndrome)
Muercke's lines	Multiple (usually double) transverse white bands, parallel to lunula; do not grow out with nail, blanch with pressure	Edema of nail bed secondary to hypoalbuminemia (prominent when serum albumin <2.2 g/dL); nephrotic syndrome; post cardiac transplantation; cardiomyopathy; ACTH-dependent Cushing's; Peutz–Jeghers syndrome with hepatic adenoma; chemotherapy
Proximal nailfold capillary abnormalities	Distortion of normal capillary architecture	Avascular portions with dilated capillary loops: scleroderma; dermatomyositis Normal vascular density with tortuous capillaries: systemic lupus erythematosus
Onychocryptosis	Ingrown nail	Trauma; neglect; highly active antiretroviral therapy (HAART) for HIV (especially indinavir, ritonavir); Rubinstein–Taybi syndrome; Turner's syndrome; chemotherapy; epidermal growth factor receptor inhibitors

367

Table 38–1 Abnormalities and associations—cont'd

Nail condition	Description	Causes/Associated disease states
Onycholysis (Plummer's nails; photo-onycholysis)	Separation of the nail plate from the nail bed	Nonspecific; trauma; contact dermatitis; infection; psoriasis; thyroid disease; porphyria; acrodermatitis continua of Hallopeau; drugs/psoralens
Onychomadesis (onychoptosis)	Shedding of the nail plate and/or separation of the nail plate from the nail bed at the proximal nailfold	Stevens–Johnson syndrome/toxic epidermal necrolysis; infection; pemphigus vulgaris; epidermolysis bullosa; Kawasaki's disease; dialysis; mycosis fungoides; alopecia universalis; critical illness; drugs; immunoglobulin class-switching recombination deficiencies
Onychomycosis/tinea unguium	Infection of the nail plate/bed with dermatophytes or other fungi	Nonspecific; immunodeficiency states (HIV/AIDS)
Onychorrhexis (see also brittle nails)	Longitudinal ridging and occasional splitting of the free nail edge	Pemphigus vulgaris; psoriasis/psoriatic arthritis; Witkop's tooth and nail syndrome; Darier's disease; palmoplantar keratoderma (punctate); drugs; gasoline exposure
Onychoschizia	Horizontal splitting of the nail plate into layers	Glucagonoma; HIV; pemphigus vulgaris; trauma; chemical exposures; hydration/dehydration
Paronychia/felon	Inflammation/infection of perionychium/periunguium	Nonspecific; Stevens–Johnson syndrome; diabetes mellitus; infection (candida, herpes, syphilis, leprosy); antiretroviral therapy for HIV
Pincer nail/Trumpet nail/ Onychoincurvatum (see also Onychocryptosis)	Sharply incurvated nail edges	Systemic lupus erythematosus; colon carcinoma; epidermolysis bullosa; Kawasaki's disease; drugs (β-blocker, SSRI); infection (tinea); psoriasis
Pitting	Small depressions in the nail plate	Nonspecific; psoriasis/psoriatic arthritis; Reiter's syndrome; lichen planus; alopecia areata; atopic dermatitis; Langerhans' cell histiocytosis; junctional epidermolysis bullosa
Proximal nail bed telangiectasia	Telangiectasias of the proximal nail bed	Diabetes mellitus
Pterygium/pterygium inversum	Triangular or 'wing' shaped deformity at proximal or distal nail edge	Proximal: lichen planus, psoriasis/psoriatic arthritis, alopecia areata; porokeratoses; lichenoid graft-versus-host disease; Marfan's syndrome; dyskeratosis congenita Distal (inverse): scleroderma; stroke; acrylate allergy
Splinter hemorrhage	Bleeding in the nail bed	Nonspecific; trauma; bacterial endocarditis (proximal may be more specific); mitral stenosis; other infection (trichinosis, fungal, septicemia); renal (dialysis, post kidney transplant, chronic glomerulonephritis); hepatic (cirrhosis, hepatitis); scurvy; anemia; atopic dermatitis; psoriasis; rheumatoid arthritis; malignancy
Terry's nails	White appearance to the nail bed, obscuring the lunula and all but the distal 1–2 mm	Liver disease (cirrhosis, hypoalbuminemia); diabetes; congestive heart failure; thyrotoxicosis; malnutrition; aging; Reiter's syndrome; leprosy; POEMS (Crow–Fukase) syndrome
Trachyonychia/ twenty nail dystrophy	Rough, linear ridging of all nails	Lichen planus; psoriasis; pemphigus vulgaris; alopecia areata; ichthyoses; sarcoidosis; drugs; punctate palmoplantar keratoderma; reflex sympathetic dystrophy (unilateral)
Triangular lunulae	Triangular shape to lunulae	Nail–patella syndrome; cirrhosis, hypoalbuminemia
Whitlow	Enlargement and erythema of the distal digit	Cold painful whitlow: digital ischemia Cold painless whitlow: metastases to bone (fingers, from pulmonary source; toes, from genitourinary source)
Yellow nails	Arrest in nail growth leading to oxidation of nail	Pulmonary (asthma, tuberculosis, pleural effusion, chronic obstructive pulmonary disease); hypoalbuminemia (hepatic disease); HIV/AIDS; malignancy (laryngeal carcinoma, non-Hodgkin's lymphoma); lymphedema/lymphatic obstruction; rheumatoid arthritis (on gold therapy)

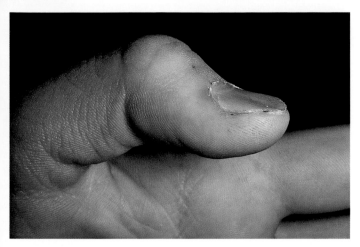

Figure 38–3 Koilonychia associated with iron deficiency anemia. (Reprinted from Callen JP, Greer KE, Paller A, Swinyer L, eds. Color atlas of dermatology, 2nd edn. Philadelphia: WB Saunders, 2000.)

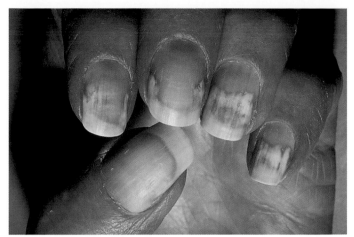

Figure 38–5 Onycholysis.

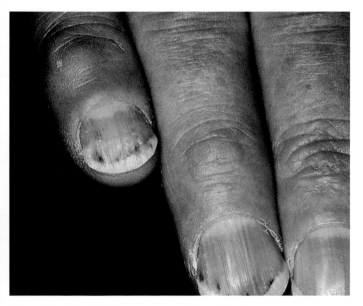

Figure 38–4 Splinter hemorrhages of the nail bed.

Nail Bed Abnormalities

Splinter Hemorrhages

Splinter hemorrhages arise from the longitudinally aligned capillaries of the nail bed and are usually the result of trauma (Fig. 38–4). However, they can be associated with systemic disease, e.g., bacterial endocarditis, particularly when they arise in multiple nails, or when they occur more proximally. Splinter hemorrhages have also been noted in association with anemia, trichinosis, chronic glomerulonephritis, vasculitis, psoriasis, scurvy, juvenile cirrhosis, high altitudes, eczematous eruptions, fungal nail infections, rheumatoid arthritis, mitral stenosis, septicemia, malignant tumors, dialysis, and following kidney transplantation.

Muehrcke's Lines

Muehrcke's lines are double white transverse bands of the nail bed that are associated with a vascular change. Unlike Mees'

lines, these disappear temporarily when the distal phalanx is squeezed, signifying nail bed and not nail plate alteration. They have been seen in patients with chronic hypoalbuminemia and vanish when the serum albumin concentration is higher than 2.2 g/100 mL. Several diseases, such as glomerulonephritis and nephrotic syndrome, cause hypoalbuminemia and are associated with Muehrcke's lines. They have also been seen in cardiomyopathy, after cardiac transplantation, and during chemotherapy. Terry's nails and half-and-half nails may be variants of the same process.

Onycholysis

Onycholysis, or separation of the nail plate from the nail bed, is often associated with trauma, irritant or allergic contact dermatitis, onychomycosis, psoriasis, or drug reactions. It is less frequently a sequela of systemic disease, e.g., thyrotoxicosis (Fig. 38–5). It also occurs with hypothyroidism, porphyria, Raynaud's disease, and the yellow nail syndrome. A number of medications, including psoralens, tetracycline, and chloramphenicol, when combined with ultraviolet light, may produce photo-induced onycholysis.

Periungual and Distal Digit Abnormalities

Clubbing

The angle between the normal nail plate and the skin of the finger at the proximal nailfold is less than 180° – usually close to 160°. Digits are regarded as clubbed if this angle is increased (≥180°). Pressure on the tissue proximal to the cuticle gives a spongy feeling in a clubbed finger. Soft tissue fibrovascular hyperplasia is the probable cause. Conditions that resemble clubbing with a slightly increased angle include curved nails, paronychia, and resorption of the distal phalanx. These are referred to as pseudoclubbing.

Simple acquired clubbing is bilateral and often related to cardiopulmonary disease. Simple acquired single-digit clubbing is most often associated with vascular lesions in the same extremity. Examples include aneurysm, arteriovenous fistula, and peripheral shunt. However, lymphadenitis, Pancoast

369

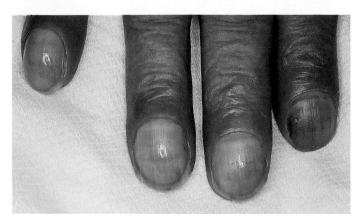

Figure 38–6 Clubbing secondary to a bronchogenic cancer.

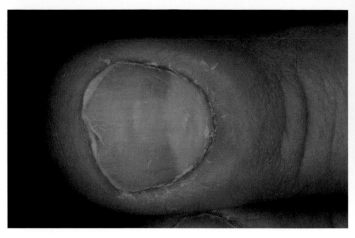

Figure 38–7 Chronic candidal paronychia in a patient with diabetes mellitus. Reproduced with permission from Mallett RB. Paronychia. In: Lebwohl et al. (eds) Treatment of Skin Disease, 3rd edn. 2009.

tumors, reflex sympathetic dystrophy, and erythromelalgia have been shown to cause unilateral clubbing. The cause is often traumatic or, less likely, congenital when only one nail is involved.

The syndrome of acquired hypertrophic pulmonary osteo-arthropathy includes simple clubbing, muscle weakness, joint pain and swelling, upper and lower extremity hypertrophy with soft tissue proliferation and sometimes edema, bone pain, proliferative periostitis, and peripheral neurovascular diseases. When all characteristics of the syndrome occur, a malignant thoracic tumor – often bronchogenic carcinoma (Fig. 38–6) – is found in more than 90% of cases.

In addition to pulmonary diseases, others less commonly associated with clubbing include processes affecting the cardiovascular, hepatic, gastrointestinal, and renal systems. Endocarditis, congestive heart failure, cirrhosis of the liver, ulcerative colitis, and chronic pyelonephritis are a few examples of the systemic diseases that may be related to acquired bilateral clubbing.

Hereditary and idiopathic clubbing may be transmitted as an autosomal dominant trait, a sex-limited trait with variable penetrance, or a simple mendelian dominant trait. These types affect both fingers and toes, are not associated with systemic disease, and usually start at puberty.

Nailfold Capillary Abnormalities

Distortions of the normal capillary architecture at the proximal nailfold may be seen in a number of connective tissue diseases. Dilated capillary loops with avascular areas are often seen with scleroderma and dermatomyositis. Tortuous capillaries with normal vascular density are more specific for systemic lupus erythematosus.

CHANGES IN SPECIFIC DISORDERS

Cardiovascular and Hematologic Systems

Red lunulae are often seen in congestive heart failure. Patients with hemochromatosis may have gray, blue, or brown nails; leukonychia; and longitudinal striations. Nail clippings may

be used to demonstrate blood groups, and therefore their sampling may have legal ramifications.

Gastrointestinal System

Blue lunulae occur in patients with Wilson's disease. Terry's nails are abnormally white, except for a distal pink zone close to the free edge known as the onychodermal band. This has been associated with cirrhosis, diabetes mellitus, congestive heart failure, thyrotoxicosis, malnutrition, and aging. Persistent hyperbilirubinemia may cause brown nails due to melanin deposition.

Cronkhite–Canada syndrome consists of nonfamilial gastrointestinal polyposis, skin pigmentation, alopecia, and nail changes. The nails are white, brittle, and often triangular. Chronic active hepatitis may cause splinter hemorrhages, clubbing, and white nails.

Endocrine System

Longitudinal pigmented bands have been seen in patients with Addison's disease. They are usually brown, and may involve the whole nail plate. Similar changes have also been described in patients having undergone bilateral adrenalectomy for Cushing's disease. These are most likely caused by melanocyte stimulation due to increased adrenocorticotropic hormone production.

Patients with acromegaly may present with short, wide, thick, and flat nails. Proximal nailbed telangiectasia with yellow nails has been described in patients with diabetes mellitus. Patients with hypothyroidism may present with brittle nails, slow nail growth, and longitudinal sulci.

Infectious Diseases

Most ungual changes in infectious diseases are nonspecific. Chronic candidal paronychia occurs often in diabetes mellitus (Fig. 38–7). Syphilis has been associated with paronychia, nail thinning, loss of the lunula, nail fragility, and fissuring of the free margin. Red lunulae have been reported in patients with lymphogranuloma venereum, and gray nails in patients with malaria. Loss of the lunula, paronychia, leukonychia, and subungual abscesses have been noted in leprosy.

Patients with acquired immunodeficiency syndrome (AIDS) may have yellowing of the nails and seem to have more frequent fungal nail infections. Zidovudine has been shown to cause longitudinal pigmented bands and yellow-brown discoloration of the nails.

Central and Peripheral Nervous Systems

Most onychopathies in association with neurologic disorders are nonspecific. Destruction of the tips of the digits occurs in Lesch–Nyhan syndrome; splinter hemorrhages and onycholysis in central nervous system disease; and Beau's lines in epilepsy. Double-edged nails are found in psychotic disease; striated leukonychia in manic–depressive disorders; and longitudinal striations in multiple sclerosis, syringomyelia, and hemiplegia. One report noted a correlation between the visibility of the nailfold subcapillary plexus and a family history of schizophrenia. This observation has been independently confirmed.

Pulmonary System

The yellow nail syndrome has been associated with many pulmonary diseases, such as asthma, pleural effusion, tuberculosis, bronchiectasis, chronic sinusitis, chronic bronchitis, and chronic obstructive pulmonary disease. The nails are thickened and yellow, with an increased transverse curvature (Fig. 38–8). The yellowish color affects both fingernails and toenails and usually the entire nail plate, although at times the proximal nail may be normal in color. The nails have a reduced growth rate, loss of the cuticle and the lunula, varying onycholysis, and periungual tissue swelling. Yellow nails resolved in a patient who had surgical removal of a carcinoma of the larynx. The yellow nail syndrome has been associated with other carcinomas, including melanoma, Hodgkin's disease, sarcoma, lymphoma, and adenocarcinoma of the endome-

trium. It has also occurred in patients receiving D-penicillamine therapy, and in women with no abnormality except unequal-sized breasts.

In Bazex's syndrome (acrokeratosis paraneoplastica), psoriasiform changes in the nails occur in association with upper gastrointestinal or upper respiratory tract carcinomas. These changes may disappear with excision of the tumor. The ungual signs consistently precede the detection of the neoplasm.

Renal System

Half-and-half nails (Lindsay's nails) exhibit a white proximal portion and a normal distal portion (Fig. 38–9). The distal part occupies 20–60% of the total nail. If less than 20% is affected this is usually referred to as Terry's nails. In 25–50% of patients the half-and-half nail has been associated with chronic renal failure.

Another group of nail findings that may accompany renal failure occurs in the nail–patella syndrome (Fig. 38–10). The signs include nail dystrophy (absence and/or discoloration),

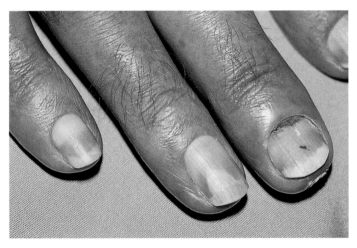

Figure 38–9 Half-and-half nails in a patient with renal failure. (Courtesy of Neil Fenske, MD, Tampa, FL.)

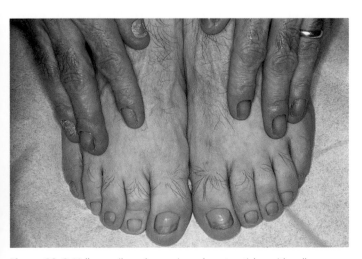

Figure 38–8 Yellow nail syndrome, i.e., absent cuticles with yellow discoloration of the nail plate.

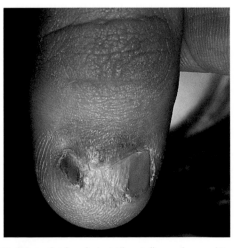

Figure 38–10 Triangular lunula in nail–patella syndrome. (Courtesy of Leonard Swinyer, MD, Salt Lake City, UT.)

triangular or poorly formed lunulae, longitudinal ridging, and koilonychia.

Splinter hemorrhages, Mees' lines, and Muehrcke's lines have been associated with renal failure. The nail bed may have an increased reddish color in relation to renal adenocarcinoma, which produces erythropoietin with erythrocytosis.

Rheumatologic Diseases

Ungual thickening, discoloration, red lunulae, longitudinal ridging with a beaded appearance, splinter hemorrhages, and periungual hemorrhagic infarcts (Bywater's lesions) are findings – some of which may be normal variants – that are reported with rheumatoid arthritis. The yellow nail syndrome has also been described in association with rheumatoid arthritis.

Systemic lupus erythematosus may also present with nail abnormalities. The proximal nailfold is often erythematous and fissured, with dilated capillary loops. Other potential findings include pitting, leukonychia striata, paronychia, splinter hemorrhages, clubbing, white nails, and onycholysis with possible secondary nail shedding. Changes secondary to distal ischemia and Raynaud's phenomenon also occur. The 'oil-spot' finding that is usually seen in psoriasis may occasionally be noted in patients with systemic lupus erythematosus.

Similar ungual abnormalities are seen in patients with dermatomyositis. In this disease, the changes include pitting, erythema, bluish-red plaques at the base of the nails, dilated tortuous capillary loops in the proximal nailfolds, and hyperkeratotic or dystrophic cuticles. Poikilodermatous skin shows different shades of red and pink, with mild atrophy and telangiectasia. These changes usually occur over the knuckles and on the proximal nailfold.

Yellowing, onycholysis, and subungual hyperkeratosis have been associated with Reiter's syndrome. Other changes may be identical to changes seen with psoriasis.

Raynaud's disease of long duration may produce significant ungual changes. The nail is often thin, with longitudinal ridging, and brittle, splitting easily. Discoloration often occurs secondary to an accumulation of debris and infection. There may be a mild reduction in the growth rate, onycholysis, and koilonychia. Excessive cold exposure can produce Beau's lines as a result of a temporary interruption of nail growth. Pterygium formation may complicate vasomotor ischemia. Patients with Raynaud's disease often have chronic paronychia, and frequently have fungal infections involving the nail.

The ungual changes in scleroderma include tightening of the skin of the digits, erythema and telangiectasia of the proximal nailfold, and infarcts of the distal digits secondary to ischemia. Pterygium inversum unguis occurs when the distal part of the nail bed and/or hyponychium adheres to the ventral surface of the nail plate. In this setting, the normal distal separation of these structures does not occur. Additional ungual findings that have been found in scleroderma include clubbing, onychorrhexis, absence of the lunula, onycholysis, ragged cuticles, vesiculation of the periungual area, hapalonychia, onychogryphosis, and deep longitudinal sulci.

Multicentric reticulohistiocytosis is another rheumatologic condition with associated ungual changes. These include brittleness, onycholysis, longitudinal ridging, atrophy, hyperpigmentation, and characteristic papules around the nailfolds ('coral beading'). The nails are wider than they are long.

Other ungual associations with rheumatic disorders include pitting with psoriatic arthritis, more rapid nail growth in acute rheumatic fever and Still's disease, and nails with absent lunulae and reduced cysteine content in chronic polyarthritis. Brittleness, leukonychia, crumbling of the nail plate, and longitudinal striations are ungual changes that have been noted in gout.

Toxicology

A variety of drug therapies, especially multidrug chemotherapies and highly active antiretroviral therapies, are associated with numerous nail changes, which are adequately discussed in other texts.

Miscellaneous

A variety of other ungual abnormalities may occur in association with systemic diseases. These include nail shedding and paronychia with Stevens–Johnson syndrome, subungual pustules in impetigo herpetiformis, onycholysis or disappearing lunulae in multiple myeloma, and leukonychia and Mees' lines in carbon monoxide poisoning. Paronychia, purpura, onycholysis, subungual hyperkeratosis, and splinter hemorrhages are noted in Langerhans' cell histiocytosis, subungual purpura in Letterer–Siwe disease, and nail shedding in toxic epidermal necrolysis and toxic shock syndrome. Nail dystrophy, including hyperkeratosis, shedding, hemorrhage, and horizontal ridging, occurs with bullous pemphigoid. Shedding of the nails may be prominent in epidermolysis bullosa, and leukonychia in cryoglobulinemia. Mees' lines have been reported in Hodgkin's disease and may be related to a poor prognosis. Leukonychia can be seen in Orthodox Jews who fast, and in patients with herpes zoster, hyperalbuminemia, and exfoliative dermatitis.

In pemphigus vulgaris the ungual findings include pitting, paronychia, discoloration, transverse lines, color changes, subungual hemorrhage, Beau's lines, subungual hyperkeratosis, fungal infection, pterygium, and onycholysis.

Onycholysis, increased fragility, brittleness, subungual thickening and striations, longitudinal ridging, and crumbling occur in amyloidosis. This may resemble lichen planus clinically.

SUGGESTED READINGS

Baran R, Dawber RPR, de Berker DAR, et al. Baran and Dawber's diseases of the nails and their management, 3rd edn. Oxford: Blackwell Science, 2001.

Baran R, Perrin C. Nail degloving, a polyetiologic condition with 3 main patterns: a new syndrome. J Am Acad Dermatol 2008; 58: 232–237.

Cutolo M, Sulli A, Secchi ME, et al. Nailfold capillaroscopy is useful for the diagnosis and follow-up of autoimmune rheumatic diseases. A future tool for the analysis of microvascular heart involvement? Rheumatology (Oxford) 2006; 45: iv43–46.

Fawcett RS, Linford S, Stulberg DL. Nail abnormalities: clues to systemic disease. Am Fam Phys 2004; 69: 1417–1424.

Haneke E. Surgical anatomy of the nail apparatus. Dermatol Clin 2006; 24: 291–296.

Hinds G, Thomas VD. Malignancy and cancer treatment-related hair and nail changes. Dermatol Clin 2008; 26: 59–68, viii.

Pappert AS, Scher RK, Cohen JL. Longitudinal pigmented nail bands. Dermatol Clin 1991; 9: 703–716.

Piraccini BM, Iorizzo M, Starace M, Tosti A. Drug-induced nail diseases. Dermatol Clin 2006; 24: 387–391.

Singh G, Haneef NS, Uday A. Nail changes and disorders among the elderly. Indian J Dermatol Venereol Leprol 2005; 71: 386–392.

Tosti A, Iorizzo M, Piraccini BM, Starace M. The nail in systemic diseases. Dermatol Clin 2006; 24: 341–347.

Tunc SE, Ertam I, Pirildar T, et al. Nail changes in connective tissue diseases: do nail changes provide clues for the diagnosis? J Eur Acad Dermatol Venereol 2007; 21: 497–503.

Oral Mucous Membranes and Systemic Disease

Pathologic changes in the oral mucous membranes can be involved in the full spectrum of systemic diseases, ranging from developmental disturbances and autoimmune diseases to infectious and neoplastic disorders (Table 39–1). A methodic inspection of the soft tissues of the oral cavity with palpation of the gutters, floor of the mouth, tongue, and major salivary glands is necessary to complete a thorough physical examination. Clues to the presenting diagnosis or significant incidental findings, such as oral carcinoma, may be disclosed. In this chapter, selected oral diseases with systemic implications are discussed and illustrated.

NEVOID BASAL CELL CARCINOMA SYNDROME(OMIM #109400)

The nevoid basal cell carcinoma syndrome (NBCCS) is an autosomal dominant trait (gene map locus 9q31, 9q22.3, 1p32) with high penetrance and variable expressivity. There is also a high spontaneous mutation rate. This condition is a result of mutations in the PTCH and/or PTCH2 genes. The major features of the nevoid basal cell carcinoma syndrome are numerous basal cell carcinomas at an early age, skeletal anomalies, palmar and plantar pits, and multiple jaw cysts. The jaw cysts, found in about 75% of affected persons, are odontogenic keratocysts (OKCs) that arise from dental lamina remnants or from basal cell components of overlying oral epithelium. They usually occur in the posterior portion of the mandible. An odontogenic keratocyst may be the first sign of the nevoid basal cell carcinoma syndrome in a child, and if there is more than one, a search for the other stigmata of this syndrome is indicated. The odontogenic keratocyst is benign, but its growth may produce lateral bone expansion, displacement of teeth, and pathologic fractures. The histologic findings of odontogenic keratocysts are specific. The cyst cavity is filled with keratin. Surgical excision is the treatment of choice, but there is a high recurrence rate (about 35%). If one or more major criteria for the diagnosis of the nevoid basal cell carcinoma syndrome besides multiple odontogenic keratocysts can be identified, genetic counseling and an aggressive program of skin cancer prevention with vigilant follow-up should be initiated.

CHEILITIS GRANULOMATOSA (MELKERSSON–ROSENTHAL SYNDROME)

Cheilitis granulomatosa is a distinct clinicopathologic entity of unknown cause that usually affects young adults and is characterized by diffuse, nontender, soft to firm, chronic swelling of one or both lips (Fig. 39–6) and other intraoral sites. Cheilitis granulomatosa is often confused with angioedema clinically, but the history of chronicity of the lip swelling is not compatible with angioedema. The biopsy specimen shows nonnecrotizing granulomas, lymphedema, and lymphangiectasia. Crohn's disease and sarcoidosis must be excluded because they also can produce granulomatous cheilitis. Cheilitis granulomatosa together with facial swelling, including periorbital skin, fissured tongue, and facial nerve palsy, constitutes the Melkersson–Rosenthal syndrome. Patients infrequently have the complete form of the syndrome, therefore the concept of orofacial granulomatosis has been accepted to include a wide array of conditions that show nonspecific granulomatous inflammation in biopsy specimens.

Patients with cheilitis granulomatosa may be treated with intralesional triamcinolone acetonide (10–20 mg/mL) injections. Patient comfort is improved by local anesthetic blocks of the lip. The response is usually favorable but temporary, and requires repeated injections at intervals of months or years. Alternative anti-inflammatory medical treatment includes hydroxychloroquine (HCl), chloroquine phosphate, sulfasalazine, methotrexate, and tumor necrosis factor (TNF)-α antagonists. Surgical reduction of the lips during a quiescent phase may correct persistent macrocheilia and improve function and appearance. Intralesional or systemic corticosteroids have been advocated to reduce the risk of recurrence after surgical treatment.

ACUTE NECROTIZING ULCERATIVE GINGIVITIS

Acute necrotizing ulcerative gingivitis (ANUG; 'trench mouth') is a fairly common oral disease of complex cause that occurs

Table 39–1 Systemic diseases with mucocutaneous manifestations

Category	Disease	Oral manifestations	Cutaneous findings
Genetic	Nevoid basal cell carcinoma syndrome	Odontogenic keratocysts	Palmar pits, multiple basal cell carcinomas
	Hereditary hemorrhagic telangiectasia (Osler–Weber–Rendu syndrome)	Mat-like telangiectases on the vermilion, tongue, buccal mucosal and palate	Mat-like telangiectasia on the perioral skin and hands, particularly the fingertips
	Multiple hamartoma syndrome (Cowden's disease)	Papillomatosis (Fig. 39–1) of the gingivae, dorsal tongue and buccal mucosal	Facial trichilemmomas, acral keratoses, and occasionally palmar or plantar pits
Inflammatory	Behçet's disease	Aphthae – recurrent and severe (Fig. 39–2)	Genital aphthae, pustular 'vasculitis', pyoderma gangrenosum-like lesions, erythema nodosum-like lesions, pathergy is common
	Inflammatory bowel disease	Oral aphthae, pyostomatitis vegetans, linear ulcers, orofacial granulomatosis	Erythema nodosum, pyoderma gangrenosum
	Lupus erythematosus	Leukoplakic patches, discoid lupus erythematosus lesions (Fig. 39–3), aphthae	Photosensitivity, discoid lupus erythematosus, subacute cutaneous lupus erythematosus, acute 'butterfly' rash
	Scleroderma (progressive systemic sclerosis)	Reduced oral aperture, mat-like telangiectasia (Fig. 39–4) (particularly in patients with CREST), xerostomia	Acral or proximal sclerosis, calcinosis cutis, Raynaud's phenomenon, mat-like telangiectasia, murine facies, hypo- or hyperpigmentation
	Wegener's granulomatosis	Gingival hyperplasia with petechiae (strawberry gingivitis), oral ulcerations, poorly healing extraction sites	Palpable purpura, cutaneous granulomatous vasculitis
	Sarcoidosis	Infiltrative lesions, orofacial granulomatosis	Papules, nodules, granulomatous lesions in scars
Infectious	Candidiasis	Thrush, angular cheilitis	—
	Oral hairy leukoplakia	Corrugated white plaques most commonly on the lateral tongue	—
Neoplastic	Kaposi's sarcoma	Blue to violaceous macular to nodular lesions (Fig. 39–5)	—
	Leukemia/lymphoma	Infiltrative lesions, boggy, friable gingival surface, erythematous to violaceous nodules of the lateral hard palate	—
Miscellaneous	Graft-versus-host disease	Reticular lichen planus-like lesions, salivary gland dysfunction, thrush, mucositis, xerostomia	Lichenoid lesions or scleroderma-like changes

in normal individuals. Contributing factors include the fuso-spirochetal oral flora, reduced host resistance, malnutrition, poor oral hygiene, smoking, and psychologic stress. ANUG occurs with increased frequency in HIV-infected patients, in whom it may evolve rapidly to stomatitis, periodontitis, and osteitis if not adequately treated. ANUG (and oral hairy leukoplakia) are significantly correlated with helper T-cell depletion.

The chief complaint is usually painful bleeding gums. The patient's breath is characteristically fetid, but the most reliable diagnostic feature of ANUG is the presence of 'punched-out' ulcerated interdental papillae. Treatment consists of thorough debridement of the involved tissue and cleaning of the teeth by a dentist, followed by chlorhexidine rinses after meals, and systemic antibiotics such as metronidazole, penicillin, or tetracycline.

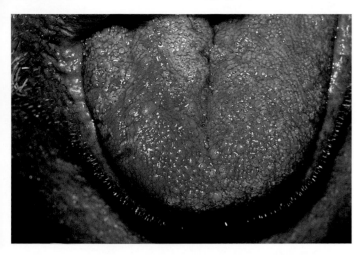

Figure 39–1 Papillomatosis of the tongue in a patient with multiple hamartomas and neoplasia syndrome.

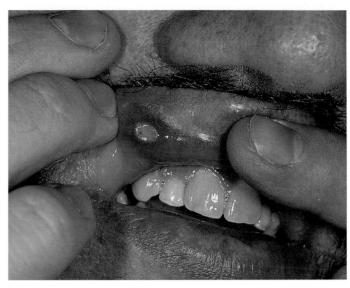

Figure 39–2 Typical major aphthous ulceration.

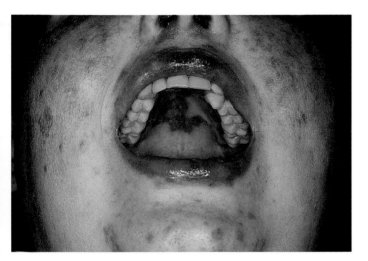

Figure 39–3 Mucosal lesion of lupus erythematosus on the palate.

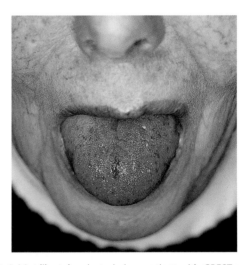

Figure 39–4 Mat-like telangiectasia in a patient with CREST syndrome. (Reprinted with permission from Color atlas of dermatology, 2nd edn. Philadelphia: WB Saunders, 2000.)

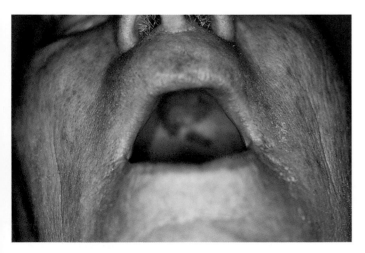

Figure 39–5 Kaposi's sarcoma on the hard and soft palates.

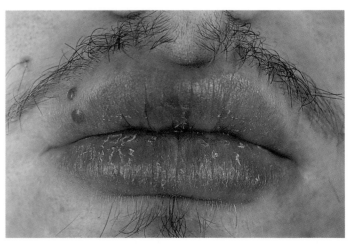

Figure 39–6 Asymmetrical swelling of the lips in cheilitis granulomatosa.

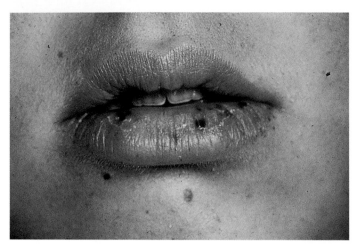

Figure 39–7 Hyperpigmented labial macules of Peutz–Jeghers syndrome.

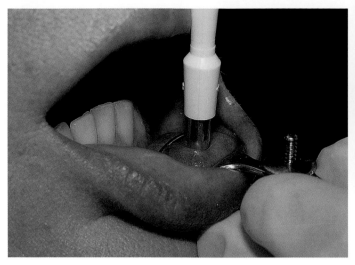

Figure 39–8 Biopsy of minor salivary glands.

ORAL PIGMENTATION

The most common form of oral hyperpigmentation is that seen distributed symmetrically in darkly pigmented individuals, although the intensity of the color is not directly related to that of the skin. Antimalarial therapy may produce a bluish-gray discoloration of the palate after long-term use. Bismuth therapy and lead intoxication produce a narrow band of bluish-black pigment along the marginal gingiva. Minocycline may discolor bone, fully developed teeth, and less commonly the oral mucosa. Cigarette smoking is associated with pigmentation of the lip and gingiva. Other causes of intraoral and cutaneous pigmentation include Addison's disease, hemochromatosis, and neurofibromatosis. Peutz–Jeghers syndrome is a highly penetrant, autosomal dominant disorder characterized by gastrointestinal hamartomatous polyps and pigmented macules around the mouth, lips, labial and buccal mucosae (Fig. 39–7), and dorsal and volar aspects of the hands and feet. The pigmentary markers of the syndrome appear early in life.

XEROSTOMIA

Xerostomia is the subjective sensation of dry mouth caused by a reduction in salivary flow. Patients with xerostomia can be recognized by their ever-present bottles of water or ice chips. A wooden tongue depressor usually sticks fast to the dorsum of the tongue. Xerostomia is one cause of glossodynia or the burning mouth syndrome. Drugs with anticholinergic effects, such as antihistamines and antidepressants, and diuretics may contribute to the problem. Xerostomia and xerophthalmia are symptoms of the sicca complex associated with primary and secondary Sjögren's syndrome. The latter group usually has the sicca complex in addition to a connective tissue disease. The tongue often has a red, parched, mammillated surface, and keratoconjunctivitis sicca may be present. Oral ulcerations may occur secondary to trauma and heal slowly. A biopsy of the labial minor salivary glands (Fig. 39–8) or the parotid gland may show foci of lymphoplasmacytic inflammation, which suggests Sjögren's syndrome.

Patients are particularly prone to dental caries; therefore, sugarless hard candies and saliva substitutes containing carboxymethylcellulose or hydroxyethylcellulose should be used. Oral pilocarpine and cevilimine are recommended for treating hyposalivation and xerostomia, but excessive sweating is the most common side effect.

GINGIVAL HYPERPLASIA

Drug-induced gingival hyperplasia is primarily fibrous and noninflammatory. It typically begins in the interdental papillae of dentate persons and overgrows the teeth. The classic drug responsible is phenytoin, but more recent culprits include cyclosporine and the antihypertensive calcium channel blockers, including nifedipine, verapamil, and amlodipine. Ironically, the latter three drugs are often used to treat hypertension caused by cyclosporine. Meticulous oral hygiene, plaque control, and professional debridement help to prevent gingival hyperplasia, and it may resolve on discontinuation of these drugs. Azithromycin in standard dosages has been shown to reduce cyclosporine-induced gingival hyperplasia.

SUGGESTED READINGS

Bhatia V, Mittal A, Parida AK, et al. Amlodipine induced gingival hyperplasia: a rare entity. Int J Cardiol 2007; 122: e23–24.

Haresaku S, Hanioka T, Tsutsui A, Watanabe T. Association of lip pigmentation with smoking and gingival melanin pigmentation. Oral Dis 2007; 13: 71–76.

Kruse-Losler B, Presser D, Metze D, Joos U. Surgical treatment of persistent macrocheilia in patients with Melkersson–Rosenthal syndrome and cheilitis granulomatosa. Arch Dermatol 2005; 141: 1085–1091.

Mirowski GW, Waibel JS. Pigmented lesions of the oral cavity. Dermatol Ther 2002; 15: 218–228.

Neville BW, Damm D, Allen C, Bouquot J. Oral and maxillofacial pathology. Philadelphia: WB Saunders, 2002.

Perez-Calderon R, Gonzalo-Garijo MA, Chaves A, de Argila D. Cheilitis granulomatosa and Melkersson–Rosenthal syndrome: treatment with intralesional corticosteroid injections. Allergol Immunopathol 2004; 32: 36–38.

Ratzinger G, Sepp N, Vogetseder W, Tilg H. Cheilitis granulomatosa and Melkersson–Rosenthal syndrome: evaluation of gastrointestinal involvement and therapeutic regimens in a series of 14 patients. J Eur Acad Dermatol 2007; 21: 1065–1070.

Shah SS, Oh CH, Coffin SE, Yan AC. Addisonian pigmentation of the oral mucosa. Cutis 2005; 76: 97–99.

Tokgoz B, Sari HI, Yildiz O, et al. Effects of azithromycin on cyclosporine-induced gingival hyperplasia in renal transplant patients. Transplant Proc 2004; 36: 2699–2702.

Treister NS, Magalnick D, Woo SB. Oral mucosal pigmentation secondary to minocycline therapy: report of two cases and a review of the literature. Oral Surg Oral Med Oral Pathol 2004; 97: 718–725.

Van der Waal RI, Schulten EA, van der Meij EH, et al. Cheilitis granulomatosa: overview of 13 patients with long-term follow-up–results of management. Int J Dermatol 2002; 41: 225–229.

Von Bultzingslowen I, Sollecito TP, Fox PC, et al. Salivary dysfunction associated with systemic diseases: systematic review and clinical management recommendations. Oral Surg Oral Med Oral Pathol 2007; 103 Suppl: S57. e1–15.

Leg Ulcerations

PREVALENCE AND ECONOMIC COST

Leg ulcerations are a common clinical problem with considerable attendant morbidity and often a dramatic negative impact on a patient's quality of life. Although marked improvements in wound healing have occurred in recent years, attributable perhaps to earlier intervention, chronic leg ulcerations remain a prevalent and costly problem.

In the UK, leg ulceration has a point prevalence rate of 0.3–0.6% and a lifetime cumulative risk of 1.0–1.8%. In the United States, the estimated prevalence of all skin ulcerations and wounds was 4.8 million in 2004. Among those aged 65 and over, an annual venous leg ulceration prevalence of 1.69 per 100 person-years has been reported. The overall incidence rate for men and women was 0.76 and 1.42 per 100 person-years, respectively. Each year, more than 50 000 patients in the United States require amputation for osteomyelitis; in most of these the osteomyelitis began as foot ulcerations caused by diabetes mellitus.

Healthcare spending on skin ulcerations and wounds has increased rapidly. In a study of the burden of skin disease in the United States in 2004, the cost of treating wounds and skin ulcerations exceeded that of all other skin diseases combined. The annual cost of skin ulcerations and wounds in 2004 was estimated at $11.9 billion (the US billion is defined as

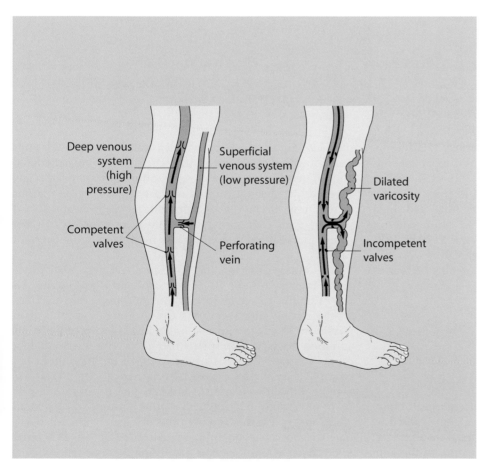

Figure 40–1 The low-pressure superficial venous system, which is protected by valves from the high-pressure deep venous system. Venous insufficiency is associated with valvular dysfunction. High pressure is thus transmitted throughout the superficial and deep venous systems. (From Phillips TJ, Dover JS. Leg ulcers. J Am Acad Dermatol 1991; 25: 965–987, with permission.)

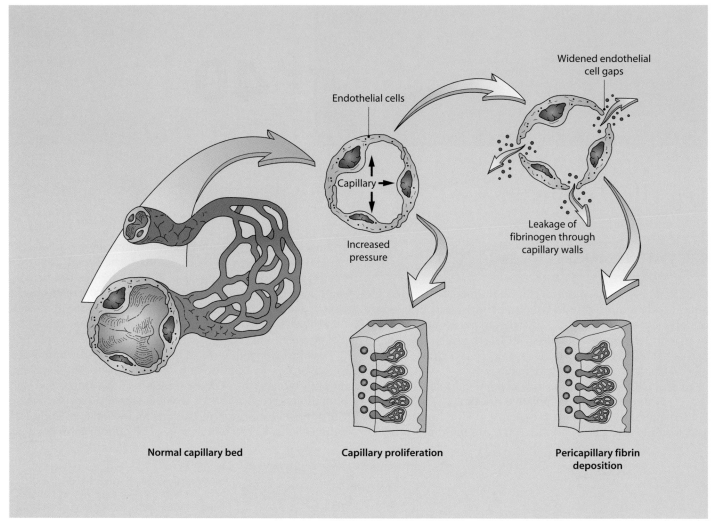

Figure 40–2 Venous insufficiency. The high venous pressure is transmitted to the capillary circulation. The endothelial pores widen, allowing the escape of fibrinogen into the extracellular fluid, with deposition around the capillaries. Capillary proliferation also occurs. (From Phillips TJ, Dover JS. Leg ulcers. J Am Acad Dermatol 1991; 25: 965–987, with permission.)

Within the figure: Endothelial cells; Widened endothelial cell gaps; Capillary; Increased pressure; Leakage of fibrinogen through capillary walls; Normal capillary bed; Capillary proliferation; Pericapillary fibrin deposition

1 000 000 000). Direct costs were approximately $9.7 billion, which comprised $8.5 billion spent on hospital inpatient costs (including $425 million on nursing home care), $157 million in hospital outpatient costs, $244 million in hospital emergency departments, $485 million in office visits, and $325 million in prescription medications. Of the $2.2 billion in lost productivity costs, the cost of lost workdays was $170 million, restricted activity was $150 million, lost caregiver workdays was $100 million, and lost future earning potential because of premature death was $1.8 billion.

PATHOPHYSIOLOGY

Overview

Although the differential diagnosis of leg ulcerations is extensive, in the western world they are most frequently caused by venous insufficiency (Figs 40–1, 40–2), arterial insufficiency, neuropathy, diabetes mellitus, or a combination of these. In

one large cohort of patients with leg ulceration, 72% of lesions were attributed to venous insufficiency, 22% to mixed arterial and venous disease, and 6% to predominantly arterial disease. A second large study showed that 54% of all leg ulcerations were venous ulcerations; this percentage rose to nearly 70% if patients with foot ulcerations only were excluded. In the elderly population, arterial disease becomes a more frequent cause.

A summary of factors that can cause and perpetuate ulcerations is given in Table 40–1. Dermatologists have a particular responsibility to recognize the less common causes of leg ulcerations because they are more thoroughly trained than physicians from other specialties in the diagnosis of these less common diseases. Appropriate therapy is critically dependent on an accurate diagnosis of the cause of the ulceration. For example, small-vessel disease associated with leg ulcerations may be difficult to recognize and may present as painful pinpoint ulcerations that heal with a white atrophic scar (livedoid vasculopathy; Fig. 40–3). Care must be taken before establishing a diagnosis of pyoderma gangrenosum (Fig. 40–4) because many other conditions can have similar presentations. Fur-

Table 40–1 Causes of leg ulcerations

Venous (see Fig. 40–10)
    Deep venous outflow obstruction
    Ineffective venous valves
    Inefficient calf muscle pumps
    Varicose leg veins
	Osteomyelitis
	    Inflammation
	        Connective tissue disease
	            Lupus erythematosus
	            Polyarteritis nodosa
	            Rheumatoid arthritis
	            Wegener granulomatosis

Ischemic
    Atherosclerosis with or without superimposed trauma
        (see Figs 40–12 and 40–13)
    Atheroemboli (cholesterol emboli)
    Arteriolar disease
    Leukocytoclastic vasculitis (vasculitis of the postcapillary venule)[a]
    Vascular occlusion
        Coagulopathy
        Livedoid vasculopathy (see Fig. 40–3)
	Panniculitis
	    Infectious
	    Noninfectious
	        Necrobiosis lipoidica
	        Pancreatic fat necrosis (malignancy pancreas)
	        α_1-Antitrypsin panniculitis
	Malignancy
	    Squamous cell carcinoma
	    Basal cell carcinoma (see Fig. 40–7)
	    Melanoma
	    Lymphoma
	    Metastatic disease
	    Sarcoma
	        Kaposi
	        Angiosarcoma

Neurotrophic (see Fig. 40–6)
    Diabetes mellitus
    Tabes dorsalis (syphilis)
    Spinal cord lesions
    Any condition associated with decreased sensation
	Metabolic
	    Diabetes mellitus
	    Gout
	    α_1-Antitrypsin deficiency
	    Calciphylaxis (see Fig. 40–15)

Nonvascular
    Trauma
        Pressure
        Injury
            External
            Self-induced or factitious (see Fig. 40–8)
            Burns (chemical, thermal, radiation)
            Cold (frostbite)
            Spider bite (brown recluse spider)
    Infection
        Bacterial
        Fungal (deep)
            Blastomycosis
            Cryptococcosis
            Coccidioidomycosis
            Histoplasmosis
        Sporotrichosis (see Fig. 40–17)
            Viral (herpes simplex)
            Mycobacterial
            Parasitic (leishmaniasis)
            Spirochetal
	Hematologic
	    Sickle cell anemia
	    Thalassemia
	    Coagulopathy (see Fig. 40–11)
	    Cryoglobulinemia
	Medication (hydroxyurea)
	Pyoderma gangrenosum
	    Ulcerative (see Fig. 40–4)
	    Bullous
	    Pustular
	    Vegetative
	Multifactorial (any combination of causes)

[a]Often caused by infection, medication, malignancy, and connective tissue disease.
From Davis MDP. Leg ulcerations. In: Rooke TW, Sullivan TM, Jaff MR, eds. Vascular medicine and endovascular interventions. Malden (MA): Blackwell Futura, 2007; 141–148, with permission.

thermore, it is important to recognize that ulcerations often have several contributing factors and different mechanisms of pathogenesis. A 'diabetic foot ulceration' is most often due to a combination of lower limb arterial insufficiency, diabetic neuropathy, and local trauma.

Pathophysiology of Chronic Ulcerations

Normal wound healing is a dynamic, integrated process that requires the interplay of numerous factors. Phases of healing are hemostasis, inflammation, proliferation, and remodeling with wound contraction (Fig. 40–5). Various factors that contribute to a nonhealing ulceration have been identified.

Chronic leg ulcerations generally appear to be anchored in the inflammatory or the proliferative phase, although they also may be due to problems in any phase of healing. Fibroblasts appear senescent, oddly shaped, and dysfunctional. Growth factors and metalloproteinases appear in excess and are associated with a state of ongoing destruction within the wound. Biofilms (communities of microorganisms in a polysaccharide matrix) can colonize the wound and form a structure that is difficult to penetrate with antibiotics. Increasing patient age, nutritional deficiency (especially protein and vitamin deficiency), chronic illness, chronic immunosuppression, hypoxia, vasculopathy, and infection all can contribute to poor wound healing.

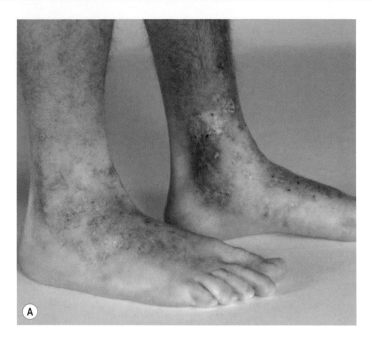
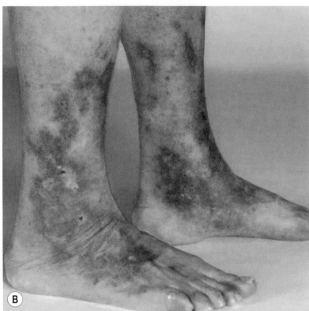

Figure 40–3 Ulceration due to livedoid vasculopathy. Shallow, pinpoint ulcerations involving the lower limbs heal with smooth, porcelain-white scars that are surrounded by punctate telangiectasia and hyperpigmentation.

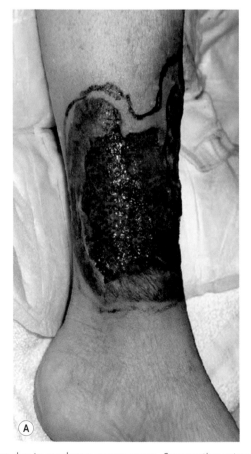
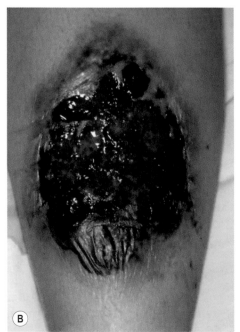

Figure 40–4 Ulceration due to pyoderma gangrenosum. Suppurative cutaneous ulcerations have edematous, boggy, blue, undermined, and necrotic borders that can progress rapidly.

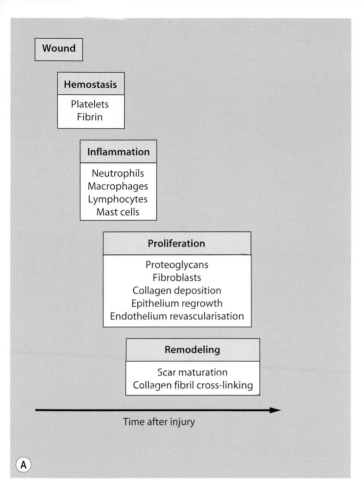

Figure 40–5 Normal wound healing. A, Time line of wound-healing events. B, Inflammatory phase (day 3). C, Re-epithelialization and neovascularization (day 5). FGF = fibroblast growth factor; IGF = insulin-like growth factor; KGF = keratinocyte growth factor; MMP = matrix metalloproteinase; PDGF = platelet-derived growth factor; TGF = transforming growth factor; t-PA = tissue plasminogen activator; u-PA = urokinase-type plasminogen activator; VEGF = vascular endothelial growth factor. (From Singer AJ, Clark RAF. Cutaneous wound healing. N Engl J Med 1999; 341: 738–746, with permission.)

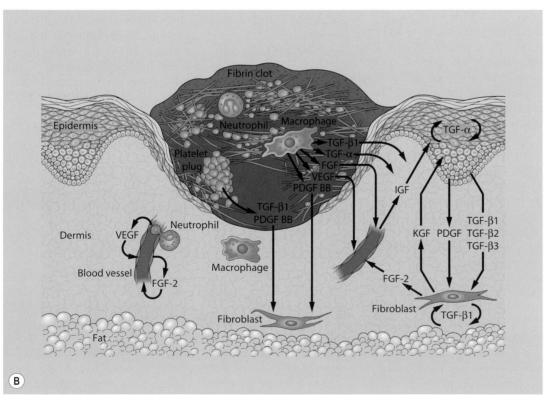

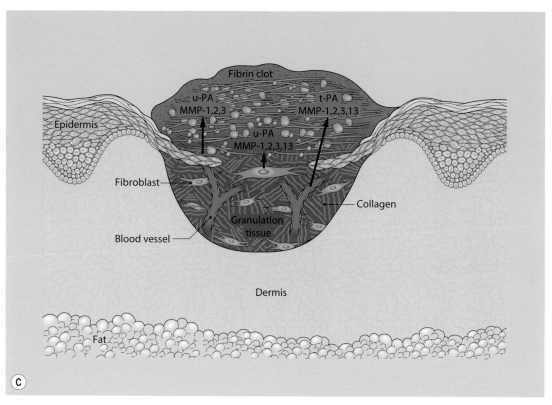

Figure 40–5 *Continued.*

Pathophysiology of Venous Ulceration

Venous blood flow in the lower extremities is dependent on the superficial, communicating, and deep venous systems. The long and short saphenous veins and their tributaries make up the superficial system. The communicating (or perforator) veins connect the superficial veins of the leg with the deep venous system. Communicating veins are equipped with one-way bicuspid valves that direct flow only into the deep system. The deep veins contain valves and are either intramuscular or intermuscular. When a person is standing, the pressure in the superficial and deep venous systems is roughly equal to the hydrostatic pressure in the legs (80 mmHg). During calf muscle contraction, when valves are functioning properly, deep veins are compressed and blood is propelled cephalad. Proper valve function ensures unidirectional flow and prevents transmission of high venous pressure to the superficial drainage system. After deep venous emptying and calf muscle relaxation, deep venous pressure decreases to 0–10 mmHg. Valves open and allow flow from the superficial system to deep venous drainage. Generally, in a healthy person, veins empty and ambulatory venous pressure decreases during exercise; this process requires intact leg veins, intact venous valves, efficient calf muscle pumps, and no deep venous outflow obstruction. In contrast, persons with venous insufficiency or dysfunction have increased ambulatory venous pressure during exercise.

Although the causes of chronic venous hypertension (venous insufficiency) seem reasonably well understood, the patho-physiology of ulceration in venous insufficiency is still unknown. One theory postulates that increased intraluminal pressure in the capillaries causes leakage of fibrinogen through capillary walls, deposition of pericapillary fibrin cuffs (shown in immunofluorescence studies), and impairment of oxygen or nutrient diffusion to tissue; together, these changes may result in tissue necrosis and ulceration. A second theory about the mechanism of injury posits that the known sludging of white blood cells in venous insufficiency causes capillary obstruction. Trapped white blood cells may become activated and release proteolytic enzymes that promote ulceration. A third theory, the 'trap' hypothesis, suggests that the leakage of fibrin and other macromolecules into the dermis traps or binds growth factors and reduces the amount available for tissue repair.

Pathophysiology of Arterial Ulceration

Arterial insufficiency results in local ulceration and digital or limb necrosis, depending on the severity of ischemia. Arterial ischemia can be caused by compression of the artery (e.g., radiation fibrosis with entrapment of the artery), wall thickening (e.g., arteriosclerosis), or intra-arterial restriction of blood flow (e.g., hyperviscosity, coagulation disorders with arterial occlusion, cholesterol embolus). Arteriosclerosis is the most common cause of arterial ischemia. In many patients with diabetes mellitus, the disease can accelerate atherogenesis, and ulceration develops as a consequence of severe arteriosclerosis.

Ulcerations due to Sensory Neuropathy and Diabetes Mellitus

Neuropathy that results in reduced sensation in the lower extremities is often associated with leg ulceration because patients may traumatize the extremity unknowingly (Fig. 40–6). Although the differential diagnosis of peripheral neuropathy is broad, the lack of sensation from any cause can lead to pressure necrosis, especially on the feet.

Diabetes mellitus is a clinically significant risk factor for foot ulcerations and is one of the most common causes of peripheral neuropathy. Although only 4% of the general population is diabetic, 46% of patients admitted to a hospital with a foot ulceration have diabetes mellitus. Moreover, half of all lower extremity amputations in hospitalized patients occur in those with diabetes mellitus. A 'diabetic ulceration' is perhaps a misnomer because such ulcerations may have multiple causes. Inadequate arterial blood flow accounts for approximately 20% of cases, diabetic neuropathy accounts for 50%, and 30% are attributable to both. Additional factors that may contribute to foot ulcerations are small-vessel disease, infection, and poor healing.

PATIENT HISTORY AND PHYSICAL EXAMINATION FINDINGS

History

An adequate history must be obtained to establish the cause of ulceration (Table 40–2). A history of ulcerations may be predictive of future ulcerations. Medications, family history, social history, and review of systems also may provide important information. For example, a longstanding, nonhealing ulceration may be associated with the development of squamous cell or basal cell carcinoma (Fig. 40–7). Contact allergies to topical medications used on the leg is a common contributory cause (up to 65% of patients in some studies). A family

history of ulcerations could be attributable to an α_1-antitrypsin deficiency. A social history of intravenous drug abuse may indicate that ulcerations could be caused by infection, or by injection of foreign material. A history of injections for cosmetic purposes may indicate a lipogranuloma. Patients may also have factitious or self-inflicted ulcerations (Fig. 40–8).

Physical Examination

Key elements of the ulceration that can provide diagnostic information are outlined in Table 40–3. The size of the ulcer should be documented at each visit with photographs and by noting dimensions of greatest length and perpendicular width and depth. Size and depth may be important prognostically because larger ulcerations are slower to heal. Any undermining, sinuses, or tunneling must be determined. The pattern of the ulcerations may also provide important clues. Characteristics of the ulcer base (color, presence of necrosis) can affect healing. The moisture level (dry, moist, or wet) and the presence or absence of an exudate help elucidate the cause of the

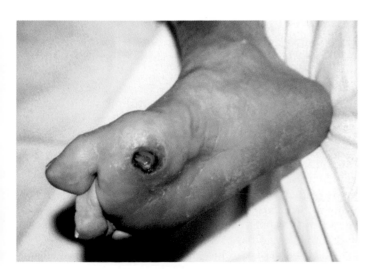

Figure 40–6 Neuropathic ulceration. A thickened callus at a site of repeated trauma or pressure disintegrates to form an ulceration on an insensate foot.

Table 40–2 Important historical features for diagnosis of ulcerations

Pain
    Usually severe when associated with ischemic ulcerations, pyoderma gangrenosum, calciphylaxis, hydroxyurea-induced ulcerations
    Less severe when associated with venous ulcerations

Rate of progression (rapid vs slow)   Pyoderma gangrenosum ulcerations progress rapidly
Duration of ulceration   Long duration of ulceration is a predictor of poor healing

Prior therapy
    Systemic
    Topical

Medical and surgical history
    History of ulcerations (predictive of future ulcerations)
    Venous disease, arterial disease, lymphedema
    Neurologic disease
    Diabetes mellitus
    Hematologic disease (sickle cell anemia, thalassemia, coagulopathy)
    Gastrointestinal tract disease (inflammatory disease may underlie pyoderma gangrenosum)
    Renal disease (calciphylaxis)
    Rheumatologic disease (connective tissue disease)
    Skin disease
    Psychiatric disease

Medications (hydroxyurea)

Family history
    Ulcerations
    Metabolic disorders
    Coagulopathy

Social history
    History of picking at skin
    Psychologic or psychiatric factors
    Smoking (exacerbates ischemic ulcerations)

From Davis MDP. Leg ulcerations. In: Rooke TW, Sullivan TM, Jaff MR, eds. Vascular medicine and endovascular interventions. Malden (MA): Blackwell Futura, 2007; 141–148, with permission.

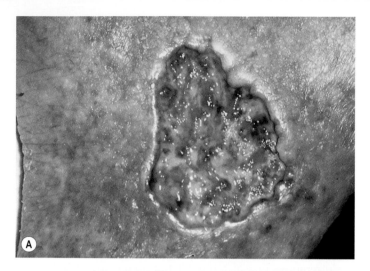

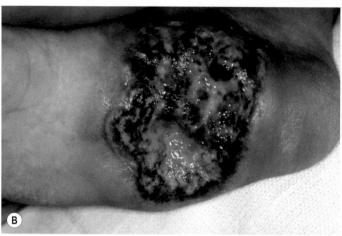

Figure 40–7 Ulceration due to malignancy. A, The rolled border of the ulceration is clinically suggestive of basal cell carcinoma. (This later was proved histologically.) B, The rolled, elevated border is suggestive of malignancy. A biopsy showed clear cell sarcoma.

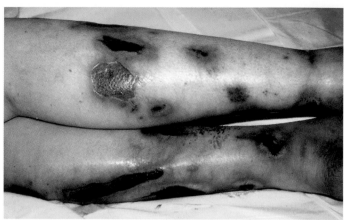

Figure 40–8 Factitious or self-inflicted ulceration. Linear, superficial ulcerations in accessible areas suggest external trauma as a cause.

ulceration and affect management decisions. The surrounding skin may suggest causes of ulceration (e.g., red, hot skin may indicate cellulitis). Screening for sensory neuropathy can be accomplished through the use of nylon monofilament (10 g). Patients who are unable to feel anything when sufficient pressure is applied to buckle the filament are at increased risk for neuropathic foot injury. Table 40–4 shows investigations that may be performed when determining the cause of leg ulcerations.

COMMON CAUSES OF ULCERATION

Venous Ulcerations

Venous ulcerations increase in prevalence with age, peaking between ages 60 and 80. The first episode of venous ulceration may occur much earlier than this, however: 13% are affected by age 30, 22% by age 40. Studies suggest a somewhat increased risk in women, with a female:male ratio of 1.6:1.

Most venous ulcerations occur in the area between the ankle and the lower calf (the gaiter area); conversely, ulcerations on the foot or the upper calf are probably nonvenous in origin. Patients with venous ulcerations typically describe aching and swelling in the legs that are exacerbated by dependency and relieved by elevation of the limb. Ulcerations themselves are classically painless but may sometimes be painful. Edema of the lower limbs is common. Brown or brown-red hemosiderin pigmentation occurs because of extravasation of red cells into the dermis, collection of hemosiderin within macrophages, and melanin deposition. Eczematous changes with erythema, scaling, pruritus, and sometimes weeping are common.

Lipodermatosclerosis or sclerosing panniculitis (woody induration and fibrosis of the dermis and subcutaneous tissue) often develops in patients with venous insufficiency, and these may precede venous ulceration. Venous ulcerations often develop over the malleoli, particularly on the medial aspect of the leg, and characteristically have an irregular, shaggy border (Figs 40–9, 40–10). Ulcerations tend to be shallow and have a yellow (fibrinous) base, but they seldom have necrotic eschar or exposed tendons. After ulceration is well established, repeat episodes of infection and cellulitis can damage the lymphatic system and result in chronic lymphedema. Ultimately, fibrous or bony ankylosis at the ankle may develop because of immobility. Hair loss on the leg may occur with venous or arterial insufficiency.

Patients may be predisposed to the development of a venous thrombosis if they have coagulation disorders (Fig. 40–11), antithrombin III deficiency, activated protein C resistance (mainly factor V Leiden mutation), antiphospholipid antibody and lupus anticoagulant, protein C or S deficiencies, prothrombin G20210A mutation, some dysfibrinogenemias, hereditary or acquired hyperhomocysteinemia, and elevated levels of procoagulant factors IX, X, and XI. A higher risk of venous thrombosis is associated with an increased risk of venous insufficiency, and patients with venous insufficiency are more likely to have venous ulceration.

Patients with venous ulcerations seem to have an increased incidence of contact dermatitis and are especially sensitive to lanolin, topical antibiotics (e.g., gentamicin, neomycin, and bacitracin), and components of Unna boots. Contact derma-

Table 40–3 Physical examination findings and clinical significance

Location
  Ulcerations in the 'gaiter' area (between the lower third of the calf and 1 inch below the malleolus) are characteristic of venous disease
  Ulcerations on the lateral malleolus, bony prominences, and distal regions are characteristic of arterial disease
  Ulcerations on pressure points of the feet (e.g., metatarsal head or heel) are characteristic of neuropathic disease
  Thigh ulcerations are characteristic of polyarteritis nodosa, calciphylaxis, or factitious causes

Size
  Smaller ulcerations (<1.5 cm) are more likely to heal within 20 weeks
  Larger ulcerations are slower to heal

Pattern
  Linear ulcerations are likely to be factitial

Base
  Color
    Beefy red appearance preferred; dusky red base may indicate poor blood supply
    Necrotic yellow or brown fibrinous slough or debris inhibits wound healing (needs débridement)
  Depth
    Superficial: likely to heal
    Deep (muscle, bone): difficult to heal
      Osteomyelitis may be suspected clinically if the ulceration reaches the bone
    Undermining: pocket of 'dead space' may be a nidus for recurrence of ulceration or infection
  Moisture level
    Moist environment: preferred for healing
    Dry or wet wounds: slow to heal
      Desiccation of tissue occurs with dry wounds
      Maceration of tissue occurs with wet wounds
  Exudate
    Clear: edema
    Yellow: infection
  Odor: fishy odor indicates likely *Pseudomonas* infection

Edges of ulceration
  Sloping: characteristic of venous ulceration
  Vertical: characteristic of arterial ulceration
  Rolled: characteristic of basal cell carcinoma
  Undermined, violaceous: characteristic of pyoderma gangrenosum
  Stellate: livedoid vasculopathy

Surrounding skin
  Skin disease
    Cellulitis
    Dermatitis: stasis, xerosis, allergic contact dermatitis
    Dry skin (asteatosis, xerosis)
    Panniculitis
    Other skin condition
  Color
    Pale: ischemic disease
    Postinflammatory hyperpigmentation
    Yellow plaques: necrobiosis lipoidica
  Edema
    Venous disease
    Lymphedema
    Systemic (cardiac, pulmonary, or renal) disease
  Induration: lipodermatosclerosis
  Patterned
    Livedo reticularis (due to polyarteritis nodosa)
    Livedoid vasculopathy

Diminished pulse: large-vessel disease

Varicose veins: predispose patients to ulceration

Abnormal sensation and motor function: neurologic disease

Modified from Davis MDP. Leg ulcerations. In: Rooke TW, Sullivan TM, Jaff MR, eds. Vascular medicine and endovascular interventions. Malden (MA): Blackwell Futura, 2007; 141–148, with permission.

Table 40–4 Investigations of leg ulcerations (if clinically indicated)

Arterial studies
 Ankle–brachial index
 Exercise ankle–brachial index
 Arterial duplex ultrasonography
 Magnetic resonance angiography
 CT angiography
 Conventional angiography
 Transcutaneous oximetry measurements
 Laser Doppler flowmetry

Venous studies
 Duplex ultrasonography to exclude deep vein thrombosis
 Contrast venography
 Functional testing (plethysmography)

Lymphatic studies
 Lymphangiogram
 Lymphoscintigraphy
 Abdominal or pelvic computed tomography or magnetic resonance
  imaging

Neurologic studies
 Electromyography
 Small-fiber nerve testing
  Autonomic reflexes (Valsalva, table tilting, quantitative
   sudomotor axon reflex test)

Blood tests to identify potential underlying disorders
 Complete blood count
 Erythrocyte sedimentation rate, C-reactive protein
 Blood chemistry (liver, kidney, thyroid function tests)
 Protein electrophoresis
 Rheumatologic investigations (antinuclear factor, antineutrophil
  cytoplasmic antibodies)
 Special coagulation studies (factor V Leiden, cryofibrinogens,
  proteins C and S, cryoglobulins, anticardiolipin antibody,
  antiphospholipid antibody screening)

Wound swab (usefulness is debated)
 Gram stain, fungal stain, acid-fast stain, *Nocardia* smear
 Culture or polymerase chain reaction assays (to identify virus,
  bacteria, mycobacteria, fungi)

Biopsy of the edge of ulceration
 Elliptical incisional biopsy (preferred over punch biopsy)
  Specimen should include edge of ulceration to depth of
   subcutaneous fat
  Routine histologic examination (hematoxylin and eosin stain)
   Special stains (Gram, methenamine silver, Fite) to detect
    microorganisms
  Culture in appropriate medium (bacteria, fungi, mycobacteria)

Radiologic studies to exclude osteomyelitis
 Radiograph of underlying bone
 Magnetic resonance image
 Bone scan

From Davis MDP. Leg ulcerations. In: Rooke TW, Sullivan TM, Jaff MR, eds. Vascular medicine and endovascular interventions. Malden (MA): Blackwell Futura, 2007; 141–148, with permission.

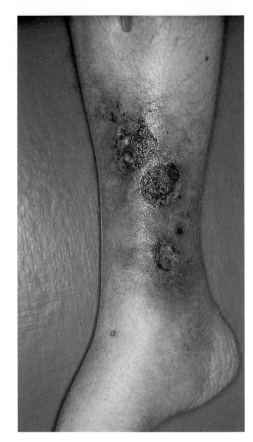

Figure 40–9 Stasis ulceration with bilateral ulcerations over the medial malleoli.

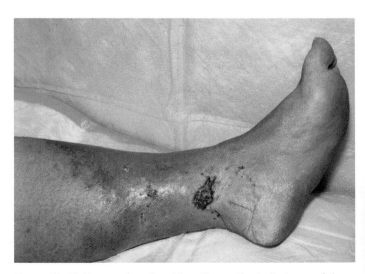

Figure 40–10 Venous ulceration. Ulceration on the 'gaiter' area of the leg shows an irregular and ill-defined border and a shallow wound bed. Ulceration is surrounded by brown pigmentation, which is characteristic of venous insufficiency.

titis can also occur with almost any of the occlusive or semi-occlusive dressings, despite improvements in wound care that were made possible with the use of such dressings.

Poor prognostic factors include a large wound area, long wound duration, poor compliance with compression, a history of venous ligation or stripping, history of knee or hip replace-ment, ankle–brachial pressure index < 0.8, and fibrin on 50% or more of the wound surface. One recent study showed that 72% of ulcerations with surface areas < 5 cm^2 at baseline had complete healing, whereas those ≥ 5 cm^2 healed at only a 40% rate using the same treatment regimen. Likewise, ulceration duration less than 1 year was associated with a 65% healing

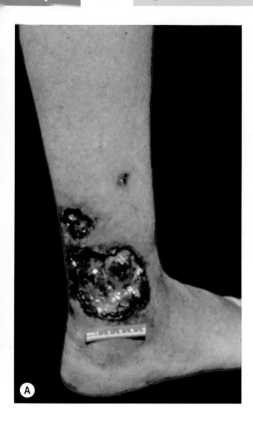

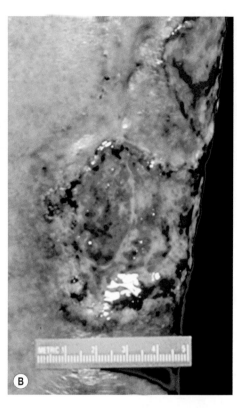

rate, and ulcerations of 1 year or longer duration healed at a rate of less than 29%.

Arterial Ulcerations

Patients with arterial ulcerations are usually older than 45. They present with symptoms of intermittent claudication and pain that initially occur with moderate exercise but are eventually present even at rest as the occlusive disease progresses. The pain from ulceration is usually severe and difficult to control, often worsening when the legs are elevated but improving with dependency. Cigarette smoking and diabetes mellitus are strong risk factors for arterial ulcerations because of atherosclerosis of the lower limbs.

Arterial ulcerations typically have a 'punched-out,' sharply demarcated border and occur over sites of pressure or trauma (e.g., bony prominences) or at distal points (e.g., toes) (Figs 40–12, 40–13). They usually appear dry and have a gray or black base that may be covered with necrotic debris. Associated findings include loss of hair on the legs, shiny and atrophic skin, and diminished or absent peripheral pulses. A prolonged capillary filling time (>4–5 seconds) and change in limb color with elevation are common findings.

Diabetic and Neuropathic Ulcerations

Neuropathic ulcerations occur commonly in patients with diabetes mellitus. They may be associated with chronic pain, dysesthesia, paresthesia, or anesthesia of the lower limb. The first sensation to be lost is light touch in the great toe, and then in the rest of the foot. The vibration sense is subsequently lost, followed by loss of the ankle jerk reflex and, finally, joint posi-

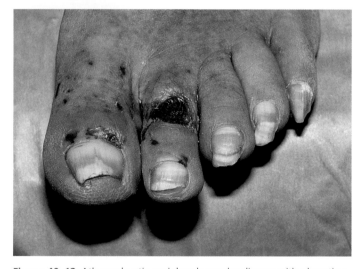

Figure 40–12 Atherosclerotic peripheral vascular disease with ulceration. (From Callen JP, Greer KE, Hood AF, et al., eds. Color atlas of dermatology. Philadelphia: WB Saunders; 1993; 231, with permission.)

tion sense. Patients are usually unaware of the precipitating trauma that commonly precedes ulceration of the heel, the plantar metatarsal area (Fig. 40–14), or the great toe. The neuropathic ulceration often is surrounded by a thick callus. Underlying osteomyelitis must be considered in patients with prolonged, purulent drainage of these ulcerations.

Patients with diabetes mellitus are predisposed to peripheral vascular disease, neuropathy, infection, and impaired healing. Of all lower limb amputations, 45–70% are performed on patients with diabetes mellitus, and 41–70% of

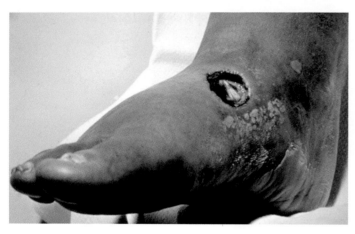

Figure 40–13 Arterial ulceration. Ulceration is round with a sharply demarcated border. Note the tendon at the base of the ulceration.

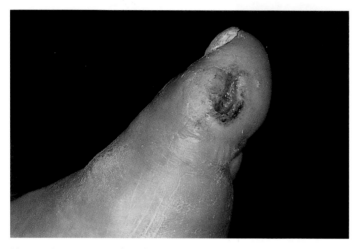

Figure 40–14 Neuropathic ulceration in a diabetic patient with peripheral neuropathy.

these patients do not survive longer than 5 years after the procedure. Early detection of neuropathy or angiopathy may prevent acceleration of complications, or even reverse the process. The exact mechanism by which diabetes mellitus causes angiopathy and neuropathy is unknown, although factors such as impaired autoregulation, a reduced hyperemic response to injury, and impaired neurogenic vasodilatation may reduce the healing potential of the skin after minor injury.

DIAGNOSTIC TESTS

Laboratory Tests

Laboratory investigations are not necessary for all patients with leg ulcerations. However, for those with nonhealing ulcers, a routine blood cell count and measurement of the blood glucose level help exclude clinically significant hematologic disorders or diabetes mellitus. A high erythrocyte sedimentation rate may indicate osteomyelitis or a connective tissue disorder. Low serum albumin or transferrin levels may suggest nutritional deficiencies. A high creatinine level may suggest

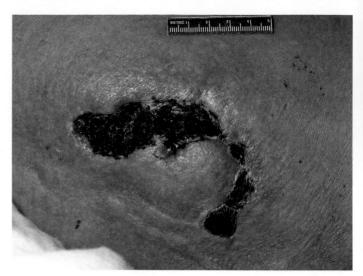

Figure 40–15 Ulceration due to calciphylaxis. Ulcerations on the thigh show taut subcutaneous tissue that is tender and hard to palpation.

calciphylaxis (Fig. 40–15). A positive antinuclear factor may be associated with ulcerations attributable to connective tissue disease.

Evaluation of underlying coagulation disorders should probably be limited to patients younger than 50 who have a history of recurrent venous thrombosis and to patients with a single thrombotic event and a positive family history of coagulopathy or recurrent venous thromboses. Coagulation testing can also be considered for patients in whom underlying coagulopathy may be present, such as livedoid vasculopathy, calciphylaxis, or other particular situations. Importantly, measurement of plasma antithrombin, protein C, protein S, or procoagulant levels may be falsely low or high within 6 months of a thrombotic event, so they should not be investigated in the acute setting. However, antiphospholipid antibodies or lupus anticoagulant can be measured immediately, and identification of gene mutations in factor V and prothrombin can be performed at any time. In rare instances, cryoglobulinemia may be a cause of leg ulcerations.

Vascular Studies

A summary of laboratory vascular tests that may be performed is given in Table 40–4.

Venous Studies

Physiologic tests and ultrasonography are used to evaluate venous disease. Currently, ultrasonography is used most frequently to assess acute and chronic venous disease. Physiologic tests are used to evaluate chronic venous disorders by measuring alterations in blood pressure, flow, and other parameters that indirectly assess the location and severity of lesions. Other tests for venous insufficiency include duplex ultrasonographic scanning, photoplethysmography, air plethysmography, strain gauge plethysmography, light reflux rheography, foot volumetry, and phlebography. Duplex ultrasonographic scanning allows direct visualization of the veins, identifies venous flow, and maps superficial and deep veins. It perhaps can be considered the diagnostic standard, but this method also requires the most technical proficiency.

Arterial Studies

The measurement of systolic blood pressure in the ankle is the most sensitive method of detecting large-vessel disease. The ankle–brachial pressure index is determined by dividing the systolic pressure in the ankle by that in the arm. Patients with moderate to severe arterial disease will have an ankle–brachial pressure index < 0.7. In patients whose peripheral pulses are not palpable, a Doppler flowmeter should be used to hear the arterial pulsations over the dorsalis pedis and posterior tibial arteries. Any patient whose Doppler studies suggest arterial disease should have arteriography and surgical assessment for the feasibility of arterial reconstruction. In patients with diabetes mellitus, noninvasive vascular studies (including the ankle–brachial pressure index) are frequently poor indicators of the severity of arteriosclerotic disease. Consequently, if ischemia is suspected in such patients, arteriography should be performed.

Patients with leg ulcerations attributable to rheumatoid arthritis or systemic sclerosis may have arterial or venous insufficiency that contributes to ulcer formation and failure to heal. A study of 15 consecutive patients with leg ulcerations together with one of these conditions showed that all but one had vascular insufficiency that markedly contributed to their ulcer formation, despite the clinical diagnosis of connective tissue disease-associated ulceration. Therefore, patients with rheumatic diseases and ulcerations that respond poorly to appropriate therapies might need vascular assessment to look for complicating disease.

Additional noninvasive tests (pulse waves from the toes and transcutaneous oximetry) may be helpful when assessing the risk of amputation in patients with skin lesions and arterial disease. Pulse waves from the toes can be recorded quickly and easily with photoplethysmography, and the wave amplitude is indicative of blood flow. These measurements may help guide decisions about arterial reconstruction.

Transcutaneous oximetry (the amount of oxygen diffusing through the skin from the capillaries) can be measured with an electrode applied to the skin surface. Oximetry can be used to predict wound healing and the most appropriate level for amputation. In one study, successful healing of below-knee amputations occurred in 96% of patients with a calf transcutaneous oxygen pressure > 20 mmHg, but successful healing occurred in only 50% of patients with a calf transcutaneous oxygen pressure of ≤20 mmHg.

Biopsy of the Edge of an Ulceration

Features of an ulceration that should prompt a biopsy include a vegetative, indurated border, a rapid increase in size, a tendency to bleed, or a failure to respond to therapy. Biopsy of all ulcerations that have not improved after 3 months of treatment should be considered to identify squamous cell carcinoma, basal cell carcinoma, vasculitis, or other inflammatory disorders as possible causes. Malignancy is identified in chronic wounds in roughly 0.33% of cases, and squamous cell carci-

noma is the most commonly cited. Squamous cell carcinoma arising in a chronic ulceration is an important reason for failure to heal. Furthermore, such carcinomas tend to behave much more aggressively with metastatic disease than with the usual skin-derived squamous cell carcinoma.

Adequate biopsy specimens are best obtained from the edge of a wound, and such a biopsy can be performed with minimal risk to the patient. An incisional wedge biopsy is preferred over a standard punch biopsy. Tissue specimens should undergo routine histologic examination and examination with special stains.

Cultures can be performed to identify bacteria, mycobacteria, and fungi from biopsy specimens, but the value of cultures obtained from wounds is debatable. Generally, tissue cultures are superior to cultures from wound swabs when determining the infectious cause of an ulceration, although a swab culture may be adequate to exclude herpes simplex virus. Bacteria are present on almost all wounds, and swabs may show only colonizing (not causative) microorganisms. Nevertheless, bacterial loads in excess of 10^5 organisms per gram of tissue are thought to impede wound healing, although other factors also affect healing.

Radiographic Studies

If bone is palpated at the base of a chronic ulceration, osteomyelitis must be suspected. Characteristic findings of osteomyelitis can be confirmed through radiographic studies (X-rays), but this method is not very sensitive. Further investigations such as a bone scan, CT scan, gallium scan, or bone biopsy may be necessary to confirm a diagnosis of osteomyelitis. The relative values of magnetic resonance imaging and three-phase bone scans have been debated, but either of these methods can be used to detect osteomyelitis.

Patch Tests

Patch tests should ideally be performed in patients with chronic leg ulcerations if contact dermatitis is suspected clinically. For patients with venous ulcerations, allergic patch test reaction rates as high as 60% have been reported; high rates probably reflect the topical medications and allergens used in wound dressings. Allergens that most commonly cause problems include neomycin, lanolin, bacitracin, formaldehyde, and parabens.

GENERAL PRINCIPLES OF WOUND CARE

The treatment of [leg ulcerations] is generally looked upon as an inferior branch of practice; an unpleasant and inglorious task, where much labour must be bestowed, and little honour gained.

On the Treatment of Ulcerated Legs,
Edinburgh Medical and Surgical Journal, 1805

Wound care is a critical part of patient management and is essential to prevent unnecessary morbidity (e.g., amputation) and death. Leg ulcerations are common (up to 2% of individuals will be affected in their lifetime), and, as outlined above, the associated costs of care are extremely high. Many factors can be associated with delayed wound healing, including vascular insufficiency, diabetes mellitus, neurologic defects, nutritional deficiencies, and local factors (e.g., pressure, infection, edema). Identification and correction of these factors is essential.

The most important aspect of wound care is recognition and appropriate management of underlying disease. For example, arterial disease should be managed with revascularization, venous disease with compression, neuropathic disease with offloading of the foot, and infectious disease with appropriate antimicrobial agents. General principles of wound care include appropriate débridement of devitalized tissue, prompt treat-

ment of any supervening wound infection, and maintenance of a moist and clean healing environment.

Débridement of Devitalized Tissue

Débridement is the removal of slough, exudate, eschar, bacterial biofilms, and callus from wound beds to permit healing (Table 40–5; Fig. 40–16). These elements generally are considered impediments to wound healing and should be removed, unless the ulceration is ischemic. (Ischemic tissues tend to desiccate after débridement and may be associated with ulcer enlargement.) In theory, débridement converts a chronic wound to an acute wound and triggers the acute wound healing

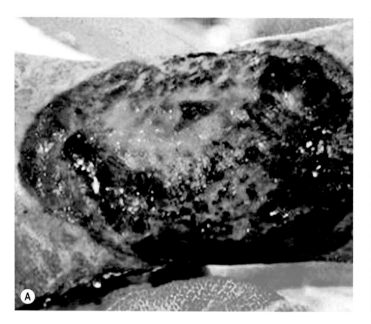

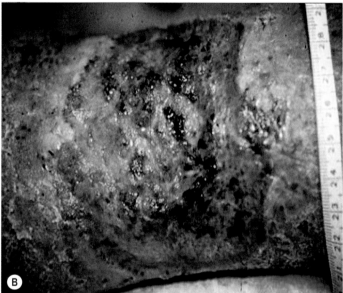

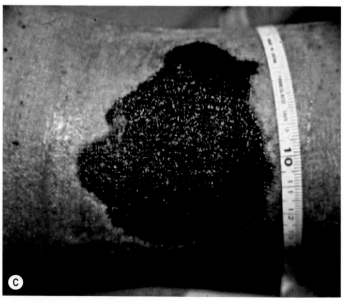

Figure 40–16 Débridement. Wet to moist dressings were used to remove the slough covering this ulceration. The beefy red granulation tissue at the base is considered optimal for wound healing.

Table 40–5 Methods of débridement

Method	Description
Surgical	Most commonly performed débridement procedure
	Uses a curette or scissors and forceps. Can be performed in the outpatient setting
	Extensive débridement is usually an inpatient procedure requiring local or general anesthesia
Mechanical	Performed by placing wet gauze on an ulceration and allowing to air dry until moist (preferred) or completely dry. Gauze and adhered debris are then removed
	Frequently changed saline dressings are safe. Wound surface remains moist, surface bacteria are removed, and ulceration surfaces are débrided
Autolytic	The body's innate enzymes separate slough and necrotic tissue from the wound bed. Best achieved in a moist wound environment
Enzymatic	Several enzymatic débriding agents are available in the United States (collagenase, papain–urea preparations). Anecdotal evidence of apparent benefit is common, but large, randomized, controlled studies are lacking
	Enzymatic débriding agents may affect adjacent healthy tissue and cause ulceration enlargement

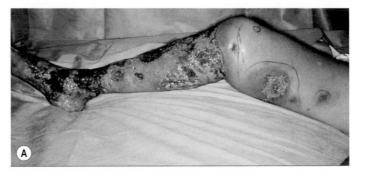
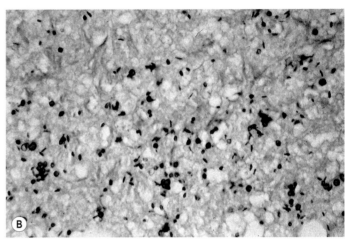

Figure 40–17 Ulceration due to infection. A, Ulcerations were initially attributed to pyoderma gangrenosum, and the patient was treated with immunosuppressive medication. However, the lymphangitic spread suggests infection. (From Byrd DR, el-Azhary RA, Gibson LE, Roberts GD. Sporotrichosis masquerading as pyoderma gangrenosum: case report and review of 19 cases of sporotrichosis. J Eur Acad Dermatol Venereol 2001; 15: 581–584, with permission.) B, A biopsy specimen showed numerous cigar-shaped bodies, consistent with *Sporothrix schenckii* (hematoxylin and eosin stain).

response. It may also directly stimulate the underlying granulation tissue by initiating bleeding.

Treatment of Infection

All open wounds are colonized by microbes. Most clinicians agree that systemic antibiotic therapy should be used if a wound has frank evidence of infection (e.g., cellulitis). Tissue biopsies are necessary to identify the infectious organism (Fig. 40–17), and the antibiotic used must specifically target the suspected organism. Empiric therapy is appropriate early in the course of care; regimens might include cephalexin, clindamycin, and fluoroquinolones.

The use of antibiotics is controversial when patients lack clear evidence of infection. Generally, it is not regarded as appropriate to treat what is grown on wound cultures because these organisms are usually colonizing the wounds. Empiric, systemic, antibiotic therapy does not necessarily diminish the microbial wound burden (colonization), nor does it reduce the progression of ulceration to amputation. Studies also have shown that topical antibiotics do not improve the probability of treatment success; in fact, topical antiseptic solutions are generally ineffective against infection and can damage granulation tissue. Still, antiseptic solutions are frequently used in the care of leg ulcerations, and recently, interest in antimicrobial dressings with slow-release iodine and silver has renewed.

To summarize, therefore, systemic antibiotic treatment should generally be started only if there is evidence of tissue infection.

Wound Dressings

For hundreds of years, therapeutic efforts focused on drying wounds, and absorptive gauzes were the mainstay of management. Nevertheless, since the 1960s, clinicians have understood that a moist wound heals more rapidly than a dry one (e.g., a wound exposed to air), and most currently available dressings are designed to maintain a moist environment for optimal healing (Table 40–6). In general, absorbent dressings (e.g., alginates, foams) are used on exudative wounds; dressings that moisturize (e.g., hydrogels, hydrocolloids) are used on dry wounds. Care must be taken to avoid an excessively moist wound, however, because the surrounding skin may macerate and result in a larger ulceration.

Dressings can do more than provide a moist environment: they can help débride the wound, change the bacterial flora,

Table 40–6 Wound dressings

Type	Description
Gauze	Most commonly used dressings, versatile. Plain cotton gauze offers good absorption. Available in pad and ribbon forms
	Many are impregnated with other materials; gauzes impregnated with petrolatum provide minimal moisturization of wounds and are less adherent
	Desiccation of the wound base may occur
Film	Thin, transparent adhesives (usually polyurethane). Slight variation in vapor permeability, strength, flexibility, and delivery systems
	Advantages include transparency, adhesiveness, and ability to serve as a bacterial barrier
	Disadvantages include problems with fluid accumulation under the film in exudative wounds, occasional difficulty in application. Adhesive on many films may strip newly formed epithelium during removal
Hydrogels	Water-based, gel-like, semitransparent, comfortable dressing material. Available in sheet and amorphous gel forms. Somewhat high cost
	Promotes autolytic débridement of slough and necrotic tissue
	Moisturizing properties help care of dry wounds but may cause maceration of surrounding skin around the wound
Hydrocolloids	Opaque, gas-impermeable absorbent dressings (hydrocolloid with a polyurethane outer coating). Adheres to the skin surrounding the wound
	Absorbs wound exudate to form a hydrophilic gel that helps maintain a moist healing environment. Can be left in place for up to 7 days or until soaked in exudate. Easy to use, cost-effective, and can successfully débride wounds
	Yellow-brown fluid that accumulates under the dressing can have an unpleasant odor (offensive to some patients)
	Can be difficult to use in cavities and may stimulate excess granulation tissue. Premature dressing removal can injure newly formed epidermis
Alginates	Highly absorbent, biodegradable dressings derived from seaweed. Forms a hydrophilic gel over the wound surface. May have an unpleasant odor. Available as ropes (twisted fibers) or pads (fibrous mats)
	Hemostatic properties are useful for exudative wounds (not helpful for dry wounds). Requires frequent dressing changes if the wound is moist. Must have a secondary dressing
Foam	Microporous, opaque dressings are made of polyurethane foam. One side is hydrophilic with a soft surface that absorbs wound exudate, the other side is hydrophobic and inhibits exudate leakage. Requires a secondary dressing
	Provides an absorbent but moist healing environment and conforms to body contours. If dressings are changed after the exudate dries, they adhere to the wound, cause pain on removal, and possibly strip away newly formed epithelium
Collagen	Available in particle and sheet form. May be derived from human, porcine, and bovine sources
	Interacts with wound exudate to form a gel over the wound. Believed to support wound healing by providing a scaffold matrix for new tissue
Antimicrobial agents	Topical antiseptics (e.g., iodine, silver, alcohols, biguanides, and chlorine) often are used to reduce microbial burden. Cadexomer–iodine preparations increasingly are used and may aid débridement and wound healing
	Some antiseptics (alcohol, chlorhexidine, hexachlorophene, and povidone–iodine) are cytotoxic for fibroblasts and may impair wound healing. Neomycin, polymyxin B, bacitracin, and gentamicin can cause sensitization, and some have triggered anaphylaxis with chronic use
	Silver ions increasingly are incorporated into wound dressing products. In bacteria, silver binds and disrupts cell walls, damages intracellular and nuclear membranes, poisons respiratory enzymes, and denatures DNA and RNA. Effective against Gram-negative bacteria and antibiotic-resistant organisms (methicillin-resistant *Staphylococcus aureus*, vancomycin-resistant *Enterococcus*)

and change the biochemical environment. Moisture-retentive dressings have the additional advantages of providing local pain relief, promoting granulation tissue formation, and reducing the frequency of dressing changes. Functionally different wound dressings are combined in commercial products (e.g., silver combined with alginate, collagen with hydrocolloid). The best combinations for exudative wounds are alginates, foams, and dry gauze. The best for dry wounds are hydrogels, hydrocolloids, and impregnated gauze.

Adjunct Wound Care Techniques

Topical Negative Pressure Therapy (Vacuum-Assisted Closure)

Vacuum-assisted closure is performed by applying open-cell foam to the wound, adding a seal of adhesive drape, and applying subatmospheric pressure (100–125 mmHg) to the wound on an intermittent or continuous basis. This method is believed to remove exudate, reduce bacteria, exert mechanical stress (causing granulation tissue formation and angiogenesis), and encourage migration of keratinocytes across wound defects. This technique is costly to perform; it is currently used by some to treat pressure ulcerations, venous ulcerations, and diabetic ulcerations. Encouraging results regarding the healing rates have been reported in the literature, but there is a relative paucity of randomized controlled trials with high patient numbers to substantiate the findings. A Cochrane review identified two small trials suggesting that vacuum-assisted closure may increase the healing rate of chronic wounds compared to the use of saline gauze dressings.

Hyperbaric Oxygen

Hyperbaric oxygen is an intermittent inhalation therapy that is sometimes administered to patients with diabetic, venous, arterial, or pressure ulcerations. During treatment the patient is sealed in a pressurized chamber and breathes pure oxygen at supra-atmospheric pressures (>1 atm). Hyperbaric oxygen therapy is based on the premise that tissue hypoxia contributes to the failure to heal of many chronic wounds; advocates suggest that tissue hypoxia may be overcome by increasing tissue oxygenation. However, the benefits for patients with chronic wounds remain controversial.

Hyperbaric oxygen therapy typically is an adjunct therapy for improving wound oxygenation, particularly when angioplasty or revascularization is not feasible. In a systematic review of randomized controlled trials involving hyperbaric oxygen for chronic wounds, the evidence suggested that the treatment reduced the risk of major amputation from 45% to 19% in patients with hypoxic, diabetic foot wounds. Wound healing also was somewhat improved (from 48% to 76%). Data are lacking for treatment of venous, arterial, or pressure ulcerations.

Hyperbaric oxygen treatments are expensive: about $400–$500 per session. Angiogenesis and infection control reportedly are achieved after 14–21 treatments. For patients with osteomyelitis, as many as 60 treatments may be necessary. Topical oxygen therapy, which involves inserting the wounded limb into an airtight, oxygenated bag, is considered ineffective.

Growth Factors

Animal models of chronic wounds have shown that growth factors can improve healing, but overall, results from clinical trials studying growth factors to accelerate wound healing have been disappointing. To date, the US Food and Drug Administration has approved only recombinant platelet-derived growth factor BB (becaplermin, in gel form) for adjunct treatment of diabetic neuropathic foot ulcerations. Efficacy studies have shown a modest benefit for patients with these ulcerations when becaplermin was combined with standard care (offloading, twice-daily dressing changes). The percentage of wounds healed at 20 weeks increased by 10–20%. In addition, becaplermin has been used to treat venous ulcerations, with variable reported benefit.

Skin Substitutes

Surgical skin grafts may be beneficial for some patients with recalcitrant ulcerations. Split-thickness and full-thickness grafts can be used, although split-thickness grafts are more common. Tissue-engineered skin equivalent and a dermal skin construct have been approved by the US Food and Drug Administration for use in treating venous ulcerations and diabetic neuropathic ulcerations. Skin substitutes are expensive but are reportedly effective in healing larger and deeper ulcerations and those that are at least 6 months old. A study of 240 patients with venous ulcerations showed that a higher proportion were healed 24 weeks after treatment with a tissue-engineered skin equivalent and compression, compared with compression alone (57% vs 40%, respectively).

Wound Care Centers

It is important to ascertain the home circumstances of each patient and determine who is available to help cleanse the ulcerations and apply dressings. Patients with recalcitrant wounds may have considerable benefit if they are referred to a multispecialty wound care or wound healing center, where many specialists and state-of-the-art therapies are available.

Pain Management

In general, pain management is an oft-neglected aspect of wound care. Many leg ulcerations are associated with disabling pain that consequently affects activities of daily living and disrupts sleep. Because chronic wounds may persist for months or years, patients can develop a chronic pain syndrome. For patients with venous ulcerations, quality-of-life measures for bodily pain, mental health, and social function are reduced compared with age-equivalent scores. A flurry of recent publications, primarily from the nursing literature, have described the inadequacy of prevalent pain management protocols and revived interest in pain management for chronic wounds. However, no evidence-based studies have been conducted to date.

Sometimes, simply covering a wound with a moisturizing dressing can reduce pain substantially. Topical analgesics such as lidocaine also may be effective. Systemic and local measures may be taken to control pain.

LEG ELEVATION. AND COMPRESSION

Elevation

Control of edema is extremely important for healing venous ulcerations. The primary role of treatment is to reverse the effects of venous insufficiency and hypertension, primarily through limb elevation and compression. The simplest method of leg elevation is to get patients off their feet and into bed when possible, and elevating the affected leg 18 cm above the level of the heart for 2–4 hours during the day and at night is most effective. If this is not possible, patients should understand that the ankle must be elevated higher than the level of the knee to be of any benefit. Even when adequate leg elevation is achieved, compression that results in partial venous occlusion at the level of the inguinal fold sometimes can impair drainage, particularly in very obese individuals. Leg elevation should be encouraged in all patients with venous insufficiency, unless they also have arterial insufficiency.

Compression

Compression is as important as elevation in the management of venous ulcerations and should be applied on arising and maintained until bedtime. The aim of compression is to overcome the effects of prolonged venous hypertension. Raising the local hydrostatic pressure and reducing the superficial venous pressure reduces the leak of solutes and fluid into the interstitial space. Compression also improves venous return. A pressure of 20–40 mmHg is recommended for venous ulcerations; most studies indicate that higher levels of compression at the ankle (35–40 mmHg) are optimal if the patient can tolerate it. A Cochrane systematic review of 22 trials determined that compression therapy was more effective than noncompressive dressings for the treatment of venous leg ulcerations. Furthermore, high-compression systems were more effective than low-compression systems. No significant differences in the effectiveness of different high-compression systems were observed.

Methods of compression include elastic and nonelastic single-layer bandages, multilayer bandages, compression stockings (alone or in combinations with bandages), and intermittent pneumatic compression. Elastic support stockings or support bandages should be comfortable and may be removed at night and before bathing or sleeping. Their major disadvantage is the difficulty of application and removal, particularly for elderly patients. However, new stockings are now available with a zipper to facilitate the process.

Unna Boot

The Unna boot is a compression bandage; it consists of a zinc oxide-impregnated gauze wrap that is applied from the toes to the knee, covered with a layer of cotton, and wrapped with an elastic compression dressing. Although the boot requires less time to apply and less patient cooperation than elastic support stockings, this treatment can cause localized purpura, cyanosis, ulceration, or necrosis of the skin if applied inappropriately. Unna boots are useful in areas where it is difficult to maintain adequate external pressure (e.g., the sides of the foot), and are especially helpful in protecting the limb from external trauma. The boot generally is worn for a week and needs to be replaced every 7–10 days. Ulcerations can be cleaned only when the boot is changed. If secondary infection occurs, infectious exudate and debris will accumulate around the ulceration, and the boot should be changed more frequently (every 3–4 days). When correctly applied, however, Unna boots are helpful in treating elderly patients, especially those with physical disabilities who have difficulty applying wound dressings. Multilayer elastic compression bandages are an alternative to the Unna boot. No clear differences in effectiveness between the different types of compression systems have been shown.

Intermittent Pneumatic Compression

Intermittent pneumatic compression devices may be used to relieve edema and may promote healing in patients with venous ulcerations. They consist of a sleeve that fits over the leg and attaches to a pump. Various pneumatic pumps with different specifications are available. This treatment is inappropriate for patients with uncontrolled congestive heart failure, patients who should not have increased venous or lymphatic return, and patients with acute inflammatory phlebitis in the limb. Intriguingly, studies comparing intermittent pneumatic compression and compressive dressings have shown no clinically significant advantage of pneumatic compression over compression dressings, assuming the patient is compliant with the latter.

Practical Issues to Consider Before Applying Compression

Before compression is considered, arterial pulses should be carefully palpated. Doppler pressure should be measured at the ankle if arterial disease is suspected clinically, because skin necrosis or even gangrene can result from compression of arterially compromised limbs. A common problem with compressive stockings occurs when leg dimensions are measured from a moderately to severely edematous leg. Patients should be strongly encouraged to elevate the leg and reduce the edema as much as possible before being fitted for stockings. Although patients may have some short-term benefit by preventing further swelling, the goal of therapy is to return the leg to its nonedematous diameter. For patients who are out of bed for part of the day, an appropriately snug elastic wrap can provide some measure of support that can be adjusted to match the shrinking leg during a period of days or weeks. Patients unable to wrap their legs properly without assistance may have better outcomes if they have fixed compression dressings applied professionally. These dressings can be sized to match the decreasingly edematous leg over time. Elastic cloth bandages can also be used.

MANAGEMENT OF CHRONIC ULCERATIONS

Ulcerations due to Stasis Dermatitis

Dermatitis is commonly associated with venous ulcerations. In patients with acute dermatitis associated with skin oozing and erosions, bed rest, frequent application of nonirritating wet dressings (e.g., saline-soaked gauze), and application of a moderate-potency corticosteroid cream for a few days may be necessary. Antibiotic coverage may be required for secondary infection of the skin. Liberal use of emollients such as white petrolatum should be recommended for patients with chronic dermatitis because pruritus and lichenification of the skin may be severe. Topical corticosteroids may be of some help in treating acute or chronic stasis dermatitis, but they are clearly less efficient than elevation and compression. High-potency corticosteroids can impair wound healing and should not be applied to the ulceration. Preparations of triamcinolone acetonide (0.025% or equivalent potency) are frequently used, although some clinicians believe that even less potent corticosteroids are indicated. Corticosteroid ointments are less likely than creams to cause contact dermatitis.

Venous Ulcerations

Large venous ulcerations may require skin grafts (usually pinch grafts or split-thickness skin grafts). Superficial venous insufficiency has been shown as the sole cause of chronic venous insufficiency in 13–38% of patients in European studies. In this group, stripping of the superficial veins can prevent ulceration recurrence.

Administration of systemic antibiotic therapy to patients with uncomplicated venous ulcerations does not markedly affect the rate of healing or influence bacterial colonization of ulcerations. Interestingly, randomized controlled trials of horse-chestnut seed extract have shown some benefit. However, the benefits of other systemic agents in the treatment of venous ulcerations are unclear. Pentoxifylline, a substituted xanthine derivative, increases fibrinolytic activity. It also reduces the risk of thrombus formation by reducing blood viscosity, increasing red cell deformability, and inhibiting platelet aggregation. Nevertheless, its effectiveness in the treatment of peripheral arterial and venous disease is controversial. The limited amount and quality of reported data describing its use in venous and arterial disease preclude a reliable estimate of its efficacy, but a Cochrane review of nine trials determined that pentoxifylline plus compression was superior to placebo plus compression for wound healing.

Arterial Ulcerations

Arterial ulcerations are due to inadequate blood supply to the skin. Atherosclerosis is the most common cause of inadequate blood supply, and, if possible, patients with arterial ulcerations should be referred to a vascular surgeon for revascularization. The patient should not smoke, and diabetes mellitus and hypertension should be well controlled. Exercise should be encouraged to promote the development of collateral circulation. The head of the patient's bed should be elevated by 4–6 inches to encourage gravity-dependent arterial flow, and limbs should be kept warm. Direct heat should not be applied, however, because of the risk of thermal injury. If the patient spends much time in bed, a sheepskin should be placed under the feet to protect bony prominences from pressure. A foot cradle to protect the toes should be used when possible. Many ischemic ulcerations are precipitated by trauma. The patient should therefore be given detailed instructions regarding care of the lower limbs. Regular use of analgesics may be required to relieve ischemic pain.

The use of systemic agents to promote healing of arterial ulcerations remains controversial. If rest pain or acute infection is present, the patient should be hospitalized and managed in close collaboration with a vascular surgeon. Cellulitis or lymphangitis should be treated with systemic antibiotics. Moist saline dressings, applied three or four times daily, are helpful when treating infected ulcerations. Débridement of dry eschar generally is not recommended for ulcerations caused by arterial insufficiency because it may promote further tissue ischemia. Arterial reconstruction should be considered for patients with arterial ulcerations, especially if rest pain or rubor is present. If arteriographic studies show vessel blockage, endarterectomy to remove localized atheromatous plaques can be performed, either alone or in combination with reconstruction to bypass occluded areas.

Cilostazol, a type III phosphodiesterase inhibitor (100 mg twice daily), can reduce pain and improve function in patients with intermittent claudication. Possible medication interactions may occur because it is metabolized by the cytochrome P450 system. Whether it helps heal arterial ulcerations is not known.

Diabetic and Neuropathic Ulcerations

Patients with diabetes mellitus have a 15–20% lifetime risk of developing a foot ulceration, usually because of neuropathy, vasculopathy, or both. Neuropathic ulcerations are most commonly observed in these patients: ulcerations often begin as thickened calluses that form at sites of repeated pressure but then break down. In patients with diabetes mellitus, healing is difficult to achieve because of nerve and vascular disease, poor tissue oxygenation, impaired immune response to injury, and a depressed immune system. Diabetic foot ulcerations are a major risk factor for limb amputation because osteomyelitis is more likely to occur.

Offloading of the affected areas is essential for healing diabetic neuropathic ulcerations. One study suggested that education and preventive measures can reduce the risk of limb ulceration and amputation by 68%. Shoe prostheses and diligent attention to reducing and redistributing pressure are essential to restore and maintain the integrity of the skin of the feet.

SUGGESTED READINGS

Bader U, Banyai M, Boni R, et al. Leg ulcers in patients with myeloproliferative disorders: disease- or treatment-related? Dermatology 2000; 200: 45–48.

Bello YM, Phillips TJ. Chronic leg ulcers: types and treatment. Hosp Pract (Minneap) 2000; 35: 101–107.

Bickers DR, Lim HW, Margolis D, et al., American Academy of Dermatology Association; Society for Investigative Dermatology. The burden of skin diseases: 2004 a joint project of the American Academy of Dermatology Association and the Society for Investigative Dermatology. J Am Acad Dermatol 2006; 55: 490–500.

Carter SA, Tate RB. The value of toe pulse waves in determination of risks for limb amputation and death in patients with peripheral arterial disease and skin ulcers or gangrene. J Vasc Surg 2001; 33: 708–714.

Choucair MM, Fivenson DP. Leg ulcer diagnosis and management. Dermatol Clin 2001; 19: 659–678.

Davis MDP. Leg ulcerations. In: Rooke TW, Sullivan TM, Jaff MR, eds. Vascular medicine and endovascular interventions. Malden (MA): Blackwell Futura, 2007; 141–148.

Dupuy A, Benchikhi H, Roujeau JC, et al. Risk factors for erysipelas of the leg (cellulitis): case–control study. Br Med J 1999; 318: 1591–1594.

Fonder MA, Lazarus GS, Cowan DA, et al. Treating the chronic wound: a practical approach to the care of nonhealing wounds and wound care dressings. J Am Acad Dermatol 2008; 58: 185–206.

Goyal S, Huhn KM, Provost TT. Calciphylaxis in a patient without renal failure or elevated parathyroid hormone: possible aetiological role of chemotherapy. Br J Dermatol 2000; 143: 1087–1090.

Hafner J, Kuhne A, Schar B, et al. Factor V Leiden mutation in postthrombotic and non-postthrombotic venous ulcers. Arch Dermatol 2001; 137: 599–603.

Hafner J, Schneider E, Burg G, Cassina PC. Management of leg ulcers in patients with rheumatoid arthritis or systemic sclerosis: the importance of concomitant arterial and venous disease. J Vasc Surg 2000; 32: 322–329.

Margolis DJ, Allen-Taylor L, Hoffstad O, Berlin JA. Diabetic neuropathic foot ulcers: the association of wound size, wound duration, and wound grade on healing. Diabetes Care 2002; 25: 1835–1839.

Nelzen O, Bergqvist D, Lindhagen A. Venous and non-venous leg ulcers: clinical history and appearance in a population study. Br J Surg 1994; 81: 182–187.

Phillips TJ. Current approaches to venous ulcers and compression. Dermatol Surg 2001; 27: 611–621.

Phillips TJ, Machado F, Trout R, et al. Prognostic indicators in venous ulcers. J Am Acad Dermatol 2000; 43: 627–630.

Robetorye RS, Rodgers GM. Update on selected inherited venous thrombotic disorders. Am J Hematol 2001; 68: 256–268.

Sarkar PK, Ballantyne S. Management of leg ulcers. Postgrad Med J 2000; 76: 674–682.

Singer AJ, Clark RA. Cutaneous wound healing. N Engl J Med 1999; 341: 738–746.

Smiley CM, Hanlon SU, Michel DM. Calciphylaxis in moderate renal insufficiency: changing disease concepts. Am J Nephrol 2000; 20: 324–328.

Valencia IC, Falabella A, Kirsner RS, Eaglstein WH. Chronic venous insufficiency and venous leg ulceration. J Am Acad Dermatol 2001; 44: 401–421.

Chapter | **41** | Susan Burgin, Stephen E. Wolverton, and Jeffrey P. Callen

Cutaneous Drug Eruptions

Cutaneous drug eruptions are common, have highly variable clinical presentations, and may at times be serious. The identification of the responsible drug presents a major challenge. The importance of understanding cutaneous drug eruptions derives from these issues and from the absence of any definitive diagnostic test that is applicable to the vast majority of clinical presentations.

This chapter includes a review of general principles, mechanisms, and clinical manifestations of cutaneous drug eruptions. The predominant focus is on immune-mediated cutaneous drug eruptions that have at least some risk of systemic complications. Each serious drug reaction is described in some detail. Diagnostic maneuvers are discussed, and an algorithm is presented to enable the clinician to attain a reasonable level of diagnostic certainty about the responsible drug.

Overall, cutaneous drug eruptions can be important dermatologic signs of systemic disease. Drug eruptions provide the clinician with an opportunity to excel in both the outpatient and the inpatient settings. Physicians must avoid errors of over-concern (erroneous blaming of a drug for a specific eruption) and under-concern (failure to identify a responsible drug, or failure to identify an eruption as potentially drug induced).

DEFINING THE PROBLEM

Dermatologic reactions are the most common manifestation of systemic drug hypersensitivity. Up to 2–3% of all hospitalized patients experience either an urticarial or an exanthematous drug eruption. Up to 5% of patients who receive certain antibiotics while hospitalized experience either urticarial or exanthematous reactions. When the combination of trimethoprim–sulfamethoxazole is given to human immunodeficiency virus (HIV)-infected patients a hypersensitivity reaction may develop in as many as 50%. The risk of severe drug eruptions such as Stevens–Johnson syndrome (SJS) and toxic epidermal necrolysis (TEN) is also increased in HIV-positive patients. Fatal anaphylaxis from intramuscular penicillin and fatal anaphylactoid reactions from radiocontrast each occur in about 1:50000 exposed patients. In hospitalized children,

cutaneous eruptions are the most common type of drug reaction seen. Around 2.5% of children receiving medication in the outpatient setting will experience a drug eruption, and this figure rises to 12% if the drug is an antibiotic.

When diagnosing a drug eruption, it is important to consider the following. Each eruption may potentially be caused by any drug a patient is taking (including prescription and over-the-counter drugs, herbal products, or even illicit drugs); may occur at any time during the administration of a drug; and may occur from any route of administration. The reaction may represent a cross-reaction from prior hypersensitivity to another chemically related drug. Pinning down the responsible drug may therefore represent a substantial challenge.

Clinically, determining the morphologic reaction pattern in a given patient is key: through this, the clinician can establish the risk of the pattern and a priority list for potential culprits. Finally, the clinical differential diagnosis must be borne in mind, such as differentiating an exanthematous drug reaction from a viral exanthem, toxin-mediated erythema, or acute graft-versus-host disease, and acute generalized exanthematous pustulosis (AGEP) from pustular psoriasis.

A further pitfall is that there is no single diagnostic test that can be employed across the board in cases of cutaneous drug hypersensitivity. This is because of the variability of pathogenetic mechanisms operating in the different morphologic variants, the possibility that drug–virus interactions were important clinically, or that nonpharmacologic additives or excipients were responsible.

Finally, the most specific clinical maneuver in the diagnosis of a cutaneous drug eruption, namely the rechallenge, is neither ideally sensitive nor specific. To rechallenge the patient with the putative responsible drug is potentially risky, particularly in those who have had more serious reaction patterns.

MECHANISMS OF CUTANEOUS DRUG ERUPTION

The patient's genetic background may be significant. HLA molecules play an important role in drug reactions, as they present antigen to T cells. Specific HLA genotypes have been shown to confer a greater susceptibility to various drug eruptions. A strong association has been seen between the presence of HLA B*1502 and carbamazepine-induced SJS, HLA B*5701 and abacavir-induced hypersensitivity syndrome, and HLA B*5801 and allopurinol-induced SJS. Furthermore, a familial predisposition to aromatic anticonvulsant and sulfonamide-induced hypersensitivity syndromes has been seen. Here, defective detoxification of reactive metabolites (with anticonvulsants, by epoxide hydroxylases) is thought to be responsible. In drug-induced lupus the acetylator phenotype is important: slow acetylators have a higher risk.

Most potentially serious cutaneous drug eruptions are idiosyncratic; therefore, by definition, they are unexpected or unpredictable. There are several cutaneous drug reactions that have well-defined specific hypersensitivity mechanisms, according to the Coombs–Gell classification. Table 41–1 lists some common examples. The delayed hypersensitivity category (type IV) has been divided into four subcategories, according to whether activation of monocytes (type IVa), eosinophils (IVb) or neutrophils (IVd) predominates, or whether there is T cell-directed apoptosis (IVc). The mechanism is still not definitively established for a number of reaction patterns.

Most drugs that induce cutaneous drug eruptions have a molecular weight of less than 1000 Daltons, therefore must serve as haptens for an immunologic response. A cell-based or soluble carrier protein is necessary for a drug of this size to become a complete antigen. In most instances, drug metabolites, and not the parent drug, induce the immunologic hypersensitivity. Most allergic (immunologic hypersensitivity) drug reactions should demonstrate the following features: (1) they occur in a small percentage of patients; (2) there is a history of prior exposure to the drug or a chemically related compound; and (3) there was a latency of 1–2 weeks between the initial exposure and the onset of the reaction and a latency of 1–2 days with rechallenge. Allergic drug reactions are not dose dependent. The reaction differs from the drug's pharmacologic effects and from other established signs of drug intolerance.

Table 41–1 Cutaneous drug eruptions with well-defined mechanisms

Immune mediated

Immediate hypersensitivity
  Urticaria, angioedema, anaphylaxis
Immune complex disease
  Cutaneous small-vessel vasculitis, serum sickness, lupus
    erythematosus
Delayed hypersensitivity (cell-mediated immunity)
  Allergic contact dermatitis, systemic allergic contact dermatitis

Metabolic idiosyncrasies

Epoxide hydroxylase deficiency
  Anticonvulsant hypersensitivity syndrome
Slow acetylators
  Lupus erythematosus

Other mechanisms

Direct mast cell degranulation
  Aspirin-, nonsteroidal anti-inflammatory drug-, codeine-, or
    radiocontrast-induced urticaria, anaphylactoid reactions
Protein C deficiency (heterozygotes)
  Warfarin-induced necrosis

The eruption should resolve with dechallenge and reappear after rechallenge with the drug in question.

Cutaneous drug eruptions that appear to occur with an allergic or hypersensitive mechanism but have no specific sensitization to a drug hapten are known as 'pseudoallergic' or anaphylactoid reactions. Drugs such as opiates and radiocontrast material directly degranulate mast cells without prior specific antigen sensitization. Aspirin and nonsteroidal anti-inflammatory drugs (NSAIDs) may induce urticaria by effects on the arachidonic acid pathway, leading to nonspecific mast cell degranulation. Idiosyncratic reactions can lead to either organ-specific (such as the skin) or generalized hypersensitivity.

Reactivation of viruses has been observed in drug reactions, especially in the drug hypersensitivity syndrome. Whether the reactivated virus further stimulates the immune system, leading to a more severe clinical course, or whether the virus is an innocent bystander that is reactivated by drug-induced immune stimulation, is controversial.

The most common mode of drug administration leading to sensitization is topical exposure. Oral exposure leads to specific sensitization more commonly than does parenteral (intramuscular or intravenous) exposure. After specific sensitization has occurred, rechallenge by parenteral routes is significantly more risky than by oral administration. Topical exposure presents the least risk of serious reactions with rechallenge.

Cross-reactions between chemically related drug groups are important to consider when assessing cutaneous drug reactions. Most notable are the many potential cross-reactions between drugs with a β-lactam nucleus, such as the original penicillins, aminopenicillins, semisynthetic penicillins, and probably cephalosporins. After the patient is sensitized to one member of this broad group of drugs, other related drugs should be considered to have a potential for cross-reaction. Aspirin and the various NSAIDs may cross-react, usually by nonallergic mechanisms. Cross-reactivity between antibacterial and non-antibacterial sulfonamides, on the other hand, is extremely unlikely based on their divergent chemical structures.

CLINICAL MANIFESTATIONS

Longitudinal studies, such as those by the Boston Collaborative Drug Surveillance Program and by investigators from Helsinki, Finland, provide a large database with regard to the most frequent cutaneous drug reaction patterns and the drugs most commonly responsible for them. A systematic review of the literature in 2001 confirmed that exanthematous reactions and urticaria are the most commonly observed categories of cutaneous reaction. The EuroSCAR project was a multinational case–control study that provided data in a number of recent publications on serious cutaneous drug reactions and their associated drugs.

The most important question with regard to the management of a patient with a cutaneous drug eruption is the following: What is the risk of serious consequences if the drug in question is either continued or restarted after discontinuation? Cutaneous drug eruptions in which the subsequent use of the responsible drug can lead to death (albeit exceedingly rarely, as has been shown by the reintroduction of abacavir after a prior abacavir-induced hypersensitivity syndrome) or significant irreversible morbidity, or those that can cause serious skin damage, are considered high-risk cutaneous drug eruption patterns. All other reaction patterns can be regarded with less concern.

The most important high-risk cutaneous drug eruptions include urticaria/angioedema, anaphylactoid reactions, SJS and TEN, vasculitis, the drug hypersensitivity syndrome, AGEP, and erythroderma. Several of these reaction patterns are significant because of the potential for the development of a more severe reaction with subsequent exposure to the responsible drug. For patients with drug-induced urticaria, the potential for subsequent anaphylaxis must always be considered. Both exanthematous reactions and erythroderma are significant because of their potential association with the drug hypersensitivity syndrome. AGEP and TEN have also been reported to coexist with this syndrome. Table 41–2 identifies the target organs potentially involved in the high-risk cutaneous drug eruptions listed earlier. Awareness of potential systemic organ involvement is important, both for diagnostic purposes after a given reaction has occurred and to characterize the risk of the specific drug eruption. Exanthematous eruptions and the fixed drug eruption are the only two moderate- to low-risk patterns that are discussed in this chapter, because of their relative frequency. Table 41–3 lists representative low-risk patterns and some higher-risk patterns that are not discussed here.

MAJOR DRUG REACTION PATTERNS

For each of the drug reaction patterns discussed, the relative frequency, cutaneous and mucosal features, underlying mechanism, potential for systemic involvement, and most common causative drugs are listed. In each of these reaction patterns it is imperative to discontinue the offending drug.

Urticaria and Angioedema

Drug-induced urticaria is usually caused by type I hypersensitivity in the Coombs–Gell system. Urticaria is frequently induced by a drug, although nondrug causes predominate with regard to urticaria in general. The significance of urticaria and angioedema derives from their potential relationship with anaphylaxis. The frequency of such severe subsequent reactions is uncertain; however, this possibility must at least be considered in clinical decision-making regarding rechallenge in cases of drug-induced urticaria.

Evanescent erythema and edema with associated pruritus characterize urticaria (Fig. 41–1). Angioedema involving the lips, tongue, and buccal mucosa is an occasional feature. Patients with anaphylaxis can have cardiovascular effects (hypotension), laryngeal edema, and bronchospasm.

Antibiotics are the most common causes of drug-induced urticaria. Clinically indistinguishable pseudoallergic reactions caused by direct mast cell degranulation by aspirin and NSAIDs are also common. Virtually any drug can cause urticaria or angioedema.

Stevens–Johnson Syndrome and Toxic Epidermal Necrolysis

Most cases of recurrent erythema multiforme (EM) are caused by herpes simplex virus infections. By contrast, SJS and TEN are typically drug-induced. Both are relatively uncommon.

The most characteristic findings in patients with EM include target lesions (three zones) and targetoid lesions (two zones). These lesions can be accompanied by features somewhat

Table 41–2 Target organs with high-risk drug eruptions	
Target	**Types of reaction**
Upper airway	Anaphylaxis, anaphylactoid reactions
Cardiovascular system	Anaphylaxis, anaphylactoid reactions, erythroderma
Lung	Anaphylaxis, anaphylactoid reactions, TEN, vasculitis
Liver	Drug hypersensitivity syndrome
Kidney	Vasculitis, serum sickness, TEN, drug hypersensitivity syndrome
Gastrointestinal system	Vasculitis, TEN
Skin (burn-like complications)	SJS/TEN, pemphigus, pemphigoid, severe photosensitivity (sepsis, fluid/electrolyte abnormalities)
Eyes	SJS/TEN
Thyroid	Drug hypersensitivity syndrome
SJS = Stevens–Johnson syndrome; TEN = toxic epidermal necrolysis.	

Table 41–3 Drug reaction patterns not discussed in this chapter
Relatively high-risk reaction patterns
Pemphigus (usually foliaceus subset) (see Chapter 12)
Bullous pemphigoid (see Chapter 12)
Linear IgA disease
Lupus erythematosus (see Chapter 1)
Dermatomyositis
Warfarin-induced necrosis
Serum sickness
Purpura (nonvasculitic)
Relatively low-risk reaction patterns
Photosensitivity
Lichenoid
Erythema nodosum
Acneiform/folliculitis
Alopecia
Hirsutism
Psoriasis
Hyperpigmentation (various types)
Pseudoporphyria
Systemic allergic contact dermatitis
Sweet's syndrome

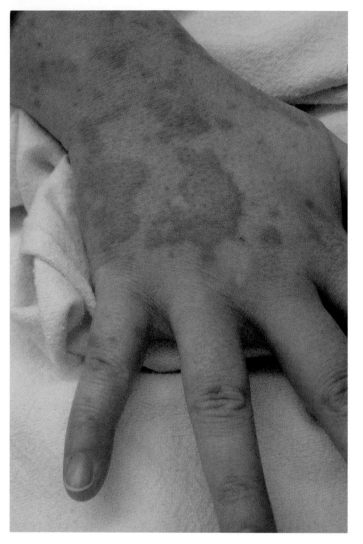

Figure 41–1 Urticaria due to NSAIDS. (Courtesy of Dr J Tan-Billet.)

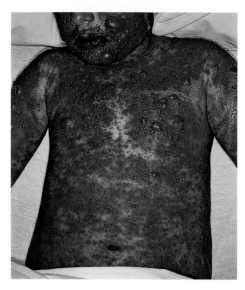

Figure 41–2 Toxic epidermal necrolysis.

similar to urticarial or exanthematous reactions. The most commonly involved sites are the oral mucosa and palms. These patients are usually systemically well.

By contrast, SJS and TEN are characterized by fever, skin pain, targetoid lesions and necrotic macules that may progress to bullae and skin denudation. Two or more mucosal sites are usually involved. The percentage of detached or detachable skin present determines whether the patient has SJS (<10%), SJS/TEN overlap (10–30%), or TEN (>30%) (Fig. 41–2).

Certain HLA types have been associated with the risk of SJS from various drugs. In TEN there is evidence that drug-specific CD8+ cells direct keratinocyte apoptosis through the perforin/granzyme B as well as the Fas/FasL pathways. Several important organ systems can be involved, with morbidity and even death related to sepsis, fluid and electrolyte abnormalities, and renal involvement manifesting as acute tubular necrosis. Gastrointestinal and pulmonary involvement can also be significant. Although presenting no risk for death, ocular involvement is of particular importance because of the potential for long-term loss of visual acuity. Historically, 25–50% of patients

with TEN died. More recently, burn unit management has significantly reduced this death rate. Although the use of intravenous immunoglobulin (IVIg) has yielded varying results in Europe, most authors in the United States feel that its institution early in the course is associated with improved survival. Unfortunately, only open-label retrospective analyses are available with historic controls, and this is not sufficient to be certain of the effectiveness of IVIg. When given, the total dose should be 3 g/kg divided over 3–4 days.

A wide variety of drugs can potentially induce SJS and TEN. Most commonly, allopurinol, anti-infective sulfonamides, the aromatic anticonvulsants (carbamazepine, phenytoin, and phenobarbital) and oxicam-NSAIDs are responsible. Nevirapine and lamotrigine have also recently emerged as major causes.

Vasculitis

Drug-induced vasculitis (also known as hypersensitivity vasculitis) is relatively uncommon. This is usually a small-vessel vasculitis. Typically, palpable purpura is present (Fig. 41–3). Commonly, these lesions are admixed with nonpalpable purpura, hemorrhagic bullae, erosions, and cutaneous infarcts with necrosis. Mucosal involvement is seldom present.

Drug-induced vasculitis results from circulating antigen–antibody immune complexes that deposit in the affected vessels and activate complement and other inflammatory mediators. Target organs include the joints, kidneys, and gastrointestinal tract, with significantly less frequent involvement of the central nervous system and lungs. Although deaths are infrequent, the risk of death is greatest when there is renal, central nervous system, or pulmonary involvement. Drugs commonly responsible include antibiotics, thiazide diuretics, furosemide, propylthiouracil, and phenytoin.

A subset of patients develop p-ANCA positivity in association with small-vessel vasculitis in the skin. Hydralazine, pro-

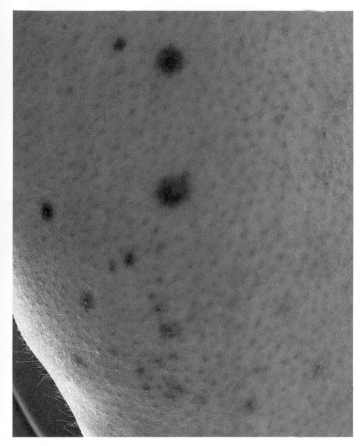

Figure 41–3 Vasculitis due to furosemide. (Courtesy of Dr J Tan-Billet.)

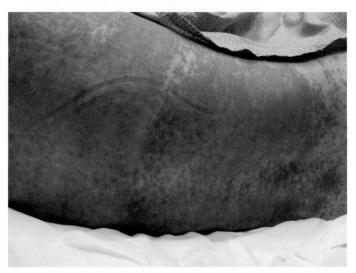

Figure 41–4 Drug hypersensitivity syndrome from ciprofloxacin. The patient had an eosinophilia of 20%, transaminitis, and prerenal failure. (Courtesy of Dr J Tan-Billet.)

pylthiouracil and allopurinol are the common offenders here, and may induce glomerulonephritis, upper respiratory tract disease, and pulmonary hemorrhage. Minocycline rarely induces p-ANCA positivity, which presents with fever, arthralgias, livedo reticularis, and subcutaneous nodules.

The Drug Hypersensitivity Syndrome

The drug hypersensitivity syndrome is also known as the hypersensitivity syndrome and drug reaction with eosinophilia and systemic symptoms, or DRESS. The aromatic anticonvulsants (phenytoin, carbamazepine, phenobarbital), lamotrigine, anti-infective sulfonamides, dapsone, minocycline, abacavir, allopurinol, and, less commonly, other drugs, can produce this syndrome. The overall incidence of the drug hypersensitivity syndrome is unknown. The incidence after exposure to antiepileptic drugs is estimated to be between 1 : 100 and 1 : 10 000.

The cutaneous features of the syndrome are variable and may include exanthematous, urticarial, and erythrodermatous (Fig. 41–4) presentations. Facial edema is commonly seen in anticonvulsant-induced reactions. Some patients with AGEP or SJS/TEN have also been found to have coexisting drug hypersensitivity syndrome. Typically, fever, pharyngitis, and prominent adenopathy are also present. Other systemic findings include a leukocytosis with eosinophilia and/or atypical lymphocytosis, and hepatitis. Interstitial nephritis, pneumonitis,

and central nervous system involvement occur more rarely. Delayed hypothyroidism has also been reported.

Genetic factors are thought to be important in the pathogenesis of this syndrome. The reactivation of viruses, particularly human herpesvirus 6, may contribute to the severity of the eruption. Systemic corticosteroids or IVIg are warranted in cases with systemic involvement. The treatment course may need to be prolonged for weeks or months to prevent relapse.

Acute Generalized Exanthematous Pustulosis (AGEP)

AGEP presents as confluent erythema with superimposed pinpoint subcorneal pustules, which typically starts on the face and progresses downwards. There is usually associated fever and leukocytosis with neutrophilia. The drug hypersensitivity syndrome has been reported in cases of AGEP. The mucous membranes are generally spared. AGEP occurs infrequently: a rate of 1–5 cases per million per year has been reported.

AGEP is a T cell-mediated reaction. There is evidence that IL-8 is produced by drug-specific CD4+ cells, and that this cytokine is responsible for the influx of neutrophils seen. The most common drug culprits include macrolides, β-lactam antibiotics, and quinolones. Terbinafine, diltiazem, and hydroxychloroquine have also been implicated.

The eruption usually resolves on discontinuation of the offending drug, but systemic corticosteroids may be necessary if the reaction is severe and extensive.

Erythroderma

Drug-induced erythroderma can be either exfoliative or nonexfoliative. The pattern can develop de novo, or as a result of a dermatitis or morbilliform eruption. The drugs that commonly cause erythroderma include gold, pyrazolone derivatives, phenytoin, dapsone, and lithium.

Cutaneous features include involvement of virtually the entire skin surface with blanchable erythema and, frequently, significant desquamation. Mucosal involvement is generally absent.

The mechanism is unknown; however, a delayed hypersensitivity mechanism may play a role. The systemic complications of erythroderma are not usually life-threatening, although high-output congestive heart failure and abnormal temperature regulation can produce significant problems. There is some question about whether this category of cutaneous drug reaction should be considered among the high-risk patterns. Certainly, the erythrodermas caused by dapsone or various anticonvulsants should be considered potentially high-risk patterns when accompanied by the previously defined hypersensitivity syndromes.

Lower-Risk Drug Reaction Patterns

Exanthematous Drug Eruptions

The exanthematous drug eruption is the most common cutaneous drug eruption, as confirmed by multiple studies. Synonyms include morbilliform, maculopapular, scarlatiniform reactions, toxic erythema, and 'drug rash.' Keratinocytes present drug antigen to T cells in conjunction with MHC class II molecules. Subsequent immune events include the secretion of both type 1 and type 2 cytokine profiles, and perforin/granzyme B-dependent mechanisms.

Generally, these reactions resolve with dechallenge and are not accompanied by significant morbidity. The skin demonstrates blanchable erythema composed of macules and papules. These lesions are initially isolated and later progress to a confluent (Fig. 41–5) and often reticulated erythema. The eruption frequently progresses from proximal to distal locations. Mucosal features are generally absent. When the exanthematous pattern is accompanied by features of the drug hypersensitivity syndrome, by signs of serum sickness, or when there is progression to an erythroderma, there is a potential systemic risk.

Virtually any drug can induce an exanthematous eruption. Previously cited studies list antibiotics (especially the β-lactams and sulfonamides) as the most common drug causes. NSAIDs are also common culprits.

Fixed Drug Eruptions

In Finnish studies, fixed drug eruptions rank in frequency below exanthematous reactions, and above urticaria and angioedema. In other series they are relatively less common. Focally recurrent erythema and edema, which takes on a completely round shape, characterize a fixed drug eruption. Plaques may have a targetoid appearance with a large central dusky zone and a surrounding annular erythematous rim, and bulla formation can occur (Fig. 41–6). Typically, the eruption recurs at sites of previous involvement and may involve new sites with each recurrence. Residual pigment remains after the reaction subsides.

There is no significant systemic risk. Cases of widespread multiple fixed drug eruption may mimic SJS or TEN, but the shape of the primary lesions is a good diagnostic clue. There

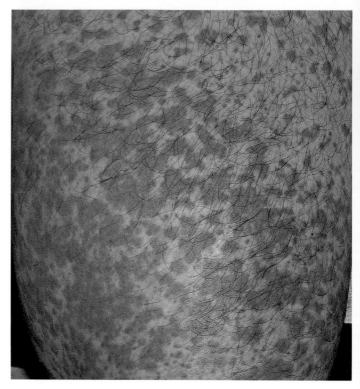

Figure 41–5 Exanthematous eruption.

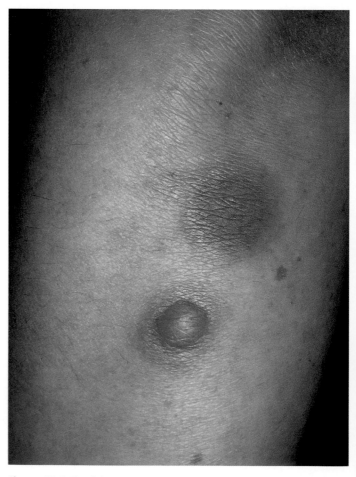

Figure 41–6 Fixed drug eruption.

are anecdotal reports of patients who develop TEN on rechallenge with the offending drug: these patients almost certainly had widespread bullous SJS or TEN initially. Responsible drugs include tetracycline and sulfonamide antibiotics, barbiturates, phenolphthalein-containing laxatives, and NSAIDs. Phenolphthalein may also be present in maraschino cherries and other nontraditional exposures.

DIAGNOSIS

Although significant advances in diagnostic testing for drug allergy have been made, few of these tests have been validated and none are 100% sensitive. In general as well, false-negative testing may be obtained with testing in cases where a virus has contributed to the eruption, such as the β-lactam eruption in cases of Epstein–Barr virus.

Table 41–4 contains a list of available in vitro and in vivo diagnostic tests for drug hypersensitivity. Specific IgE assays, such as the radioallergosorbent test (RAST), are the most commonly employed for evaluating type I hypersensitivity reactions. These include urticaria, angioedema, and anaphylaxis. Only a few drugs can be tested this way, such as the β-lactams and insulin. Although IgE assays are still less sensitive than scratch tests, they should be used together with scratch testing in patients at risk for anaphylaxis. The basophil activation test uses flow cytometry to detect markers of response to drug allergens. It has been employed in cases of immediate hypersensitivity to β-lactams, muscle relaxants, and NSAIDs.

The lymphocyte transformation test (LTT) measures the proliferative response of a patient's T cells in vitro to a suspected drug culprit. It has been reported to be more sensitive for diagnosis than patch testing, but has some limitations. First, although it has been found to be positive in the majority of cases of exanthematous reactions, the drug hypersensitivity syndrome, and AGEP, it is only rarely positive in cases of TEN, fixed drug eruption, and vasculitis. Second, timing of the test is important, with cases of the drug hypersensitivity syndrome showing a negative test in the first few weeks after onset of the eruption. Finally, the test is not available at most clinical centers.

Prick tests have been found to be a useful diagnostic tool in cases of sensitivity to β-lactams and muscle relaxants used in anesthesia. Intradermal testing can be performed when prick tests are negative. To date, penicillin is the most widely used systemic drug for which intradermal skin testing is significantly reliable. Patients with the majority of important drug reactions, including SJS and TEN, exanthematous reactions, vasculitis, and erythroderma, should not undergo this form of testing.

Patch testing for cutaneous drug reactions has been studied the most vigorously of all the skin tests. Sensitivity varies depending on the type of reaction, the putative drug, the concentration of drug tested, and, for fixed drug eruptions, the site at which the patch is placed. Positive results have been obtained in cases of exanthematous reactions, fixed drug eruption, AGEP, and the drug hypersensitivity syndrome. Sensitivity has varied between 30% and 50%. The specificity and negative predictive value have not been determined.

Histopathologic findings may help clarify the drug reaction pattern, but they do not identify the responsible drug. Histopathologic examination can confirm the diagnosis of EM, fixed drug eruption, vasculitis, and erythroderma, and may support the clinical diagnosis of urticarial or morbilliform drug reactions. Eosinophils are widely believed to be major participants in many cutaneous drug reactions. The microscopic presence of eosinophils certainly suggests a drug cause; however, the absence of eosinophils does not exclude a drug as a possible etiologic agent.

Diagnostic Clinical Algorithm

Through a defined clinical algorithm, the clinician can readily and often accurately determine the cause of most cutaneous drug eruptions. This process involves four major steps: challenge, dechallenge, rechallenge, and exclusion. Three of these steps are prospective, whereas the challenge is a retrospective step in the diagnostic process. This process is still the gold standard for identifying a putative drug in the absence of the aforementioned tests, or when they yield negative results or are not validated.

Challenge

Of the steps listed in Table 41–5, characterization of the drug reaction pattern and focusing on drugs started during the previous month (particularly the previous 1–2 weeks) are the most important steps. There are a number of potential pitfalls here. Improper characterization of the reaction pattern can lead to an inaccurate determination of the systemic risk and likely drug causes. The patient's ability to recall previous drug reactions accurately is frequently suspect. A great deal of potentially misleading anecdotal single-case experience is quoted in the literature. Most case reports do not reach a high level of certainty regarding the diagnostic clinical algorithm described here.

It is important to avoid diagnostic errors related to the 'bad kid in the classroom' concept. When a drug gets a 'bad' reputation as a cause of a given reaction type, it is increasingly likely that that drug will be falsely implicated in the clinical setting and in subsequent literature citations. A single case report does not dramatically increase the likelihood that a specific drug caused a given reaction in clinical practice.

Table 41–4 Diagnostic tests used selectively in drug reactions

In vitro tests

IgE assays: radioallergosorbent test (RAST), immunoenzymatic assays
Basophil activation test
Lymphocyte transformation test
Lymphocyte activation test

In vivo tests

Prick, scratch, or intradermal skin tests
Epicutaneous patch test
Histopathologic examination
Rechallenge/provocation

Table 41–5 Clinical diagnosis algorithm to determine the responsible drug

Challenge circumstances (retrospective step)
Characterize reaction pattern
Evaluate patient history of prior reactions
Review literature experience with drugs in question
Focus on drugs started during past month
Dechallenge
Most reactions fade in next few weeks after drug discontinuation
Rechallenge
Intentional selective rechallenge
Unintentional (accidental) rechallenge
Reverse rechallenge
Exclusion
Systemic involvement with certain reactions
Nondrug precipitators of same reaction pattern

Likelihood a specific drug is cause
(given positive (+) challenge circumstances)
Definite = (+) dechallenge, (+) rechallenge, and (+) exclusion
Probable = (+) dechallenge and (+) exclusion (no rechallenge)
Possible = (+) dechallenge or (+) exclusion only
Unlikely = (+) challenge circumstances only

Table 41–6 Criteria for intentional drug rechallenge with potentially serious drug reactions

Drug in question is essential for treatment of the specific medical condition
No suitable alternative drug(s) is available
Illness to be treated is potentially serious
Rechallenge occurs ideally at least 1–2 months after reaction subsides
Appropriate informed consent is obtained
Undertaken in hospital setting, preferably with an oral form of the drug in question
Pretreatment with corticosteroids, antihistamines, or desensitization protocol, if applicable, is considered

Dechallenge

Most cutaneous drug eruptions that occur as a result of hypersensitivity resolve promptly within 1–2 weeks after discontinuation of the responsible drug. Drugs can mimic or exacerbate a number of independently existing diseases. Many of these diseases can wax and wane; therefore, a drug given coincidentally near the time of the disease flare can be falsely blamed for the reaction. Conversely, it is well documented that certain cutaneous reactions can resolve in spite of continuation of the drug in question.

Discontinuation of drug therapy and resumption of therapy with the drug in question at a later time may allow immunologic effector mechanisms to 'recharge' fully, making large-scale discontinuation of all drugs the patient is receiving worthy of careful scrutiny. The potential for the disease being treated to worsen after drug discontinuation has to be considered in dechallenge decisions. Each case should be handled individually, with a consideration of the risks and benefits of discontinuing drug therapy.

Rechallenge

In managing patients with high-risk reaction patterns, rechallenge with the drug in question should be carried out only in very rare circumstances, when the need to know the responsible drug exceeds the risk of a severe reaction with the rechallenge. Intentional rechallenge can be performed only when a clinical presentation meets the criteria in Table 41–6. Reports of patients with accidental rechallenge provide useful informa-

tion on drug causes, but it is essential to avoid such accidental rechallenge. It is important to note that rechallenge is not optimally sensitive or specific. Despite these limitations, rechallenge, when indicated, is the best way to identify accurately the causative drug in the clinical setting. The presence or absence of drug–drug and drug–virus interactions should always be considered in this diagnostic step.

The technique of 'reverse challenge' seems most reasonable and practical when there is one drug of high suspicion and several others of lower suspicion that were started simultaneously prior to the cutaneous drug eruption. The failure to reproduce the reaction when the patient receives the low-suspicion drugs increases the likelihood that the high-suspicion drug (which is not rechallenged) is responsible for the drug reaction. This method essentially clears from responsibility the drugs that were actually rechallenged.

A negative result with oral rechallenge can mean that the drug tested was not responsible for the reaction; that it was perhaps administered at too low a dose; or that the rechallenge did not reproduce all the clinical conditions for the prior cutaneous drug eruption. A positive rechallenge can be regarded with reasonable certainty as indicating that the drug tested was responsible for the cutaneous drug reaction. Again, rechallenge is not endorsed for high-risk drug reaction patterns, except in the most exceptional circumstances.

Exclusion

The exclusion step of the clinical algorithm has two components. The clinician should use appropriate historic and physical examination findings, along with well-directed laboratory tests, to exclude (to a reasonable degree of certainty) nondrug causes for the reaction pattern present. Most commonly, a variety of infectious agents can mimic the majority of cutaneous drug eruptions discussed. In addition, the clinician should attempt to define the degree of systemic involvement in the high-risk reaction patterns.

LITERATURE RESOURCES

Table 41–7 lists a number of resources to assist the clinician in the identification of drugs that are commonly responsible

Table 41 7 Sources for information on specific cutaneous drug eruptions and responsible drugs

Dermatology texts

General dermatology texts
Specific monographs on drug reactions
    Kauppinen K, Alanko K, Hannuksela M, et al. Skin Reactions to Drugs. Informa Healthcare, 1998
    Breathnach SM, Hintner H. Adverse Drug Reactions and the Skin. Oxford: Blackwell Scientific Publications, 1992
    Litt JZ. Drug Eruption Reference Manual Including Drug Interactions, 14th edn. Informa Healthcare, 2008

Major clinical studies

Boston Collaborative Drug Surveillance Program
Finnish studies (see Suggested Readings)
EuroSCAR studies (see Suggested Readings)

Periodicals

The Medical Letter on Drugs and Therapeutics
WHO Pharmaceuticals Newsletter
WHO Drug Information

Other resources

FDA Medwatch (http://www.fda.gov/medwatch/)
Package insert for a given drug
PDR Guide to Drug Interactions, Side Effects and Indications, 2008. Thompson Healthcare (updated yearly)
Pharmaceutical company data
USP DI. Drug Information for the Health Care Professional. Greenwood Village, CO: Thomson Micromedex (published annually)

Table 41–8 Drug categories most commonly responsible for cutaneous drug eruptions

Antibiotics

β-Lactam
Penicillins
Semisynthetic penicillins (e.g., dicloxacillin)
Aminopenicillins (e.g., ampicillin or amoxicillin)
β-Lactamase inhibitor (e.g., amoxicillin/clavulanate)
Extended-spectrum penicillins (e.g., carbenicillin)
Cephalosporins, all four generations
Monobactams (e.g., aztreonam)
Penems (e.g., imipenem)

Sulfonamides and related drugs

Sulfamethoxazole/trimethoprim combination
Sulfapyridine
Sulfasalazine
Sulfones (e.g., dapsone)

Anti-inflammatory agents

Aspirin
Nonsteroidal anti-inflammatory drugs
Antimalarials
Gold
D-Penicillamine
Allopurinol

Anticonvulsants

Phenytoin
Phenobarbital
Carbamazepine
Lamotrigine

Antiretroviral drugs

Abacavir
Nevirapine

for various cutaneous drug reaction patterns. The Boston Collaborative Drug Surveillance Program and the series of articles from Finnish investigators presented data collected only from 1982 to 1985. The latest data from the EuroSCAR study was published in 2008. Several sources identified in Table 41–7 are the best resources when a recently released drug is in question.

There are several categories of drug responsible for the majority of common and serious reaction patterns (Table 41–8). Antibiotics, anti-inflammatories, and anticonvulsants are the drug categories most frequently responsible for cutaneous drug eruptions.

The diagnosis of the cutaneous drug eruption pattern and the most likely drug cause are most optimally determined with the clinical algorithm previously described. With high-risk drug reaction patterns, it is important to avoid future use of drugs with a 'possible' and 'probable' likelihood of responsibility. The rapidly growing number of drugs available to treat various medical conditions gives the clinician more latitude to substitute chemically unrelated drugs than was previously possible.

MANAGEMENT ISSUES

The most difficult step of drug reaction management is the identification of the responsible agent. The easier decisions involve symptomatic management of the cutaneous drug eruption. The clinician should consider discontinuing all but the essential drugs required for the patient's care. The clinician should substitute medications with the same pharmacologic effects, but with different chemical structures from those of the drugs in question.

SUGGESTED READINGS

Alanko K, Stubb S, Kauppinen K. Cutaneous drug reactions: clinical types and causative agents. A five year survey of inpatients (1981–1985). Acta Dermatol Venereol (Stockh) 1989; 69: 223–226.

Bahna SL, Khalili B. New concepts in the management of adverse drug reactions. Allergy Asthma Proc 2007; 28: 517–524.

Barbaud A. Drug patch testing in systemic cutaneous drug allergy. Toxicology 2005; 209: 209–216.

Bigby M. Rates of cutaneous reactions to drugs. Arch Dermatol 2001; 137: 765–770.

Halevy S, Ghislain P-D, Mockenhaupt M, et al. Allopurinol is the most common cause of Stevens-Johnson syndrome and toxic epidermal necrolysis in Europe and Israel. J Am Acad Dermatol 2008; 58: 25–32.

Kauppinen K, Stubb S. Drug eruptions: causative agents and clinical types. A series of in-patients during a 10 year period. Acta Dermatol Venereol (Stockh) 1984; 64: 320–322.

Knowles SR, Shear NS. Recognition and management of severe cutaneous drug reactions. Dermatol Clin 2007; 25: 245–253.

Mockenhaupt M, Viboud C, Dunant A, et al. Stevens–Johnson syndrome and toxic epidermal necrolysis: asssessment of medication risks with emphasis on recently marketed drugs. The EuroSCAR study. J Invest Dermatol 2008; 128: 35–44.

Pichler WJ. Delayed drug hypersensitivity reactions. Ann Intern Med 2003; 139: 683–693.

Romano A, Demoly P. Recent advances in the diagnosis of drug allergy. Curr Opin Allergy Clin Immunol 2007; 7: 299–303.

Segal AR, Doherty KM, Leggott J, et al. Cutaneous reactions to drugs in children. Pediatrics 2007; 120: e1082–e1086.

Thong BYH, Blanca M. Risk factors and diagnostic tests in drug allergy. Curr Opin Allergy Clin Immunol 2007; 7: 297–298.

Valeyrie-Allanore L, Sassolas B, Roujeau JC. Drug-induced skin, nail and hair disorders. Drug Safety 2007; 30: 1011–1030.

Systemic Therapy for Cutaneous Disease

Although the subject of systemic drug therapy for dermatologic conditions is vast, in this chapter we will review the important general principles that guide its safe use. Supporting concepts and important clinical examples follow each principle. Two broad categories overriding these principles are drug selection and monitoring.

PRINCIPLES OF DRUG SELECTION

Principle 1. Systemic drugs with an element of risk are essential in the management of numerous dermatoses

Many dermatologic therapies are administered through relatively safe topical routes. In addition, there are a number of systemic drugs for which there are few significant risks and which therefore require little or no routine monitoring for adverse effects (Table 42–1). This chapter focuses on the systemic drugs with a significant element of risk that are commonly used to treat more serious dermatologic conditions (Table 42–2).

Principle 2. It is important initially to make a reasonable estimation of the cutaneous disease's 'severity'

There are a number of dermatologic conditions in which the disease's severity and associated risks are self-evident. Blistering diseases, such as pemphigus vulgaris, have well-established risks. Malignancies that are multicentric at the outset, such as cutaneous T-cell lymphoma (mycosis fungoides), represent another example of high-risk dermatoses. At times, the dermatologic risk is a function of the systemic findings associated with the dermatologic signs of internal disease. Systemic lupus erythematosus, sarcoidosis, and dermatomyositis are appropriate examples. The severe irreversible ocular mucosal morbidity with cicatricial pemphigoid also presents a noteworthy risk.

It is more difficult to determine disease severity and risk in conditions without life-threatening potential and without severe irreversible morbidity. Dermatologists are commonly confronted with the psychosocial risk and/or functional impairment presented by patients with severe acne vulgaris or psoriasis. At best, it is a judgment call to determine which of these patients warrant appropriate systemic drug therapy with an element of risk.

Dermatologic conditions in which the morbidity results in a loss of work can also justify potentially risky systemic therapy. Pyoderma gangrenosum is an example of such a condition.

Principle 3. 'Risk–risk' analysis is performed by comparing the risk(s) of a given disease (as defined earlier) with the inherent risk(s) of the proposed systemic drug therapy. The treatment risks should not exceed the inherent untreated disease risk

The risk–risk analysis may be preferable to the risk–benefit ratio, which is traditionally discussed. Even after considering conditions deemed severe by the criteria cited earlier, in general, dermatologists face conditions with less risk of death and severe morbidity than do most other specialists in medicine. Generally, there is a significant subjective element to this risk–risk analysis. The patient has a central role in this decision-making process.

Principle 4. It is important to be aware of a given drug's official Food and Drug Administration (FDA)-approved indications, and the generally accepted but 'unapproved' or 'off-label' indications for that drug

Official FDA approval means that there has been an application for a specific use of a drug and that sufficient safety and efficacy data have been presented to warrant use of the drug for that specific disease indication. Safety data are usually applicable to generally accepted but off-label indications. What is lacking in these off-label indications is efficacy data officially submitted by the pharmaceutical company to the FDA. Considerable expense is associated with applications for each 'new use.' Usually, there is either significant personal or widespread literature experience to justify drug use for the various off-label indications.

Table 42–1 Some systemic agents used in dermatology that require little or no routine monitoring

Antibiotics

Penicillins
Cephalosporins
Tetracycline
Erythromycins
Fluoroquinolones

Antivirals

Acyclovir
Valacyclovir
Famciclovir

Antifungal

Griseofulvin

Antihistamines

Vasoactive drugs

Pentoxifylline
Nifedipine
Aspirin
Dipyridamole

Miscellaneous

Potassium iodide
Niacinamide

Table 42–2 Some important dermatoses selectively requiring systemic medications with an element of risk*

Psoriasis – acitretin, anti-IL-12/23 agents cyclosporine, methotrexate, PUVA, T-cell modulating agents, tumor necrosis factor (TNF)-α antagonists

Acne vulgaris – isotretinoin, minocycline

Vasculitis – azathioprine, colchicine, corticosteroids, dapsone

Lupus erythematosus – antimalarials (hydroxychloroquine, chloroquine, quinacrine), azathioprine, corticosteroids, cyclosporine, dapsone, methotrexate, mycophenolate mofetil, retinoids, thalidomide

Pyoderma gangrenosum – adalimumab, anti-TNF-α agents, corticosteroids, cyclosporine, dapsone, infliximab, intravenous immunoglobulin, mycophenolate mofetil, thalidomide

Pemphigus vulgaris – azathioprine, corticosteroids, cyclosporine, intravenous immunoglobulin, mycophenolate mofetil, rituximab

Bullous pemphigoid – azathioprine, corticosteroids, cyclosporine, dapsone, methotrexate, rituximab

Dermatitis herpetiformis – dapsone, sulfapyridine

Mycosis fungoides – bexarotene, methotrexate, PUVA, retinoids

Disorders of keratinization – retinoids

Atopic dermatitis, severe – azathioprine, corticosteroids, cyclosporine, mycophenolate mofetil, PUVA

*The drugs listed under each heading are those on which this chapter focuses and are not an exhaustive list of therapeutic options. The listing of drugs is alphabetic, and does not imply a therapeutic sequence.
PUVA = psoralen–ultraviolet A therapy.

Systemic drug therapy is commonly associated with some element of risk. The patient ideally should be notified when the drug will be used for an off-label indication. This communication is of growing importance because of the recent increased FDA interest in policing such off-label uses of medications.

Principle 5. The priority sequence of systemic drug choices should be individualized for each specific patient. Factors such as drug cost, simplicity of the therapeutic regimen, inherent drug risk, and patient preference enter into the decision

When all other factors are equal, a drug that is relatively inexpensive, simple to use, and relatively safe should be prescribed. Ideally, such a drug should be supported by an FDA indication or sufficient clinical data and experience to justify its use. If such therapy is not appropriate or is not successful, more costly, complicated, or novel treatments with an element of risk can be tried. Frequently, patient preferences are shaped by logistics, such as drug cost, patient income, time, travel, and the patient's tolerance of risk.

Principle 6. Be cognizant of important drug–drug interactions when prescribing systemic therapy for cutaneous diseases

An increasing number of patients who present to the dermatologist are already receiving a wide variety of systemic medica-

tions for nondermatologic medical problems. An awareness of the patient's complete medication profile helps enhance the safety of prescribing systemic drugs, particularly for patients who are receiving cyclosporine or methotrexate. The risk of erythromycin or itraconazole interacting with the nonsedating antihistamines terfenadine or astemizole is of historic interest, as these nonsedating antihistamines are no longer available, but the interaction with cyclosporine remains an issue. A systematic way of recording the patient's complete medication profile helps minimize the risk of these potential interactions. Therefore it is our suggestion that current drug therapy be monitored and recorded at each patient visit.

MONITORING PRINCIPLES

Principle 1. Informed consent is a communication process and not merely a signature on a piece of paper. Appropriately thorough informed consent is an essential step toward the safe use of systemic drugs

There is an important medicolegal basis for informed consent. This communication is usually documented by noting that the patient is aware of the risks, benefits, and alternatives to the proposed therapy. Generally, chart documentation of this discussion by the physician is sufficient. Only with experimental protocols is a signed consent form imperative. In addition, consent forms for the use of isotretinoin in both men and women are recommended by Roche, Inc., and the FDA.

The medical basis for the informed consent communication process is even more important. This discussion enables the patient to be more aware of specific areas of risk and the patient's role in reporting important signs and symptoms. Occasionally, a patient decides not to use a specific drug after learning about the risks. This is probably preferable to treating a patient who continually focuses on the potential risks of therapy, however remote.

Principle 2. A patient information handout specific to the drug being prescribed can be an important measure to reinforce all aspects of the monitoring process

A patient information handout should reinforce all elements of the informed consent process described earlier. More importantly, a clear listing of the signs and symptoms the patient should report allows the patient to know when to be concerned regarding problems that may arise later in therapy. These patient information handouts should clarify the follow-up visits required, and laboratory testing, X-ray procedures, and nondermatologist specialty examinations required for a given drug therapy.

Sources of such handouts include the American Academy of Dermatology, National Psoriasis Foundation, American College of Rheumatology, various pharmaceutical companies, the patient (lay) volume of the USP DI annual drug information booklet, and the American Medical Association Patient Medical Instruction sheets. Clinicians with sufficient experience with a given drug can develop their own patient information handouts.

Principle 3. Monitoring for adverse effects associated with systemic drugs used in dermatology is largely based on risk reduction through detecting drug-induced abnormalities at an early reversible stage

The complete elimination of risks from systemic drugs is not possible, although more favorable 'risk–risk' ratios, as defined previously, are definitely achievable. The monitoring process is most important when there are subclinical findings that have serious potential consequences. A classic example is the low-grade fibrosis and potential for subsequent cirrhosis in patients receiving long-term methotrexate therapy. In addition, mild asymptomatic leukopenia or transaminase elevations may herald serious complications if left undetected. Lastly, corticosteroid-induced osteoporosis should be detected early with DEXA scans and treated with vitamin D, calcium, and bisphosphonates.

Principle 4. Virtually all tests and examinations to be used in the monitoring process should have a baseline determination

Baseline laboratory testing can often aid in the following issues:

- To determine which patients should not receive a given drug.
- To determine which patients are at high risk and require closer subsequent surveillance.
- To allow the clinician to avoid assigning blame to the drug therapy for an existing condition(s).
- To serve as a basis of comparison for subsequent follow-up testing.

Principle 5. 'Critical toxicities' are defined as any drug-induced adverse effect that may result in either loss of life or potentially irreversible significant morbidity. These adverse effects receive the highest priority in systemic drug monitoring

The following adverse effects meet this definition of 'critical toxicities:'

- Hepatotoxicity
- Hematologic toxicity (agranulocytosis, aplastic anemia, or thrombocytopenia)
- Induction of malignancy
- Teratogenicity
- Pneumonitis
- Opportunistic infections (such as reactivation or dissemination of tuberculosis)
- Hypothalamopituitary–adrenal axis suppression
- Growth suppression
- Renal toxicity
- Hyperlipidemia
- Ocular toxicity (retinopathy, cataracts)
- Bone toxicity (osteoporosis or osteonecrosis).

Principle 6. Risk reduction can be optimized through the use of well-defined monitoring guidelines

Both patient and physician benefit when consistent monitoring guidelines are used. Systematic ordering of laboratory tests, X-ray procedures, and specific examinations minimizes the potential for oversights leading to inadequate monitoring. Recording the test results on an appropriate flow sheet can be helpful in following patients receiving relatively high-risk drugs. A well-trained nurse can assist in the tracking and recording of these values.

Specific guidelines can be found in the reference cited in the Suggested Reading section. These guidelines were derived from consensus articles that discussed single or multiple drugs, and from pharmaceutical company or FDA guidelines proposed for specific drugs.

Principle 7. Monitoring guidelines are based on data from low-risk patients with normal test results. More frequent surveillance is necessary for high-risk patients and for those patients with significantly abnormal test results

An example of a high-risk patient is an individual who might be receiving methotrexate and who has any of the following: mildly abnormal baseline liver function test results, increased probability of fatty changes (as a result of obesity, ethanol abuse, or diabetes mellitus), prior hepatitis, renal disease, or immunosuppression. Patients at very high risk should usually not receive the drug at all.

Subsequent abnormal test results also warrant more frequent surveillance. An example would be mild to moderate retinoid-induced elevations of triglycerides. Mild to moderate dapsone-induced hemolysis is another example.

Principle 8. Particularly close follow-up is required for critical toxicities that are idiosyncratic and have a potential for rapid and severe changes in the patient's status

Toxic hepatitis and agranulocytosis are two critical toxicities that stand out in this regard. Toxic hepatitis may be preceded by mild to moderate asymptomatic elevations of liver transaminase levels, whereas agranulocytosis may be preceded by relatively mild leukopenia. Significant laboratory abnormalities of either type require careful follow-up and, in many cases, drug discontinuation. Drugs prescribed by dermatologists that are most likely to induce toxic hepatitis include methotrexate, azathioprine, itraconazole, dapsone, and minocycline. Dapsone and methotrexate present the greatest risk of agranulocytosis among the systemic dermatologic drugs. Azathioprine may also produce significant depression of the white blood cell count, although this effect is much more likely to be predictable by measuring thiopurine methyltransferase levels and avoiding concomitant use of allopurinol.

These toxicities can be significantly contrasted with low-grade indolent changes that may have significant implications. Examples include cirrhosis from low-dose methotrexate, ocular toxicity from antimalarials, and the risk of nonmelanoma and melanoma skin cancer in patients treated with photochemotherapy (psoralen with UVA light). Long-term surveillance through special examinations and procedures is used when prescribing these drugs.

Principle 9. Share the responsibility of monitoring for adverse effects with other appropriate specialists

The practice of medicine is in many instances a team effort, requiring coordinated management by various physicians. Monitoring for adverse effects of systemic drugs frequently requires the application of this principle. Ophthalmologic consultation for patients receiving antimalarial therapy is an example. Consultation with an appropriate specialist is important both for the liver biopsy procedure and for decisions regarding abnormal liver function test results in patients receiving methotrexate. The patient's primary care physician plays a significant role in monitoring for potential malignancy induction from immunosuppressive therapy.

Less well clarified is the need for co-management with dermatologists from an academic center. We believe that in many situations systemic drug therapy with an element of risk can be orchestrated through an academic dermatologist, with the patient's primary dermatologist playing the major role in the ongoing surveillance process.

Principle 10. Minimize the risk of systemic drug therapy through adjunctive therapy with other systemic drugs and topical or local therapy, and by modifying disease precipitators when possible

The classic addition of corticosteroid-sparing agents, such as azathioprine and methotrexate, serves to reduce the dose and the associated risk of systemic corticosteroid therapy. A combination of oral retinoids and PUVA therapy for patients with psoriasis is another example of systemic drug combination therapy with a lower overall treatment risk.

In situations requiring systemic corticosteroid therapy, concomitant use of topical and/or intralesional corticosteroid therapy may reduce the systemic corticosteroid dose requirement. Modifying disease precipitators in patients with psoriasis, atopic dermatitis, and acne may improve the efficacy and safety of systemic drug therapy.

SUGGESTED READING

Wolverton SE, ed. Comprehensive dermatologic drug therapy, 2nd edn. Philadelphia: WB Saunders, 2007.

Index

Please note that page references relating to non-textual content such as Figures or Tables are in *italic* print